Diagnosis and classification in psychiatry

Diagnosis and classification in psychiatry
A critical appraisal of DSM-III

Edited by
GARY L. TISCHLER, M.D.

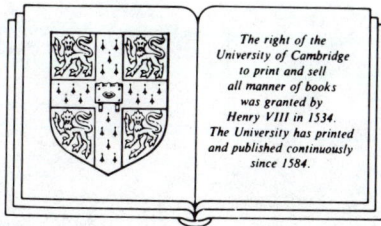

The right of the
University of Cambridge
to print and sell
all manner of books
was granted by
Henry VIII in 1534.
The University has printed
and published continuously
since 1584.

CAMBRIDGE UNIVERSITY PRESS

Cambridge
New York   New Rochelle   Melbourne   Sydney

Published by the Press Syndicate of the University of Cambridge
The Pitt Building, Trumpington Street, Cambridge CB2 1RP
32 East 57th Street, New York, NY 10022, USA
10 Stamford Road, Oakleigh, Melbourne 3166, Australia

First published 1987

Printed in the United States of America

Library of Congress Cataloging-in-Publication Data
Diagnosis and classification in psychiatry.
Based on a conference held Oct. 13–15, 1983 and
sponsored by the American Psychiatric Association's
Committee to Evaluate DSM-III.
1. Diagnostic and statistical manual of mental
disorders. 2. Mental illness – Classification – Con-
gresses. 3. Mental illness – Diagnosis – Congresses.
I. Tischler, Gary L. II. American Psychiatric
Association. Committee to Evaluate DSM-III.
[DNLM: 1. Mental Disorders – classification – congresses.
2. Mental Disorders – diagnosis – congresses.
WM 141 D53653 1983]
RC455.2.C4D53 1987 616.89′0012 86-33397

British Library Cataloguing-in-Publication Data
Diagnosis and classification in psychiatry:
a critical appraisal of DSM-III.
1. Psychology, Pathological – Classification
2. Mental illness – Diagnosis
I. Tischler, Gary L.
616.89′0012 RC455

ISBN 0 521 32366 5

Contents

viii   *Contents*

Preface

Diagnosis and classification are essential elements of medical practice. Their importance to a medical subspecialty generally varies as a function of their power to inform and facilitate clinical practice. If the therapeutic armamentarium of a subspecialty is limited, rigorous demarcations between disease categories have little practical import. As treatment options expand and differential responses to specific therapeutic interventions are identified, accurate and precise delineation of pathological conditions becomes crucial. Such is the current state of affairs within the fields of psychiatry.

Beginning in the late 1950s, advances in psychopharmacology and biological psychiatry highlighted limitations of the diagnostic schema and classification systems then in use. Psychiatrists had difficulty in achieving diagnostic consensus when reviewing the same clinical material. Syndromes within a particular class of disorders were not sharply demarcated from one another. The treatment responses and long-term outcomes for specific psychiatric syndromes showed considerable variation. Faced with a growing need for more precise and rigorous descriptions of clinical phenomena, the field responded by developing more objective methods for describing psychopathology. These efforts demonstrated the utility of the descriptive approach as a mode of inquiry that could substantially advance psychiatric practice. The past decade witnessed further confirmation of its value as a mode of inquiry. Refinements in diagnostic instrumentation together with improved techniques for testing diagnostic reliability facilitated the development of criteria-based diagnostic typologies. These typologies, in turn, opened new avenues for research in behavioral genetics, epidemiology, and clinical psychopathology.

Perhaps the most striking testimony to the impact of the descriptive approach has been its use as the cornerstone for the official classification system adopted by the American Psychiatric Association. The third edition of the *Diagnostic and Statistical Manual of Mental Disorders (DSM-III)* was published by the American Psychiatric Association in 1980. Over 400 pages long, it contains detailed descriptions of diagnostic categories that set forth the essential and commonly associated features of a disorder. Textual material is included on incidences of disorders, sex ratios, familial patterns, predisposing factors, usual age at onset, clinical courses, complications, and levels of impairment. A discussion of differential diagnosis is also provided. New diagnostic categories have been introduced, and some older categories have been extensively revised or deleted. For the first time, a criteria-oriented typology, with fixed decision rules providing guidelines for confirming diagnoses, and a multiaxial approach to diagnostic evaluation are incorporated into an official classification system for mental disorders.

It is not unusual for the introduction of a new classification system to elicit discussion. The major innovations in substance and format characterizing *DSM-III*, however, generated a good deal of debate even before it was formally adopted, and that led the Board of Trustees of the American Psychiatric Association to establish a Committee to Evaluate *DSM-III*. As part of its evaluation, the committee sponsored a three-day conference that addressed a broad range of topics relevant to an assessment of *DSM-III*. The proceedings of that conference form the nucleus of this volume. The contributors include the authors of the various chapters as well as the conference participants, whose comments are summarized in an overview for each section – in all, some 65 contributors.

Detailed consideration of a broad range of issues central to diagnoses and classification in psychiatry underscores the premise advanced in the introduction to *DSM-III* (third edition): " . . . DSM-III is only one still frame in the ongoing process of attempting to better understand mental disorders." The first seven sections of the volume address the clinical syndromes. The relevant research literature is reviewed, and recommendations are set forth concerning how to improve and refine our approach to diagnosis and classification. The section on nosologic principles and diagnostic hierarchies provides an overview of conflicting objectives of classification systems designed for administrative, clinical, and research purposes, issues involved in constructing classification systems, and steps being taken to revise *DSM-III*. Separate sections are devoted to assessing the multiaxial approach and to evaluating the applicability of *DSM-III* to clinical practice, psychiatric education, and administrative uses.

We live in an era in which the growth of knowledge and the diversification of practice have created a need for a more highly differentiated diagnostic framework. *DSM-III* represents one response to that need. A classification system such as that of *DSM-III*, however, both reflects and exposes the limits of current knowledge and understanding. Significant modifications in diagnostic systems and our approach to classification will undoubtedly occur as our knowledge base continues to expand. The commentaries provided by the contributors to this volume represent an excellent point of departure as we move toward *DSM-IV*.

Gary L. Tischler

Contributors

Hagop S. Akiskal, M.D.
Department of Psychiatry
University of Tennessee
66 North Pauline Street, Suite 633
Memphis, TN 38163

Nancy C. Andreasen, M.D.
Professor, Department of Psychiatry
University of Iowa Hospitals & Clinics
500 Newton Road
Iowa City, IA 52242

David H. Barlow, Ph.D.
Department of Psychology
State University of New York – Albany
1400 Washington Avenue
Albany, NY 12222

James Barrett, M.D.
Research Professor of Psychiatry &
Community and Family Medicine
Dartmouth Medical School
Hanover, NH 03756

Jeffrey H. Boyd, M.D., M.P.H.
Psychiatrist
Waterbury Hospital
Waterbury, CT 06721

Jack D. Burke, Jr., M.D.
Deputy Director, Division of Clinical
Research
National Institute of Mental Health
5600 Fishers Lane, Room 10-105
Rockville, MD 20857

Gabrielle A. Carlson
Director of Child Psychiatry
Department of Psychiatry & Behavioral
Sciences
State University of New York – Stony
Brook
Putnam Hall – South Campus
Stony Brook, NY 11794-8790

Paul Chodoff, M.D.
Clinical Professor of Psychiatry
George Washington University Medical
School
1904 R Street, N.W.
Washington, DC 20009

Paula J. Clayton, M.D.
Chair, Department of Psychiatry
University of Minnesota
420 Delaware Street, S.E.
Minneapolis, MN 55455

C. Robert Cloninger, M.D.
Department of Psychiatry
Washington University School of Medicine
4940 Audubon Avenue
St. Louis, MO 63110

Arnold M. Cooper, M.D.
Professor of Psychiatry & Director of
Education
The New York Hospital – Cornell Medical
Center
525 East 68th Street
New York, NY 10021

William H. Coryell, M.D.
Professor, Department of Psychiatry
University of Iowa College of Medicine
500 Newton Road
Iowa City, IA 52242

Jean Endicott, Ph.D.
Research and Assessment Training Unit
New York State Psychiatric Institute
722 West 168th Street
New York, NY 10032

Horacio Fabrega
Western Psychiatric Institute & Clinic
3811 O'Hara Street
Pittsburgh, PA 15213-2593

Jan A. Fawcett, M.D.
Professor & Chairman
Department of Psychiatry
Rush Medical College
Marshall Field IV Health Center
1720 West Polk Street
Chicago, IL 60612

Richard M. Finn, M.D.
Associate Professor
Department of Psychiatry
Psychiatric Hospital
University of Iowa Hospitals & Clinics
500 Newton Road
Iowa City, IA 52242

Allen J. Frances, M.D.
Professor of Psychiatry
Payne Whitney Clinic
Cornell University Medical College
525 East 68th Street
New York, NY 10021

Linda K. George, Ph.D.
Professor of Medical Sociology
Duke University Medical Center
Box 3003
Durham, NC 27710

Ernest M. Gruenberg, M.D.
Professor Emeritus of Mental Hygiene
& of Psychiatry
Johns Hopkins University
5225 Pooks Hill Road, Apt. S-222
Bethesda, MD 20814

John E. Helzer, M.D.
Professor of Psychiatry
Washington University School of Medicine
4940 Audubon Avenue
St. Louis, MO 63110

Robert Hirschfeld, M.D.
Chief, Affective & Anxiety Disorders
Research Branch
National Institute of Mental Health
Parklawn Building, Room 10C-24
5600 Fishers Lane
Rockville, MD 20857

Charles E. Holzer III, M.D.
Associate Professor of Psychiatry
Department of Psychiatry
University of Texas Medical Branch
321 Administration Annex I
Galveston, TX 77550

Marvin Karno, M.D.
Department of Psychiatry
University of California – Los Angeles
760 Westwood Plaza
Los Angeles, CA 90024

Martin B. Keller, M.D.
Assistant Professor of Psychiatry
Massachusetts General Hospital
15 Parkman Street, Room 707
Boston, MA 02114

Kenneth S. Kendler, M.D.
Associate Professor
Departments of Psychiatry & Human
Genetics
Medical College of Virginia Hospitals
Box 710
Richmond, VA 23298

Martha J. Kirkpatrick, M.D.
Associate Clinical Professor of Psychiatry
988 Bluegrass Lane
Los Angeles, CA 90049

Gerald L. Klerman, M.D.
The New York Hospital – Cornell Medical
Center
Westchester Division
21 Bloomingdale Road
White Plains, NY 10605

Maria Kovacs, Ph.D.
Professor of Psychiatry
University of Pittsburgh School of Medicine
Western Psychiatric Institute & Clinic
3811 O'Hara Street
Pittsburgh, PA 15213

David J. Kupfer, M.D.
Professor & Chair, Department of
Psychiatry
University of Pittsburgh School of Medicine
Western Psychiatric Institute & Clinic
3811 O'Hara Street
Pittsburgh, PA 15213

Philip J. Leaf, Ph.D.
Research Scientist
Director, Center for Mental Health
Services Research
Yale University School of Medicine
350 Congress Avenue
New Haven, CT 06519

Contributors xiii

Larry McEvoy, M.A.
Statistical Data Analyst
Washington University School of Medicine
4949 Barns Hospital Plaza
St. Louis, MO 63110

David P. McWhirter, M.D.
4545 Park Boulevard, Suite 207
San Diego, CA 92116

Kathleen R. Merikangas, Ph.D.
Depression Research Unit
Department of Psychiatry
Yale University School of Medicine
350 Congress Avenue
New Haven, CT 06519

Ada C. Mezzich, Ph.D.
Western Psychiatric Institute & Clinic
3811 O'Hara Street
Pittsburgh, PA 15213-2593

Juan E. Mezzich, M.D., Ph.D.
Western Psychiatric Institute & Clinic
3811 O'Hara Street
Pittsburgh, PA 15213-2593

Robert Michels, M.D.
Chairman, Department of Psychiatry
Cornell University Medical College
Psychiatrist-in-Chief
The New York Hospital
525 East 68th Street
New York, NY 10021

Jerome K. Myers, Ph.D.
Professor, Department of Sociology
Yale University
140 Prospect Street
New Haven, CT 06520

Judy Nath, Ph.D.
Trenton State College
Hillwood Lake, CN 4700
Trenton, NJ 08650

John C. Nemiah, M.D.
Professor of Psychiatry Emeritus
Harvard Medical School
Professor of Psychiatry
Dartmouth Medical School
4 Rayton Road
Hanover, NH 03755

Gerald Nestadt, M.D., Ph.D.
Department of Psychiatry
Johns Hopkins University School of
  Medicine
Meyer Building, Room 228
600 North Wolfe Street
Baltimore, MD 20215

Donald S. Rae, M.A.
Division of Clinical Research
National Institute of Mental Health
5600 Fishers Lane, Room 10C-09
Rockville, MD 20857

Darrel A. Regier, M.D., M.P.H.
Director, Division of Clinical Research
National Institute of Mental Health
5600 Fishers Lane, Room 10-105
Rockville, MD 20857

Lee J. Robins, Ph.D.
Professor of Sociology in Psychiatry
Department of Psychiatry
Washington University Medical School
4940 Audubon Avenue
St. Louis, MO 63110

Bruce J. Rounsaville, M.D.
Director of Research
Substance Abuse Treatment Unit
Department of Psychiatry
Yale University School of Medicine
904 Howard Avenue, Suite 2E
New Haven, CT 06519

William A. Scheftner, M.D.
Department of Psychiatry
Rush Medical College
1725 West Harrison, Suite 1072
Chicago, IL 60612

Steven S. Sharfstein, M.D.
Clinical Professor, University of Maryland
Vice-President & Medical Director
The Sheppard & Enoch Pratt Hospital
P.O. Box 6815
Baltimore, MD 21285-6815

Larry J. Siever, M.D.
Director, Outpatient Clinic
Bronx Veterans Administration Medical
  Center
130 West Kingsbridge Road
Bronx, NY 10468

Richard C. Simons, M.D.
Professor of Psychiatry
Department of Psychiatry, Box C-249
University of Colorado Health Science
  Center
4200 East 9th Avenue
Denver, CO 80262

Denise Snyder, Ph.D.
Trenton State College
Hillwood Lake, CN 4700
Trenton, NJ 08650

Robert L. Spitzer, M.D.
Biometric Research Department
New York State Psychiatric Institute
722 West 168th Street
New York, NY 10032

Roger K. Stoltzman, M.D.
King's Daughters Medical Center
2200 Lexington Avenue
Ashland, KY 41101

Michael Alan Taylor, M.D.
Professor & Chairman
Department of Psychiatry & Behavioral
  Sciences
UHS/The Chicago Medical School,
  Building 50
3333 Green Bay Road
North Chicago, IL 60064

Michael E. Thase, M.D.
Western Psychiatric Institute & Clinic
3811 O'Hara Street
Pittsburgh, PA 15213-2593

Gary L. Tischler, M.D.
Professor & Chairman, Department of
  Psychiatry
Yale University
25 Park Street, Room 619
New Haven, CT 06519

Gary J. Tucker, M.D.
Professor & Chairman
Department of Psychiatry & Behavioral
  Sciences
University of Washington, RP-10
Seattle, WA 98195

George E. Vaillant, M.D.
Raymond Sobel Professor of Psychiatry
Dartmouth Medical School
Hanover, NH 03756

Lynn Waterhouse, Ph.D.
Director, Child Behavior Study
Holman Hall 341
Trenton State College
Hillwood Lakes, CN 4700
Trenton, NJ 08625-4700

Myrna M. Weissman, Ph.D.
Director, Depression Research Unit
Department of Psychiatry
350 Congress Avenue
New Haven, CT 06519-8068

Thomas A. Widiger, Ph.D.
Associate Professor, Psychology
  Department
University of Kentucky
Lexington, KY 40506-0044

Janet B. W. Williams
Biometric Research Department
New York State Psychiatric Institute
722 West 168th Street
New York, NY 10032

Normund Wong, M.D.
Department of Psychiatry
Box 1195
Letterman Army Medical Center
San Francisco, CA 94129

Lyman C. Wynne, M.D., Ph.D.
University of Rochester Medical Center
300 Crittenden Boulevard, Wing R
Rochester, NY 14642

PART I

The affective disorders

It is quite appropriate to begin a consideration of diagnosis and classification in psychiatry with a review of recent findings on the utility and validity of the classification of affective disorders set forth in *DSM-III*. The affective disorders are among the disorders with the highest prevalence and have constituted a major focus of recent clinical and epidemiologic studies in adults and in children. These studies, all of which are still ongoing, include the following: the NIMH Collaborative Study on the Psychobiology of Depression, which has both a clinical component and a biological component; the NIMH Treatment Study of Depression, comparing two types of psychotherapy (interpersonal and cognitive) against imipramine in outpatients with major depression; the NIMH Collaborative Study on the Maintenance Drug Treatment of Depression, comparing lithium and/or imipramine in patients with recurrent major depression; the NIMH Epidemiologic Catchment Area (NIMH–ECA) study, which is being conducted in five United States centers and has epidemiologic data on rates and risk factors for the affective disorders; several studies of children at high risk for major depression by virtue of having a parent with an affective disorder, as well as family studies of the first-degree relatives of probands with major depression or bipolar disorder. Much of the data from these studies, though still unpublished, is quite pertinent to this topic. In Part I, some preliminary results based on follow-up, family aggregation, and treatment studies are presented and discussed.

The initial chapter by Gerald Klerman and his colleagues provides a conceptual framework for the approaches to validating the definitions of the affective disorders adopted by the NIMH Collaborative Study on the Psychobiology of Depression and describes results based primarily, but not exclusively, on the clinical data from the NIMH Collaborative Study. Next, the validity of the definition of major depression from a psychobiological perspective is discussed by David Kupfer in a comprehensive review of biological studies that either support or fail to support the nosologic independence of major depression. Paula Clayton focuses on bipolar disorders and schizoaffective disorders, and Hagop Akiskal discusses the border between the affective disorders and the personality disorders, including atypical subtypes, temperamental variants, and schizoaffective disorders. In the "Overview," we review the affective and other disorders from the perspective of the NIMH–ECA study and the family-genetic studies of adults and children that are currently being conducted by the Yale group. We also provide a summary of issues that were raised during discussion of the preceding chapters.

Myrna M. Weissman

1   *Major depression and related affective disorders*

GERALD L. KLERMAN,
ROBERT M. A. HIRSCHFELD,
NANCY C. ANDREASEN, WILLIAM CORYELL,
JEAN ENDICOTT, JAN FAWCETT,
MARTIN B. KELLER, AND
WILLIAM A. SCHEFTNER

The third edition of the *Diagnostic and Statistical Manual of Mental Disorders (DSM-III)* represents a major advance in the field of affective disorders. It is the first official diagnosis and classification system to create a separate category for affective disorders. The decision to create that category recognized the findings from increasingly sophisticated research involving epidemiology, family and genetic studies, clinical course, psychopathology, and therapeutics in this group of psychiatric conditions.

In previous editions of the *DSM* and the World Health Organization (WHO) *International Classification of Diseases (ICD)* the various affective disorders were not grouped together in a separate category, but were assigned to the psychotic and neurotic categories. The *DSM-III* decision not to continue that division between neurotic and psychotic affective disorders was based on a number of considerations. Foremost was the intention that *DSM-III* be as free as possible of assumptions regarding etiology, causation, and pathogenesis for those disorders in which causes were not firmly established by available scientific evidence. The psychotic–neurotic distinction carried the connotation that psychotic conditions are due to biological factors, whereas neurotic conditions are due to intrapsychic conflict, personality abnormalities, or psychosocial and behavioral factors.

From the National Institute of Mental Health–Clinical Research Branch Collaborative Program on the Psychobiology of Depression: Clinical Studies. This was completed with the cooperation and participation of the Collaborative Program Investigators: G. L. Klerman, M.D. (Chairperson) (Boston); R. M. A. Hirschfeld, M.D. (Project Director and Co-Chairperson) and B. H. Larkin, B.A. (Coordinating Protocol Monitor) (NIMH); M. B. Keller, M.D., and P. Lavori, Ph.D. (Boston); J. Fawcett, M.D., W. A. Scheftner, M.D., G. Winokur, M.D., and P. Wasek, B.A. (Iowa City); J. Endicott, Ph.D., and P. McDonald-Scott, M.A. (New York); J. Rice, Ph.D., S. Guze, M.D., T. Reich, M.D., and D. Altis, B.A. (St. Louis). Other contributors include P. J. Clayton, M.D., J. Croughan, M.D., M. M. Katz, Ph.D., E. Robins, M.D., R. W. Shapiro, and R. Spitzer, M.D.

In general, *DSM-III* takes an atheoretical position with regard to the causes of most disorders. The organic disorders and substance-abuse disorders are the notable exceptions, because evidence regarding the causes of these conditions is very good. For the category of affective disorders, in which the evidence regarding causes is inconclusive, the criteria for classifying depressive and manic conditions together are based on phenomenology and clinical description.

As a whole, *DSM-III* cannot be atheoretical, because every classification has its assumptions and preconceptions. The phenomenologic and descriptive approach adopted by *DSM-III* represents a general theoretical position with regard to the nature of psychopathology, disorders, and psychiatry (Cooper and Michels, 1981; Klerman, 1983). However, with regard to the causation of the affective disorders, individually or as a group, an atheoretical position, sometimes called "agnostic," is adopted (Carroll, 1981).

This chapter reviews the evidence for the reliability and validity of the classes of affective disorders in *DSM-III*. The review is based mainly on the experience of the NIMH Collaborative Study, as well as a review of the literature. For each disorder there is a brief review of the background of the concept, followed by a discussion of the evidence for reliability and validity, as available.

The general approach to determining reliability and validity is summarized in Table 1.1. The basic principle is that in the absence of conclusive evidence regarding etiology or pathogenesis, the validity of a diagnostic class is established by (1) careful description, (2) demonstration of the reliability of diagnostic judgments, and (3) demonstration of its relevance. The validity category is divided into internal and external validity. The most powerful sources of evidence for justifiability are external validations, that is, correlations of the clinical picture with other domains of evidence: epidemiologic rates and covariation with age and sex; familial aggregation and genetic transmission; correlation with psychosocial factors such as personality, life events, and social supports; response to treatments, both psychopharmacologic and psychotherapeutic; clinical course and outcome; biochemical and neurophysiologic studies.[1] In addition, following Kendell (1982), attention must be given to boundary problems – the degree of separation between the disorder in question and related conditions.

NIMH Collaborative Program on the Psychobiology of Depression

Most, but not all, of the material reviewed in this chapter derives from the NIMH–Clinical Research Branch (CRB) Collaborative Program on the Psy-

---

[1] Because the chapter by Kupfer and Thase in this volume deals comprehensively with biochemical and neurophysiologic studies, these validators are not reviewed in this chapter.

Table 1.1. *Criteria for establishing the validity of individual classes of affective disorders*

A. Reliability
B. Internal validity
C. External validity
   1. Epidemiology
   2. Familial aggregation and genetic transmission
   3. Psychosocial factors: personality, social support, and life events
   4. Response to treatment
   5. Clinical course and outcome
   6. Biochemical and neurophysiological studies
D. Boundary problems: degree of separation between the disorder and related conditions

chobiology of Depression (CPPD): Clinical Studies (Katz and Klerman, 1979; Katz et al., 1979). This program was initiated following the 1968 Williamsburg Conference (Williams, Katz, and Shield, 1972). In the early 1970s, two collaborative programs were undertaken by NIMH: One was entitled the Biology of Affective Disorder, and the other Clinical Studies.

The Clinical Studies program involves five university centers in Boston, New York, Chicago, St. Louis, and Iowa City. The major goal of the clinical studies is to establish the comparative validities of alternative nosologic systems for affective disorders. In addition, there is a large family-genetic study and also a follow-up of the probands and of the relatives to determine factors related to natural history and clinical course in affective disorders. The sample of patients includes 957 probands admitted to the five institutions with diagnoses of depression or manic episodes. Findings regarding clinical symptoms, reliability, and follow-up have been reported (Katz and Klerman, 1979).

To study the comparative validity of nosology it was considered necessary to use a structured diagnostic interview. For this purpose, the Schedule of Affective Disorders and Schizophrenia (SADS) was developed and its reliability established (Endicott and Spitzer, 1978). In addition, a set of algorithms for operational diagnostic criteria for 22 disorders was developed and codified in the Research Diagnostic Criteria (RDC) (Spitzer, Endicott, and Robins, 1978). The RDC was based in large part on the Washington University criteria (Feighner et al., 1972).

In many respects, the RDC is a precursor to the approach taken by *DSM-III*. This not only was conceptual but also was based on the roles played by a number of individuals (Drs. Spitzer, Endicott, Andreasen, and Clayton) who served on the *DSM-III* committee and were also involved in the NIMH Collaborative Study.

BIPOLAR DISORDER[2]

Background

The concept "manic-depressive insanity" was proposed by Kraepelin in 1895. In this nosologic category, a large number of clinical states described in the nineteenth century, including *folie "circulaire,"* mania, melancholia, and involutional melancholia, were combined based on their similar clinical courses. In 1959, Leonhard proposed separating patients with Kraepelin's manic-depressive insanity into two groups: patients with a history of both depressive and manic episodes, whom he called "bipolar," and those with only depressive episodes or only manic/hypomanic episodes, whom he called "monopolar." As subsequent usage evolved, the category of bipolar disorder came to include patients with a history of episodes of both depression and mania, as well as those uncommon patients with one or more episodes of only mania or hypomania, and the term "unipolar" came to be applied to patients with recurrent episodes of depression but without a history of episodes of hypomania or mania. The concept of bipolar disorder gained rapid acceptance within the research and clinical communities in the 1970s. Controversy, however, continued around the concept of unipolar illness and its criteria and relation to other disorders, particularly neurotic depression.

The *DSM-III* adopted the concept of bipolar illness as a replacement for the *DSM-II* manic-depressive illness. It did not include "unipolar illness," but subsumed what most clinicians called "unipolar" within the category of major depression.

Reliability

The evidence for reliability in defining bipolar disorder is good. In the NIMH Collaborative Study, the results from joint interviews, test–retest, and intercenter reliability determinations were excellent (Andreasen et al., 1982).

Internal validity

The diagnostic criteria for depressive episodes are widely accepted. A number of researchers have observed that the clinical picture of depressive episodes in bipolar patients includes hypersomnia and increased appetite (Beigel and Murphy, 1971).

The diagnostic criteria for mania are also widely accepted. Factor-analytic studies have demonstrated a manic-excitement factor in psychiatric hospitalized patients (Lorr, 1963). However, disagreement exists as to which particular

---

[2] Bipolar disorder is not discussed in great detail in this chapter because it is covered in the chapter by Clayton.

symptom set is most useful. The inclusion of irritability as one of the key diagnostic symptoms has been criticized (Young, 1983).

External validity

The validity of the category bipolar disorder has been widely accepted. There are excellent correlations with clinical course and familial aggregation, suggestive of genetic transmission, and there is good response to treatment, particularly with lithium.

Boundary problems

Disagreement exists as to three boundaries for bipolar disorder: (1) with milder nonpsychotic forms, (2) with other psychotic states, particularly schizophrenia and schizoaffective disorder, and (3) with unipolar depression.

Bipolar II. A number of investigators have proposed distinctions between bipolar I and bipolar II (Dunner, 1983). This category does not appear in *DSM-III* but does appear in the RDC. Bipolar II features less severe forms of symptoms, without delusions or other psychotic features, and without need for hospitalization. Reliability studies indicate low reliability for defining bipolar II disorder (Coryell et al., 1984a; Endicott et al., 1985).

Other psychotic states. The other significant boundary problem occurs in patients with marked overactivity, delusional thinking, and grandiosity. The problem of determining the boundary between schizophrenia and schizoaffective states continues to plague the field (Pope and Lipinski, 1978).

Are bipolar and unipolar disorders separate? An unresolved issue is whether bipolar disorder and nonbipolar major depression (unipolar illness) are separate forms of disorder or whether they form a continuum. A number of efforts have applied genetic models using multiple-threshold liability statistics (Gershon, 1983; T. Reich, pers. commun.). The answers are not yet clear.

Discussion

There is wide agreement regarding the validity and utility of the category bipolar illness. Unresolved questions center around the symptom set for defining patients, the symptomatic quality of the depression associated with bipolar illness, and the boundary problems, particularly the possible heterogeneity within bipolar disorder and the necessity to establish boundaries with schizophrenia and schizoaffective states.

The major theoretical issue is whether unipolar and bipolar illnesses represent a single disorder or whether they represent two disorders, or more likely two groups of disorders. Pending further information on this, separation of these disorders on clinical grounds seems justified.

MAJOR DEPRESSION

Background

Major depression, a new category in *DSM-III,* brings together a number of conditions, including psychotic depressive disorder, psychoneurotic depressive reaction, and nonbipolar forms of recurrent manic-depressive insanity.

Major depression is the subject of much controversy. It represents a significant departure from previous nomenclatures and from current clinical usage in Western Europe. The distinction is made between the endogenous–psychotic and the neurotic forms of depression as codified in *ICD-9.* This distinction is based on presumed causes rather than clinical psychopathology and symptoms. In European centers, "endogenous depression" refers to depressions with presumed biological causes as manifested by a pattern of symptoms during a given episode and by the phasic course of the illness.

In addition to the differences between American and European views, two groups of American clinicians and investigators have differing views. Many psychodynamically oriented psychiatrists are dissatisfied with the elimination of "neurotic depression," whereas many biological psychiatrists view the criteria as too broad, the symptom set too general, and the criterion of two weeks' duration of symptoms too brief. Consequently, they conclude that many patients diagnosed as having major depression are experiencing states of demoralization and/or having transient responses to situational stress and/or to chronic adverse social circumstances, such as poverty or persistent marital discord, rather than a "true," i.e., biological, depression.

Reliability

Studies have reported excellent reliability for the RDC definition of major depressive disorder. Because the *DSM-III* and the RDC criteria are so close, we can assume that this also applies for the *DSM-III* definition of major depression. The reliability in diagnosing major depression is indirectly corroborated by findings from the NIMH Epidemiologic Catchment Area (ECA) study. Rates of depression among age and sex groups have been similar across the three participating sites, New Haven, Baltimore, and St. Louis, suggesting that the reliability of the diagnosis is consistent in these three locales (Myers et al., 1984).

Internal validity

Factor-analytic and cluster-analytic studies have generated a general factor for rating the severity of illness and the depressive syndrome (Katz and Hirschfeld, 1978; Andreasen, Grove, and Maurer, 1980).

External validity

Epidemiology

Rates. Epidemiologic studies have shown an incidence of about 4% per year (Weissman and Myers, 1978).

Age. There is evidence of a cohort effect (Klerman, 1976; Klerman et al., 1985). For patients from the most recent cohorts, there appears to be a younger age of onset and fewer male–female differences than reported for previous cohorts (Klerman, 1983; Murphy et al., 1984).

Sex. Almost all studies have indicated a higher incidence among females than among males.

Familial aggregation and genetic transmission. Family studies, although indicating a high familial aggregation, have indicated less familial aggregation than for bipolar disorder. Investigators using familial aggregation techniques have looked more carefully at subtypes, particularly psychotic depression and melancholia (see later sections).

Psychosocial factors: personality, social support, and life events

Personality. Numerous hypotheses have been proposed to describe the relationship of personality attributes and patterns to the predisposition for major depression. Various theoretical approaches have been applied to depression, including psychoanalystic, interpersonal, behavioral, and cognitive. No consistent personality pattern has been reliably associated with depression using systematic techniques. These have been reviewed by Hirschfeld and Klerman (1979) and Akiskal, Hirschfeld, and Yerevanian (1983).

Social support. A number of hypotheses have been proposed linking a lack of social support to predisposition to acute episodes of depression (Brown and Harris, 1978). Henderson (Henderson et al., 1978), one of the early proponents of the social-support hypothesis, has recently presented new data indicating that social support does not operate independently of personality and other predisposing factors and that when these factors are controlled, the power of social support as a risk factor is markedly diminished.

Life events. Early childhood loss has been hypothesized as an antecedent life event predisposing to adult depression. However, the results of this research are still inconclusive (Tennant, Bebbington, and Hurry, 1980).

Adverse life events in the 6 to 12 months preceding the onset of depression have been shown to increase the risk for acute depression (Paykel, 1978). Comparative studies have indicated that the increased risk following adverse life events is greater for depression than for schizophrenia (Paykel et al., 1969). However, life events by themselves cannot account for all depressions, and most observers have concluded that there is an interaction of life events with vulnerability factors based on familial background.

Response to treatment

Treatment of acute episodes. Partial validation of the concept of major depression has come from the numerous studies indicating a beneficial response of the depressive syndrome to a number of classes of compounds, particularly the tricyclic antidepressants and the monoamine oxidase (MAO) inhibitors. In addition, electroconvulsive therapy (ECT) has a high degree of efficacy. However, response to treatment has more often been advocated as being a validator for specific subtypes, such as melancholia, than for the category as a whole. The *DSM-III* definition of major depression has not been widely used as a criterion for selection of patients in clinical trials. Most clinical trials have used variations of *DSM-II* criteria or the investigator's own classifications.

Long-term treatment. Another aspect of the treatment response that serves as a validator concerns the differential effects of long-term treatment on relapse and recurrence for unipolar patients and bipolar patients. The NIMH studies (Prien, Klett, and Caffey, 1973) have demonstrated that for bipolar patients, treatment with tricyclics alone is deleterious, in that a substantial proportion of bipolar patients will be "pushed over" into mania. This has also been reported for MAO inhibitors and for a number of the newer antidepressants. For bipolar patients, therefore, maintenance therapy with lithium is the most effective treatment. For nonbipolar patients, who fall within the *DSM-III* category major depression, elsewhere called unipolar, the evidence is that two classes of drugs, lithium and tricyclics, provide the best treatment, and recent studies have indicated a slight advantage for the tricyclics over lithium for prevention of recurrence and relapse.

Psychotherapy. A number of controlled clinical trials have indicated value in some forms of brief psychotherapy for ambulatory depressed, nonpsychotic, nonbipolar patients (Rush, 1982; Weissman, 1984).

Clinical course and outcome. A number of outcomes are relevant for establishing the validity of the category major depression. These include the following:

1. *Recovery from the acute episode.*
2. *Tendency to relapse and recurrence.* The majority of patients with major depressive disorder have one episode (Robins and Guze, 1972). About 50% of patients will experience one or more recurrences. The likelihood of recurrence increases with each successive episode (Lavori, Keller, and Klerman, in press).
3. *Suicide.*
4. *Stability of the diagnosis of affective disorder.* A significant percentage of patients who present with major depression later develop manic episodes. Attempts to predict the characteristics of patients initially diagnosed as having major depressive disorder who will subsequently shift to bipolar disorder are

now under way. A number of such factors have been identified, including a previous history of mild hypomanic swings, a family history of bipolar illness in first-degree relatives, and hypomanic responses to tricyclic and MAO medication (Akiskal, 1981).

5. *Change in bipolarity.* A substantial percentage (approximately 10%) of patients with major depressive disorder are likely to subsequently develop a manic or hypomanic episode (switch in polarity), requiring a change in subsequent diagnosis from major depression to bipolar disorder.

6. *Quality of intermorbid functioning* in psychosocial activities and personality.

Boundary problems: degree of separation between the disorder and related conditions

There are three major boundary problems for major depression:

1. *Bipolar disorder.*[3]
2. *Anxiety disorders.* A substantial percentage of patients with depression (approximately 60%) will have symptoms of anxiety, often of sufficient intensity and duration to meet the criteria for generalized anxiety disorder. The hierarchical principle in *DSM-III* subsumes these under major depression. A certain percentage, as yet uncertain, of patients will also have panic attacks and other anxiety disorders. With respect to the boundary for anxiety disorders, many observers point to the high rate of anxiety symptoms among patients with a diagnosis of depression (approximately 60%). Use of discriminant-function analysis has contributed to separation of depression from anxiety states (Downing and Rickels, 1974; Prusoff and Klerman, 1974). Contributing to the complexity of the problem is the increased incidence of anxiety disorders among relatives of patients with depressive disorders (Leckman et al., 1985).
3. *Axis II personality disorders.*

The overlap with personality disorders is a considerable problem, particularly for dysthymia. The *DSM-III* encourages simultaneous diagnosis of axis I and axis II disorders. Recent studies indicate that about 40% of patients who meet the *DSM-III* criteria for major depression also have some axis II diagnosis (Shea, 1983).

Discussion

As indicated, two types of dissatisfaction have been expressed regarding the general concept of major depressive disorder. Many psychoanalytically oriented investigators propose to reinstate the concept of neurotic depression or to introduce a category of "reactive or situational depression." This is also an issue in the interchange between North American and Western European investigators, among whom the endogenous–neurotic distinction is widely accepted.

Many other clinicians and investigators, particularly those with a biological orientation, have criticized the *DSM-III* definition of major depressive disorder

---

[3] The boundary with bipolar disorder was discussed earlier.

as too broad and have proposed various restrictions on the diagnostic symptom set and the duration criteria. Gershon, Angst, and others have proposed more stringent impairment criteria requiring some evidence of hospitalization or occupational role impairment.

A number of proposals have been made for additional subtypes within the category of major depression, including return of the concept of reactive or situational depression and of concepts related to "atypical depression." These proposals are discussed in later sections.

MAJOR DEPRESSION, MELANCHOLIA

Background

The creation in *DSM-III* of the category of major depression, melancholia, was the response of the *DSM-III* task force to the debate over "endogenous depression." Whereas the European concept, as described earlier, involves widespread etiologic assumptions, research using the criteria based exclusively on symptomatic expression during a current episode has shown evidence for reliability and validity. By using the term "melancholia," *DSM-III* attempted to remove any presumption of cause from the diagnosis of "endogenous depression," and following the RDC, the *DSM-III* definition of melancholia relies entirely on symptom patterning, assessed cross-sectionally during an acute episode.

Reliability

Studies have indicated high reliability for the RDC definition of endogenous depression (Andreasen et al., 1982; Keller et al., 1983).

Internal validity

Numerous factor-analytic studies (Mendels and Cochrane, 1968) have consistently demonstrated an entity with symptoms of diurnal impairment, early morning awakening, insomnia, appetite disturbance, loss of weight, loss of interest, and so on. Klein (1974) has proposed that his symptom complex be called "endogenomorphic."

Several alternative sets of symptom criteria have been established. These include the RDC endogenous, the *DSM-III* melancholic, and the symptom set in autonomous depression (Nelson, Charney, and Quinlan, 1981). Hirschfeld has presented data indicating a high degree of overlap among patients diagnosed concurrently by these three systems. This has been called the polydiagnostic approach (Berner and Katschnig, 1983). The *DSM-III* criteria cast the widest net. The autonomous depression criteria, which emphasize the nonreactive clinical course after entrance into treatment, select the narrowest group. The RDC criteria for endogenous depression are intermediate.

External validity

Epidemiology

> *Rates.* Epidemiologic studies have shown an incidence of about 4% per year (Weissman and Myers, 1978).
>
> *Age.* There is evidence of a cohort effect (Klerman, 1976; Klerman et al., 1985). For patients from the most recent cohorts, there appears to be a younger age of onset and fewer male–female differences than reported for previous cohorts (Klerman, 1983; Murphy et al., 1984).
>
> *Sex.* Almost all studies have indicated a higher incidence among females than among males.

Familial aggregation and genetic transmission. Two recent family studies using RDC or *DSM-III* criteria did not find evidence of increased familial aggregation of depression among relatives of patients diagnosed as having melancholia (R. Hirschfeld and T. Reich, unpublished data; Leckman et al., 1984). These findings are surprising in view of the assumption among most biological psychiatrists that among all the subtypes of depression, patients with melancholia or endogenous depression are the most likely to show a genetic-familial, that is, endogenous or constitutional, basis (Kiloh and Garside, 1963).

Psychosocial factors: personality, social support, and life events. Attempts to test hypotheses regarding personality correlates have not proved successful (Hirschfeld and Klerman, 1979). The relationship involving melancholic symptom patterns and life events is complicated. The classic view of endogenous depression presumes that precipitating life events are not to be found. Recent studies in the United States using RDC (Klerman et al., 1979) and studies in Austria (H. Katschnig, per. commun.) have indicated that about 50% of patients with RDC endogenous depression also have had demonstrable adverse life events when the life-events assessment is made by standardized techniques and collected independently of the clinical-symptoms picture. Therefore, the presence or absence of recent life events cannot be used as either a diagnostic or validating criterion.

Response to treatment. The conventional wisdom among clinicians and investigators is that the melancholic symptom pattern is predictive of responses to drugs, particularly tricyclics, and to ECT. This has not been established by controlled clinical trials with random assignment to endogenous versus alternative treatment groups. Nevertheless, that remains the consensus (Bielski and Friedel, 1977). Differential responses of melancholic patients to drugs and poor responses to psychotherapy have been reported (Prusoff and Klerman, 1974).

Clinical course and outcome. Most of the research relevant to melancholia was conducted on the concepts of endogenous depression prior to *DSM-III*. Assuming equivalence of *DSM-III* melancholia with endogenous depression, the hypothesis would be that melancholia is more prone to a phasic course, that is, clearly demarcated episodes with discernible periods of recovery and wellness between episodes. Moreover, patients with this subtype are hypothesized to be prone to multiple recurrences over a lifetime. Meanwhile, relationships to other outcomes (i.e., shift to bipolarity, suicide, social adjustment) have not been well established. The classic concept of endogenous depression predicts good return to premorbid adjustment and a relatively normal intermorbid state. However, the concept of normality used in previous studies focused on affective symptoms and mental functioning. Relatively less attention was given to interpersonal relations, work performance, and measures of self-esteem and personal satisfaction.

Boundary problems: degree of separation between the disorder and related conditions

There is a continuing debate, particularly in the United Kingdom and Continental centers, as to the endogenous–neurotic distinction. As reviewed in great detail by Kiloh and Garside, this extensive debate has pitted the Newcastle School, associated with Roth (Cambridge, England) and Kiloh (Australia), against the London Group. Various attempts to use factor analysis in multivariate techniques have not resolved this problem.

Discussion

There is wide agreement on the utility of the concept of melancholic depression. Further research is needed to determine the most efficient set of symptom criteria with the best validity. Further efforts to establish the validity, particularly predictive validity with respect to treatment assignment, are called for. Attempts to reconcile U.K. and European concepts concerning endogenous–reactive depression with American concepts regarding major depression and melancholia are needed and are under way in many settings.

MAJOR DEPRESSION, PSYCHOTIC

Background

The nature of psychotic depression has been controversial for many decades. The *DSM-II* category of psychotic depressive reaction subsumed patients whose depressions were of psychotic quality and intensity but did not fit into the manic-depressive category, usually because they were judged by clinicians to be precipitated by life events. Different criteria for psychotic depression were used inconsistently:

1. Some criteria were based on symptoms of impairment of higher mental functioning, specifically delusions, hallucinations, or confusion. This is the "narrow" definition relying exclusively on cross-sectional psychopathology.

2. The psychoanalytic concept of psychotic states (Fenichel, 1945) defined psychosis on the basis of the level of regression and the degree of impairment of ego functions, rather than evidence of specific psychopathology or level of impairment of social functioning.
3. Many U.S. clinicians equated psychotic depression with severity of impairment, particularly of social functioning, and the term "psychotic" came to mean severely ill. In the RDC, the category of incapacitating depression was created to separate this entity from depression with delusions and hallucinations.
4. Many clinicians and investigators used the term "psychotic" as if it were synonymous with "endogenous," implying a biochemical or genetic cause. The RDC restricted the category of psychotic depression to patients with delusions and hallucinations and included a category of incapacitating depression.
5. The *DSM-III,* in the subcategory of major depression, for psychotic features relies exclusively on evidence of delusions and hallucinations without any presumptions as to cause, life events, degree of social incapacity, or psychodynamic ego regression.

Reliability

Coryell and associates (1984b) have reviewed the evidence for reliability and have found high overall reliability, although low reliability for the individual delusions.

Internal validity

High internal consistency has been demonstrated when the presence of delusions has constituted the essential clinical picture. These symptoms are often correlated with suicidal intent, low levels of social functioning, and the clinician's judgment of the need for hospitalization. There is controversy about whether or not mood-incongruent delusions should be included (Brockington, Kendell, and Wainwright, 1980). Many researchers regard mood-incongruent delusions as a major indication for a diagnosis of schizoaffective, depressed, as separate from major depressive disorder, psychotic.

External validity

Epidemiology

Rates. Psychotic depression is relatively uncommon. Only about 10% of inpatient samples meet this criteria, and a very small percentage of outpatient samples. Data on risk factors are not available.

Familial aggregation and genetic transmission. Studies indicate that there is a slightly increased familial aggregation of delusional depression among first-degree relatives of probands with delusional depression (Charney and Nelson, 1981; Coryell et al., 1984b; Leckman et al., 1984; Endicott et al., 1985).

Psychosocial factors: personality, social support, and life events. Psychosocial factors have not been widely investigated for delusional depression. Brown has hypothesized that loss of a parent before the age of 11 predisposes to psychotic features in adult episodes of depression (Brown and Harris, 1978). This hypothesis has not been confirmed.

Response to treatment. Treatment-response studies also indicate the validity of this diagnosis. Patients with delusional features do not respond well to tricyclics alone (Sweeney et al., 1978; Glassman and Roose, 1981), but they do respond to a combination of tricyclics and neuroleptics (Spiker, 1979) or to ECT. Quitkin, Rifkin, and Klein (1976) have reanalyzed their data following a 20-year study by Klein and do not agree that delusional depressions are always unresponsive to tricyclics. Delusional features in a depressed person also increase the likelihood of suicide.

Clinical course and outcome. The best evidence for the validity of this concept comes from follow-up studies. Coryell et al. (1982) have reviewed the evidence for the predictive validity of delusions in the course of depression and found that delusions influenced the short-term course, but not the long-term course, such that the presence of delusions means that it will take a longer time to recover.

Boundary problems: degree of separation between the disorder and related conditions

A major problem exists concerning the boundary between psychotic depression and schizoaffective, depressed, disorder. This has been addressed by Coryell and associates (1984b). Some investigators advocate that the criteria for psychotic depression be restricted to mood-congruent delusions and that the use of criteria of mood-incongruent delusions be reserved for making a diagnosis of schizoaffective, depressed, disorder.

Discussion

The subcategory of psychotic depression seems to exhibit reliability and validity. The main area of disagreement concerns the importance to be given to the distinction between mood-congruent and mood-incongruent delusions. This symptom seems to provide a distinction between the category of major depression, psychotic, and that of schizoaffective, depressed, disorder.

CYCLOTHYMIC DISORDER

Background

In almost all diagnostic nomenclatures prior to *DSM-III,* cyclothymia was grouped with the personality disorders. "Cyclothymic personality" referred to individuals who had long-standing patterns, sometimes cyclical and periodic, of fluctuations between depressive and hypomanic states, but not severe enough to meet the criteria for major affective disorder. Because of the similarities between its symptom pattern and those of other affective disorders, cyclothymic disorder was included in the affective disorders in *DSM-III*.

Many theorists and clinicians consider cyclothymia to be a variant of bipolar illness. Kraepelin, in his original monograph on manic-depressive insanity, described a number of temperaments, one of which was similar to the current definition of cyclothymic personalities; these temperaments were considered by Kraepelin to be formes frustes of the manic-depressive insanity predisposition. This concept was widely accepted in European psychiatry, particularly in the writings of Kretschmer and Schneider.

Reliability

Reliability data are available from two studies: the NIMH Collaborative Study and the field trial for the *DSM-III*. These indicate reasonably good reliability for the definition of cyclothymic disorder, but at lower levels than for major depressive disorder or bipolar disorder.

Internal validity

There have been two recent reports of studies of reasonably large groups of patients diagnosed as having cyclothymic personality (Akiskal et al., 1977; Dunner, 1983). Those two reports agree on the existence of the phenomenon in clinical practice and describe its symptoms and clinical course as similar to those of bipolar disorder. There are differences in terminology: Dunner refers to cyclothymia as equivalent to bipolar II disorder.

External validity

Epidemiology. No community epidemiologic studies have had large enough samples to report risk factors associated with age, sex, or social class.

> *Rates.* The only community study of the incidence of cyclothymia has been the New Haven study, which reported a rate of 0.4.

Familial aggregation and genetic transmission. Family-history data suggest major overlap between cyclothymic disorder and bipolar I disorder (Akiskal et al., 1977; Angst, Felder, and Lohmeyer, 1980; Weissman et al., 1984).

Psychosocial factors: personality, social support, and life events. The relationship is not clear. R. Depue, at the University of Minnesota Department of Psychology, has developed a personality-trait inventory predictive of bipolar disorder. There have been no studies of life events or social supports as they relate to bipolar disorder.

Response to treatment. Akiskal (1981) and Dunner (1983) have reported good responses to lithium.

Clinical course and outcome. Many clinicians have reported that the clinical course and follow-up results often parallel those for bipolar illness.

Boundary problems: degree of separation between the disorder and related conditions

A number of problems exist with respect to hysterical personality, borderline personality, and the concept of bipolar II disorder. These have been discussed by Akiskal and associates (1977), who reported various boundary problems, particularly with hysterical personality disorder and with other forms of personality disorders. Clinical differentiation between cyclothymic disorder and other forms of affective disorders, particularly bipolar I and bipolar II, is often difficult.

Discussion

Further research is needed to clarify the boundaries between cyclothymia and other disorders. Proposals have been made to move cyclothymic disorder to the category of bipolar disorder and consider it a subcategory of bipolar disorder.

DYSTHYMIC DISORDER

Background

Dysthymic disorder is a new diagnostic category first appearing in *DSM-III*. The term "dysthymia" appears in the nineteenth-century literature and refers to unpleasant mood. The inclusion of this category in *DSM-III* was in recognition of the large numbers of individuals with chronic, low-grade distress, usually over two years in duration, who are increasingly being seen by psychiatrists and other health professionals. Because of the duration of their symptoms, these patients have been referred to by various terms: "neurotically depressed" (Klerman et al., 1979), "depressive personality," or "characterologic depression" (Spitzer, Williams, and Skodal, 1980; Akiskal, 1983). However, unlike patients with personality disorders, dysthymic individuals experience their illness as distressing (ego-alien), whereas those with personality disorders consider their behavior as ego-syntonic and not a source of distress to themselves. The combination of distress and predominant depressive symptoms led to the inclusion of dysthymia as a new category among *DSM-III* affective disorders. The RDC included categories of chronic intermittent and chronic minor depression.

Reliability

The only reliability data available are from the field trial for *DSM-III*. The RDC categories of chronic intermittent and chronic minor depression have relatively low reliability.

Internal validity

The symptom set involved in dysthymia is very similar to that for major depression. The main boundary problem is with major depressive disorder, particularly the chronic form. There is also a boundary problem with personality disorder, particularly cyclothymic and borderline personality disorders. The coexistence of acute episodes of major depression superimposed on dysthymia has led to the concept of "double depression" (Keller and Shapiro, 1982).

External validity

Epidemiology. No data on social class or other risk factors are available.

> *Rates.* Data from the NIMH-ECA study indicate a high incidence for this disorder, about 4% (about equal to the rate for major depressive disorder).
> *Age.* Preliminary findings suggest that patients fall into two groups, one group hypothesized to have an early age of onset, in childhood or adolescence, and another group that has a later age of onset, in adulthood.
> *Sex.* Females predominate.

Familial aggregation and genetic transmission. No family or genetic studies have been reported.

Psychosocial factors: personality, social support, and life events. No studies have been reported.

Response to treatment. There have been uncontrolled trials reporting responses to treatment with tricyclics, MAO inhibitors, and psychotherapy. However, in the absence of controlled trials, no definitive conclusions can be stated.

Clinical course and outcomes. Akiskal (1983) reported that a substantial percentage of dysthymic patients with onset in young adulthood or adolescence have a "switch in polarity" to bipolar illness. This has not been confirmed by other investigators. It appears that individuals with dysthymic disorder are at greater risk for acute episodes of major depressive disorder. The NIMH Collaborative Study has found that a substantial percentage of patients with chronic depression experience acute episodes (i.e., double depression).

Boundary problems: degree of separation between the disorder and related conditions

The most serious boundary problems for dysthymia are with major depression and with personality disorders. With regard to major depression, the NIMH Collaborative Study has reported the phenomenon of double depression, in which a substantial percentage of patients with dysthymia have superimposed episodes of acute depression that meet the criteria for major depression. In this situation, both diagnoses should be given. Whether this represents a single disease or two separate diseases is uncertain.

More complicated problems arise in considering the boundaries with personality disorders. Because of the duration of the problems encountered by patients with dysthymia and the enduring quality of their problems with self-esteem, guilt, and poor interpersonal relations, they often are considered to be "characterologic depressions" or are simultaneously diagnosed as axis II personality disorders, particularly dependent personality disorder, avoidant personality disorder, borderline personality, and narcissistic personality disorder. Depending on the theoretical orientation of the research or the clinician, varying degrees of emphasis will be placed on axis I or axis II.

Discussion

Akiskal (1983) has recommended a subclassification of dysthymic disorder between the early-onset and late-onset forms. Clarification is needed concerning the diagnostic status of patients with acute episodes of major depressive disorder who do not remit. These patients can be considered either to have major depressive disorder, chronic or unremitted, or to be dysthymic, or both.

The situation for dysthymic disorders as one form of chronic depression is unclear. It appears that there are two pathways to chronicity: one for patients with an early onset whose dysthymic symptoms have been present since adolescence and have persisted for many years, the other for patients who become chronic because their acute episodes of major depressive disorder fail to resolve fully (Klerman, 1980; Keller et al., 1982). Approximately 15% of patients with acute episodes of major depressive disorder have only partially remitted at one to two years. Given successive cohorts of acute episodes of major depressive disorder, this 15% residual produces a "silting" in the population contributing to the large reservoir of patients who have been diagnosed as dysthymic. The ECA reported an incidence of about 4% (Myers et al., 1984).

ATYPICAL AFFECTIVE DISORDER

The *DSM-III* includes the category of atypical affective disorder within the larger category of affective disorders. There is considerable confusion about this diagnostic category. Although systematic evidence is not available, experience indicates that the category of atypical affective disorder is used in three ways:

1. Some clinicians and investigators use this designation to refer to patients with depressive or bipolar features who do not meet the criteria of intensity of symptoms and/or duration and/or impairment. This use has similarities to terms such as "subclinical" or "borderline" conditions.
2. Other clinicians and investigators use this designation to refer to the presence of mixed symptoms and a mixed clinical course.
3. Others refer to a specific constellation of signs and symptoms often considered to be responsive to MAO inhibitors. It is this latter use that has the most clinical and research precedence.

Atypical depression

Many clinicians follow the British use of atypical depression to refer to patients whose symptom pattern does not meet the conventional criteria for endogenous depression, similar to *DSM-III* melancholia. It is widely believed that certain of these symptom classes are predictive responses to MAO inhibitors rather than to tricyclics. The original work derived from the group at St. Thomas's Hospital in London, including West and Dally (1959) and Sargent (1960). They used the term "atypical" to refer to a symptom pattern that featured the absence of vegetative signs, the absence of diurnal variation, and the presence of anxiety and phobic symptoms. This concept is well described by Davidson and associates (1982) and also by Quitkin, Rifkin, and Klein (1979) and Liebowitz and associates (1981). Partial support for this view comes from studies of predictors of responses to MAO inhibitors conducted by Robinson and associates (1973) in the United States and Paykel and associates (1979) in the United Kingdom.

Klein, Quitkin, Liebowitz, and their associates at the New York State Psychiatric Institute have developed operational criteria for "atypical depression" and have reported preliminary findings from a controlled clinical trial comparing responses of such patients to MAO inhibitors, tricyclics, and placebo.

Hysteroid dysphoria

Klein (1974) has also described a group of patients with what he calls "hysteroid dysphoria" – mainly women with atypical depressive features who are especially prone to feelings of rejection and sensitivity and who respond to MAO inhibitors (Liebowitz et al., 1981).

SCHIZOAFFECTIVE DISORDERS[4]

Background

The *DSM-III* handles schizoaffective disorders by putting them in a residual category. No specific symptom set or other diagnostic criteria are described, but the designation is used to refer to patients who have a mixture

---

[4] This is not discussed in great detail because it is reviewed in the chapter by Clayton.

of affective and schizophrenic symptoms. The category of schizoaffective disorders has a long and complicated history in twentieth-century psychiatry. The concept emerged as a response to the apparent consensus developed after Kraepelin's distinction between manic-depressive insanity and dementia praecox. Schizoaffective disorders remain matters of controversy. Historically, there have been different approaches to these disorders:

1. The term "schizoaffective disorder" was first used by Kasanin (1933), who described a group of patients with acute onset, following good premorbid adjustment, with a strong mixture of affective symptoms, including depression, anger, and fear. This description is similar to that of the Scandinavian concept of psychogenic or reactive psychosis. Kasanin emphasized the role of precipitating events. This was to distinguish these patients from those with classic dementia praecox, which involved insidious onset, no apparent precipitating event, absence of affect, and poor premorbid adjustment.

2. Another group of investigators has given prominence to the criterion of mood-incongruent delusions. The *DSM-III* criteria for psychotic depression allow for both mood-incongruent and mood-congruent delusions. Brockington and associates (1980) and Coryell, Tsuang, and McDaniel (1982) have reported different prognostic significance for delusions that are mood-congruent or mood-incongruent. These investigators would place depressed or manic patients with mood-incongruent delusions in this schizoaffective group.

3. Other investigators have emphasized the pattern of the clinical course rather than the specific psychopathology. In this view, the acute episode has schizophrenic and psychotic features, but there is usually a return to premorbid functioning in the interval between episodes. Although there may be recurrences, the intervals between recurrences are symptom-free, with good adjustment, a pattern considered characteristic of affective disorder.

4. Perris (1974) and his associates, following Leonard, have emphasized this as a separate disorder, the third psychosis, which they call "cycloid psychosis." This concept has not gained much attention in the United States.

A number of workers, including Clayton (1982b), who has analyzed the NIMH Collaborative Study data, have emphasized the importance of distinguishing within the schizoaffective group as to whether the presenting episode is manic or depressive. Following that suggestion, the remainder of this discussion is divided into two categories: schizoaffective, manic, and schizoaffective, depressed.

Schizoaffective, manic

Reliability data from the field trial for *DSM-III* and from the NIMH Collaborative Study indicate reasonably good reliability. The most convincing evidence for the validity of this distinction comes from family studies and studies of clinical course and follow-up.

Family studies have been reported by Clayton (1982b) and Angst and associates (1980), among others. These studies suggest that schizoaffective, manic patients have a strong familial aggregation along with that of bipolar illness. Gershon and associates (1982) have applied the multiple-threshold liability model, developed by Kidd and Reich, and proposed that schizoaffective patients are part of a continuum with bipolar and unipolar patients. Reich and Rice have applied this modification of statistical analysis to the NIMH Collaborative Study data and suggested the occurrence of a manic familial spectrum.

No systematic studies are available with regard to psychosocial factors, such as personality, social support, and life events.

The situation with regard to response to treatment is not clear. The few controlled studies have suggested that patients with schizoaffective, manic, illness respond in a manner similar to the way bipolar patients respond. It is likely that these patients will respond to neuroleptics and/or lithium during acute symptomatic episodes. No long-term studies with lithium have been done to demonstrate the preventive value of this treatment.

Follow-up studies, particularly those by Brockington and associates (1983) and by Coryell, have supported the view that patients with schizoaffective, manic, disorder have similarities in clinical course to patients with bipolar disorder, but with more severe impairment.

Schizoaffective, depressed

Having separated out schizoaffective, manic, disorders, uncertainty exists regarding the status of schizoaffective, depressed. Here, the boundary problems are with major depressive disorder, psychotic subtype, with major depression, and with schizophrenia. Data from the NIMH Collaborative Study regarding this problem have been reviewed by Coryell and associates (1984a).

Familial-aggregation studies have suggested an increase in schizophrenia among the families of probands with schizoaffective, degressed, disorder as compared with schizoaffective, manic, and with major depression. This excess of schizophrenia has also been reported by Stroeber and Carlson (1982) among the families of adolescents hospitalized with severe affective disorder.

No consistent data are available regarding personality, life events, and social supports.

The numbers of controlled clinical trials have been insufficient to indicate any response to treatment.

Most of the studies of schizoaffective disorders have not divided them into depressive and manic subtypes. However, the suggestion is that patients with schizoaffective, depressed, disorder have a clinical course intermediate between that for major depression and that for schizophrenia in terms of severity of impairment, frequency of recurrence, and suicide.

Clayton has suggested that schizoaffective disorder be considered a variant of bipolar illness.

AFFECTIVE DISORDERS CLASSIFIED AS OTHER THAN AFFECTIVE DISORDERS IN *DSM-III*

There are three other affective disorders included in the *DSM-III* that appear in categories other than affective disorders: (1) adjustment reaction with depressed mood, (2) uncomplicated grief, and (3) organic affective disorders.

Adjustment disorder with depressed mood

There has been only one report on validation of the concept of adjustment reaction (Andreasen and Hoenk, 1982). The concept of childhood adjustment disorder with depressed mood was tested recently in a group of prepubertal children presenting with depressive symptoms. Kovacs reported that adjustment disorder with depressed mood can be diagnosed in children before puberty with high reliability and that they have much better prognoses than patients with dysthymia or with major depressive disorder. Children with adjustment disorder with depressed mood are less likely to have recurrences; they have shorter episodes and do not develop dysthymia.

The relationship between adjustment disorder with depressed mood and reactive and/or situational depression is discussed in a later section.

The boundary between adjustment disorder with depressed mood and post-traumatic stress disorder (PTSD) is unclear. In regard to symptoms, most patients with PTSD exhibit anxiety and fearfulness rather than sadness and other depressive symptoms.

Uncomplicated grief

Uncomplicated grief is included in the *DSM-III* to recognize the frequent occurrence of depressive symptoms following death and bereavement. The majority of persons experiencing uncomplicated grief recover (Lazare, 1979; Clayton, 1982a; Klerman, 1984). Although many persons experiencing uncomplicated grief are distressed and may seek medical attention, most societies do not regard the grieving person as ill or worthy of the sick role, but rather designate them a special role, that of grieving person.

Empirical studies are needed to document the categories of abnormal grief, such as delayed grief, absence of grief, anniversary reactions, and pathologically intense grieving. These categories have been suggested as complications of grief, but they have not been subjected to empirical studies to establish their reliability and validity.

Organic affective disorders

It is widely accepted that a large variety of diseases of the central nervous system (CNS) will produce affective syndromes. This is sometimes called secondary affective disorder, although, as noted in a later section, the St. Louis criteria for secondary affective disorder did not include medical illnesses or neurologic conditions. Clinicians must exercise a good deal of judgment in determining if a person who has a medical or neurologic disease, particularly if it is life-threatening, and who also has symptoms of depression should be regarded as having two disorders (the medical-neurologic disorder plus major depression) or should be coded as having an organic affective disorder. Other clinicians would regard this as a form of adjustment disorder with depressed mood and would consider that the stress involved is that of the medical condition.

The criteria of *DSM-III* should be reviewed with special attention to systemic medical conditions, CNS disorders, and reactions to drugs such as reserpine and steroids.

PROPOSED CATEGORIES OF AFFECTIVE DISORDERS NOT IN *DSM-III*

In any evaluation of *DSM-III*, attention should be given to proposed categories not currently included in *DSM-III*. For affective disorders, there are five categories that merit attention.

Primary and secondary affective disorders

Distinguishing between primary and secondary depression was first proposed by Robins and Guze (1972). Their intent was to define homogeneous samples for research, particularly for research on diagnostic criteria and on familial-genetic factors.

The most common preexisting conditions leading to secondary depression are alcoholism, panic and other related anxiety disorders, and schizophrenia. The status of affective disorders associated with personality conditions remains obscure. The question is whether or not these should be regarded as forms of secondary depression.

Krauthammer and Klerman (1978) have proposed the concept of secondary mania and secondary bipolar disorder related to drugs and medical illness. In this concept, mania and bipolar disorder can occur in association with neurologic disease, certain drugs, and also alcoholism and antisocial personality.

Situational or reactive depression

For many years, clinicians have described depressive reactions following acute stress. These have variously been called neurotic depression, reactive depression, or situational depression. In order to clarify this, the RDC created a category of situational depression. The reliability and validity of this concept have been discussed by Hirschfeld (1981).

Among the patients diagnosed clinically as having reactive depression will be some patients appropriate for the *DSM-III* category of adjustment disorder with depressed mood. Other patients who meet the criteria for *DSM-III* major depressive disorder (MDD) should be jointly classified as having MDD on axis I and acute stress on axis IV. There have been proposals to create a subcategory of MDD, situational, parallel to the subcategories of MDD, melancholia, and delusional MDD. However, given the apparently low reliability for this diagnosis, this proposal should be delayed until further research is completed.

Demoralization

The concept of demoralization has been proposed to encompass patients reacting not only to acute episodes of distress (who would meet the criteria for adjustment disorder with depressed mood) but also to lifetime or enduring adverse circumstances. The concept was originally proposed by Frank (1973) in his writings on psychotherapy, but it has recently been amplified and expanded by DeFigueiredo (1983), Dohrenwend and Dohrenwend (1982), and Klein (1974). The concept encompasses a group of patients, usually of lower socioeconomic class, who experience symptoms of pessimism, hopelessness, and frustration closely allied with adverse life circumstances. Some question whether or not these patients are "truly" psychiatrically ill. This work has been criticized by Murphy and associates (1984).

Winokur's system

Winokur and associates (1978) have proposed a diagnostic system based on family history. This involves three categories: pure depressive disorder, in which patients have a family history of depression, including a depressed first-degree family member; depressive spectrum disorder, in which there is a history of alcoholism and/or antisocial personality in the family; and sporadic depressive disorder. Schlesinger and associates have reported evidence from dexamethasone suppression tests (DST) supportive of the distinction. The diagnostic significance of a history of alcoholism in the family remains to be determined. Whether or not there is an increased incidence of alcoholism in the families of depressives is controversial. Studies using case–control methods have not always demonstrated this.

Mixed anxiety and depression

Attention has already been given to the high overlap between depression and anxiety. Many clinicians have attempted to describe the characteristics of patients with mixed anxiety and depression, especially as seen among outpatients, as a possible separate category, particularly for drug-efficacy research (Downing and Rickels, 1974; Prusoff and Klerman, 1974).

CONCLUSIONS

On the whole, the *DSM-III* classification of affective disorders can be considered a successful innovation. It has brought together a group of disorders, previously separated into psychotic and neurotic categories, and focused attention on the importance of manifest symptoms as the common feature in many of these disorders. Reasonable reliability has been achieved for defining most disorders, with the notable exceptions of certain forms of bipolar illness and schizoaffective disorder.

Certain problems of validity remain, and extensive research is now under way to establish the validity of various concepts and categories, particularly dysthymic and schizoaffective disorders. Various proposals for modifying diagnostic criteria and for making other changes merit consideration, particularly as new research evidence becomes available.

REFERENCES

Akiskal, HS: Subaffective disorders: dysthymic cyclothymic and bipolar II disorders in the "borderline" realm. Psychiatr Clin North Am 4:25–46, 1981

Dysthymic disorder: psychopathology of proposed chronic depressive subtypes. Am J Psychiatry 140:11–20, 1983

Akiskal, HS, Djenderedjian AH, Rosenthal RH, et al: Cyclothymic disorder: validating criteria for inclusion in the bipolar affective group. Am J Psychiatry 134:1227–1232, 1977

Akiskal HS, Hirschfeld RMA, Yerevanian BI: The relationship of personality to affective disorders. Arch Gen Psychiatry 40:801–810, 1983

Andreasen NC, Grove WM, Maurer R: Cluster analysis and the classification of depression. Br J Psychiatry 137:256–265, 1980

Andreasen NC, Hoenk PR: The predictive value of adjustment disorders: a follow-up study. Am J Psychiatry 139:584–590, 1982

Andreasen NC, McDonald-Scott P, Grove WM, et al: Assessment of reliability in a multicenter collaborative research using a videotape approach. Am J Psychiatry 139:7, 1982

Angst J, Felder W, Lohmeyer B: Course of schizoaffective psychoses: results of a follow-up study. Schizophr Bull 6:579–584, 1980

Beigel A, Murphy DL: Unipolar and bipolar affective illness. Arch Gen Psychiatry 24:215–220, 1971

Berner P, Katschnig H: Improving the quality of diagnostic systems: multiaxiality and polydiagnostic approach, in Proceedings of the VIIth World Congress of Psychiatry, 11–16 July 1983, Vienna. Edited by Berner P, et al. New York, Plenum, pp 31–43

Bielski RJ, Friedel RO: Subtypes of depression – diagnosis and medical management. West J Med 126:347–352, 1977

Brockington IF, Hillier VF, Francis AF, et al: Definitions of mania: concordance and prediction of outcome. Am J Psychiatry 140:435–439, 1983

Brockington IF, Kendell RE, Wainwright S: Depressed patients with schizophrenic or paranoid symptoms. Psychol Med 10:665–675, 1980

Brown GW, Harris T: The Social Origins of Depression. London, Tavistock, 1978

Carroll B: Letter to the editor: from the researcher's perspective. Am J Psychiatry 138:705–707, 1981

Charney DS, Nelson CJ: Delusional and non-delusional unipolar depression: further evidence for distinct subtypes. Am J Psychiatry 138:328–333, 1981

Clayton PJ: Bereavement, in Handbook of Affective Disorders. Edited by Paykel E. London, Churchill Livingstone, 1982a

Schizoaffective disorders. J Nerv Ment Dis 170:646–650, 1982b

Cooper AM, Michels R: DSM-III: an American view. Am J Psychiatry 138:128–129, 1981

Coryell W, Endicott J, Reich T, et al: A family study of bipolar II disorder. Br J Psychiatry 145:49–54, 1984a

Coryell W, Lavori P, Endicott J, et al: Outcome in schizoaffective, psychotic and nonpsychotic depression: course over a six to twenty-four month follow-up. Arch Gen Psychiatry 41:787–791, 1984b

Coryell W, Tsuang MT, McDaniel J: Psychotic features in major depression: is mood congruence important? J Affect Dis 4:227–236, 1982

Davidson JRT, Miller RD, Turnbull CD, et al: Atypical depression. Arch Gen Psychiatry 39:527–535, 1982

DeFigueiredo JM: The law of sociocultured demoralization. Social Psychiatry 18:73–78, 1983

Dohrenwend BP, Dohrenwend BS: Perspectives on the past and future of psychiatric epidemiology: the 1981 Rema Lapouse Lecture. Am J Public Health 72:1271–1279, 1982

Downing RW, Rickels K: Mixed anxiety-depression: fact or myth? Arch Gen Psychiatry 30:312–317, 1974

Dunner DL: Subtypes of bipolar affective disorder with particular regard to bipolar II. Psychiatr Dev 1:75–86, 1983

Endicott J, Nee J, Andreasen N, et al: Bipolar II: combine or keep separate? J Affect Dis 8:17–28, 1985

Endicott J, Spitzer RL: A diagnostic interview: the Schedule for Affective Disorders and Schizophrenia. Arch Gen Psychiatry 135:837–844, 1978

Feighner JP, Robins E, Guze SB, et al: Diagnostic criteria for use in psychiatric research. Arch Gen Psychiatry 26:57, 1972

Fenichel O: The Psychoanalytic Theory of Neurosis. New York, Norton, 1945

Frank J: Persuasion and Healing: A Comparative Study of Psychotherapy. Baltimore, Johns Hopkins Press, 1973

Gershon ES: The genetics of affective disorders, in Psychiatry Update, Vol II. Edited by Grinspoon L. Washington, DC, American Psychiatric Press, 1983

Gershon ES, Hamovit J, Guroff JJ, et al: A family study of schizoaffective, bipolar I, bipolar II, unipolar and normal control probands. Arch Gen Psychiatry 39:1157–1167, 1982

Glassman A, Roose SP: Delusional depression. Arch Gen Psychiatry. 38:424–427, 1981

Hirschfeld RMA: Situational depression: validity of the concept. Br J Psychiatry 139:297–305, 1981

Hirschfeld RMA, Klerman GL: personality attributes and affective disorders. Am J Psychiatry 136:67–70, 1979

Kasanin J: The acute schizo-affective psychoses. Am J Psychiatry 13:97–126, 1933

Katz MM, Hirschfeld RMA: Phenomenology and classification of depression, in Psychopharmacology: A Generation of Progress. Edited by Lipton MA, DiMascio A, Killam KF. New York, Raven Press, 1978, pp 1185–1195

Katz MM, Klerman GL: Overview of the clinical studies program. Am J Psychiatry 136:49–70, 1979

Katz MM, Secunda SK, Hirschfeld RMA, et al: NIMH-Clinical Research Branch Collaborative Program on the Psychobiology of Depression. Arch Gen Psychiatry 36:765–771, 1979

Keller MB, Klerman GL, Lavori PW, et al: Treatment received by depressed patients. JAMA 248:1848–1855, 1982

Keller MB, Lavori P, McDonald-Scott P, et al: The reliability of retrospective treatment reports. J Psychiatry Res 9:81–88, 1983

Keller MB, Shapiro RW: Double depression: superimposition of acute depressive episodes on chronic depressive disorders. Am J Psychiatry 139:438–442, 1982

Kendell RE: The choice of diagnostic criteria for biological research. Arch Gen Psychiatry 39:1334–1339, 1982

Kiloh L, Garside R: The independence of neurotic depression and endogenous depression. Br J Psychiatry 109:451, 1963

Klein DF: Endogenomorphic depression: a conceptual and terminological revision. Arch Gen Psychiatry 31:447–454, 1974

Klerman GL: Age and clinical depression: today's youth in the twenty-first century. J Gerontol 31:318–323, 1976

Other specific affective disorders, in Comprehensive Textbook of Psychiatry. Vol. III. Edited by Kaplan HI, Freedman AM, Sadock BJ. Baltimore, Williams & Wilkins, 1980, pp 1332–1339

The significance of DSM-III in American psychiatry, in International Perspectives on DSM-III. Edited by Spitzer RL, Williams JB, Skodal AE. Washington, DC, American Psychiatric Press, 1983, pp 3–25

Klerman GL, Endicott J, Spitzer R: Neurotic depressions: a systematic analysis of multiple criteria and meanings. Am J Psychiatry 136:57–61, 1979

Klerman GL, Lavori P, Rice J, et al: Birth cohort effect on rates of major depression in relatives of patients with affective disorder. Arch Gen Psychiatry 42:689–693, 1985

Krauthammer C, Klerman GL: Secondary mania: manic syndromes associated with antecedent physical illness or drugs. Arch Gen Psychiatry 35:1333–1339, 1978

Lavori PW, Keller MB, Klerman GL: Relapse in affective disorders: a reanalysis of the literature using life table methods. J Psychiatr Res (in press)

Lazare A: Unresolved grief, in Outpatient Psychiatry: Diagnosis and Treatment. Edited by Lazare A. Baltimore, Williams & Wilkins, 1979, pp 498–512

Leckman JF, Weissman MM, Merikangas KR, et al: Major depression and panic disorder: a family study perspective. Psychopharmacol Bull 21:543–545, 1985

Leckman JF, Weissman MM, Prusoff BA, et al: Subtypes of depression: family study perspective. Arch Gen Psychiatry 41:833–838, 1984

Liebowitz MR, Quitkin FM, Stewart JW, et al: Phenelzine and imipramine in atypical depression. Psychopharmacol Bull 17:159–161, 1981

Lorr M: Syndromes of Psychosis. New York, Pergamon, 1963

Mendels J, Cochrane C: The nosology of depression: the endogenous reactive concept. Am J Psychiatry 124:1, 1968

Murphy J, Sobol AM, Neff RK, et al: Stability of prevalence. Arch Gen Psychiatry 41:990–997, 1984

Myers JK, Weissman MM, Tischler GL, et al: The prevalence of psychiatric disorders in three communities: 1980–1982. Arch Gen Psychiatry 41:959–967, 1984

Nelson JC, Charney DS, Quinlan DM: Evaluation of the DSM-III criteria for melancholia. Arch Gen Psychiatry 38:555–559, 1981

Paykel ES: Contribution of life events to causation of psychiatric illness. Psychol Med 8:245–253, 1978

Paykel ES, Myers JR, Dieneit MN, et al: Life events and depression: a controlled study. Arch Gen Psychiatry 21:753–760, 1969

30   GERALD L. KLERMAN ET AL.

Paykel ES, Parker RR, Penrose RJJ, et al: Depressive classification and prediction of response of phenelzine. Br J Psychiatry 134:572–581, 1979

Perris C: Study of cycloid psychosis. Acta Psychiatr Scand [Suppl. 253] 1974

Pope HG, Lipinski JF: Diagnosis in schizophrenia and manic-depressive illness: a reassessment of the specificity of "schizophrenia" symptoms in the light of current research. Arch Gen Psychiatry 35:811–828, 1978

Prien RF, Klett CJ, Caffey EMJ: Prepublication report no. 94. Central Neuropsychiatric Research Laboratory, VA Cooperative Studies in Psychiatry, VA Hospital, Perry Point, Md, 1973

Prusoff B, Klerman GL: Differentiating depressed from anxious, neurotic outpatients: use of discriminant function analysis for separation of neurotic affective states. Arch Gen Psychiatry 30:302–309, 1974

Quitkin F, Rifkin A, Klein DF: Imipramine response to deluded depressed patients. Am J Psychiatry 135:806–811, 1976

Monoamine oxidase inhibitors: a review of antidepressant effectiveness. Arch Gen Psychiatry 36:749–760, 1979

Robins E, Guze SB: Classification of affective disorders: the primary-secondary endogenous-reactive, and neurotic-psychotic concepts, in Recent Advances in the Psychobiology of Depressive Illness. Edited by Williams TA, Katz MM, Shield JA Jr. DHEW publication HO (HSM) 79-9053. Washington, DC, US Government Printing Office, 1972

Robinson DS, Nies A, Ravaris CL, et al: The monoamine oxidase inhibitor, phenelzine, in the treatment of depressive-anxiety states. Arch Gen Psychiatry 29:407–413, 1973

Rush AJ (ed): Short-Term Psychotherapies for Depression. New York, Guilford Press, 1982

Sargent W: Some newer drugs in the treatment of depression and their relation to other somatic treatments. Psychosomatics 1:14–17, 1960

Shea T: Unpublished paper presented at the Society for Psychotherapy Research, Sheffield, England, June 1983

Spiker D: Schizoaffective disease and atypical psychosis. Presented at a meeting of the American College of Neuropsychopharmacotherapy, San Juan, Puerto Rico, December 12, 1979

Spitzer RL, Endicott J, Robins E: Research diagnostic criteria: rationale and reliability. Arch Gen Psychiatry 35:773–782, 1978

Spitzer RL, Williams JBW, Skodol AE: DMS-III: the major achievements and an overview. Am J Psychiatry 137:151–164, 1980

Stroeber M, Carlson G: Bipolar illness in adolescents with major depression. Arch Gen Psychiatry 39:549–555, 1982

Sweeney D, Nelson C, Bowers M, et al: Delusional versus nondelusional depression: neurochemical differences. Lancet 2:100–101, 1978

Tennant C, Bebbington P, Hurry J: Parental death in childhood and risk of adult depressive disorders: a review. Psychol Med 10:289–299, 1980

Weissman MM: The psychological treatment of depression: an update of clinical trials, in Psychotherapy Research: Where Are We Going and Where Should We Go? Edited by Spitzer RL, Williams JBW. New York, Guilford Press, 1984

Weissman MM, Gershon ES, Kidd KK, et al: Psychiatric disorders in the relatives of probands with affective disorders: the Yale-NIMH Collaborative Family Study. Arch Gen Psychiatry 41:13–21, 1984

Weissman MM, Myers JK: Affective disorders in a U.S. urban community: the use of Research Diagnostic Criteria in an epidemiological survey. Arch Gen Psychiatry 35:1304–1311, 1978

West ED, Dally PJ: Effect of iproniazid in depressive syndromes. Br Med J 1:1491–1494, 1959

Williams TA, Katz MM, Shield JA Jr (eds): Recent Advances in the Psychobiology of the Depressive Illnesses. DHEW publication HO (HSM) 70-9053. Washington, DC, US Government Printing Office, 1972

Winokur G, Behar D, Vanvalkenburg C, et al: Is a familial definition of depression both feasible and valid? J Nerv Ment Dis 166:764, 1978

Young M: Establishing diagnostic criteria for mania. J Nerv Ment Dis 171:676–682, 1983

2 Validity of major depression

A psychobiological perspective

DAVID J. KUPFER AND MICHAEL E. THASE

This chapter considers the validity of the *DSM-III* category of major depression from a psychobiological perspective. Such a review is timely, given the proliferation of research on the biological aspects of the major affective syndromes since the publication of *DSM-III* in 1980. After a brief summary of the classification issues that shaped the *DSM-III* format for diagnosis of affective disorders, we focus on biological studies that either support or fail to support the nosologic independence of major depression. Studies employing measurements of neurotransmitters and their metabolites, receptor function, neuroendocrine regulation, and neurophysiological methods are reviewed. Attention is given to the psychobiological heterogeneity of the broad major depression grouping, particularly with respect to evidence supporting differentiation of discrete subtypes of affective disorders. Conversely, extension of applicable findings to certain "boundary" diagnoses, such as schizoaffective disorder and borderline personality disorder, is briefly addressed. Finally, conclusions drawn from these psychobiological studies are used to formulate recommendations for future research directed toward further refinement of diagnoses of affective disorders.

DSM-III CLASSIFICATION OF AFFECTIVE DISORDERS

A major task accomplished by *DSM-III* has been development of a widely acceptable, objective, and reliable set of diagnoses for the affective disorders (Spitzer, Williams, and Skodol, 1980). Such achievements were largely accomplished by revision and modification of *DSM-II* categories with respect to empirical findings, use of more detailed descriptive and phenomenological presentations of conditions, and use of operationalized criteria for inclusion and exclusion of cases (Spitzer et al., 1980; American Psychiatric Association, 1980). With regard to affective disorders, *DSM-III* is a direct descendant of the research classification system developed by Feighner and associates (1972) and

Preparation of this chapter was supported in part by National Institute of Mental Health grants MH-30915, MH-24652, and MH-16804, as well as by a grant from the John D. and Catherine T. MacArthur Foundation Research Network on the Psychobiology of Depression.

subsequently expanded and revised into the Research Diagnostic Criteria (RDC) by Spitzer, Endicott, and Robins (1978). In fact, major depression, according to *DSM-III*, is nearly identical with major depressive disorder, as defined by the RDC, and shares a high degree of concordance with primary depression as diagnosed by the criteria of Feighner and associates (1972).

The *DSM-III* criteria for major depression are summarized in Table 2.1. It is apparent that any two patients with major depression may manifest markedly different symptom profiles. In fact, several sets of symptoms are rather mutually exclusive (i.e., insomnia/hypersomnia, weight gain/weight loss, agitation/retardation). Nevertheless, each of the symptoms and signs has been shown to occur relatively frequently in depression (Nelson and Charney, 1981), and many have at least some value in predicting responses to antidepressant therapy (Bielski and Friedel, 1976). However, it is important to keep in mind that no sign or symptom is pathognomonic; rather, a constellation of signs and symptoms that are relatively severe and persistent (and are not superimposed on selected non-affective conditions) defines the syndrome.

In terms of *DSM-III* major depression, this means that a patient must report depressed mood and/or loss of interest "nearly every day for the past two weeks," as well as manifest at least four other symptoms from Table 2.1, in order to meet the criteria for the syndrome. Moreover, the patient cannot have a preexisting diagnosis of schizophrenia or dementia or an underlying medical-neurological syndrome known to cause depression (e.g., pancreatic carcinoma or hypothyroidism).

A flowchart for *DSM-III* affective disorders is presented in Figure 2.1. Major depression can be divided initially into bipolar and nonbipolar subtypes. Although some controversy exists concerning this dichotomy (Taylor and Abrams, 1980), it is generally accepted to be useful. Patients considered to have bipolar II depression according to the RDC (i.e., a history of brief hypomanias, but no full-blown manic episodes) are classified as having an atypical bipolar affective disorder in *DSM-III*. Chronic subsyndromal conditions punctuated by mood swings are diagnosed as cyclothymic disorder. Nonbipolar major depression can be subdivided into recurrent- and single-episode types and further categorized as melancholic or delusional. This latter distinction is somewhat unfortunate in that most delusional depressives are also melancholic (Nelson and Charney, 1981). Regardless, there is considerable agreement with the decision to subtype the heterogeneous nonbipolar major depression grouping in this fashion (Kendell, 1976; Van Praag, 1982). Chronic, subsyndromal nonbipolar dysphorias are diagnosed as dysthymic disorder or atypical depression. Finally, acute mild depressions clearly related to an environmental precipitant can be diagnosed as an adjustment disorder only if the syndromal criteria for major depression are not met.

The *DSM-III* classification system for affective disorders is essentially pragmatic and atheoretical. This is partly reflected in the use of the term "disorder," rather than "illness" or "disease" (American Psychiatric Association, 1980; Spitzer et al., 1980). Threshold criteria may seem arbitrary in some cases, but

Table 2.1 *Diagnostic criteria for major depressive episode*

A. Dysphoric mood or loss of interest or pleasure in all or almost all usual activities or pastimes. The dysphoric mood is characterized by symptoms such as the following: depressed, sad, blue, hopeless, low, down in the dumps, irritable. The mood disturbance must be prominent and relatively persistent.

B. At least four of the following symptoms have each been present nearly every day for a period of at least two weeks:
    1. Poor appetite or significant weight loss (when not dieting) or increased appetite or significant weight gain.
    2. Insomnia or hypersomnia.
    3. Psychomotor agitation or retardation (but not merely subjective feelings of restlessness or being slowed down).
    4. Loss of interest or pleasure in usual activities, or decrease in sexual drive not limited to a period when delusional or hallucinating.
    5. Loss of energy, fatigue.
    6. Feelings of worthlessness, self-reproach, or excessive or inappropriate guilt (either may be delusional).
    7. Complaints or evidence of diminished ability to think or concentrate, such as slowed thinking, or indecisiveness not associated with marked loosening of associations or incoherence.
    8. Recurrent thoughts of death, suicidal ideation, wishes to be dead, or suicide attempts.

C. Neither of the following dominates the clinical picture when an affective syndrome is absent (i.e., symptoms in criteria A and B above):
    1. Preoccupation with a mood-incongruent delusion or hallucination.
    2. Bizarre behavior.

D. Not superimposed on schizophrenia, schizophreniform disorder, or a paranoid disorder.

E. Not due to any organic mental disorder or uncomplicated bereavement.

this is a reasonable compromise for enhanced reliability at this time. Inspection of *DSM-III* nomenclature reveals a careful selection of terms to avoid confusion with previous theoretically based but less standardized classifications, such as the neurotic–psychotic or reactive–endogenous dichotomies. The importance of long-standing "neurotic" or characterological difficulties can be addressed by employing multiple psychiatric diagnoses, if indicated, on axes I and II. Similarly, the global impact of psychosocial stressors also may be rated on a separate diagnostic axis.

Despite the considerable overlap among the criteria of *DSM-III*, RDC, and Feighner and associates for affective disorders, several notable differences exist. First, *DSM-III* does not employ the primary–secondary dichotomy for major depression, beyond use of the several exclusionary diagnoses already mentioned. The net effect of this practice is to broaden *DSM-III* major depression

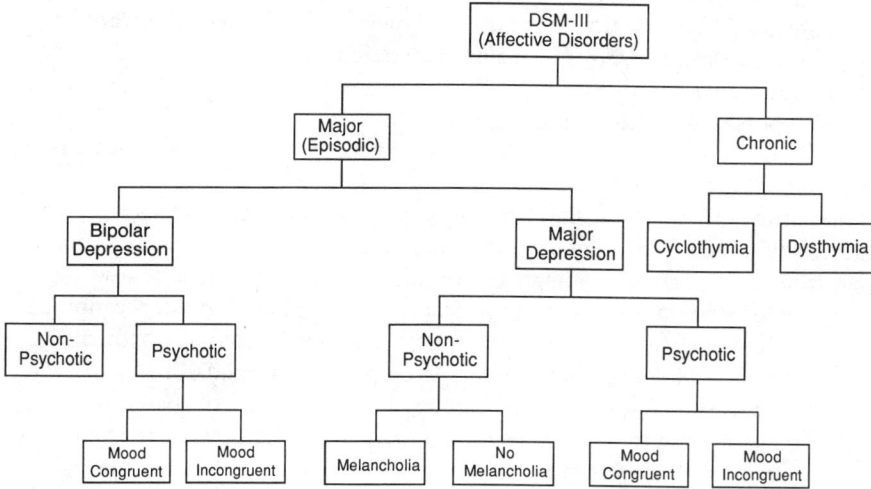

Figure 2.1. Flowchart for *DSM-III* affective disorders.

by grouping patients with antecedent, nonaffective disorders (such as alcoholism, somatization disorder, agoraphobia, etc.) together with patients with uncomplicated depression. This practice can be justified on clinical grounds, because few symptomatic or treatment-outcome differences reliably separate primary and secondary depression (Andreasen and Winokur, 1979; Clayton and Lewis, 1981); however, it does increase the heterogeneity of the category of major depression. Second, the *DSM-III* subtype of melancholia is more restrictive than the corresponding RDC diagnosis of endogenous depression (Nelson, Charney, and Quinlan, 1981). Most cases of "probable endogenous depression" and a number of "definite" cases defined by RDC are considered nonmelancholic according to *DSM-III*. Thus, by tightening criteria for melancholia, the nonmelancholic major depression grouping is further broadened. Finally, *DSM-III* does not use impairment in social role or treatment-seeking as criteria for major depression. Whereas this difference is essentially irrelevant in clinical settings (by definition, patients have sought treatment), it may further broaden the definition of the disorder for nonpatients surveyed in epidemiological studies.

VALIDITY OF MAJOR DEPRESSION

General issues

Establishing reliable diagnostic criteria for affective disorders is a necessary first step, but it does not guarantee that the diagnoses will be valid. The validity of medical diagnoses traditionally has been tested against several lines of evidence: clinical phenomenology, longitudinal course (natural history), family history, treatment response, and, if available, laboratory studies (Akiskal,

1980). A substantial body of clinical, longitudinal, genetic, and treatment-response data supports the diagnostic independence of affective disorders. In psychometric terms, *DSM-III* major depression can be considered to have "face" validity in that the criteria directly relate to the disorder being defined and also possess a considerable degree of concurrent, predictive, and discriminant validity (Klein et al., 1980; Andreason, 1982; Coryell and Winokur, 1982; Matarazzo, 1983).

Identification of replicable laboratory parameters that characterize major depression would help establish construct validity (Akiskal, 1980). Of course, identification of reliable biological correlates of affective states is also highly desirable to better understand the pathophysiology underlying depression and to aid in development of more efficacious, theoretically derived treatments.

In order for a biological abnormality to be useful as a validator of a disorder, the validity of the abnormality itself must first be established. Essentially, this means that the finding must be replicated by independent research groups and must occur in a reasonable percentage of patients with the index disorder. This latter requirement corresponds to the sensitivity of a laboratory test. Furthermore, the abnormality must be fairly specific to the disorder in question (i.e., not be present in most normal individuals or patients with nonaffective psychopathological conditions). Of course, identification of a very uncommon but highly specific biological abnormality may herald discovery of a previously undetected subtype of depression. However, such a finding may easily be missed in grouped data and, depending on the rarity, may be quite difficult to replicate. Finally, it is crucial to ascertain if an apparent biological correlate is actually more directly related to an extraneous factor than to the disorder in question. Examples of such potentially confounding factors include age, weight loss, diet, use of medication, sex, menstrual phase, and hospitalization status. Closely matched control groups are needed to minimize the influence of such extraneous and potentially confounding variables. In this regard, recommendations for psychobiological research on depression have recently been published (Kupfer and Rush, 1983).

Once an abnormality has been recognized and replicated, it is heuristically important to ascertain whether the potential "marker" is intimately related to the pathophysiology of the disorder or more simply reflects either a biological amplification of a symptom or an epiphenomenon of the disorder. Examples of the latter markers are presented later in this chapter. Although such markers may prove clinically useful, abnormalities that are subsequently found to be intimately related to more basic pathophysiological mechanisms are of greater theoretical interest than those that amplify symptoms.

It is also necessary to determine if an abnormality is present only when a patient is experiencing an episode of depression (i.e., a state marker) or is also present during periods of remission. Abnormalities that are present prior to the onset of the initial episode of illness or that persist in recovered patients are usually termed "trait" markers. Of course, such abnormalities are not necessarily inherited, as in the strictest sense of the term "trait." Moreover, prohibitively expensive longitudinal studies of never-ill, high-risk individuals (i.e., first-degree relatives) are necessary to properly test the relationship between a biological abnormality and vulnerability. Nevertheless, identification of abnormalities that persist in remitted patients may have important implications for prediction of relapse or for maintenance antidepressant treatment. A more detailed discussion of the various types of state and trait markers is presented elsewhere (Kupfer, 1982).

With these issues in mind, investigators have doggedly pursued a variety of biological paradigms over the past two decades in search of biological correlates of affective disorders. Convergent observations pertaining to neurovegetative symptom profiles, familial (genetic) associations, and relatively specific responses to somatic treatment in patients with clinical (major) depression have fueled such investigations, because it is apparent that some form or forms of biological abnormalities ought to underlie these disorders. Despite a number of false leads, progress is being made, especially as this process becomes facilitated by the development of more refined laboratory methods and acceptance of standardized diagnostic nomenclature.

Psychobiological investigations

Investigations employing a variety of psychobiological paradigms for patients with depressive disorders are reviewed in the following sections. In particular, we focus on investigations of monoaminergic, cholinergic, neuroendocrine, neurophysiological, and circadian abnormalities as possible correlates of major depression. For each proposed abnormality we review pertinent experimental data with respect to (1) the frequency of the proposed abnormality in major depression, (2) the degree of specificity of this abnormality to affective disorders, and (3) clinical correlates of the abnormality within the major depression grouping. We also attempt to summarize the extent to which each biological abnormality supports the construct validity of major depression.

Monoamine studies. Interest in the potential roles of monoamines (norepinephrine, serotonin, and dopamine) in the pathophysiology of depression was sparked by early observations of the effects of agents such as reserpine (amine-depleting) and iproniazid, imipramine, and amphetamine (amine-enhancing), as well as growing knowledge of the importance of these substances as neurotransmitters. Several investigators (Bunney and Davis, 1965; Schildkraut, 1965) advanced amine hypotheses for affective disorders in which clinical depression was predicted to be associated with low levels of monoamines in the synaptic cleft. It is important to keep in mind that even in these early hypotheses, biological heterogeneity was anticipated (Bunney and Davis, 1965).

The original amine hypotheses stimulated nearly 20 years of research activity. Methods developed for those studies included measurement of renal excretion of norepinephrine metabolites, determination of plasma concentrations of monoamines and their substrates and/or metabolites, measurement of enzymes involved in monoamine synthesis or degradation, determination of serotonin uptake in platelets as a peripheral physiological model of the neuronal membrane, direct assay of monoamines in tissues obtained postmortem (usually following suicide), measurement of monoamine metabolites in cerebrospinal fluid (CSF) (with and without probenecid to enhance metabolite accumulation), and pharmacologic challenges using monoamine precursors or false transmitters.

Despite such extensive investigations, little conclusive evidence has emerged; many promising leads have been followed by equal or greater numbers of contradictory reports. For a time it appeared that determination of 24-hour urinary 3-methoxy-4-hydroxyphenylglycol (MHPG) excretion might identify a subgroup of major depression with a low-norepinephrine condition (Maas, 1975; Schildkraut, 1982). In particular, "low" MHPG excretion was found predominantly in patients with bipolar and schizoaffective depressions, as well as a subset (25%–40%) of nonbipolar patients (Maas, 1975; Schildkraut, 1982). These findings seemed particularly exciting because "low" MHPG excretion was reported to predict subsequent responses to imipramine, relative to "serotonergic" antidepressants such as amitriptyline, mianserin, and chlorimipramine (Maas, 1975; Schatzberg et al., 1981; Gaertner et al., 1982; Schildkraut, 1982).

Unfortunately, continued study in this area has revealed a number of methodological and conceptual problems that do not permit the use of urinary MHPG as a marker for major depression. First, a number of negative reports have been published, as reviewed by Kelwala, Jones, and Sitaram (1983). Beyond the problems in replication, perhaps the most limiting concern is that "low" MHPG excretion is a relative term; in most cases, "low" values actually do not fall outside the normal range (Hollister, 1981; Kelwala et al., 1983). Thus, low MHPG excretion is not specific to major depression and may be seen in normals or other patient populations. Furthermore, variables such as diet, psychomotor activity, and anxiety level greatly influence urinary MHPG excretion; marked day-to-day variations in excretion levels are reported (Kelwala et al., 1983). It is conceivable that psychomotor retardation, a clinical variable that is common in bipolar depression and is predictive of an imipramine response (Nelson and Charney, 1981), may account for a considerable amount of the variance. Finally, studies measuring MHPG in plasma and CSF (i.e., more direct measurements of central noradrenergic activity) have yielded conflicting results (Kelwala et al., 1983; Schatzberg et al., 1983). More recent investigations have actually suggested noradrenergic overactivity in a substantial number of depressed patients (Koslow et al., 1983).

There is some suggestion of a central serotonergic deficiency in major depression on the basis of low levels of 5-hydroxyindoleacetic acid (5-HIAA) in the CSF (Asberg, Traskman, and Thoren, 1976; Van Praag, 1980a). Van Praag (1980a) estimates that about 40% of "vital" (i.e., melancholic) depressives have low 5-HIAA levels, and he has nicely summarized pharmacologic data that support the validity of this subgrouping. Unfortunately, a number of contradictory reports exist, and the potential influencing factors such as sex and age have not been fully controlled (Kelwala et al., 1983; Koslow et al., 1983). An earlier report (Asberg et al., 1976) of bimodal distribution of 5-HIAA in vital depression was not confirmed in a recent study (Koslow et al., 1983). Furthermore, the use of probenecid to enhance accumulation of monoamine metabolites may introduce experimental artifact (Kelwala et al., 1983). Nevertheless, some evidence points to an association of low CSF 5-HIAA levels with risk of relapse (Van Praag, 1980a) and violent suicidal behavior (Asberg and Traskman, 1981). However, low 5-HIAA levels also appear to be related to violent or suicidal behavior in individuals who do not meet the diagnostic criteria for depression (Asberg and Traskman, 1981; Traskman et al., 1981). It is conceivable that such patients have "masked" depression, although it is also possible that a low 5-HIAA level can be associated with a more nonspecific clinical state. These interesting findings merit further attention, but they do not provide biological validation for major depression at this time. This is particularly true if one considers that in many settings only a minority of major depressives would be considered to have vital depression.

Likewise, little conclusive evidence exists to support the role of a dopamine deficiency (Van Praag, 1980b). Several groups have documented low postprobenecid levels of homovanillic acid (HVA), a dopamine metabolite (Van Praag and Korf, 1971; Bank, 1977; Van Praag, 1980b). These findings appear to be related to motor retardation. It is noteworthy that administration of L-dopa does not produce an antidepressant response, but may precipitate a transient hypomania in bipolar depressives or increased psychomotor activity levels in nonbipolar patients (Van Praag, 1980b).

Extensive studies of various enzymes involved in the synthesis or degradation of monoamines have also failed to produce any "markers" for major depression (Baldessarini, 1975; Van Praag, 1980b). Platelet levels of monoamine oxidase (MAO) may be low in some bipolar patients, but this finding is neither specific nor widely replicated (Rotman, 1983). Conversely, high platelet MAO levels have been reported in nonbipolar major depressives and have been linked to anxiety, hypochondriac and somatic symptoms, and dexamethasone nonsuppression (Gudeman et al., 1982; Schatzberg et al., 1983). Again, such findings have not been widely replicated and may reflect the clinical state rather than a specific relationship to nonbipolar major depression.

In summary, there is little direct evidence of specific monoamine deficits to validate the diagnosis of major depression. Evidence of noradrenergic or dopaminergic abnormalities may be most closely related to the clinical state (motor retardation) and have not been conclusively replicated. Serotonergic deficiency may indeed exist, but this finding appears to be limited to a relatively small group of the most severely ill patients.

Within the last five years, attention has shifted somewhat away from measurement of monoamine metabolites in favor of study of monoamine receptor characteristics. Investigation of the binding of ^{3}H-imipramine to platelet membranes from human plasma suggested the presence of high-affinity sites analogous to those demonstrated in rat brain (Paul et al., 1980, 1981a). Subsequent work related these high-affinity sites to the serotonin-uptake receptor; specifically, the potency of tricyclics to inhibit reuptake of serotonin was found to correlate with their ability to inhibit binding of ^{3}H-imipramine (Paul et al., 1981a).

More recently, comparison of the numbers of such imipramine-binding sites in major depressives, psychiatric controls, and normal individuals indicated that the numbers of receptor sites are significantly lower in patients with affective disorders (Briley et al., 1980; Paul et al., 1981b). One recent study (Suranyi-Cadotte et al., 1983) found significantly lower ^{3}H-imipramine binding in major depressives than in controls with schizophrenia, schizoaffective disorder, or no psychiatric conditions. Antidepressant treatment resulted in significant elevations in ^{3}H-imipramine inhibition (Suranyi-Cadotte et al., 1983), indicating that prior treatment did not produce the abnormality and that the marker may be state-dependent. The affinities of imipramine receptors are identical in depressives and controls (Briley et al., 1980; Paul et al., 1981b). Moreover, the maximum velocity (V_{max}) of ^{14}C-serotonin uptake, an alternative measure of the number of serotonin receptor sites, has also been found to be significantly decreased in inpatients with major depression or schizoaffective disorder (Meltzer et al., 1981, 1983). Such a decrease in platelet serotonin receptors appears to be associated within families with a history of affective illness and may persist in recovered patients, indicating that this abnormality may ultimately prove useful as a trait marker of major depression (Meltzer et al., 1983). However, a recent study by Meltzer and associates (1983) found that only 45% of a sample of depressed patients had V_{max} values that fell outside of the normal range.

Although further clinical correlation of this abnormality is needed, Meltzer and associates (1983) found decreased numbers of platelet serotonin receptors in both endogenous and nonendogenous subtypes of major depression (defined by RDC). Moreover, analogous measurements using ^{3}H-imipramine have shown reduced numbers of receptor sites in similar proportions of nonbipolar and bipolar major depressives (Paul et al., 1981b).

In summary, there is growing evidence of reduced numbers of serotonin-uptake sites in a sizable proportion of patients with major depression. Although more extensive replication obviously is needed to confirm these relatively new findings, it appears that this abnormality may be applicable across the diagnostic subtypes of major depression. In particular, research is needed to confirm that the decrease in platelet serontonin-uptake sites is relatively specific to major depression before these findings can be used to validate the independence of the disorder itself.

Cholinergic hyperactivity. Over a decade ago, Janowsky and associates (1972) expanded the original monoamine hypothesis to include the "balancing" influence of cholinergic activity. As extended over the past 10 years (Janowsky, Risch, and Gillin, 1983), this hypothesis is based on observations of the clinical effects of cholinergic agonists in normals, depressives, and manic patients, as well as growing knowledge of the subtle interrelationships between acetylcholine and monoaminergic neurotransmitters in the central nervous system (CNS)

(Carroll et al., 1980; Janowsky et al., 1983). Unfortunately, accurate measurement of acetylcholine and its metabolites has not yet been possible; and evidence of a hypercholinergic state must be inferred from indirect models. As discussed later in more detail, investigations employing neuroendocrine (Carroll et al., 1980) and electroencephalographic (EEG) sleep (Sitaram et al., 1982) strategies do support the possible existence of a functional state of cholinergic hyperactivity in some patients with major depression. Further, the work of Sitaram and associates (1982) using REM-sleep-induction tests suggests that cholinergic hypersensitivity may indeed prove to be a useful trait marker for bipolar depression. Replication in nonbipolar major depressives is necessary. Further, no evidence of increased muscarinic binding in the brains of suicide victims as compared with tissues from closely matched, nondepressed controls has been found (Van Praag, 1986). Although further investigations in this area are necessary, it can be concluded at this time that there is not sufficient evidence of a cholinergic hypersensitivity state to validate the construct of major depression.

Neuroendocrine studies. Neuroendocrine strategies have been widely used in research for the past decade, and there is every indication that this trend will continue. Such studies have the advantage of providing objective data concerning neuroendocrine abnormalities in major depression and mania, in addition to offering an indirect method for assessing altered neurotransmitter function in states of neuroendocrine dysregulation. Such an approach is particularly relevant to hypothalamic–pituitary–end organ (adrenal cortex, thyroid, or gonad) interactions. Further, because investigators have hypothesized that dysfunction in the limbic system is present in major depression, neuroendocrine strategies provide a rather direct window into the functional integrity of this complex system.

Abnormalities in the hypothalamic–pituitary–adrenal cortex (HYPAC) axis have been extensively studied in psychopathological states. Two basic paradigms have emerged: One study concerns basal and diurnal secretions of cortisol in major depressives, normal controls, and patients with other psychopathological conditions; the other involves the dexamethasone suppression test (DST).

Sachar (1982) has reviewed the evidence supporting the presence of abnormalities of cortisol secretion in major depression. A majority of hospitalized patients with endogenous depression (according to RDC) exhibit hypercortisolemia, especially during the evening and night. This latter finding may be viewed as a blunting of the normal diurnal rhythm of cortisol secretion. However, the diagnostic specificity of such measurements has been questioned, particularly relative to the more qualitative DST (Carroll, Curtis, and Mendels, 1976; Carroll et al., 1982). Nevertheless, studies of cortisol hypersecretion continue to show promise as a research method, particularly when measurements are combined with sleep recordings and other neuroendocrine parameters (Jarrett, Coble, and Kupfer, 1983).

Perhaps the most dramatic development in biological psychiatry to emerge in the past five years has been the use of the DST as a state marker of depression. The rationale, historical development, and methodological issues pertaining to use of the DST in psychiatry have been extensively reviewed elsewhere (Kalin et al., 1981; Carroll, 1982). Briefly, observations of relatively nonspecific elevations in plasma cortisol and urinary steroid metabolites in depressed patients, as well as blunting of the normal circadian pattern of cortisol secretion, led investigators to employ a low-dose (1 or 2 mg) DST to assess the integrity of the feedback-inhibition mechanism of the HYPAC axis. It was subsequently determined that, in contrast to the hypercortisolemia detected in mildly stressed volunteers or nonaffective psychiatric patients, a significant number of patients with major depression fail to suppress cortisol values normally over the next 24 hours following dexamethasone administration (Kalin et al., 1981; Carroll, 1982; Carroll et al., 1982). This basic finding has been extensively replicated, with the majority of studies reporting higher rates of DST nonsuppression in depressed patients relative to normal controls or patients with other psychiatric conditions (Kalin et al., 1981; Carroll, 1982; Carroll et al., 1982). More recent studies have begun to address various factors which invalidate the DST, such as marked weight loss (i.e., > 10 kg) (Edelstein et al., 1983), recent alcohol withdrawal (Newsom and Murray, 1983), and advanced age (Spar and La Rue, 1983). Because each of these factors has some relationship to the natural history of clinical depression, it is unclear at this time what proportion of DST nonsuppression is epiphenomenal. Moreover, extreme exertion, fever, intercurrent medical illnesses, primary endocrinopathies (especially Cushing's disease, uncontrolled diabetes, and hypothyroidism), and use of selected medications are known to invalidate the DST (Kalin et al., 1981; Carroll, 1982). As a result, careful exclusion criteria are needed to ensure accurate use of the test.

After it was established that DST nonsuppression does indeed occur in a number of patients with major depression, clinical correlation led to several observations:

1. The percentage of depressed patients manifesting DST nonsuppression may range from 15% to 80%, depending on the characteristics of the patient group studied and the methods employed.
2. Bipolar and nonbipolar major depressives may manifest this abnormality.
3. DST nonsuppression is highest in patients with the most severe and persistent depressive disorders.
4. Relatively few (i.e., zero to 15%) normal individuals manifest DST nonsuppression (Kalin et al., 1981; Carroll, 1982; Carroll et al., 1982).

DST nonsuppression is more likely in patients diagnosed as having the melancholic or delusional subtype of major depression than in patients with less severe forms of the disorder, although several groups have not found this relationship (Berger et al., 1982; Coryell, Gaffney, and Burkhardt, 1982; Stokes et al., 1983). DST abnormalities frequently normalize with recovery, indicating that cortisol nonsuppression is a state-limited phenomenon. However, DST nonsuppression has not been shown conclusively to predict responses to somatic antidepressant interventions (Hirschfeld, Koslow, and Kupfer, 1983).

Such findings, coupled with the relative ease and low cost of the DST, led to its rather premature use in clinical practice as a laboratory test for depression. Indeed, in closely controlled research settings employing multiple postdexamethasone cortisol determinations, standardized test procedures, careful assessment to rule out patients with complicating and potentially invalidating conditions, and delimitation of clinical samples to consider only melancholic depressives, the DST performed with acceptable sensitivity (40%–67%) and high specificity (85%–98%) (Kalin et al., 1981; Carroll, 1982; Carroll et al., 1982). Carroll (1982) has noted that such a level of performance is on a par with a number of conventional laboratory tests employed in general medicine. However, as the use of this test has expanded to less rigorously controlled clinical and research settings, its performance has suffered (Kupfer, 1983; Hirschfeld, Koslow, and Kupfer, 1985).

It must be kept in mind that *DSM-III* major depression includes most patients considered to have secondary depression according to the criteria of Feighner and associates (1972) and the RDC (Spitzer et al., 1978). A number of studies have documented relatively low rates of nonsuppression in secondary depressives (Carroll, 1982). Similarly, it is important to reiterate that major depression is not synonymous with melancholia; the latter is a restricted subset of the former. Thus, in settings in which nonmelancholic major depression predominates (i.e., ambulatory clinics), rates of DST nonsuppression may be markedly lower (Amsterdam et al., 1982; Rabkin et al., 1983; Rush et al., 1983). In essence, dexamethasone nonsuppression is a useful research tool that helps establish the validity of major depression (particularly its more restrictive subtypes), but it is not a laboratory test for major depression.

Attempts to relate DST nonsuppression to neurochemical mechanisms have to date been limited by the complex regulatory mechanisms governing the HYPAC axis. It is possible for either functional deficiencies of monoamines (norepinephrine or serotonin) or cholinergic hypersensitivity to produce DST nonsuppression (Kalin et al., 1981; Carroll, 1982). Administration of cholinergic agonists will induce nonsuppression in normals (Carroll et al., 1980), whereas pharmacologic challenges with agents like amphetamine will elicit a blunted cortisol response in depressives suggestive of noradrenergic deficiency (Sachar et al., 1981). Conversely, preliminary evidence links low CSF 5-HIAA levels, dexamethasone nonsuppression, and suicidal behavior (Banki and Arato, 1983). Obviously, much work remains to be done to clarify these promising leads. Measurement of ACTH levels, before and after dexamethasone administration, should help investigators further localize the abnormalities underlying nonsuppression. However, some recent studies measuring ACTH levels have reported conflicting results (Fang et al., 1981; Kalin, Weisler, and Shelton, 1982).

Of particular interest with respect to the amine hypothesis are recent reports of high rates of DST nonsuppression in patients with mania (Graham et al., 1982; Stokes et al., 1983). Because an inverse neurochemical disturbance is often hypothesized to differentiate mania from depression (Bunney and Davis, 1965; Schildkraut, 1965), further research is needed to better understand the implications of this interesting finding. Conversely, high rates of DST non-suppression in patients with obsessive–compulsive disorder (Insel et al., 1982b), bulimia or anorexia (Gwirtsman et al., 1983), dementia (Spar and Gerner, 1982), or schizophrenia (Targum, 1983b) and nondepressed patients with borderline personality disorder (Carroll et al., 1981; Soloff, George, and Nathan, 1982) raise questions regarding specificity. Whether or not such observations reflect a psychobiological commonality with affective disorders requires further verification. The use of biological markers to study selected conditions on the boundaries of the affective disorders is discussed later in this chapter in more detail.

Over the same time period, investigators have also studied the functional integrity of the hypothalamic–pituitary–thyroid axis. Again, initial observations of transient, nonspecific elevations in thyroid hormone levels during acute depression fueled interest in the possibility of some form of neuroendocrine dysregulation. Moreover, hypothyroidism was also well known to produce an organic affective syndrome often indistinguishable from major depression. Identification and synthesis of the hypothalamic neuropeptide thyrotropin-releasing hormone (TRH) and development of sensitive assay methods for thyroid-stimulating hormone (TSH) enabled investigators to directly test regulation of this system. The result of these efforts led to standardization of the TRH stimulation test, which has now been widely studied in affective states, as recently reviewed by Loosen and Prange (1982) and Kirkegaard (1981).

To summarize briefly, a minority of patients with major depression (15%–40%) reflect a blunting of TSH secretion following administration of a test dose of TRH (Kirkegaard, 1981; Loosen and Prange, 1982). This suggests some form of dysregulation of the thyroid axis, in terms of increased overriding inhibitory tone, excess endogenous TRH (i.e., hypothalamic disinhibition), or diminished anterior pituitary receptor sensitivity. It is hypothesized that a blunted TSH response to TRH is indicative of a central noradrenergic deficiency (Loosen and Prange, 1982). However, this hypothesis is not yet supported by empirical findings in studies of depressed patients (Davis et al., 1981; Sternbach et al., 1983).

As in the case of the DST, a number of extraneous factors must be controlled to assure a valid study, but the results do not appear to be solely attributable to medication usage, activity level, diet, or history of alcoholism (Kirkegaard, 1981; Loosen and Prange, 1982). Rates of TSH blunting are higher in patients with major depression than in normal controls and patients with several other nonaffective psychopathological conditions, indicating some degree of test specificity. However, determination of the degree of specificity requires more extensive investigation. TSH blunting has been found in similar proportions of patients with chronic alcoholism (Loosen et al., 1983), borderline personality disorder (Garbutt et al., 1983), mania (Loosen and Prange, 1982), and schizophrenia (Langer et al., 1983). In the case of alcoholism, TSH blunting may persist despite years of abstinence (Loosen et al., 1983). Again, the issue of test specificity versus psychobiological overlap of a boundary condition is not resolved.

There is some evidence suggesting higher rates of TRH–TSH abnormalities in nonbipolar depression as compared with bipolar depression, although this finding has not been widely replicated (Kirkegaard, 1981; Loosen and Prange, 1982). It does appear that patients with more severe endogenomorphic or vital depressions are more likely to have blunted TRH tests than nonmelancholic major depressives (Kirkegaard, 1981; Rush et al., 1983), although it is not yet possible to state with certainty that this abnormality is specific to the melancholic subtype of major depression.

More recent studies have identified a small number of patients with depression and an exaggerated TSH response (Sternbach et al., 1983; Targum et al., 1983). Such patients are likely to have normal thyroid function studies but to appear to be in the earliest stages of thyroid failure (Sternbach et al., 1983). Preliminary evidence indicates that these patients may not fully benefit from tricyclic antidepressant therapy without adjunctive thyroid supplementation (Targum et al., 1983).

Of specific interest is the finding that TSH blunting is not statistically related to dexamethasone nonsuppression. The two findings may coexist, but only at a frequency expected by chance alone (Kirkegaard and Carroll, 1980; Gold et al., 1981; Rush et al., 1983). Thus, the underlying mechanisms responsible for these abnormalities are (1) independent and (2) not mutually exclusive. Given this degree of independence, combination of the two tests in the form of a battery will enhance the yield of cases correctly identified (Gold et al., 1981; Sachar et al., 1981; Amsterdam et al., 1983).

Blunted TSH responses may normalize with recovery or may persist despite remission. It has been suggested that persistent blunting may serve as a vulnerability marker for relapse (Kirkegaard, 1981). This observation also has been made for persistent DST nonsuppression (Carroll, 1982; Yerevanian et al., 1983). Obviously, although these findings are important, they are applicable only to patients who initially manifest the abnormality. Moreover, treatment with electroconvulsive therapy (ECT) may produce a transient normalization of the DST that is not predictive of the short-term outcome (Coryell and Zimmerman, 1983). It remains to be seen if the presence of persistent abnormalities on the DST or the TRH stimulation test can be used prospectively to improve the efficacy of maintenance treatment strategies.

To summarize, TSH blunting occurs in a minority of major depressives, although it may be premature to conclude that it is a fairly specific abnormality. Such findings help support the construct validity of major depression, while at the same time providing further evidence of biological heterogeneity within the syndrome. Although further confirmation is needed, TSH blunting may be most characteristic of patients with the more severe or restrictive subtypes of affective disorder.

Other neuroendocrine abnormalities. Among other potential neuroendocrine correlates of major depression, the rates of secretion of growth hormone and prolactin have been increasingly studied. Investigations include measurement of basal levels of these hormones, as well as various pharmacologic challenge strategies. Again, as in the case of most other neurotransmitter and neuroendocrine studies, the effects of age, nutritional status, sex, and menstrual phase need to be closely controlled.

With respect to growth hormone, it is fairly well established that a large number of patients with endogenous major depression (according to RDC) exhibit diminished responses to insulin-induced hypoglycemia (Gruen et al., 1975; Koslow et al., 1982). Parallel blunting of growth-hormone responses to *d*-amphetamine (Langer et al., 1976), desipramine (Laakman, 1980), and clonidine (Checkley, Slade, and Shur, 1981) has been observed, although these findings are more preliminary. Neither L-dopa nor apomorphine appears to elicit a blunted growth-hormone response, which suggests that such an effect is related to a functional deficit.

Several groups have reported abnormal basal secretion patterns for prolactin in depression (Halbreich, Grunhaus, and Ben-David, 1979; Sachar, 1982). Prolactin responses to TRH (Mendlewicz, Linkowski, and Brauman, 1980; Winokur et al., 1983) and methadone (Judd et al., 1982) are also blunted in some patients with major depression. These promising preliminary findings merit more extensive investigation with larger samples and matched controls (both nonaffective psychiatric patients and normals). Because daytime prolactin secretion is inhibited by dopamine, and stimulation of prolactin secretion is most likely mediated by serotonergic mechanisms (Brown and Seggie, 1980), several alterations in neurotransmitter function may be implicated.

More recent work has begun to focus on possible abnormalities in gonadotropin regulation (Amsterdam et al., 1981) and melatonin secretion (Lewy et al., 1985) and on the role of beta-endorphin (Risch, 1982) in major depression. Although these preliminary investigations certainly add to our knowledge of the complexity of neuroendocrine dysfunction in depression, more extensive study will be necessary before such findings can be used to validate the diagnosis of major depression.

Review of recent neuroendocrine studies in patients with major depression leads to several conclusions. First, multiple neuroendocrine abnormalities are observed in variable numbers of patients with major depression. Second, such findings are most likely to be seen in patients with an endogenomorphic or melancholic major depressive syndrome. Neuroendocrine dysregulation in nonmelancholic major depression is not so well established. Third, at least with respect to the DST and the TRH stimulation test, responses may be relatively independent. Thus, there are not two broad groups of major depression (i.e., patients with normal profiles and those with multiple abnormalities). Finally, the weight of evidence collected to date from neuroendocrine studies provides compelling evidence that some form of psychobiological abnormality exists in a considerable number of patients with the more severe forms of major depression. More longitudinal investigations are indicated to approach state-versus-trait issues.

More extensive studies using batteries of neuroendocrine tests also are in order. Evidence from several groups (Gold et al., 1981; Amsterdam et al., 1983;

Rush et al., 1983; Targum, 1983a) suggests that diagnostic sensitivity is greatly enhanced by application of several tests. Use of multiple tests is particularly important in better understanding the interrelationships of neuroendocrine abnormalities.

Neurophysiological studies. Neurophysiological paradigms entail recordings of psychomotor activity levels (Greden and Carroll, 1981), measurement of electrodermal (Iacono et al., 1983) or EMG (Schwartz et al., 1976) activity, determinations of colonic motility (Lechin et al., 1983), use of the EEG in both wakefulness (D'Elia and Perris, 1974; Perris and Monakhov, 1979) and sleep (Kupfer and Thase, 1983), recordings of specific EEG evoked potentials (Buchsbaum, 1979), and newer techniques that allow direct imaging of the brain under static (Reider et al., 1983) and physiological (Buchsbaum et al., 1982) conditions.

Several of these methods may be viewed as involving biological amplifications of the symptoms of major depression. For example, monitoring of psychomotor activity and EMG measurements of the facial musculature provide objective assessments of behavior that also can be directly observed by examiners. Amplification and objective recording of such phenomena may increase reliabiity (Greden and Carroll, 1981) and thus add to clinical assessment. Changes in these recordings may also occur in a desynchronized fashion because of cognitive or affective improvements during treatment, providing additional information about responses (Greden and Carroll, 1981). Despite such promising applications, however, it must be noted that measurements of psychomotor activity and EMG recordings have not been widely used. Moreover, extensive studies of diagnostic accuracy have not been completed.

At the simplest level, all-night EEG sleep studies also provide an objective, independent measure of patients' reports of insomnia or hypersomnia. Such investigations have confirmed that nearly all hospitalized patients with major depression exhibit some form of sleep disturbance, with a majority experiencing sleep-continuity disturbance (70%–80%) and a minority experiencing hypersomnia (15%–25%). Moreover, correlations between reported sleep disturbances and analogous EEG sleep parameters are generally rather low (Weis, McPartland, and Kupfer, 1973), indicating the limitations of patients' reports and clinical assessments. However, measurements of sleep-continuity disturbances, decreased slow-wave sleep, and early morning awakening have not proved to be particularly useful for discriminating between depression and other psychopathological or medical-neurologic conditions without the aid of data on REM-sleep abnormalities (Kupfer and Thase, 1983; Thase and Kupfer, in press).

Beyond the verification of symptomatic reports, however, EEG sleep studies are rapidly gaining acceptance as an important research tool for study of affective syndromes (Kupfer and Thase, 1983; Thase and Kupfer, in press). In particular, a shortened latency to the first REM-sleep period (i.e., less than 60 minutes), increased REM density, and shifting of REM distribution into the first several hours of sleep have now been widely replicated in major depression (Kupfer and Thase, 1983; Thase and Kupfer, in press). As is the case for most neuroendocrine parameters, such findings are most common in patients with prominent endogenomorphic symptoms (Feinberg et al., 1982; Rush et al., 1982; Thase and Kupfer, in press).

Diagnostic application of EEG sleep studies has led to several conclusions:

1. Shortened latency to REM sleep occurs in 60%–90% of moderately to severely depressed patients, compared with only 10%–30% of normals and patient controls (Gillin et al., 1979; Akiskal et al., 1982; Feinberg et al., 1982; Rush et al., 1982; Kupfer and Thase, 1983; Thase and Kupfer, in press).
2. Application of several EEG sleep variables generally results in improved classification relative to the use of a single variable such as REM latency (Coble, Foster, and Kupfer, 1976; Kupfer et al., 1978, 1982; Gillin et al., 1979; Feinberg et al., 1982; Reynolds et al., 1983).
3. Conditions such as narcolepsy (Reynolds et al., 1983), drug- or alcohol-withdrawal states (Kupfer and Thase, 1983), or dementia (Kupfer et al., 1982) may be associated with false-positive shortened REM latency values.

The specificity of shortened REM latency used alone may be questioned, because a subset of patients with schizophrenia, obsessive–compulsive disorder, anorexia, dysthymia or atypical depression, and borderline personality disorder manifest REM latencies less than 60 minutes (Kupfer and Thase, 1982). The implications of such findings are discussed later in this chapter. The relationship between age and REM latency requires more extensive study, particularly with respect to development of age-adjusted norms for use in differential diagnosis. Different combinations of EEG variables also may be needed for various differential diagnostic applications (Coble et al., 1976; Kupfer et al., 1978, 1982; Gillin et al., 1979; Feinberg et al., 1982; Reynolds et al., 1983). Inclusion of milder cases of secondary depression within the major depression classification may lower the diagnostic accuracy of EEG sleep studies (Coble et al., 1976; Kupfer et al., 1978). However, secondary depressives with more severe, endogenomorphic syndromes are likely to evince characteristic EEG sleep abnormalities (Thase, Kupfer, and Spiker, 1984).

Within the major depression grouping, several EEG sleep variables appear to differentiate between subtypes (Kupfer and Thase, 1983; Thase and Kupfer, in press). For example, nondelusional bipolar depressives frequently exhibit hypersomnia or lesser degrees of sleep-continuity disturbance than unipolar patients, while having similarly shortened REM latencies (Thase and Kupfer, in press). This finding parallels motor-activity and symptomatic differences between these clinical subtypes and thus may prove to be an epiphenomenon. Conversely, delusionally depressed patients experience significantly greater sleep-continuity disturbances and are more likely to have extremely shortened REM latencies (i.e., less than 20 minutes) as compared with nondelusional major depressives (Kupfer and Thase, 1983; Thase and Kupfer, in press). Again, there are parallels with the clinical features that support the contention of independence of delusional depression; namely, age, severity, persistence of the syndrome, and relative resistance to tricyclic antidepressants (Thase and Kupfer, in press). Finally, as previously noted, patients with the melancholic subtype of major depression are more likely to evince shortened REM latency and increased REM density than are nonmelancholic patients (Feinberg et al., 1982; Kupfer and Thase, 1983).

Such characteristic EEG sleep changes are well-documented state markers of major depression. Preliminary evidence indicates that when patients recover, there is a strong trend toward normalization, although some residual abnormalities may persist (Kupfer, 1982; Thase and Kupfer, in press). Administration of the cholinergic agonist arecholine may prove useful in provoking an exaggerated shortening of REM latency in remitted depressives (Sitaram et al., 1982). Obviously, more detailed investigations of EEG sleep in remitted patients will be necessary to clarify state–trait issues.

Several concurrent comparisons of EEG sleep patterns, neurotransmitter metabolite or enzyme concentrations, and neuroendocrine tests have been completed. Although compelling evidence for EEG-sleep/monoamine-deficiency relationships has not been forthcoming (Thase and Kupfer, in press), cholinergic mechanisms have been indirectly implicated (Sitaram et al., 1982; Thase and Kupfer, in press). Growing evidence also links shortened REM latency with hypercortisolemia or dexamethasone nonsuppression. Cortisol abnormalities are most likely to be seen in patients with the shortest REM latencies (i.e., less than 40 minutes) (Carroll, 1982; Feinberg et al., 1982; Rush et al., 1982, 1983; Thase and Kupfer, in press). Clinical correlations with age, illness severity, and the presence of delusions appear likely. A practical implication of this finding is that EEG sleep studies appear to perform with higher sensitivity for major depression than does the DST, particularly for milder forms in ambulatory populations (Thase and Kupfer, in press). Further work is needed to confirm observations that this increased sensitivity is at the expense of inclusion of a greater number of false-positive cases (Rush et al., 1982). Studies involving EEG sleep patterns and multiple neuroendocrine parameters are under way. One recent study found that whereas shortened REM latency characterized patients with DST nonsuppression or TSH blunting, REM latency was a more sensitive marker for endogenous depression than were both neuroendocrine tests combined (Rush et al., 1983). With respect to growth hormone and prolactin, such research is of particular interest given the relationship between hormonal secretions and specific stages of sleep.

Studies of waking EEG patterns in depression are also of interest. Although no gross waking EEG abnormalities characterize depression, more sophisticated studies employing quantitative and topographic measurements of EEG amplitude and frequency have revealed some interesting, albeit conflicting, findings. For example, abnormal lateralization of EEG rhythms was found in several studies (D'Elia and Perris, 1974; Matousek, Capone, and Okawa, 1981), although this finding has not been widely replicated (Perris and Monakhov, 1979; Shagass, Roemer, and Straumanis, 1982). It is interesting that Schaffer,

Davison, and Saron (1983) found such hemispheric asymmetry in a very mildly depressed nonpatient sample. Thus, such differences may relate to emotional state rather than to the major depression syndrome per se. Studies employing measurements of regional cerebral blood flow in major depression suggest bihemispheric abnormalities (Uytdenhoff et al., 1983). Conflicting results have also been reported using quantitative EEG measurements of mean frequency and amplitude in depressives versus controls or nonaffective patient samples (Shagass et al., 1982). Moreover, even if discrete quantitative EEG differences exist between groups, they do not appear to be robust enough to permit application for diagnostic discrimination (Shagass et al., 1982).

Use of neuroradiologic tests in psychiatric research is also increasing. Computerized tomography (CT) scans particularly have been of interest because of evidence indicating cortical atrophy in a subset of patients with chronic schizophrenia. However, several recent studies have detected cortical atrophy in a number of patients with affective syndromes (Standish-Barry et al., 1982; Kellner et al., 1983; Reider et al., 1983), indicating that this marker may be more closely related to chronicity or age than to any particular disorder. One small study has related hypercortisolemia to atrophy shown on CT scans (Kellner et al., 1983). Of course, the relationship that embraces increasing age, severity of illness, and the melancholic form of major depression may account for this finding.

Positron-emission tomography (PET) scanning has recently received extensive publicity as a tool for psychiatric research. Preliminary evidence, based on a small number of carefully selected cases, suggests a relative increase in non-dominant-hemisphere glucose metabolism in affective disorders, as compared with patients with schizophrenia or normal controls (Kling et al., 1983). Obviously, research using this extremely expensive tool is in its infancy, and the findings require replication in larger numbers of patients and controls before any conclusions can be drawn.

Circadian abnormalities. Clinical variables, such as early morning awakening and diurnal mood variation, as well as a seasonality in the incidence of depression, led several investigators to hypothesize that major depression is pathogenetically related to a phase advancement of normal circadian rhythms (Wehr and Goodwin, 1981; Wehr and Wirz-Justice, 1982). Elevated nocturnal cortisol levels, reduced latency of nocturnal cortisol secretion, and shortened REM latency may be viewed as supporting this hypothesis. Wehr and Goodwin (1981) have summarized other lines of evidence that suggest a phase advancement in major depression. However, a review of recent studies indicates that blunted amplitude of the nadir of various circadian rhythms may account for nocturnal temperature elevation (Avery, Wildschiodtz, and Rafaelsen, 1982) and hypercortisolemia (Sachar, 1982) in depression, rather than an actual shifting or phase advance of the rhythm. Moreover, shortened REM latency, elevated nocturnal temperature, and hypercortisolemia appear closely interrated (Avery et al., 1982; Jarrett et al., 1983). Increased levels of evening psychomotor activity (agitation), frequent arousals during sleep, or a diminished amount of slow-wave sleep occurring in melancholic depression thus may account for such findings. Regardless, identification of disrupted or normal circadian parameters in depression graphically supports the broader notion of core psychobiological disturbances underlying major depression.

APPLICATION OF VALIDATORS TO BOUNDARY CONDITIONS

In addition to the use of biological variables to validate the independence of a disorder, such markers can be applied to test for commonalities between related conditions. Of course, simultaneous use of clinical methods (i.e., phenomenology, longitudinal course, family history, and treatment response) is also important in these endeavors. Moreover, similarity on one validator is not sufficient to establish a relationship. We would suggest that the diagnostic marker be extensively replicated and standardized.

Such methods have recently been applied with respect to several diagnostic conditions: schizoaffective disorder, dysthymic disorder, "characterological" disorders (particularly borderline personality disorder), anxiety disorders, chronic pain syndromes, obsessive–compulsive disorder, and eating disorders such as bulimia and anorexia nervosa (Carroll, 1982; Akiskal and Lemmi, 1983; Kupfer and Thase, 1983). It appears that a number of patients with each of these conditions will manifest either DST nonsuppression (Carroll et al., 1981; Carroll, 1982; Insel et al., 1982; Soloff et al., 1982; Spar and Gerner, 1982; Gwirtsman et al., 1983; Targum, 1983) or shortened REM latency (Insel et al., 1982a; Akiskal, 1983; Kupfer and Thase, 1983).

With the possible exception of the DST in borderline personality disorder (Carroll et al., 1981; Soloff et al., 1982), the presence of a relatively persistent and clinically significant depressive syndrome is perhaps the best predictor of which "boundary" disorder patient will cross over into an affective disorder grouping (Carroll, 1982; Thase and Kupfer, in press). It can be argued that such complicated patients actually have two conditions: a chronic nonaffective disorder and a more acute episode of major depression. The psychobiological abnormality may then simply reflect the second, more acute, condition. Thus, identification of accurate trait markers for major depression or subtypes of the disorder is needed to determine whether such patients have an episode of depression superimposed on a primary nonaffective disorder or have a primary condition that is actually a variant of affective disorder. A more rigorous interpretation would be to conclude that biological abnormalities such as shortened REM latency and DST nonsuppression are rather nonspecific correlates with limited diagnostic utility. Extensive longitudinal studies of patients with "boundary" conditions are needed to determine which conclusion is more accurate. Nevertheless, when biological markers are invoked to validate an affective disorder in a complicated case, caution is needed. Features of the patient's disorder, such as weight loss or considerable (and often unreported) substance abuse, may invalidate the test in question. Conversely, the limited sensitivities of our best-studied markers do not allow their use to rule out a diagnosis of major depression.

CONCLUSIONS

Major depression is a heterogeneous condition, when viewed from either a clinical or a psychobiological perspective. The diagnosis is now made with acceptable reliability; the major subtypes account for a good deal of the clinical variability within the broader grouping. Although no single biological parameter has emerged to support the notion that a common biological substrate underlies major depression, there is growing documentation of a number of abnormalities. In particular, shortened REM latency, DST nonsuppression, and a blunted TSH response to TRH have received the closest scrutiny. Each of these abnormalities occurs in a considerable number of patients with major depression, although the diagnostic sensitivities of the DST and TRH stimulation test are rather low in milder disorders among ambulatory patients. Shortened REM latency is observed in a substantially higher proportion of major depressives, although again this finding is most likely to occur in patients with endogenomorphic or melancholic symptoms. Strategies employing a battery of tests appear to yield the highest sensitivity. However, reliance on such combination strategies to confirm the diagnosis of major depression will not help clarify the pathogenetic alterations producing such psychobiological heterogeneity.

There is less conclusive evidence documenting the existence of specific biochemical subtypes of major depression. Methodological issues have undoubtedly limited progress, although our level of sophistication is increasing. A diminished number of platelet serotonin-uptake receptor sites is a potentially valuable finding; more research is certainly indicated. Although studies employing quantitative EEG methods, regional cerebral blood flow, and brain imaging techniques may ultimately be shown to be of considerable value, it is premature to judge their merit at this time.

There is some question regarding the utility of the diagnosis of nonbipolar, nonmelancholic, nondelusional major depression. Indeed, only a few of the psychobiological studies reviewed in this chapter employed samples that would approximate this residual grouping. In most cases, biological markers of depression are less applicable to these patients than to patients with the more restrictive subtypes. Thus, the major depression grouping includes a number of patients for whom it is possible that no biological abnormality will be demonstrated.

The implications of this conclusion may vary as a function of the setting. For example, in inpatient research settings, a high percentage of major depressives also will meet the criteria for melancholic, bipolar, recurrent (unipolar), or delusional subtypes. Application of findings from such a setting to milder disorders among ambulatory populations may be like comparing apples and oranges. For example, competently administered structured, short-term psychotherapies appear to match the effects of tricyclics in certain ambulatory research clinics (Weissman, 1979; Thase, 1983), but they are likely to prove to be of only adjunctive use in more severely ill populations (Rush, 1983). It has been suggested that the presence of a state marker of depression, such as DST non-suppression or shortened REM latency, may define the limits of application for psychosocial treatments (Rush, 1983; Thase, 1983). This interesting hypothesis requires empirical confirmation. Conversely, results from psychosocial-treatment studies indicate that the threshold for identification of major depression appears to be too low to define the absolute need for a somatic intervention.

If major depression is supposed to reflect (1) a high probability of some form of biological disturbance and (2) the need for a somatic form of therapy, then the current classification is too broad. Thus, the validity suffers. However, if a more general syndromal category is desired, and subtypes of the disorder are employed to account for the more severe clinical forms, then the current classification is quite appropriate.

These issues merit further attention and will undoubtedly require some degree of resolution before publication of *DSM-IV*. We suggest that for clinical purposes, the current broad classification will suffice, provided that importance of diagnosing the subtypes of major depression is recognized. In future research, it will be useful to focus more on identification of discrete biological subtypes of major depression, particularly with respect to genetic and treatment-response correlations. Such subtypes may not necessarily correspond to established clinical groupings, for even a relatively discrete classification such as bipolar disorder ultimately may prove to be biologically heterogeneous. Greater emphasis is needed regarding the use of carefully matched controls, particularly with respect to important biological variables such as age, medication status, sex, phase of menstrual cycle, and weight loss. Finally, simultaneous study of multiple biological parameters should help clarify the interrelationships and independence of these variables.

Considerable progress has been made over the past two decades in our knowledge of the psychobiology of major depression. Such advances have led to greater understanding of the complexity of the CNS and away from more simplistic models. Nevertheless, with continued and persistent effort, it is not unreasonable to expect further advances that ultimately will lead to a more refined and useful classification of the depressive disorders.

REFERENCES

Akiskal HS: Dysthymic disorder: psychopathology of proposed chronic depressive subtypes. Am J Psychiatry 140:11–20, 1983

External validating criteria for psychiatric disorders: their application in affective disorders. J Clin Psychiatry 41:6–15, 1980

Akiskal HS, Lemmi H: Clinical, neuroendocrine, and sleep diagnosis of "unusual" affective presentations: a practical review. Psychiatr Clin North Am 6:69–83, 1983

Akiskal HS, Lemmi H, Yerevanian B, et al: The utility of the REM latency test in psychiatric diagnosis: a study of 81 depressed outpatients. Psychiatr Res 7:101–110, 1982

American Psychiatric Association: Diagnostic and Statistical Manual of Mental Disorders, third edition. Washington, DC, APA, 1980

Amsterdam JD, Winokur A, Caroff S, et al: Gonadotrophin release after administration of GnRH in depressed patients and healthy volunteers. J Affect Dis 3:367–380, 1981

The dexamethasone suppression test in outpatients with primary affective disorder and healthy control subjects. Am J Psychiatry 139:287–292, 1982

Amsterdam JD, Winokur A, Lucki I, et al: A neuroendocrine test battery in bipolar patients and healthy subjects. Arch Gen Psychiatry 40:515–521, 1983

Andreasen NC: Concepts, diagnosis and classification, in Handbook of Affective Disorders. Edited by Paykel ES. New York, Guilford Press, 1982

Andreasen NC, Winokur G: Secondary depression: familial, clinical, and research perspectives. Am J Psychiatry 136:62–66, 1979

Asberg M, Traskman L: Studies of CSF 5-HIAA in depression and suicidal behavior. Adv Exp Med Biol 133:739–752, 1981

Asberg M, Traskman L, Thoren P: 5-HIAA in the cerebrospinal fluid. Arch Gen Psychiatry 33:1193–1197, 1976

Avery D, Wildschiodtz G, Rafaelsen O: REM latency and temperature in affective disorder before and after treatment. Biol Psychiatry 17:463–470, 1982

Baldessarini RJ: The basis of the amine hypotheses in affective disorders: a critical evaluation. Arch Gen Psychiatry 32:1087–1093, 1975

Banki CM: Correlation between cerebrospinal fluid amine metabolites and psychomotor activity in affective disorders. J Neurochem 29:255–257, 1977

Banki CM, Arato M: Amine metabolites and neuroendocrine responses related to depression and suicide. J Affect Dis 5:223–232, 1983

Berger M, Doerr P, Lund R, et al: Neuroendocrinological and neurophysiological studies in major depressive disorders: are these biological markers for the endogenous subtype? Biol Psychiatry 17:1217–1241, 1982

Bielski RJ, Friedel RO: Prediction of tricyclic antidepressant response. Arch Gen Psychiatry 33:1479–1489, 1976

Briley MS, Langer SZ, Raisman R, et al: Tritiated imipramine binding sites are decreased in platelets of untreated depressed patients. Science 209:303–305, 1980

Brown GM, Seggie J: Neuroendocrine mechanisms and their implications for psychiatric research. Psychiatr Clin North Am 3:205–221, 1980

Buchsbaum MS: Neurophysiological reactivity stimulus intensity modulation and the depressive disorders, in The Psychobiology of the Depressive Disorders. Edited by Depue RA. New York, Academic Press, 1979

Buchsbaum MS, Ingvar DH, Kessler R, et al: Cerebral glucography with positron tomography. Arch Gen Psychiatry 39:251–259, 1982

Bunney WE, Davis JM: Norepinephrine in depressive reactions: a review. Arch Gen Psychiatry 13:483–494, 1965

Carroll BJ: The dexamethasone suppression test for melancholia. Br J Psychiatry 140:292–304, 1982

Carroll BJ, Curtis GC, Mendels J: Neuroendocrine regulation in depression, II: discrimination of depressed from nondepressed patients. Arch Gen Psychiatry 33:1051–1058, 1976

Carroll BJ, Feinberg M, Greden JF, et al: A specific laboratory test for the diagnosis of melancholia. Arch Gen Psychiatry 140:292–304, 1982

Carroll BJ, Greden JF, Feinberg M, et al: Neuroendocrine evaluation of depression in borderline patients. Psychiatr Clin North Am 4:89–99, 1981

Neurotransmitter studies of neuroendocrine pathology in depression. Arch Psychiatr Scand [Suppl 280] 61:183–200, 1980

Checkley SA, Slade AP, Shur E: Growth hormone and other responses to clonidine in patients with endogenous depression. Br J Psychiatry 138:51–55, 1981

Clayton PJ, Lewis CE: The significance of secondary depression. J Affect Dis 3:25–35, 1981

Coble PA, Foster FG, Kupfer DJ: Electroencephalographic sleep diagnosis of primary depression. Arch Gen Psychiatry 33:1124–1127, 1976

Coryell W, Gaffney G, Burkhardt PE: *DSM-III* melancholia and the primary–secondary distinction: a comparison of concurrent validity by means of the dexamethasone suppression test. Am J Psychiatry 139:120–122, 1982

Coryell W, Winokur G: Course and outcome, in Handbook of Affective Disorders. Edited by Paykel ES. New York, Guilford Press, 1982

Coryell W, Zimmerman M: The dexamethasone suppression test and ECT outcome. A six-month follow-up. Biol Psychiatry 18:21–27, 1983

Davis KL, Hollister LE, Mathe AA, et al: Neuroendocrine and neurochemical measurements in depression. Am J Psychiatry 138:1555–1562, 1981

D'Elia G, Perris C: Cerebral functional dominance and memory functions: an analysis of EEG integrated amplitude in depressive psychotics. Acta Psychiatr Scand [Suppl 255] 50:143–157, 1974

Edelstein CK, Roy-Byrne P, Fawzy FI, et al: Effects of weight loss on the dexamethasone suppression test. Am J Psychiatry 140:338–341, 1983

Fang VS, Tricou BJ, Robertson A, et al: Plasma ACTH and cortisol levels in depressed patients. Life Sci 29:931–938, 1981

Feighner JP, Robins E, Guze SB, et al: Diagnostic criteria for use in psychiatric research. Arch Gen Psychiatry 26:57–63, 1972

Feinberg M, Gillin JC, Carroll BJ, et al: EEG studies of sleep in the diagnosis of depression. Biol Psychiatry 17:305–316, 1982

Gaertner HJ, Kreuter F, Scharek G, et al: Do urinary MHPG and plasma drug levels correlate with response to amitriptyline therapy? Psychopharmacology 76:236–239, 1982

Garbutt JC, Loosen PT, Tipermas A, et al: The TRH test in patients with borderline personality disorder. Psychiatr Res 9:107–113, 1983

Gillin JC, Duncan W, Pettigrew KD, et al: Successful separation of depressed, normal, and insomniac subjects by EEG sleep data. Arch Gen Psychiatry 36:85–90, 1979

Gold MS, Pottash ALC, Extein I, et al: Diagnosis of depression in the 1980's. JAMA 245:1562–1564, 1981

Graham PM, Booth J, Boranga G, et al: The dexamethasone suppression test in mania. J Affect Dis 4:201–211, 1982

Greden JF, Carroll BJ: Psychomotor function in affective disorder: an overview of new monitoring techniques. Am J Psychiatry 138:1441–1448, 1981

Gruen PH, Sachar EJ, Altman N, et al: Growth hormone response to hypoglycemia in postmenopausal depressed women. Arch Gen Psychiatry 32:31–33, 1975

Gudeman JE, Schatzberg AF, Samson JA, et al: Toward a biochemical classification of depressive disorders, VI: platelet MAO activity and clinical symptoms in depressed patients. Am J Psychiatry 139:630–633, 1982

Gwirtsman HE, Roy-Byrne P, Yager J, et al: Neuroendocrine abnormalities in bulimia. Am J Psychiatry 140:559–563, 1983

Halbreich U, Grunhaus L, Ben-David M: Twenty-four hour rhythm of prolactin in depressive patients. Arch Gen Psychiatry 36:1183–1186, 1979

Hirschfeld RMA, Koslow SH, Kupfer DJ: The clinical utility of the dexamethasone suppression test in psychiatry. JAMA 250:2172–2174, 1983

Clinical utility of the dexamethasone suppression test, in Proceedings of a National Institute of Mental Health workshop. U.S. Department of Health and Human Services, No. (ADM) 85–1318, 1985

Hollister LE: Excretion of 3-methoxy-4-hydroxyphenylglycol in depressed and geriatric patients and normal persons. Int Pharmacopsychiatry 16:138–143, 1981

Iacono WG, Lykken DT, Peloquin LJ, et al: Electrodermal activity in euthymic unipolar and bipolar affective disorders. Arch Gen Psychiatry 40:557–565, 1983

Insel TR, Gillin JC, Moore A, et al: The sleep of patients with obsessive–compulsive disorder. Arch Gen Psychiatry 39:1372–1377, 1982a

Insel TR, Kalin NH, Guttlmacher LB, et al: The dexamethasone suppression test in patients with obsessive–compulsive disorder. Psychiatr Res 6:153–160, 1982b

Janowsky DS, El-Yousef MK, Davis JM, et al: A cholinergic-adrenergic hypothesis of mania and depression. Lancet 2:632–635, 1972

Janowsky DS, Risch SC, Gillin JC: Adrenergic-cholinergic balance and the treatment of affective disorders. Prog Neuro-Psychopharmacol Biol Psychiatry 7:297–307, 1983

Jarrett DB, Coble PA, Kupfer DJ: Reduced cortisol latency in depressive illness. Arch Gen Psychiatry 40:506–511, 1983

Judd LL, Risch SC, Parker DC, et al: Blunted prolactin response. Arch Gen Psychiatry 39:1413–1416, 1982

Kalin NH, Risch SC, Janowsky DS, et al: Use of the dexamethasone suppression test in clinical psychiatry. J Clin Psychopharmacol 1:64–69, 1981

Kalin NH, Weisler SJ, Shelton SE: Plasma ACTH and cortisol concentrations before and after dexamethasone. Psychiatr Res 7:87–92, 1982

Kellner CH, Rubinow DR, Gold PW, et al: Relationship of cortisol hypersecretion to brain CT scan alterations in depressed patients. Psychiatr Res 8:191–197, 1983

Kelwala S, Jones D, Sitaram N: Monoamine metabolites as predictors of antidepressant response: a critique. Prog Neuro-Psychopharmacol Biol Psychiatry 7:229–240, 1983

Kendell RE: The classification of depressions: a review of contemporary confusion. Br J Psychiatry 129:15–28, 1976

Kirkegaard C: The thyrotropin response to thyrotropin-releasing hormone in endogenous depression. Psychoneuroendocrinology 6:189–212, 1981

Kirkegaard C, Carroll BJ: Dissociation of TSH and adrenocortical disturbances in endogenous depression. Psychiatr Res 3:253–264, 1980

Klein DF, Gittelman R, Quitkin R, et al: Diagnosis and Treatment of Psychiatric Disorders, second edition. Baltimore, Williams & Wilkins, 1980

Kling AS, Kuhl DE, Metter EJ, et al: Positron computer tomography and CT scans in schizophrenia and depression. Paper presented at the New Research section of the annual meeting of the American Psychiatric Association, New York, May 5, 1983

Koslow SH, Maas JW, Bowden CL, et al: CSF and urinary biogenic amines and metabolites in depression and mania. Arch Gen Psychiatry 40:999–1010, 1983

Koslow SH, Stokes PE, Mendels J, et al: Insulin tolerance test: human growth hormone response and insulin resistance in primary unipolar depressed, bipolar depressed and control subjects. Psychol Med 12:45–55, 1982

Kupfer DJ: EEG sleep as biological markers in depression, in Biological Markers in Psychiatry and Neurology. Edited by Hanin I, Usdin E. New York, Pergamon Press, 1982

Kupfer DJ, Foster FG, Coble PA, et al: The application of EEG sleep for the differential diagnosis of affective disorders. Am J Psychiatry 135:69–74, 1978

Kupfer DJ, Reynolds CF, Ulrich RF, et al: EEG sleep, depression and aging. Neurobiol Aging 3:351–360, 1982

Kupfer DJ, Rush AJ: Recommendations for depression publications. Arch Gen Psychiatry 40:1031, 1983

Kupfer DJ, Thase ME: The use of the sleep laboratory in the diagnosis of affective disorders. Psychiatr Clin North Am 5:3–25, 1983

Laakman G: Mechanisms of HGH response to DMI in volunteers and depressed patients, in Abstracts of the 12th CINP Congress. Edited by Radouco-Thomas C, Garcia F. New York, Pergamon Press, 1980

Langer G, Aschauer H, Koinig G, et al: The TSH response to TRH: a possible predictor of outcome to antidepressant and neuroleptic treatment. Prog Neuro-Psychopharmacol Biol Psychiatry 7:335–342, 1983

Langer G, Heinze G, Reim B, et al: Reduction of growth hormone response in endogenous depressive patients. Arch Gen Psychiatry 33:1451–1457, 1976

Lechin F, Van der Dijs B, Acosta E, et al: Distal colon motility and clinical parameters in depression. J Affect Dis 5:19–26, 1983

Lewy AJ, Nurnberger JI, Wehr TA, et al: Supersensitivity to light: possible trait marker for manic-depressive illness. Am J Psychiatry 142:725–727, 1985

Loosen PT, Prange AJ Jr: The serum thyrotropin response to thyrotropin-releasing hormone in psychiatric patients: a review. Am J Psychiatry 139:405–416, 1982

Loosen PT, Wilson IC, Dew B, et al: Thyrotropin-releasing hormone (TRH) in abstinent alcoholic men. Am J Psychiatry 140:1145–1149, 1983

Maas JW: Biogenic amines and depression: biochemical and pharmacological separation of two types of depression. Arch Gen Psychiatry 32:1357–1361, 1975

Matarazzo JD: The reliability of psychiatric and psychological diagnosis. Clin Psychol Rev 3:103–145, 1983

Matousek M, Capone C, Okawa M: Measurement of the interhemispheral differences as a diagnostic tool in psychiatry. Adv Biol Psychiatry 6:76–80, 1981

Meltzer HY, Arora RC, Baber R, et al: Serotonin uptake in blood platelets of psychiatric patients. Arch Gen Psychiatry 38:1322–1326, 1981

Meltzer HY, Arora RC, Tricou BJ, et al: Serotonin uptake in blood platelets and the dexamethasone suppression test in depressed patients. Psychiatr Res 8:41–47, 1983

Mendlewicz J, Linkowski P, Brauman H: Reduced prolactin release after thyrotropin-releasing hormone in manic depression. N Engl J Med 302:1091–1092, 1980

Nelson JC, Charney DS: The symptoms of major depressive illness. Am J Psychiatry 138:1–13, 1981

Nelson JC, Charney DS, Quinlan DM: Evaluation of the DSM-III criteria for melancholia. Arch Gen Psychiatry 38:555–559, 1981

Newsom G, Murray N: Reversal of dexamethasone suppression test nonsuppression in alcohol abusers. Am J Psychiatry 140:353–354, 1983

Paul SM, Rehavi M, Rice K, et al: Does high affinity ³H-imipramine binding label serotonin reuptake sites in brain and platelet? Life Sci 28:2253–2260, 1981a

Paul SM, Rehavi M, Skolnick P, et al: Demonstration of specific high affinity binding sites for ³H-imipramine on human platelets. Life Sci 26:953–959, 1980

Depressed patients have decreased binding of tritiated imipramine to platelet serotonin "transporter." Arch Gen Psychiatry 38:1315–1317, 1981b

Perris C, Monakhov K: Depressive symptomatology and systemic analysis of the EEG, in Hemisphere Asymmetries of Function in Psychopathology. Edited by Gruzelier J, Flor-Henry P. Amsterdam, Biomedical Press, 1979

Rabkin JG, Quitkin FM, Stewart JW, et al: The dexamethasone suppression test with mildly and moderately depressed outpatients. Am J Psychiatry 140:926–927, 1983

Reider RO, Mann LS, Weinberger D, et al: Computed tomographic scans in patients with schizophrenia, schizoaffective and bipolar affective disorder. Arch Gen Psychiatry 40:735–739, 1983

Reynolds CF, Christiansen CL, Taska LS, et al: Sleep in narcolepsy and depression: does it all look alike? J Nerv Ment Dis 171:290–295, 1983

Risch SC: Beta-endorphin hypersecretion in depression: possible cholinergic mechanisms. Biol Psychiatry 17:1071–1079, 1982

Rotman A: Blood platelets in psychopharmacological research. Prog Neuro-Psychopharmacol Biol Psychiatry 7:135–151, 1983

Rush AJ: Cognitive therapy of depression: rationale, techniques, and efficacy. Psychiatr Clin North Am 6:105–127, 1983

Rush AJ, Giles DE, Roffwarg HP, et al: Sleep EEG and dexamethasone suppression test findings in outpatients with unipolar major depressive disorder. Biol Psychiatry 17:327–341, 1982

Rush AJ, Schlesser MA, Roffwarg HP, et al: Relationships among the TRH, REM latency, and dexamethasone suppression test: preliminary findings. J Clin Psychiatry 44:23–29, 1983

Sachar EJ: Endocrine abnormalities in depression, in Handbook of Affective Disorders. Edited by Paykel ES. New York, Guilford Press, 1982

Sachar EJ, Halbreigh U, Asnis G, et al: Paradoxical cortisol responses to dextroamphetamine in endogenous depression. Arch Gen Psychiatry 38:1113–1117, 1981

Schaffer CE, Davison RJ, Saron C: Frontal and parietal electroencephalogram asymmetry in depressed and nondepressed subjects. Biol Psychiatry 18:753–762, 1983

Schatzberg AF, Orsulak PJ, Rosenbaum AH, et al: Toward a biochemical classification of depressive disorders, III: pretreatment urinary MHPG levels as predictors of response to treatment with maprotiline. Psychopharmacology 75:34–38, 1981

Schatzberg AF, Orsulak PJ, Rothschild AJ, et al: Platelet MAO activity and the dexamethasone suppression test in depressed patients. Am J Psychiatry 140:1231–1233, 1983

Schildkraut JJ: The catecholamine hypothesis of affective disorder: a review of supporting evidence. Am J Psychiatry 122:509–522, 1965

The biochemical discrimination of subtypes of depressive disorders: an outline of our studies on norepinephrine metabolism and psychoactive drugs in the endogenous depressions since 1967. Pharmakopsychiatrie 15:121–127, 1982

Schwartz GE, Fair PL, Salt P, et al: Facial expression and imagery in depression: an electromyographic study. Psychosom Med 38:337–347, 1976

Shagass C, Roemer RA, Straumanis JJ: Relationships between psychiatric diagnosis and some quantitative EEG variables. Arch Gen Psychiatry 39:1423–1435, 1982

Sitaram N, Nurnberger JI, Gershon ES, et al: Cholinergic regulation of mood and REM sleep: potential model and marker of vulnerability to affective disorders. Am J Psychiatry 139:571–576, 1982

Soloff PH, George A, Nathan RS: Dexamethasone suppression test in patients with borderline personality disorder. Am J Psychiatry 139:1621–1623, 1982

Spar JE, Gerner R: Does the dexamethasone suppression test distinguish dementia from depression? Am J Psychiatry 139:238–240, 1982

Spar JE, La Rue A: Major depression in the elderly: DSM-III criteria and the dexamethasone suppression test as predictors of treatment response. Am J Psychiatry 140:844–847, 1983

Spitzer RL, Endicott J, Robins E: Research diagnostic criteria. Arch Gen Psychiatry 34:773–782, 1978

Spitzer RL, Williams JBW, Skodol AE: DSM-III: the major achievements and an overview. Am J Psychiatry 137:151–164, 1980

Standish-Barry HMAS, Bouras N, Bridges DK, et al: Pneumo-encephalographic and computerized axial tomography scan changes in affective disorders. Br J Psychiatry 141:614–617, 1982

Sternbach HA, Kirstein L, Pottash ALC, et al: The TRH test and urinary MHPG in unipolar depression. J Affect Dis 5:233–237, 1983

Stokes PE, Stoll P, Koslow H, et al: Pretreatment DST and hypothalamic-pituitary-adreno-cortical function in depressed patients and comparison groups. Arch Gen Psychiatry 41:257–267, 1984

Suranyi-Cadotte BE, Wood PL, Schwartz G, et al: Altered platelet ³H-imipramine binding in schizoaffective and depressive disorders. Biol Psychiatry 18:923–927, 1983

Targum SD: The application of serial neuroendocrine challenge studies in the management of depressive disorder. Biol Psychiatry 18:3–19, 1983a

Neuroendocrine dysfunction in schizophreniform disorder: correlation with six-month clinical outcome. Am J Psychiatry 140:309–313, 1983b

Targum SD, Greenburg R, Harmon R, et al: Adjunctive thyroid hormone in refractory depression. Paper presented at the New Research section of the annual meeting of the American Psychiatric Association, New York, May 3, 1983

Taylor MA, Abrams R: Reassessing the bipolar-unipolar dichotomy. J Affect Dis 2:195–217, 1980

Thase ME: Cognitive and behavioral treatments for depression: a review of recent developments, in Affective Disorders Reassessed: 1983. Edited by Ayd FJ, Taylor IJ, Taylor BT. Baltimore, Md, Ayd Medical Communications, 1983

Thase ME, Kupfer DJ: Current status of EEG sleep in the assessment and treatment of depression, in Advances in Human Psychopharmacology. Edited by Burrows GD, Werry JS. Greenwich, Ct, JAI Press (in press)

Thase ME, Kupfer DJ, Spiker DG: EEG sleep in secondary depression: a revisit. Biol Psychiatry 19:805–814, 1984

Traskman L, Asberg M, Bertilsson L, et al: Monoamine metabolites in CSF and suicidal behavior. Arch Gen Psychiatry 38:631–636, 1981

Uytdenhoff P, Portelange P, Jacquy J, et al: Regional cerebral blood flow and lateralized hemispheric dysfunction in depression. Br J Psychiatry 143:128–132, 1983

Van Praag HM: Central monoamine metabolism in depressions, I: serotonin and related compounds. Compr Psychiatry 21:30–43, 1980a

Central monoamine metabolism in depressions, II: catecholamines and related compounds. Compr Psychiatry 21:44–54, 1980b

A transatlantic view of the diagnosis of depressions according to DSM-III, I: controversies and misunderstandings in depression diagnosis. Compr Psychiatry 23:315–329, 1982

Biological suicide research: outcome and limitations. Biol Psychiatry 21:1305–1323, 1986

Van Praag HM, Korf J: Retarded depression and dopamine metabolism. Psychopharmacology 19:199–203, 1971

Wehr TA, Goodwin FK: Biological rhythms and psychiatry, in American Handbook of Psychiatry, vol 7. Edited by Arieti S, Brodie HKH. New York, Basic Books, 1981

Wehr TA, Wirz-Justice A: Circadian rhythm mechanisms in affective illness and in antidepressant drug action. Pharmacopsychiatry 15:31–39, 1982

Weis BL, McPartland RJ, Kupfer DJ: Once more: the inaccuracy of non-EEG estimations of sleep. Am J Psychiatry 130:1282–1285, 1973

Weissman MM: The psychological treatment of depression. Arch Gen Psychiatry 36:1261–1269, 1979

Winokur A, Amsterdam JD, Oler J, et al: Multiple hormone responses to protirelin (TRH) in depressed patients. Arch Gen Psychiatry 40:525–531, 1983

Yerevanian BI, Olafsdottir H, Milanese E, et al: Normalization of the dexamethasone suppression test at discharge from hospital. J Affect Dis 5:191–197, 1983

3   *The boundaries of mood disorders*

Implications for defining temperamental variants, atypical subtypes, and schizoaffective disorder

HAGOP SOUREN AKISKAL

New nosologic rubrics for mood disorders were added to *DSM-III* (American Psychiatric Association, 1980) in recognition that a large number of affectively ill patients fell below the threshold of the major mood disorders, or presented with manifestations deemed in some way atypical. Many of these patients are seen in ambulatory settings, raising questions in regard to differentiating between their conditions and nonspecific dysphoria or the misery that often is part of the human condition; more important for the clinician, this raises questions regarding the relationships between these low-grade and atypical affective conditions and the more classic or more typical forms of affective disorders. The advent of community psychiatry, the availability of a large armamentarium of potent treatments for combating mood disorders, and the decreased stigmatization associated with affective diagnoses are bringing large numbers of mildly dysphoric individuals to the offices of mental health practitioners (Akiskal and Cassano, 1983). It is therefore relevant to inquire if the affective malaise experienced by some or many of these individuals represents precursors or variants of major affective syndromes or if these patients would more appropriately be classified in the characterologic domain. Such inquiries are also of major relevance to research efforts designed to identify individuals at risk for major affective disorders.

Atypical presentations of affective syndromes also involve the classic question of the boundaries between psychotic affective and schizophrenic disorders. The major issue here is whether so-called schizoaffective disorders constitute variants of affective or schizophrenic psychoses or constitute a distinct "third psychosis" that is neither schizophrenic nor affective.

All of these questions relate to the boundaries between mood disorders and normality, on the one hand, and nonaffective disorders, on the other. In this chapter I first discuss methodological issues concerning these boundaries before considering the relationships between specific *DSM-III* nonmajor affective sub-

Supported in part by a contract with the Tennessee Department of Mental Health and Mental Retardation and by grants MH-05931 and MH-06147 from the National Institute of Mental Health. Dr. James Seymour provided research assistance, and Christy Wright provided editorial assistance.

61

types and major mood disorders. In this endeavor I draw heavily on previously published reviews (Akiskal, 1983b; Akiskal and Webb, 1983; Akiskal and Lemmi, 1983) and summarize work conducted in our mood clinic and elsewhere on many of the unresolved questions concerning the interface between affective and nonaffective disorders.

METHODOLOGIC ISSUES

The problems facing nosologists in erecting boundaries between affective and nonaffective conditions were most eloquently summarized by Kendell (1976) in his review of the confusion regarding the classification of depression:

What constitutes a depressive illness is itself subject to dispute and disagreement: the boundaries between depression and sadness, between affective psychosis and schizophrenia, and between recurrent depression and personality disorder are all arbitrary and ill-defined.

The clinical overlap of mood disorders with these various conditions is large indeed, and both mathematical and clinical arguments have been advanced for continuity – and discontinuity – between them. Kendell pointed out that this debate is part of a wider unresolved discussion about the nature of disease. The Hippocratic approach conceptualized disease as an outgrowth of premorbid characteristics; hence, disease states were not sharply demarcated from health, and each case was viewed as unique. By contrast, the rival Platonic school believed that diseases should be categorized into "ideal" forms, distinct from one another.

The dimensional approach, though seemingly "fuzzy," has intuitive clinical appeal to members of the psychoanalytic and Meyerian schools of thought. The categorical or typologic approach, exemplified by Kraepelin and neo-Kraepelinian biological psychiatry, appears more "scientific," but must account for the symptomatologic overlap among the various psychiatric disorders. According to Robins (1976), these two approaches represent different phases in the scientific study of diseases. Initially, clinical investigators make use of the categorical approach to describe the fundamental characteristics of a given syndrome and to investigate etiologically relevant factors. As more is learned about the syndrome, the stage is set for extending its boundaries to delineate atypical variants or attenuated forms. It is in this light that one should view the developments of the Washington University criteria (Feighner et al., 1972), the Research Diagnostic Criteria (RDC) (Spitzer, Endicott, and Robins, 1978), and the *DSM-III* criteria: They represent tools to explore the largely uncharted universe of mental illness.

The categorical approach has heuristic value in the beginning phases of a young clinical field like psychiatry. The dimensional strategy, though useful in clinical formulation, may prove scientifically sterile unless it is coupled with its categorical counterpart. For instance, the concept of a continuum from bipolar psychosis to cyclothymia would not have developed without a rigorous categorical definition that set manic-depressive psychosis apart from schizophrenic and personality disorders. This approach permitted delineation of the essential features of bipolar disorder and the subsequent description of its attenuated forms as cyclothymic and related temperaments.

The dimensional approach to mood disorders must also contend with the fact that qualitative jumps take place at the tail of what may seem to be normal distributions of "moods" and "moodiness." For instance, although clinical depression may have features in common with the "blues," the clinical disorder is often autonomous and has a distinct quality different from everyday depression. Yet the threshold for defining the clinical disorder is somewhat arbitrary and depends on the definition's projected uses. For instance, the broad RDC definition for probable depression (dysphoria and four depressive symptoms of at least one week's duration) may be desirable in certain epidemiologic studies of symptomatic volunteers (Barrett, 1981), whereas the more restrictive Feighner definition (dysphoria and five symptoms lasting over four weeks) may be preferable for genetic studies (Coryell, Winokur, and Andreasen, 1981). An intermediate threshold, such as that in *DSM-III* (dysphoria and four symptoms sustained for two weeks), may suffice for general clinical purposes. This elasticity of the boundary between normal and morbid is not unique to psychiatry; similar questions arise in assessing hypertension, coronary artery disease, and cirrhosis.

According to Kendell, mathematical models have generally been unsuccessful in resolving the boundary issues between affective illness and its subtypes, on the one hand, and normality, on the other. Approaches to the validation of psychiatric entities originally developed by Robins and Guze (1970) to evaluate schizophrenia have been extended to all psychiatric disorders (Akiskal, 1980). They include (1) phenomenologic and associated features, (2) premorbid and longitudinal course, (3) family history, (4) treatment response, (5) neuroendocrine findings, and (6) neurophysiologic findings. Current *DSM-III* criteria are largely based on the first two approaches; family history is not included in the definitions of syndromes, presumably because it represents a departure from the "atheoretical" framework of *DSM-III*. Yet many recent proposals for affective-disorder subtyping have used the family-history strategy (Fieve and Dunner, 1975; Winokur, 1979; Akiskal, 1983a,b). From the clinician's standpoint, treatment response may represent the most important validator of an affective subtype; predicting which patient will respond to what treatment and assessing prognosis are the very reasons for assigning patients to diagnostic subtypes. For instance, the *DSM-III* category of dysthymic disorder could be considered invalid from this standpoint, because it encompasses an unwieldy heterogeneity of conditions with different treatment and prognostic implications (Akiskal, 1983d).

Ideally, the validity of a given diagnosis should be supported by pathogenetic understanding (construct validity). This is rarely possible in psychiatric disorders, with the exception of organic psychiatric syndromes. Although depression associated with conditions such as hypothyroidism, systemic lupus erythematosus, and carcinoma of the head of the pancreas can be considered as organic affective syndromes (Akiskal, 1982a), in many other conditions, such as reserpine-induced depression (Goodwin and Bunney, 1971), it appears that the drug is merely precipitating a clinical depression to which the patient is predisposed by personal or family history (Akiskal and Tashjian, 1983). We have insufficient systematic data on most depressions occurring in the setting of medical diseases to determine which of these diseases can cause de novo affective episodes, as opposed to nonspecific precipitation in otherwise vulnerable individuals. For this reason – and because the term "organic affective syndrome" implies that other mood disorders are not organic – I prefer the designation of "symptomatic depression." An alternative would be to code all cases meeting the syndromal criteria for major depression on axis I irrespective of organic etiologic concomitants. This would not result in any loss of clinical information, because *DSM-III* explicitly requires the coding of relevant medical conditions on axis III. This approach would be analogous to acknowledging relevant psychosocial concomitants on axis IV. In this respect, the APA diagnostic manual would be more consistent in coding both biological and psychosocial factors relevant to the causes of mood disorders on axes other than axis I. (The same remarks apply to organic anxiety syndromes, drug-induced psychoses, and organic schizophreniform syndromes in general.) By splitting off organic affective or schizophreniform syndromes from those of undetermined causes, we risk losing ground every time organic causes are established for a given area, culminating in the ridiculous situation of defining psychiatry as that branch of medicine that concerns itself with behavioral disorders of unknown causes (Akiskal, 1978). More dangerous is the message that nonphysician mental health workers might read into this: Because discrete biologic causes have not been conclusively established for most of the "functional" psychiatric disorders, psychiatrists' professional "jurisdiction" over mental disorders might be questioned.

As we move toward *DSM-IV*, the emerging biological technology – neuroendocrine and sleep electroencephalographic (EEG) batteries – may prove useful in providing construct validity for the various affective subtypes and in distinguishing them from bordering conditions. Indeed, laboratory procedures are beginning to provide validity for distinctions between various affective and nonaffective conditions. The relevance of these approaches to the psychobiology of major depressions is reviewed elsewhere in this volume (see Chapter 2). This chapter focuses on their joint application with more traditional clinical indices in resolving boundary questions in the area of affective disorders.

DISTINCTION BETWEEN NORMAL AND CLINICAL DEPRESSION

Sadness and joy, like fear, are part of the normal human emotional repertoire. How, then, does one draw the line between, for example, an adaptive depressive response to loss and clinical depression?

Measurement of pharmacologic responses is one useful approach. Morbid depression is often alleviated by tricyclic antidepressants, whereas ordinary sadness is unaffected. By contrast, stimulants with immediate mood-elevating properties have no long-term benefit in clinical depression. These pharmacologic factors are often overlooked by those who view clinical depression and the "blues" as being on a continuum. Recent studies have shown that depressive symptoms falling short of syndromal criteria ("minor" and "intermittent" depressions) are prevalent in the community, even in untreated populations, and are highly represented among symptomatic volunteers (Blumenthal and Dielman, 1975; Barrett et al., 1978). Unlike the "blues," which by definition are short-lived, these conditions tend to pursue a fluctuating course. At least one study has shown some response to tricyclic antidepressants in these "noncases" of so-called minor or intermittent depression (Nandi et al., 1976), suggesting some affinity with morbid depression.

Table 3.1 presents proposed criteria that may assist in determining when depressive manifestations indicate mood disorder worthy of clinical attention (Akiskal, 1983b). The first two are self-explanatory; the others deserve further comment.

Clinical or major depression is usually incapacitating. Hitherto, much attention has been paid to interpersonal consequences. Recent evidence from Cassano and associates (1977) indicates that measurable deficits in work performances are also often early manifestations. Clinically depressed individuals are unable to benefit from leisure; hence the well-known futility of "prescribing" vacations (Cassano and Akiskal, 1984). Other work has shown that depressives who seek clinical attention differ from those who do not in that they manifest vegetative and anxiety symptoms (Hogarty and Katz, 1971; Weissman, Prusoff, and Pincus, 1975). The clinical subjects were behaviorally incapacitated and unable to cope with their conditions, whereas the "depressed normals" – who had more subjective depression – attributed their mental states to realistic external circumstances and were able to cope with those states.

Bipolarity – whether mild or pronounced, spontaneous or pharmacologically occasioned – is another indicator of clinically significant mood disorder (Nandi et al., 1976; Akiskal et al., 1983b). Likewise, a family history of bipolar disorder should prompt consideration of clinical depression in an individual who may otherwise appear to be experiencing an adjustment disorder with depressed mood (Akiskal et al., 1983b).

A consecutive-generation family history of affective disorder – especially when "loaded" – is even more characteristic of primary affective illness. For instance, in a University of Tennessee prospective study of "minor" or "neurotic" depressives, it was found that such pedigrees predicted the development of major episodes (Akiskal et al., 1979b). This study also provided evidence that many primary depressions had their onset in mild dysphoric states phenomenologically indistinguishable from "unhappiness."

Finally, recurrence – especially periodicity (seasonality or regular recurrence) – is characteristic of mood disorder (Akiskal, 1983a).

Requiring the presence of several of these characteristics will restrict the

Table 3.1. *Suggested criteria to set the threshold for clinical depression*

1. Sustained syndromal depression at some phase of the disorder
2. The presence of marked vegetative and psychomotor disturbances in addition to psychological symptoms
3. Functional incapacitation
4. Bipolar course – either spontaneous or pharmacologically mobilized
5. Family history of bipolar disorder
6. Recurrences, especially periodicity or seasonality
7. Loaded family pedigrees – especially in consecutive generations – for treated affective disorders

operational meaning of major depressions to their appropriate clinical "territory" (i.e., disorders above the threshold of clinical significance).

DISTINCTION BETWEEN GRIEF AND CLINICAL DEPRESSION

Uncomplicated bereavement is an exclusion criterion for the diagnosis of major depression, because many individuals undergoing normal bereavement exhibit most of the features listed under major depression. It would be desirable to make the distinction more explicit by requiring features not seen in normal bereavement, such as psychomotor retardation, guilt of commission, delusional lowering of self-esteem, persistent suicidal ideation, "mummification," and severe anniversary reaction (Clayton et al., 1974).

Although the dexamethasone suppression test and REM latency test have revealed few false positives among nonpsychiatric controls, these measures have not yet been fully tested for their usefulness in differentiating normal grief and morbid depressions. However, sleep EEG studies have failed to show pathological shortening of REM latency in grieving monkeys (Reite and Short, 1978) and in transiently dysphoric subjects (Cartwright, Stephen, and Trenholm, 1982), indicating that this measure may help in separating clinical depressions from normative reactions to loss. A preliminary report from our sleep laboratory has also shown that patients with *pathological* grief (i.e., those bereaved subjects seeking medical or psychiatric attention) have sleep EEG characteristics (including shortened REM latency) similar to those of primary depressives.

DISTINCTION BETWEEN "HAPPINESS" AND MORBID ELATION

Clinical differentiation between normal elation and morbid euphoria or hypomanic states is particularly difficult because hypomania is often socially and vocationally adaptive, and such individuals rarely seek help. Unfortunately, social disasters sometimes provide the first clue to the presence of a morbid process. *DSM-III* has not defined the clinical threshold at which elation can be considered pathologic: The *DSM-III* text simply states that hypomania is a milder form of mania. This may explain why the diagnosis of "atypical bipolar disorder" (in which excited periods are deemed to be on a lower plane of severity than in mania) is generally considered unreliable. In our mood clinic (Akiskal, 1983b), we have found that hypomania:

1. can be dysphoric in its drivenness,
2. tends to be labile,
3. may lead to substance abuse,
4. can impair social judgment,
5. is often preceded or followed by retarded depression,
6. typically springs from a positive familial background for classic bipolar disorder,
7. finally, tends to recur – happiness does not!

These features may serve as guidelines to set the threshold for *clinical* hypomania.

We have also developed criteria (Akiskal, 1983b) for setting the threshold at which hypomania can be said to have reached manic proportions:

1. Pleasant euphoria gives way to irritable belligerence, even violence.
2. Delusional grandiosity, other delusions, and transient hallucinatory phenomena occur.
3. Frenzied physical activity, sleep loss, and loss of social judgment usually dictate hospitalization.

Such a degree of disturbance is rarely reached until the illness has persisted for two weeks, whereas hypomanic levels of disturbance may build up within one week, at which time it can be considered "definite." At least two days of hypomanic behavior (probable hypomania) are necessary to define the subtle hypomanic periods seen in what Dunner (1983) refers to as bipolar II disorder (the precursor of the *DSM-III* atypical bipolar category). This disorder, which accounts for half of all bipolar outpatients, as discussed later, occurs in three forms (Akiskal, Khani, and Scott-Strauss, 1979):

1. major depression superimposed on cyclothymic disorders
2. recurrent hypersomnia-retarded depressions, with infrequent spontaneous hypomanic episodes that do not require clinical attention
3. pharmacologically mobilized hypomanic episodes in hypersomnia-retarded depressions.

This last group, sometimes referred to as unipolar II (Fieve and Dunner, 1975) or bipolar III (Klerman, 1981; Akiskal, 1983a) – in view of a bipolar family history, which lowers its threshold for pharmacologic hypomania – has been shown to be at risk for spontaneous hypomanic episodes during prospective observation (Akiskal et al., 1983b).

As proposed elsewhere (Akiskal, 1983a, b), it would be desirable to distinguish recurrent major depressions with a bipolar family history from the heterogeneous universe of major depressions without such a history. They differ not only in course but also in terms of responses to lithium carbonate versus tricyclics (Kupfer et al., 1975); indeed, unipolar-II/bipolar-III depressives are at risk for rapid cycling when exposed to tricyclic antidepressants (Wehr and Goodwin, 1979; Grof, 1980). Because predictive validity is the most important function of a clinical diagnostic manual, revisions of *DSM-III* should consider taking account of bipolar family history and pharmacologically mobilized hypomania in the classification of depressive disorders. This approach, modified from earlier work (Akiskal, 1983a,b), is summarized in Table 3.2.

DISTINCTION BETWEEN ANXIETY AND DEPRESSIVE STATES

The relationship between anxiety and depression is reflected in the high correlation between anxiety and depression rating scales (Mendels, Weinstein, and Cochrance, 1972) and is sanctioned in the hybrid nosologic concept of "anxious depression" in the psychopharmacologic literature (Overall et al., 1966). Anxiety symptoms are often reported by depressed patients, and depression, often of syndromal depth, commonly complicates anxiety disorders. Distinguishing between these two alternatives on strictly clinical grounds can prove difficult, but differential pharmacologic responsiveness argues for the importance of this effort (Ayd, 1980). Although some anxiety states respond to imipramine-type drugs, and monoamine oxidase inhibitors (MAOIs) may be useful in both types of disorders, sedatives and standard anxiolytic agents not only fail to ameliorate primary depressive states but often make them worse. Further, the "wrong" prescription may also supply the depressed patient with a lethal dose of sedative-hypnotics (Murphy, 1975).

Roth and Mountjoy (1982) have recently summarized the differentiating clinical characteristics of depressive and anxiety disorders. These include such traditional clinical indices as early morning awakening, self-denigration, psychomotor retardation, feelings of hopelessness, and suicidal tendencies in depression, and somatic tension, panic attacks, and compulsions in anxiety disorders. Such differences tend to acquire greater prominence on long-term follow-up: Depressives tend to remit, whereas many patients with anxiety disorders continue to exhibit marked tension, phobias, panic attacks, vasomotor instability, derealization, perceptual distortions, transient paranoid and hypochondriacal ideas, histrionic behavior, and aggressive outbursts. However, such contrasts in symptom profiles, though differentiating the two groups of disorders at a statistically significant level, may not be of great help in individual cases. Further, family history and twin data, which have given rise to conflicting results, have failed to resolve the differential diagnostic dilemma (Noyes et al., 1978; Cloninger et al., 1981; Curtis, Cameron, and Nesse, 1982; Crowe et al., 1983; Leckman et al., 1983; Torgerson, 1983; Van Valkenburg et al., 1983).

More persuasive evidence for sharpening the boundaries between depressive

Table 3.2. *Proposed classification of major affective disorders*

I. *Clinical depression* (sustained for at least four weeks, although shorter duration may suffice if typical features develop acutely); it is useful to distinguish among three varieties:

   A. *Symptomatic depression* – induced by medical disease; recurrences unlikely

   B. *(Major) depressive disorder* – "naturally" occurring; single episode, recurrent, or chronic

   C. *Melancholia* – autonomous and anhedonic, with marked vegetative and psychomotor disturbance; may be of psychotic proportions, including occasional mood-incongruent hallucinations and delusions; melancholic depressions can be further subdivided into unipolar and bipolar subtypes:

      1. *Unipolar I* – no bipolar family history, and no personal history for hypomanic and manic episodes; onset usually after age 30; psychomotor agitation is common; tendency for chronicity

      2. *Unipolar II* (or *bipolar III*) – family history for bipolar disorder; activation of hypomania by pharmacologic challenge only; onset is commonly in teens, 20s, and 30s; psychomotor retardation is characteristic; typically recurrent; may be precursor of bipolar II or I

      3. *Bipolar II* – adaptive hypomanic episodes of spontaneous occurrence in addition to depressive episodes; typically recurrent

      4. *Bipolar I* – at least one episode of mania; typically recurrent

II. *Clinical hypomania and manic psychoses* (sustained for at least two weeks, although shorter duration will suffice if typical symptoms develop more acutely); two subtypes can be recognized:

   A. *Recurrent mania* – notoriously noncompliant to lithium treatment; chronicity common; may progress to bipolar I

   B. *Symptomatic mania*[a] – induced by medical disease; recurrence unlikely

---

[a]Concept discussed by Krauthammer and Klerman (1978) and Akiskal (1983a).

and anxiety states has recently come from laboratory investigations. Two studies have recently shown that REM latency is shortened (and REM percentage increased) in primary depressive illness, whereas the numbers of awakenings and stage shifts are significantly higher in anxiety states (Reynolds et al., 1983; Akiskal et al., 1984). Furthermore, our laboratory (Akiskal et al., 1984) has shown that the anxiety group has tremendous variability in sleep measures from night to night, whereas primary depressives tend to maintain the same degree of disturbance across nights, suggesting autonomy from the sleep-laboratory environment.

Another study from our program (Van Valkenburg et al., 1983) comparing various groups of anxious and depressed subjects has suggested that depressive states occurring in the setting of a preexisting anxiety disorder – whether dysthymic or of major syndromal severity – are perhaps best viewed as part of the symptomatic picture of the anxiety disorder. Other research (Dube et al., 1985) has shown that arecoline REM induction does not occur in these mixed anxious-depressed patients, in contrast to the situation for primary major depressives. Furthermore, these "depressives" may not respond to tricyclic antidepressants (Sheehan, Ballenger, and Jacobson, 1981; Zitrin, Woerner, and Klein, 1981), even after the panic disorder is controlled, suggesting that they may reflect long-term complications of an incapacitating, demoralizing, and longstanding neurotic illness. It is widely believed – although not by all investigators – that MAOIs are more useful in alleviating these admixtures of anxiety and depression (Quitkin, Rifkin, and Klein, 1979; Tyrer, 1979; Nies and Robinson, 1982). However clinical experience testifies to the fact that unmistakable melancholias – even bipolar episodes – may, on occasion, complicate the course of an anxiety disorder; such an illness, if of psychotic proportions, may require the use of electroconvulsive therapy.

To summarize, there are some biological differences between depressive and anxiety states that support the view that these are distinct entities. However, considerable symptomatologic and familial overlap exists, reflected in the clinical colloquialism "anxious depression." The value of this rubric may be prognostic (i.e., the coexistence of the two disorders produces an unfavorable outcome) (Van Valkenburg et al., 1983). The implications of these findings for *DSM-III* revisions are not entirely clear. Although it has been proposed that when panic disorders and major depression coexist, both conditions should be diagnosed (Curtis et al., 1982; Torgerson, 1983; Van Valkenburg et al., 1983), it is possible that this joint clinical picture – except in elderly subjects – may simply indicate a more severe variant of panic disorder. In the British literature (West and Dally, 1959; Sargent, 1962; Tyrer, 1979; Nies and Robinson, 1982), and more recently in work by Klein's group (Quitkin et al., 1983), anxious depressions are subsumed under the rubric of "atypical depression" (used in a different sense from that in *DSM-III*). My preference, based on the evidence reviewed here, would be to subsume them under atypical anxiety disorder.

DISTINCTION BETWEEN PERSONALITY AND AFFECTIVE DISORDERS

Affective symptoms, as well as full-blown episodes, not uncommonly complicate the courses of patients with conditions variously referred to as passive-aggressive, dependent, histrionic, emotionally unstable, and borderline personalities. This area represents another controversial boundary of affective disorder.

As conceptualized elsewhere, personality disorders may predispose to, modify the clinical expression of, or result from mood disorders (Akiskal, Hirschfeld, and Yerevania, 1983). *DSM-III* has taken the "atheoretical" position that personality disorders and illness can coexist in an orthogonal fashion without necessarily having a causal relationship; hence the decision to record them on separate axes.

Psychoanalytic theory has long considered the personality disorder to be the "real" illness; affective breakdowns are regarded merely as symptomatic phases. The Kraepelinian position, which postulates hypomanic, cyclothymic, irritable, and depressive temperaments as representing the premorbid and intermorbid substrates of affective psychoses, tends to concur. Yet clinical lore views affective disorders as episodic and personality disorders as chronic (indeed, "chronic" is often used synonymously with "characterologic"). This may be due to an overinterpretation of Kraepelin's description of affective disorders as remitting disorders; Kraepelin was referring to the remission of psychotic episodes, not the temperamental foundations of the disorder that often persist between episodes (Kraepelin, 1921).

The intermittent chronicity and characterologic "masks" of cyclothymia led to it being classified in the personality section of *DSM-II* (American Psychiatric Association, 1968), obscuring its relationship to major affective episodes. Cyclothymics often present to mental health facilities with such disturbances as episodic promiscuous behavior, repeated conjugal failure, an uneven work or school record, dilettantism, alcohol and drug abuse, and geographic instability (Akiskal et al., 1977). The possibility that these features could be secondary to mild but chronic bipolar illness has been supported by the readiness with which hypomanic responses can be elicited in such patients by tricyclic antidepressants, the occurrence of more classic affective episodes during prospective follow-up, and the familial loading for bipolar illness. Accordingly, *DSM-III* has reclassified cyclothymic disorder under the affective disorders section.

The central feature of cyclothymia is its biphasic course, (i.e., mini–depressive episodes alternating with hypomania) (Akiskal et al., 1979a). Predominantly depressed forms of cyclothymia are the most common forms in psychiatric settings. By contrast (as discussed later), a predominantly hyperthymic form is rare in psychiatric settings (less than 10% in our series). Depue and associates (1981), who incorporated many of the clinical features described in the Tennessee studies into a self-report inventory to identify a noncase (college student) population of cyclothymics, concurred on the relative incidences of subtypes. Although only 13% of the 126 subjects studied had received outpatient treatment for psychiatric reasons, histories in the group as a whole had been complicated by interpersonal, academic, and civic disturbances as the subjects had entered early adulthood. About a third of the sample had a bipolar family history, again comparable to the proportion in the Tennessee studies. In brief, the study of Depue and associates extended the Tennessee findings to nonclinical subjects who were 10 years younger and who had accumulated psychosocial liabilities as they had moved from adolescence to adulthood. These findings underscore the importance of criteria that set cyclothymia apart from overlapping axis II conditions.

The *DSM-III* criteria could be sharpened even more to distinguish cyclothymia from character disorder (Table 3.3). It would first be necessary to specify criteria that would set the stage for identifying an early-onset subsyndromal disorder (we have seen no onsets after age 15 years) with short cycles fluctuating over a lifetime and with little discernible relationship to psychosocial antece-

Table 3.3. *Modified criteria for cyclothymic disorder*

I. *General*
    A. Onset typically in teens; cardinal manifestations obvious before age 25
    B. Disorder is probably lifelong and, for definite diagnosis, should have lasted for a minimum of two years in adults (one year in children and adolescents)

II. *Signs and symptoms*
    A. Short cycles (days), which are recurrent in an irregular fashion, with infrequent euthymic periods
    B. May not attain full syndrome for depressive and hypomanic phases during any one cycle, but entire range of affective manifestations occurs at various times
    C. Abrupt and unpredictable change, from one phase to another, often unrelated to external circumstances
    D. Biphasic manifestations
        (a) Subjective manifestations
            1. Lethargy alternating with eutonia
            2. Pessimism and brooding alternating with optimism and carefree attitudes
            3. Mental confusion alternating with sharpened and creative thinking
            4. Shaky self-esteem alternating between low self-confidence and grandiose overconfidence
        (b) Behavioral manifestations (carry greater diagnostic weight)
            1. Hypersomnia alternating with decreased need for sleep
            2. Introverted self-absorption alternating with uninhibited people-seeking
            3. Decreased verbal output alternating with talkativeness
            4. Unexplained tearfulness alternating with excessive punning and jocularity
            5. Marked unevenness in quantity and quality of productivity, often associated with unusual working hours

III. *Exclusion criteria:* not explained by alternating abuse of stimulants and depressant drugs

---

dents. Next, it would be necessary to give greatest weight to those biphasic manifestations – criteria under D(b) in Table 3.3 – that have a reasonable chance of being directly observed by the clinician or verified by significant others (Akiskal et al., 1979a).

In subaffective dysthymic disorder, hypomanic periods are even more subtle than in cyclothymia and may not be evident unless pharmacologically mobilized (Akiskal, 1983d). ["Subaffective" in this context is used to convey the meaning of the attenuated temperamental form of primary mood disorder (Akiskal, 1983c).] I have elsewhere detailed suggestions for identifying such a disorder within the broader *DSM-III* category of dysthymia (Akiskal, 1983d). Prospective work in our clinic has shown that the offspring of bipolars may manifest such a pattern as early as late childhood (Akiskal et al., 1985b). The course fluctuates over many years, but the patient is rarely free of depressive manifestations for more than a few weeks at a time. Although the symptom profile is subsyndromal, the full range of depressive symptoms occurs at various times, and may even crystallize into short superimposed syndromal episodes; this pattern has been described as "double depression" by other investigators (Keller et al., 1983). Hypersomnia was present in 60% of the probands we studied. Most of our patients were habitually introverted, with brief periods of extraversion sometimes seen in relatively "euthymic" periods; this tendency was further activated into transient hypomanic episodes when patients were given secondary amine tricyclics (Akiskal et al., 1980). As expected, up to 30% of these dysthymic patients had a bipolar familial background (Rosenthal et al., 1981). Brief extraversion was also noted by Liebowitz and Klein (1979) in their description of hysteroid dysphoric patients, who apparently can also be pushed into hypomania by MAOI therapy. However, unlike the more "volatile" hysteroid dysphoric group, the dysthymics we studied conformed to the masochistic-depressive personality. Indeed, they exhibited many of the Schneiderian depressive personality traits (Schneider, 1958), and unfounded lowering of self-esteem was one of the hallmarks of the disorder. To summarize, the description given herein applies to temperamental dysthymias that, like cyclothymia, represent formes frustes of primary affective illness (Akiskal, 1983c) and exclude the residual chronic phase of an adult-onset major depressive disorder, as well as nonspecific dysphorias that are part of the clinical picture of incapacitating nonaffective disorders (Akiskal, 1983d).

Current *DSM-III* criteria for dysthymia identify a large universe of low-grade dysphoric manifestations common to many psychiatric disorders. The residual chronic phase of a major depressive disorder does not deserve separate nosologic status distinct from major depressive disorder, unless preceded by dysthymic manifestations. These chronic residuals are best conceptualized as extensions of the very processes – genetic, psychologic, or neurophysiologic – that underlie unipolar illness (Akiskal, 1982b). When major unipolar depression does not fully remit within two years (a common occurrence in late-onset illness), the qualifying phrase "residual chronic" is appropriate. Furthermore, in approaching the diagnosis of dysthymia as a distinct affective disorder, the exclusionary clause in *DSM-III* to the effect that the dysthymic disposition "by virtue of its intensity or effect on functioning, can be clearly distinguished from the individual's usual mood" should be more fully qualified. To paraphrase Aubrey Lewis (1936), most severe neurotic disorders – and many other incapacitating psychiatric disorders – are depressing. Such manifestations as fluctuating dysphoric symptoms, lowered self-esteem, feelings of hopelessness, suicidal ideas, fatigue, and decreased interest are part of the clinical picture in many nonaffective disorders. In brief, to diagnose a primary dysthymic disorder distinct from the large universe of chronic neurotic abnormalities, it is necessary to require that dysthymic manifestations not be explainable by another major nonaffective disorder. (One possible exception is substance abuse, which may complicate the early course of dysthymia.) Low-grade dysphoric manifestations are also commonplace in histrionic, sociopathic, schizotypal, and related "primitive" personality disorders. These "depressions" are unrelated to primary mood disorders and rarely progress to major episodes (Akiskal et al., 1980, Reveley and Reveley, 1981). Hence the proposal to limit the nosologic territory of dysthymia to introverted individuals with unfounded lowering of self-esteem (Akiskal, 1983d) who fit Schneider's description of the depressive personality, as operationally defined in our Clinical Data Questionnaire on Affective Disorders (Akiskal et al., 1979a). This description, summarized in Table 3.4, represents a minor modification of recently published criteria (Akiskal, 1983d).

There exists another form of affective temperament whose differentiation from personality disorders is problematic – hyperthymic disorder. Hyperthymic subjects – who are overrepresented among successful professionals and businessmen – are rarely seen in psychiatric practice unless manic episodes supervene. They are more likely to be encountered in sleep-disorder clinics, where they may seek help because of insomnia (Akiskal, 1982c). This may explain why such a disorder was not included in *DSM-III*. Our experience in a sleep-disorder center (Akiskal, 1984) has suggested the usefulness of recognizing such a category (Table 3.5). In the diagnostic approach to hyperthymia, it is important to emphasize that cheerfulness is not invariable and that irritable or labile moods are common. Decreased need for sleep is often a lifetime trait (and perhaps a hallmark of the disorder); yet, during rare depressive dips, hypersomnia of a few days' duration may occur. Finally, it is necessary to ensure that the clinical picture is not due to another condition like stimulant abuse or adult-attention-deficit disorder.

As proposed elsewhere, hyperthymic, cyclothymic, and dysthymic temperaments appear to lie on a familial-genetic continuum (Akiskal, 1983a). This conclusion was based on the bipolar familial history in all three groups and considerations of courses. Hypomania occurs spontaneously in hyperthymic and cyclothymic groups, but usually requires pharmacologic challenge in the dysthymic group. Furthermore, recent sleep polygraphic data suggest that a common neurophysiologic abnormality – shortened REM latency – underlies phenomenologically "opposite" manifestations like hyperthymia and dysthymia (Akiskal, 1984).

Many patients with hyperthymic, dysthymic, cyclothymic, and bipolar II disorders as defined in this chapter will also meet the criteria for borderline personality. A discussion of the validity of this controversial *DSM-III* axis II term is beyond the scope of the present review (see Chapter 17). However, a common thrust in the current literature is that some borderline personalities may actually represent borderline manic-depressive psychosis (Stone, 1980; Akiskal, 1981). Findings with DST, REM latency, and TSH blunting following TRH administration have also supported this affinity with affective disorder (Akiskal, 1981; Carroll et al., 1981; Garbutt et al., 1983). The borderline rubric, as defined in *DSM-III*, may be more a reflection of clinicians' need to label highly unstable patients with complicated diagnoses than a reflection of a specific nosologic

Table 3.4. *Dysthymia conceived as a subaffective disorder*

I. *General*
  A. Indeterminate onset in childhood or teens; cardinal manifestations obvious before 25 years
  B. Fluctuating course over at least two years (one year in children and adolescents), but typically not free of depressive manifestations for more than a few weeks at a time

II. *Signs and symptoms*
  A. Habitually subsyndromal, although the full range of depressive symptoms may occur at various times
  B. At least two of the following:
    1. Psychomotor inertia
    2. Hypersomnia
    3. Anhedonia
    4. Diurnal variation (worse in morning)

III. *Personality attributes*
  A. Unfounded lowering of self-esteem
  B. Habitual introversion, with brief periods of extraversion sometimes seen during relatively "well" periods
  C. Presence of a minimum of five of Schneider's depressive personality traits:
    1. Gloomy, pessimistic, humorless or incapable of fun
    2. Quiet, passive, and indecisive
    3. Skeptical, hypercritical, or complaining
    4. Brooding and given to worry
    5. Conscientious or self-disciplining
    6. Self-critical, self-reproaching, and self-derogatory
    7. Preoccupied with inadequacy, failure, and negative events to the point of morbid enjoyment of one's failures

IV. *Exclusion criteria:* clinical picture not explained by another major nonaffective disorder such as obsessive–compulsive disorder, agoraphobia, somatization disorder, anorexia nervosa, transsexualism, or schizophrenia

---

entity. It appears to be the final common pathway of many conditions – high-episode-frequency affective, polysymptomatic neurotic, histrionic, and minimal brain damage – all of which preclude the development of a coherent sense of self (Akiskal et al., 1985a). Hence, as sanctioned by Kernberg's usage of the term, it is most appropriately reserved for an intermediate stage of ego development between neurosis and psychosis, rather than being a discrete axis II personality type (Kernberg, 1976).

A final boundary question to be considered involves depressive disorders with somatic presentations, which are often confused with histrionic personalities, especially those with somatization disorder. A recent study in our sleep laboratory has shown that the criterion of shortened REM latency can successfully

Table 3.5. *Toward a definition of hyperthymic disorder*

I. *General*
  A. Onset before age 25
  B. Disorder is probably lifelong and, for a definite diagnosis, should have lasted for a minimum of two years in adults (one year in children and adolescents)

II. *Signs and symptoms*
  A. Hypomanic subsyndromal features on an intermittent basis with rare periods of euthymia (not lasting more than a few weeks at a time)
  B. Habitually short sleeper, although occasional periods of hypersomnia may supervene
  C. Although depression is rarely admitted, irritability and labile mood are common features

III. *Personality attributes:* at least five of the following Schneiderian hyperthymic traits:
  1. Cheerful, overoptimistic, or exuberant
  2. Naive, overconfident, self-assured, boastful, bombastic, or grandiose
  3. Vigorous, full of plans, improvident, rushing off with restless impulse
  4. Overtalkative
  5. Warm, people-seeking, or extroverted
  6. Overinvolved and meddlesome
  7. Uninhibited, stimulus-seeking, or promiscuous

IV. *Exclusion criteria:* not explained by stimulant abuse or residual attention-deficit disorder

separate the two disorders (Akiskal, 1982d). Such depressives, who often deny subjective depressive symptoms and may even exhibit the "conversion V" on the MMPI, are at high risk for being labeled "crocks" or "hypochondriacs." These so-called masked depressions, which tend to pursue intermittent or chronic courses, are commonly seen in primary-care medical settings and are among the more prevalent forms of affective disorders in the community. Whereas some will admit to irritability and loss of interest, others vehemently deny any subjective mood change. As a result, they would be excluded from *DSM-III*-defined major depression. The requirement of dysphoric mood change and/or loss of interest (criterion A for major depression) has thus created the untenable situation of relegating one of the most common forms of depressive illness into the "atypical" depressive category.

To conclude, certain types of personality disturbances either are attenuated expressions of mood disorders or are secondary to high-episode-frequency illness that prevents optimum ego maturation. The clinician should generally refrain from making a characterologic diagnosis during the delicate recovery phase of an affective episode, when transient interpersonal maladjustments are commonly seen. Postdepressive personality complications – which may at times reflect accentuation of premorbid traits – are most frequent in the course of recurrent affective disorders (Cassano, Maggini, and Akiskal, 1983). When prominent and persistent, these disturbances can be coded on an orthogonal axis, distinct from the affective axis. However, this double coding – intended to bring therapeutic attention to the personality disturbances seen in high-episode-frequency primary mood disorders – should not obscure the fact that the observed personality disturbances represent affective manifestations as much as do changes in mood and derangements in the somatic, psychomotor, or cognitive sphere (Akiskal, 1984).

DISTINCTION BETWEEN AFFECTIVE AND SCHIZOPHRENIC PSYCHOSES

Differentiation of affective and schizophrenic disorders is the prototype of a boundary dispute in psychiatry. Because this topic has been extensively reviewed elsewhere (Akiskal, 1983a,b; Akiskal and Puzantian, 1979), only major nosologic issues will be highlighted here.

Although there are lingering doubts about Kraepelin's two-entities model, the thrust of evidence has generally supported the distinction between affective and schizophrenic psychoses:

1. They are genetically discriminable in that schizophrenia is not seen in twin pairs discordant for affective disorders, and vice versa (Coryell and Winokur, 1980).
2. Lithium alone is generally of little therapeutic help in schizophrenic disorders (Dunner and Fieve, 1978), and when treated with neuroleptics, the affectively ill appear to be at higher risk for tardive dyskinesia (Baldessarini et al., 1980).
3. Measures of REM latency, the DST, and the TSH response to TRH are rarely, if ever, positive in schizophrenic disorders, but are often so in the affective psychoses, including those formerly classified under schizoaffective states (Kupfer et al., 1979, 1980; Schlesser, Winokur, and Rush, 1981; Extein et al., 1982).
4. MHPG is lowered in many bipolar, psychotic, and "schizoaffective" depressives, but not in schizophrenia (Schildkraut et al., 1978).

It does not appear that many "schizoaffectives," especially those with bipolar courses (Clayton et al., 1981), belong in the group of affective disorders. Furthermore, current evidence indicates that the presence of occasional Schneiderian signs does not justify a schizophrenic diagnosis, nor do the two major Bleulerian A's (associative slippage and blunted affect), unless present on repeated examinations (Andreasen and Akiskal, 1983). Indeed, the cross-sectional mental status of a psychotic episode seems less important than its longitudinal course (e.g., bipolarity) in differential diagnosis. Although recent work has reaffirmed what had long been known about the frequency of minor depressive states occurring in the setting of well-established schizophrenic disorders: Their existence is best explained as a neuroleptic side effect or existential demoralization in intelligent schizophrenic subjects rather than as a separate schizoaffective entity, as reviewed elsewhere (Akiskal, 1983a).

The *DSM-III* classification of the affective, schizophrenic, and schizoaffective psychoses was based in part on the massive review undertaken by Pope and Lipinski (1978), which concluded that "traditional" schizophrenic symptoms were of little diagnostic value. As a result, the *DSM-III* concepts of these disorders are largely polythetic – relying more on symptom clusters over time than on detailed phenomenologic study of individual symptoms. This approach tends to disregard the contributions of such authorities as Jaspers (1950), Fish (Hamilton, 1974), and Wing, Cooper, and Sartorius (1974), who attempted to lay down phenomenologic rules for faithful description of the subjective experiences of psychotic patients. The late Vahe Puzantian (who had studied under Frank Fish in Edinburgh) and I have elsewhere elaborated on these phenomenologic principles (Akiskal and Puzantian, 1979). The most important implication of these principles for the proposed revision of *DSM-III* concerns situations in which an affective psychosis may develop mood-incongruent perceptual and thinking disturbances. Examples include such premorbid features as introverted personality and mental retardation, concurrent medical disease and substance abuse, mixed states, and subcultural factors. A more detailed analysis of these factors can be found in our original report (Akiskal and Puzantian, 1979). In that report we concluded that the diagnosis of schizoaffective disorder should not be contemplated unless such processes as could account for mood incongruence were first excluded by phenomenologic analysis.

In summary, only when one excludes the depressive states occurring in well-established schizophrenic disorders and "explainable" mood incongruence occurring in the setting of a bipolar affective psychosis can one legitimately enter the territory of the schizoaffective psychoses. Suggested operational criteria, modified from a previous proposal (Akiskal, 1983a), are provided in Table 3.6.

RELATIVE INCIDENCES OF PROPOSED *DSM-III* AFFECTIVE SUBTYPES

Table 3.7 lists the diagnoses of 200 subjects, randomly selected and followed up for a minimum of six months, who had sought help in a community mental health center; these diagnoses, representing the dominant and often the chronologically primary disorder, were made according to the principles outlined in this chapter for resolving boundary questions in affective disorders. Perhaps the most striking finding is that when the threshold for major depression is set rigorously, unipolar and bipolar depressions will have equal rates, very much like the findings in the Amish study (Egeland, 1983). Within the bipolar group, types I and II also have equal rates, indicating that so-called atypical bipolars are, at least from a statistical point of view, as much the norm as the "classic" forms. Finally, dysthymic and schizoaffective disorders – when appropriate exclusions are made – emerge as uncommon disorders.

Table 3.6. *Proposed criteria for schizoaffective disorder*

A. *Exclusion criteria*
  1. Depression in the setting of a well-established schizophrenic illness
  2. Mood-incongruent psychotic features in an affective disorder that can be accounted for by certain premorbid and concurrent conditions known to produce such features
  3. Mixed states with bipolar course

B. *Inclusion criteria*
  1. Acute onset
  2. Confusion and disorientation
  3. Schizophrenic and affective symptoms are apparent at the onset of psychosis
  4. Affective and schizophrenic syndromes coexist during each episode
  5. Remitting course

Table 3.7. *Affective disorders and "bordering" conditions in a random sample of adult (>18 years) referrals to a community mental health center (N = 200) followed prospectively for a minimum of six months*

Diagnosis	N	Diagnosis	N
Bipolar disorder (B-I)	12	Multiple personality	1
Atypical bipolar disorder (B-II)	12	Histrionic personality[a]	3
Cyclothymia	3	Antisocial personality[a]	11
Dysthymia (Akiskal criteria)	4	Borderline personality[a]	3
Unipolar II (B-III)	4	Brief reactive psychosis	1
Major depression (Feighner)	30	Schizoaffective disorder	1
Symptomatic depression	1	Schizophreniform disorder	2
Adjustment disorder	36	Schizophrenia	9
Generalized anxiety disorder	3	Paranoia	1
Panic disorder, uncomplicated	5	Alcohol abuse/dependence	15
Panic disorder with agoraphobia	4	Drug abuse/dependence	5
Obsessive–compulsive disorder	1	Alcohol & drug abuse/dependence	4
Ego-dystonic homosexuality	6	Alcohol/drug psychosis	2
Inhibited sexual excitement		Attention deficit, residual	1
(impotence)	2	Mental retardation	2
Psychogenic pain disorder	2	Dementia	2
Somatization disorder	4	Undiagnosed	5
Factitious disorder, psychological	1	No mental disorder	2

[a]No axis I diagnosis.

SUMMARY

It is apparent from the foregoing presentation that the manifestations of mood disorders are multifaceted and interface with the "blues," bereavement reactions, anxiety states, personality disorders, and schizophrenia. Another boundary area, not discussed in this chapter, is represented by dementiform or pseudodemented depressions, where cognitive impairment raises questions of differential diagnosis from true dementia. These considerations suggest that the manifestations of affective disease embrace a wide range of disturbances in the somatic, psychomotor, emotional, cognitive, and characterologic spheres. It is for this reason that boundary questions often arise between affective and other psychiatric conditions. The challenge for future research is to determine why different subtypes of mood disorders manifest different mixtures of disturbances in each of these areas. A diagnostic manual, if it is to be used by clinicians, must do justice to the heterogeneity of affective conditions seen in clinical practice and must provide faithful descriptions of individual subtypes.

As we near *DSM-IV*, emerging biological markers may enhance the predictive and construct validity of phenomenologically defined affective subtypes and aid in distinguishing them from bordering conditions (Akiskal and Webb, 1978).

REFERENCES

Akiskal HS: The joint use of clinical and biological criteria for psychiatric diagnosis, I: a historical and methodological review, in Psychiatric Diagnosis: Exploration of Biological Predictors. Edited by Akiskal HS, Webb WL. New York, Spectrum, 1978, pp 103–132

External validating criteria for psychiatric diagnosis: their application in affective disorders. J Clin Psychiatry 41:6–14, 1980

Subaffective disorders: dysthymic, cyclothymic, and bipolar II disorders in the "borderline" realm. Psychiatr Clin North Am 4:25–46, 1981

Affective disorders, in Merck Manual of Diagnosis and Therapy, Fourteenth edition. Edited by Berkow R. Rahway, NJ, Merck Sharp and Dohme Research Laboratories, 1982a, pp 1448–1462

Factors associated with incomplete recovery in primary depressive illness. J Clin Psychiatry 43:266–271, 1982b

Hypomanic personality: clinical and sleep EEG study. Presented at annual meeting of the American Psychiatric Association, Toronto, Canada, May 1982c

Masked depression: a variant of melancholia. Presented at Society of Biological Psychiatry annual convention, Toronto, May 1982d

The bipolar spectrum: new concepts in classification and diagnosis, in Psychiatry Update: The American Psychiatric Association Annual Review, Vol II. Edited by Grinspoon L. Washington, DC, APA, 1983a, pp 271–292

Diagnosis and classification of affective disorders: new insights from clinical and laboratory approaches. Psychiatr Dev 1:123–160, 1983b

Dysthymic and cyclothymic disorders: a paradigm for high-risk research in psychiatry, in The Affective Disorders. Edited by Davis JM, Maas JW. Washington, DC, American Psychiatric Press, 1983c, pp 211–231

Dysthymic disorder: psychopathology of proposed chronic depressive subtypes. Am J Psychiatry 140:11–20, 1983d

Characterologic manifestations of affective disorders: toward a new conceptualization. Integrat Psychiatry 2:83–88, 1984

Akiskal HS, Cassano GB: The impact of therapeutic advances in widening the nosologic boundaries of affective disorders: clinical and research implications. Pharmacopsychiatry 16:111–118, 1983

Akiskal HS, Chen SE, Davis GC, et al: Borderline: an adjective in search of a noun. J Clin Psychiatry 46:41–48, 1985a

Akiskal HS, Djenderedjian AH, Rosenthal RH, et al: Cyclothymic disorder: validating criteria for inclusion in the bipolar affective group. Am J Psychiatry 134:1227–1233, 1977

Akiskal HS, Downs J, Jordan P, et al: Affective disorders in the referred children and younger siblings of manic-depressives: mode of onset and prospective course. Arch Gen Psychiatry 42:996–1003, 1985b

Akiskal HS, Hirschfeld RMA, Yerevanian BI: The relationship of personality to affective disorders: a critical review. Arch Gen Psychiatry 40:801–810, 1983a

Akiskal HS, Khani MK, Scott-Strauss A: Cyclothymic temperamental disorders. Psychiatr Clin North Am 2:527–554, 1979a

Akiskal HS, Lemmi H: Clinical, neuroendocrine, and sleep EEG diagnosis of "unusual" affective presentations: a practical review. Psychiatr Clin North Am 6:175–192, 1983

Akiskal HS, Lemmi H, Dickson H, et al: Chronic depressions, part 2: sleep EEG differentiation of primary dysthymic disorders from anxious depressions. J Affect Dis 6:287–295, 1984

Akiskal HS, Puzantian VR: Psychotic forms of depression and mania. Psychiatr Clin North Am 2:419–439, 1979

Akiskal HS, Rosenthal RH, Rosenthal TL, et al: Differentiation of primary affective illness from situational, symptomatic and secondary depressions. Arch Gen Psychiatry 36:635–643, 1979b

Akiskal HS, Rosenthal TL, Haykal RF, et al: Characterological depressions: clinical and sleep EEG findings separating "subaffective dysthymias" from "character-spectrum" disorders. Arch Gen Psychiatry 37:777–783, 1980

Akiskal HS, Tashjian R: Affective disorders, part II: recent advances in laboratory and pathogenetic approaches. Hosp Community Psychiatry 34:822–830, 1983

Akiskal HS, Walker PW, Puzantian VR, et al: Bipolar outcome in the course of depressive illness: phenomenologic, familial and pharmacologic predictors. J Affect Dis 5:115–128, 1983b

Akiskal HS, Webb WL: Affective disorders, part I: recent advances in clinical conceptualization. Hosp Community Psychiatry 34:695–702, 1983

(eds): Psychiatric Diagnosis: Exploration of Biological Predictors. New York, Spectrum, 1978

American Psychiatric Association: Diagnostic and Statistical Manual of Mental Disorders, second edition. Washington, DC, APA, 1968

Diagnostic and Statistical Manual of Mental Disorders, third edition. Washington, DC, APA, 1980

Andreasen NC, Akiskal HS: The specificity of Bleulerian and Schneiderian symptoms: a critical re-evaluation. Psychiatr Clin North Am 6:41–54, 1983

Ayd FJ: Is it anxiety or depression? A crucial differential diagnosis, in Clinical Depressions: Diagnostic and Therapeutic Challenges. Edited by Ayd FJ. Baltimore, Ayd Medical Communications, 1980, pp 33–46

Baldessarini RJ, Cole JO, Davis JM, et al: Tardive dyskinesia. Task Force report 18. Washington, DC, American Psychiatric Association, 1980

Barrett J: Psychiatric diagnosis (research criteria) in symptomatic volunteers. Arch Gen Psychiatry 38:153–157, 1981

Barrett J, Hurst MW, Di Salla C, et al: Prevalence of depression over a 12-month period in a nonpatient population. Arch Gen Psychiatry 35:741–744, 1978

Blumenthal MD, Dielman TE: Depressive symptomatology and role function in a general population. Arch Gen Psychiatry 32:958–991, 1975

Carroll BJ, Greden JF, Feinberg M, et al: Neuroendocrine evaluation of depression in borderline patients. Psychiatr Clin North Am 4:89–99, 1981

Cartwright R, Stephen L, Trenholm I: Dream differences during divorce and after in moderately and highly depressed women. Presented at the 22nd annual meeting of the Association for the Psychophysiological Study of Sleep, San Antonio, Texas, June 1982

Cassano GB, Akiskal HS: Work and leisure in depressive illness: significance for the practitioner, in Common Errors in Managing Depression [German]. Edited by Kielholz P. Bern, Hans Huber, 1984, pp 59–69

Cassano GB, Castrogiovanni P, Ghiozzi M, et al: Standard assessment of social and environmental data by means of a self-administered questionnaire [in Italian]. Presented at the 23rd Congresso Nazionale della Societa Italiana di Psichiatria, Napoli, Italy, October 29 to November 2, 1977

Cassano GB, Maggini C, Akiskal HS: Short-term subchronic and chronic sequelae of affective disorders. Psychiatr Clin North Am 6:55–67, 1983

Clayton P, Endicott J, Coughan J, Rice J: Schizoaffective disorders divided by polarity. Presented at the III World Congress of Biological Psychiatry, Stockholm, Sweden, June 1981

Clayton PJ, Herjanic M, Murphy GE, et al: Mourning and depression: their similarities and differences. J Can Psychiatr Assoc 19:309–312, 1974

Cloninger CR, Martin RL, Clayton P, et al: A blind follow-up and family study of anxiety neurosis: preliminary analysis of the St. Louis 500, in Anxiety: New Research and Changing Concepts. Edited by Klein DF, Rabkin JG. New York, Raven Press, 1981, pp 137–154

Coryell W, Winokur G: Diagnosis, family and follow-up studies, in Mania: An Evolving Concept. Edited by Belmaker RH, Van Praag HM. New York, Spectrum, 1980

Coryell W, Winokur G, Andreasen NC: Effect of case definition on affective disorder rates. Am J Psychiatry 138:1106–1109, 1981

Crowe RR, Noyes R, Pauls DL, et al: A family study of panic disorders. Arch Gen Psychiatry 40:1065–1069, 1983

Curtis GC, Cameron OG, Nesse RM: The dexamethasone suppression test in panic disorder and agoraphobia. Am J Psychiatry 139:143–146, 1982

Depue RA, Slater JF, Welfstetter-Kausch H, et al: A behavioral paradigm for identifying persons at risk for bipolar depressive disorders: A conceptual framework and five validation studies. J Abnorm Psychol [Suppl 90], 1981, pp 381–438

Dube S, Kumar N, Ettedgui E, et al: Cholinergic REM induction response: separation of anxiety and depression. Biol Psychiatry 20:408–418, 1985

Dunner DL: Sub-types of bipolar affective disorder with particular regard to bipolar II. Psychiatr Dev 1:75–85, 1983

Dunner DL, Fieve RL: The lithium ion: its impact on diagnostic practice, in Psychiatric Diagnosis: Exploration of Biological Predictors. Edited by Akiskal HS, Webb WL. New York, Spectrum 1978, pp 233–246

Egeland JA: Bipolarity: the iceberg of affective disorders. Compr Psychiatry 24:337–344, 1983

Extein I, Pottash ALC, Gold MS, et al: Using the protirelin test to distinguish mania from schizophrenia. Arch Gen Psychiatry 39:77–81, 1982

Feighner JP, Robins E, Guze SB, et al: Diagnostic criteria for use in psychiatric research. Arch Gen Psychiatry 26:57–63, 1972

Fieve RR, Dunner DL: Unipolar and bipolar affective states, in The Nature and Treatment of Depression. Edited by Flach FF, Draghi SC. New York, Wiley, 1975, pp 145–166

Garbutt JC, Lossen PT, Tipermas A, et al: The TRH test in patients with borderline personality disorders. Psychiatr Res 9:107–113, 1983

Goodwin F, Bunney WE Jr: Depression following reserpine, a re-evaluation. Semin Psychiatry 3:435–448, 1971

Grof P: Continuation and maintenance antidepressant drug treatment, in Clinical Depressions: Diagnostic and Therapeutic Challenges. Edited by Ayd F. Baltimore, Ayd Medical Communications, 1980, pp 132–144

Hamilton M (ed): Fish's Clinical Psychopathology. Bristol, John Wright & Sons, 1974

Hogarty GE, Katz MM: Norms of adjustments and social behavior. Arch Gen Psychiatry 25:470–480, 1971

Jaspers K: General Psychopathology. University of Chicago Press, 1950

Keller MB, Lavori PW, Endicott J, et al: "Double depression": two year follow-up. Am J Psychiatry 140:689–694, 1983

Kendell RE: The classification of depressions: a review of contemporary confusion. Br J Psychiatry 129:15–28, 1976

Kernberg OF: Borderline Conditions and Pathological Narcissism. New York, Jason Aronson, 1976

Klerman GL: The spectrum of mania. Compr Psychiatry 22:11–20, 1981

Kraepelin E: Manic-Depressive Insanity and Paranoia. Edinburgh, Livingstone, 1921

Krauthammer C, Klerman GL: Secondary mania. Arch Gen Psychiatry 35:1333–1339, 1978

Kupfer DJ, Broudy D, Coble PA, et al: EEG sleep and affective psychoses. J Affect Dis 2:17–25, 1980

Kupfer DJ, Broudy D, Spider DG, et al: EEG sleep and affective psychoses, I: schizoaffective disorders. Psychiatr Res 1:173–178, 1979

Kupfer DJ, Pickard D, Himmelhock HM, et al: Are there two types of unipolar depression? Arch Gen Psychiatry 32:866–871, 1975

Leckman JF, Weissman MM, Merikangas J, et al: Panic disorder increases risk of depression, alcoholism, panic and phobic disorder in families of depressed probands. Arch Gen Psychiatry 40:1055–1066, 1983

Liebowitz MR, Klein DF: Hysteroid dysphoria. Psychiatr Clin North Am 2:555–575, 1979

Mendels J, Weinstein N, Cochrance C: The relationship between depression and anxiety. Arch Gen Psychiatry 27:649–653, 1972

Murphy GE: The physician's responsibility for suicide, I: an error of commission. Ann Intern Med 82:301–304, 1975

Nandi DN, Ajmay S, Gangoli H, et al: A clinical evaluation of depressives found on a rural survey in India. Br J Psychiatry 128:523–527, 1976

Nies A, Robinson DS: Monamine oxidase inhibitors, in Handbook of Affective Disorders. Edited by Paykel ES. New York, Guilford Press, 1982, pp 246–261

Noyes R, Clancy J, Crowe R, et al: The familial prevalence of anxiety neurosis. Arch Gen Psychiatry 35:1057–1059, 1978

Overall JE, Hollister LE, Johnson M, et al: Nosology of depression and differential response to drugs. JAMA 195:162–164, 1966

Pope HG Jr, Lipinski JF Jr: Diagnosis in schizophrenia and manic depressive illness. Arch Gen Psychiatry 35:811–828, 1978

Quitkin F, Rifkin A, Klein DF: Monoamine oxidase inhibitors: a review of antidepressant effectiveness. Arch Gen Psychiatry 36:749–760, 1979

Quitkin F, Schwartz D, Liebowitz JR, et al: Atypical depressives: a preliminary report of antidepressant response, sleep patterns, and cortisol secretion, in Treatment of Depression: Old Controversies and New Approaches. Edited by Clayton PU, Barret JE. New York, Raven Press, 1983

Reite M, Short RA: Nocturnal sleep in separated monkey infants. Arch Gen Psychiatry 35:1247–1253, 1978

Reveley AM, Reveley MA: The distinction of primary and secondary affective disorders. J Affect Dis 3:273–279, 1981

Reynolds CF, Shaw DH, Newton TF, et al: EEG sleep in outpatients with generalized anxiety: a preliminary comparison with depressed outpatients. Psychiatr Res 9:81–89, 1983

Robins E: Categories versus dimensions in psychiatric classification. Psychiatr Ann 6:39–55, 1976

Robins E, Guze SB: Establishment of diagnostic validity in psychiatric illness: its application to schizophrenia. Am J Psychiatry 37:138–139, 1970

Rosenthal TL, Akiskal HS, Scott-Strauss A, et al: Familial and developmental factors in characterological depressions. J Affect Dis 3:183–192, 1981

Roth M, Mountjoy Q: The distinction between anxiety states and depressive disorders, in Handbook of Affective Disorders. Edited by Paykel ES. New York, Guilford, 1982, pp 70–92

Sargent W: The treatment of anxiety states and atypical depressions by the monoamine oxidase inhibitor drugs. J Neuropsychiatry 3:96–103, 1962

Schildkraut JJ, Orsulak PJ, Schatzberg AF, et al: Toward a biochemical classification of depressive disorders. Arch Gen Psychiatry 35:1427–1433, 1978

Schlesser MA, Winokur G, Rush AJ: Dexamethasone suppression test in schizoaffective psychosis. Presented at the III World Congress of Biological Psychiatry, Stockholm, Sweden, June 1981

Schneider K: Psychopathic Personalities. Translated by Hamilton MW. London, Cassell, 1958

Sheehan DV, Ballenger J, Jacobson G: Relative efficacy of monamine oxidase inhibitors and tricyclic antidepressants in the treatment of endogenous anxiety, in Anxiety: New Research and Changing Concepts. Edited by Klein DF, Rabkin JG. New York, Raven Press, 1981, pp 47–62

Spitzer RL, Endicott J, Robins E: Research diagnostic criteria: rationale and reliability. Arch Gen Psychiatry 35:773–782, 1978

Stone MH: The Borderline Syndrome: Constitution, Personality, and Adaptation. New York, McGraw-Hill, 1980

Torgerson S: Genetic factors in anxiety disorder. Arch Gen Psychiatry 40:1085–1089, 1983

Tyrer P: Clinical use of monoamine oxidase inhibitors, in Psychopharmacology of Affective Disorders. Edited by Paykel ES, Coppen A. Oxford University Press, 1979, pp 159–178

Van Valkenburg C, Akiskal HS, Puzantian VR, et al: Anxious depressions: clinical, family history, and naturalistic outcome comparisons with panic and major depressive disorders. J Affect Dis 24:287–295, 1983

Wehr TA, Goodwin FE: Rapid cycling in manic-depressives induced by tricyclic-antidepressants. Arch Gen Psychiatry 36:555–559, 1979

Weissman MM, Prusoff B, Pincus C: Symptom patterns in depressed patients and depressed normals. J Nerv Ment Dis 160:15–23, 1975

West ED, Dally PJ: Effects of iproniazid in depressive syndromes. Br Med J 1:1491–1494, 1959

Wing JK, Cooper JE, Sartorius N: The Measurement and Classification of Psychiatric Symptoms. Cambridge University Press, 1974

Winokur G: Unipolar depression: is it divisible into autonomous subtypes? Arch Gen Psychiatry 36:47–57, 1979

Zitrin CM, Woerner MG, Klein DF: Differentiation of panic anxiety from anticipatory anxiety and avoidance behavior, in Anxiety: New Research and Changing Concepts. Edited by Klein DF, Rabkin JG. New York, Raven Press, 1981, pp 27–42

4   *Bipolar and schizoaffective disorders*

PAULA J. CLAYTON

The affective disorders are divided into *major* affective disorders, in which a full affective syndrome is present, *other* affective disorders, in which a partial affective syndrome of two years' duration is present, and *atypical* affective disorders, in which affective disorders that cannot be classified elsewhere are recorded. The major affective disorders are divided into bipolar disorder and major depression. The bipolar subdivision subsumes unipolar mania and the more common cyclic disorder of bipolar affective disorder. It is possible to sub-classify bipolar disorder in the fourth digit as mixed, manic, or depressed, and in the fifth digit as (2) without psychotic features, (4) with mood-congruent psychotic features, (7) with mood-incongruent psychotic features, or (6) in remission. If the current episode cannot be classified, the fifth digit is listed as zero. The criteria for the diagnosis of a manic episode are shown in Table 4.1. Bipolar II (major depression with a past history of hypomania) is classified in DSM-III as atypical affective disorder. This is discussed in a separate section.

BIPOLAR DISORDER

One minor correction in *DSM-III* is suggested. Although the summary page of the *DSM-III* classification lists, under affective disorders, bipolar and major depression, the text that deals with the former diagnostic category does not so label it. Thus, we have a description (p. 206) of "manic episode" that should read "bipolar disorder, manic episode," and "diagnostic criteria for a manic episode" (p. 208) that should read "diagnostic criteria for bipolar disorder, manic episode."

A recent study by Brockington and associates (1983) looked at the definitions of mania used in three psychotic British samples who were followed up. They assigned six definitions (CATEGO, the project or hospital diagnosis, Feighner criteria, RDC, *DSM-III*, and Leff) to patients from these three samples. In the Camberwell series (psychotic first admissions), the mean κ coefficient for these six pairwise concordances was .75. In the Netherne Hospital series (consecutive psychotic admissions), the mean κ coefficient for these six pairwise concor-

This work was supported in part by U.S. Public Health Service grant MH-25430.

Table 4.1. *Criteria for diagnosis of a manic episode*

Differential diagnosis: organic affective syndromes; schizophrenia, paranoid type; schizoaffective disorder; cyclothymic disorder

Diagnostic criteria:

A. One or more distinct periods with a predominantly elevated, expansive, or irritable mood; the elevated or irritable mood must be a prominent part of the illness and relatively persistent, although it may alternate or intermingle with depressive mood

B. Duration of at least one week (or any duration if hospitalization is necessary), during which, for most of the time, at least three of the following symptoms have persisted (four if the mood is only irritable) and have been present to a significant degree:
   1. increase in activity (either socially, at work, or sexually) or physical restlessness
   2. more talkative than usual or feeling pressure to keep talking
   3. flight of ideas or subjective experience that thoughts are racing
   4. inflated self-esteem (grandiosity, which may be delusional)
   5. decreased need for sleep
   6. distractibility, i.e., attention too easily drawn to unimportant or irrelevant external stimuli
   7. excessive involvement in activities that have a high potential for painful consequences that is not recognized, e.g., buying sprees, sexual indiscretions, foolish business investments, reckless driving

C. Neither of the following dominates the clinical picture when an affective syndrome (i.e., criteria A and B above) is not present; that is, before it developed or after it has remitted:
   1. preoccupation with a mood-incongruent delusion or hallucination
   2. bizarre behavior

D. Not superimposed on schizophrenia, on schizophreniform disorder, or on paranoid disorder

E. Not due to any organic mental disorder, such as substance intoxication

Note: A hypomanic episode is a pathological disturbance similar to, but not as severe as, a manic episode.

dances was .56. In the schizoaffective series, the concordance between RDC schizoaffective mania and the nearest *DSM-III* equivalent (mood-incongruent psychotic mania) was .75. When they compared RDC mania with *DSM-III* mood-congruent mania, the concordance was .67. Although there were large differences in the numbers of patients diagnosed, ranging from 17 to 55, the ranges in the three series were much smaller than the ranges for schizophrenia, and the concordance was better. They looked at outcome measures with all sets of criteria. Using the *DSM-III* criteria for mania, there were no differences in general-outcome scores between nonpsychotic manics, mood-congruent manics, and mood-incongruent manics, although the mood-incongruent patients showed more psychopathology (mania, depression, schizophrenia, and paranoid symptoms) than the other two groups in the follow-up period. Using RDC criteria for mania and schizoaffective mania, the results were similar, although the schizoaffective manics showed less time in the hospital and lower social-involvement scores in the follow-up period. *DSM-III* criteria provide for patients to be rated as nonpsychotic versus psychotic, as well as mood-congruent and mood-incongruent. Thus, it allows for a tripartite division, which other classifications do not. Their conclusion was that because there were striking and enduring symptomatic differences in the manic patients divided by clinical symptoms at intake, these patients should continue to be separated in the hope of finding either etiologic or treatment differences. In an earlier version of their report they recommended the continued use of the *DSM-III* definitions, which recognize the three subclasses of mania.

The only other follow-up that has dealt with manic and schizoaffective manic patients as well as schizophrenic patients was by Pope and associates (1980). Their follow-up showed no differences in outcome between manic and schizoaffective manic patients, but marked differences from schizophrenic patients. The manic and schizoaffective manic patients for the most part received vigorous and prolonged lithium treatment. This probably accounts for the differences in follow-up outcome between the two studies.

Walker (1981), studying patients with RDC diagnoses of schizophrenia, schizoaffective disorder, and other affective disorders, assessed attentional and neuromuscular functions for these patients. Both in the schizoaffective group and in the affective group, she had a mixture of manic and depressive patients. Approximately 75% of the patients were medicated at the time of study. Many of the RDC schizoaffectives had diagnoses by the hospital physicians of schizophrenia and were receiving antipsychotic medication at dosages comparable to those for the RDC schizophrenics. Previous research, however, had shown that medication is not related to the occurrence of neurologic "soft" signs in psychiatric patients. Walker performed a series of neuromotor tests and attentional assessment and found with regard to both assessments that schizoaffectives were distinguishable from schizophrenics, but not from other patients with affective disorder. She concluded by saying:

Of course, the absence of specific behavioral, family history, biologic, and treatment response differences between schizoaffectives and other affective patients does not preclude etiologic differences. Nevertheless, as Pope et al. (1980) pointed out, diagnostic subtypes should undergo rigorous screening for validity before accepted into clinical use. Until it is established that a schizoaffective disorder differs from affective disorders on a dimension other than subclinical symptoms, this diagnostic category will only have descriptive meaning.

Many investigators dividing patients by RDC definitions into groups with mania and schizoaffective mania have found minimal differences between these groups in regard to demographic variables and responses to treatment (Clayton, 1982). Abrams and Taylor (1981) studied pure manics versus those with one and two or more schizophrenic symptoms and again found no differences in any of the variables mentioned. They had no follow-up data, only improvement at discharge. Again, many of their patients in all groups were treated with lithium.

Almost all investigators found that schizoaffective manics, compared with manics, had equal or greater numbers of bipolar relatives (Clayton, 1982; Gershon et al., 1982). Even a recent study by Kendler and Hays (1983) dividing *DSM-III*-diagnosed schizophrenics on the basis of family history (no affective disorder, unipolar affective disorder, and bipolar affective disorder) showed that in five years of follow-up, schizophrenics with bipolar relatives were more depressed during the prodrome, were more elated and catatonic when actively psychotic, had fewer residual symptoms when remitted, and were more likely to have a manic syndrome develop during the follow-up period. The family data and this interesting last study justify the inclusion of the more psychotic group of patients in the *DSM-III* definition of bipolar disorder and speak against changing the *DSM-III* category of schizoaffective disorders.

To my knowledge, no one has used the *DSM-III* definition of mania that would divide patients on the basis of euphoric mood versus irritable mood to determine whether or not there are differences in terms of course, outcome, family history, or treatment response.

BIPOLAR II DISORDER

Bipolar II disorder is a syndrome first defined by Fieve and Dunner in 1975. In their definition, the bipolar II patient is one who has been hospitalized for a depressive disorder that may or may not be recurrent but who has a past history of hypomania that did not require hospitalization. Dunner and associates and Akiskal (1981) have collected interesting data on this condition. However, this definition of bipolar II disorder is not universal. RDC criteria require that the patient meet the RDC definition of major depression (less stringent than Feighner criteria for depression) or minor depression or intermittent depression and have two days of hypomanic symptoms. Reliability studies using the RDC definition have shown that the reliability of the diagnosis is far from satisfactory. Andreasen and associates (1981), in collaborative studies, examined the reliability of SADS–L–RDC lifetime diagnoses in 50 relatives and/or controls in a test–retest paradigm. The initial diagnosis versus the follow-up diagnosis of bipolar II disorder had an intraclass R value of .06, and the items for hypomania and cyclothymia were also unreliably rated. The authors mentioned that Mazure and Gershon (1979) reported similar results for minor depression. This suggests that both sets of minor symptoms are not reliable over time. Keller and associates (1981), using collaborative-study patients, also found the lifetime diagnosis of hypomania to be unreliable. In this case the raters could not reach consensus on current hypomania. Although in all these studies the base rates for bipolar II disorder were small, the recurring finding is striking. One must conclude that the SADS–L–RDC definition of bipolar II disorder cannot be recommended. More rigorous criteria, perhaps as Akiskal (1981, 1983) suggests, are necessary.

REFERENCES

Abrams R, Taylor MA: Importance of schizophrenic symptoms in the diagnosis of mania. Am J Psychiatry 138:658–661, 1981

Akiskal HS: Subaffective disorders: dysthymic, cyclothymic and bipolar II disorders in the "borderline" realm. Psychiatr Clin North Am 4:25–46, 1981
   The bipolar spectrum: new concepts in classification and diagnosis, in Psychiatry Update, Vol II. Edited by Grinspoon L. Washington, DC, American Psychiatric Press, 1983

Andreasen NC, Grove WM, Shapiro RW, et al: Reliability of lifetime diagnosis: a multicenter collaborative perspective. Arch Gen Psychiatry 38:400–405, 1981

Brockington IF, Hillier VF, Francis AF, et al: Definitions of mania: concordance and prediction of outcome. Am J Psychiatry 140:435–439, 1983

Clayton PJ: Schizoaffective disorders. J Nerv Ment Dis 170:646–650, 1982

Fieve RR, Dunner DL: Unipolar and bipolar affective states, in The Nature and Treatment of Depression. Edited by Flach F, Draghi S. New York, Wiley, 1975

Gershon ES, Hamovit J, Guroff JJ, et al: A family study of schizoaffective, bipolar I, bipolar II, unipolar, and normal control probands. Arch Gen Psychiatry 39:1157–1167, 1982

Keller MB, Lavori PW, McDonald-Scott P, et al: Reliability of lifetime diagnoses and symptoms in patients with a current psychiatric disorder. J Psychiatr Res 16:229–240, 1981

Kendler KS, Hays P: Schizophrenia subdivided by the family history of affective disorder. Arch Gen Psychiatry 40:951–955, 1983

Mazure C, Gershon ES: Blindness and reliability in lifetime psychiatric diagnosis. Arch Gen Psychiatry 36:521–525, 1979

Pope HG, Lipinski JF, Cohen BM, et al: "Schizoaffective disorder": an invalid diagnosis? A comparison of schizoaffective disorder, schizophrenia, and affective disorder. Am J Psychiatry 137:921–927, 1980

Walker E: Attentional and neuromotor functions of schizophrenics, schizoaffectives, and patients with other affective disorders. Arch Gen Psychiatry 38:1355–1358, 1981

5   Overview

MYRNA M. WEISSMAN,
KATHLEEN R. MERIKANGAS, PHILLIP J. LEAF,
CHARLES E. HOLZER, JEROME K. MYERS, AND
GARY L. TISCHLER

Before summarizing the varied issues that emerged during discussion of the chapters in this section, we would like to add findings that are relevant to *DSM-III* and are derived from recent genetic and epidemiologic studies. The material presented is based on recent data from the Epidemiologic Catchment Area study (Regier et al., 1984) and from the Yale–NIMH collaborative study on the genetics of affective disorders (Weissman, Kidd, and Prusoff, 1982; Weissman et al., 1984a,b,c). The recommendations suggested should be reviewed in the light of the fact that many of the findings are preliminary or have not yet been replicated in other studies.

EPIDEMIOLOGIC DATA CITED IN *DSM-III*

At various points in the descriptive portions of diagnoses in *DSM-III*, reference is made to the prevalence of specific disorders in the community and to the characteristics of individuals manifesting these disorders. It is not clear where these descriptions were obtained. Given our limited knowledge of the distributions of psychiatric disorders in the community, it might be useful to stress the variability in rates of disorders or the confidence bounds of the estimates. Many probably are "best guesses" that have appeared in the literature and then have been referenced repeatedly as if based on scientific evidence. These descriptions should be updated as new data from the Epidemiologic Catchment Area (ECA) program and other sources become available. For example, preliminary analysis of the ECA data suggests that the mean age of onset for major depression may be earlier than previously thought, and onset may not be evenly distributed throughout adult life as noted in *DSM-III*.

CASE DESCRIPTIONS

The descriptions of usual cases in *DSM-III* have been derived from studies of treated populations. It is not yet clear how the characteristics of patients in various types of treatments differ from each other or from those of nontreated populations. Current evidence suggests that there may be significant differences, because factors other than symptoms may influence help-seeking behavior. Data from the ECA study may soon help to clarify the full clinical picture of disorders independent of help-seeking. If differences are found, it may be useful to update the clinical descriptions.

EXCLUSIONS AND HIERARCHIES

Although *DSM-III* is multiaxial within axis I and to a lesser degree axis II, clinicians are encouraged to make decisions concerning what is due to what. At a minimum, the intention of this exercise needs to be clarified. Our research suggests that if clinicians focus on the nature of a current episode of a disorder in developing a strategy for providing treatment, they may miss significant information concerning the existence of previous episodes of that or another disorder. Further, they may fail to uncover important information about seemingly unrelated symptoms that may have occurred in the past.

We do not underestimate the difficulty of obtaining accurate accounts of previously occurring or co-occurring illness episodes. We are sure that most clinicians forgo undertaking extensive clinical histories and find structured interviews constraining, in part because they have legitimate questions about the interpretations that can be applied to these data. On the other hand, *DSM-III* as it now stands discourages collection of these data in two ways. Because it emphasizes exclusion criteria, physicians may feel that they do not need to collect detailed information about syndromes that will not contribute to the primary diagnosis. Thus, the use of exclusion criteria and hierarchies discourages the clinician from keeping track of those syndromes and symptoms that do not fit in with current conceptions of the illness. Second, even when a complete psychiatric history is obtained, details of specific symptoms and syndromes may be expunged from the record because the illness is seen as being due to other causes.

Another problem in the exclusion issue is the fact that there are exclusionary criteria that are not precisely defined. There is the possibility that even when the criteria for a major disorder are met, an additional exclusion criterion can force reversion to "no diagnosis." These issues occur at several points in the system. The first is the "uncomplicated" bereavement exclusion for major depression. The occurrence of uncomplicated bereavement can exclude major depression, but the criteria for moving from uncomplicated bereavement to "complicated" bereavement (major depression?) are not very precise. Specification of the number of symptoms or duration would be helpful.

Analyses from our genetic study of major depression (Weissman et al., 1982) also support the notion that at least some diagnostic hierarchies tend to obscure meaningful clinical distinctions. In this study we found that rates of major depression were elevated among relatives of probands with major depression and an anxiety disorder, regardless of whether the anxiety disorder occurred temporally separate from or concomitant with the depressive episode (Leckman et al., 1983a). Furthermore, the presence of panic disorder in a depressed proband conveyed additional risk for both depression and anxiety disorders both in adult relatives and in the proband's children (ages 6–17 years) (Leckman et al., 1983b; Weissman et al., 1984b).

Based on these data, it would seem advisable that an individual be given every diagnosis whose criteria the individual meets, either currently or in the past. Until the relationships between the various diagnostic categories are more fully understood, failure to classify patients according to all of the syndromes that they may have will obscure important sources of variation in diagnoses. Judgments about the underlying versus contributing causes of disease cannot be made until all such sources of variation are more fully explored.

NUMBER OF SYMPTOMS

Recent data presented by Angst and Dobler-Mikola (1984) suggest that depression may have different presentations in males and females. Given the same level of social impairment, males report fewer symptoms than females. Furthermore, males are more likely to forget the presence of symptoms (particularly loss of interest, worthlessness and appetite disturbance) than females, who tend to have accurate recall for symptoms of depression. This finding raises an important question about the *DSM-III* requirement of a specified number of symptoms, despite equal levels of social impairment. Use of the rule of a specified number of symptoms may produce a bias in favor of females that may actually be an artifact of reporting.

We have only begun to investigate in the ECA data the problem of differential reporting of symptoms and possible correlates of symptoms confounding diagnosis. Attention needs to be paid to determining the extent to which subclinical cases of disorders are subclinical only in terms of symptom counts. Although it will not be possible to make any specific recommendations concerning this point until additional data analysis has been conducted, the issue of the number of symptoms required for a particular diagnosis is one that usually warrants further study.

SOCIAL IMPAIRMENT

A related issue concerns the requirement that there be social impairment in order to make certain diagnoses. Substantiation for the presence of this requirement for some disorders and not for others is not evident in *DSM-III*. The degree of social impairment can vary widely, given a constant number of symptoms or similar severities of clinical disease. It has been shown that social adjustment and symptomatic severity are separate components of psychiatric illness (Merikangas, Bromet, and Spiker, 1983). For example, if one person with diabetes is able to go to work and perform reasonably well, whereas another at a similar stage of the disease cannot function, we do not deny that both individuals have diabetes. It seems appropriate to raise the question whether or not the same principle should be applied to psychiatric illness before further introducing such requirements into a diagnostic system.

In our attempts to apply the *DSM-III* criteria for Diagnostic Interview Schedule (DIS) computer programs, we have had particular difficulty in determining the extent to which impairment should be filtered into diagnostic decisions. It is not clear from *DSM-III* to what extent there is a minimum threshold of impairment, dysfunction, or dissatisfaction that is required in addition to the existence of symptom clusters. This problem appears to be greatest in the diagnosis of phobias, in which both our epidemiologic instruments and the clinicians participating in our validity studies appear to be finding a higher rate of *DSM-III* phobia than our earlier community studies found using the RDC. These data are in the process of being analyzed, and more information will be forthcoming.

DISTINCTION BETWEEN BIPOLAR DISORDER AND MAJOR DEPRESSION

Data from our epidemiologic study (ECA) and from our genetics study support previously reported findings on rates of bipolar disorder and major depression by sex. In both studies, the sex ratios were equal for bipolar disorder, but females had a higher prevalence of major depression. These epidemiologic differences between bipolar disorder and major depression provide further support for the distinction between these disorders (Weissman et al., 1982; Myers et al., 1984).

SUBTYPES OF MAJOR DEPRESSION

Data from our family-genetic study, which has as one of its goals the validation of subtypes of depression, lead to the following suggestions regarding differentiated depressed probands (as compared with depressed probands without the specific subtype):

1. *Melancholia* in the depressed proband does not increase the risk for major depression among first-degree relatives.
2. The *delusional subtype* in the depressed proband does increase the risk for major depression, as well as for delusional and endogenous depression and bipolar disorder, among first-degree relatives.
3. An *early age of onset* (under 30 years) of major depression in the proband does increase the risk for major depression, as well as early-onset major depression, among first-degree relatives of all ages. In fact, probands with onset of depression after the age of 40 years showed little familial transmission as compared with normals.
4. *Major depression* plus an *anxiety disorder* does increase the risk for major depression, as well as any anxiety disorder, among both adult and child first-degree relatives. The increased risk for relatives was found whether the anxiety disorder occurred in association with or separate from the depression in probands. This observation is the basis for our recommending the elimination of that hierarchy.

Although *DSM-III* should not be revised on the basis of one study, attention should be given to these findings if they are replicated. If replicated, they suggest that, at least in terms of familial transmission, melancholia may not be a discriminating subtype.

The findings also suggest the validity of the psychotic depression subtype, the possibility that psychotic depression may be related to bipolar disorder, the importance of diagnosing anxiety disorders in depressed persons regardless of the order of their occurrence, and the importance of determining the age of onset of depression. Even now we would recommend that clinicians determine the age of onset of major depression.

ATYPICAL DEPRESSION

The concept of atypical depression as now included in *DSM-III* is confusing. This concept implies something unusual or irregular, when indeed it may be a result of insufficient information or may be applied to someone who falls just below the threshold of criteria specification. Classification of hypomania as an atypical affective disorder provides a good example. This diagnosis has been plagued by a lack of reliability for numerous reasons, such as the lack of clear-cut onset of episodes. To classify this as atypical reflects our inability to quantify the symptoms and course, rather than an unusual course of illness. Confusing the unusual presentation of a disorder and the amount of information and/or impairment available on which to base the diagnosis should be carefully considered in future revisions of *DSM-III*.

We would recommend that the diagnosis of atypical depression be saved for unusual presentations of a disorder and that a category of insufficient information and/or probable disorder be added. Hypomania or bipolar II probably should be added as a subgroup of bipolar disorder.

OTHER SPECIFIC AFFECTIVE DISORDERS

Our data support the inclusion of cyclothymia and dysthymia as affective disorders rather than personality disorders. Weissman and associates (1984b) demonstrated that cyclothymia aggregates in first-degree relatives of bipolar probands, but not in relatives of probands with major depression; depressive personality (dysthymia) aggregates in the relatives of probands with major depression. Thus, on the basis of our data, cyclothymia should be classified with bipolar disorder, and dysthymia with major depression. Also, a distinction probably should be made between early onset and late onset in these disorders, following the work of Akiskal and Winokur.

DIAGNOSIS IN CHILDREN

Our studies support the use of current diagnostic criteria for major depression and the anxiety disorders in children (Weissman et al., 1984b). We have found strong familial aggregation of major depression among the children, ages 6–17, of probands with major depression. In addition, depression and panic appear to be transmitted to children of probands with both disorders (Weissman et al., 1984b). Thus, the onset of these disorders appears to be early, and they appear to be diagnosable in children. Our data give partial support for the diagnosis of separation anxiety in children and its relationship to adult panic disorders. More than one-third of the children of probands with panic disorder and depression also had separation anxiety.

Again, no one study can stand alone. However, there are several researchers studying depressed children (Michael Strober, UCLA; Maria Kovacs and Joaquim Puig-Antich, University of Pittsburgh) who have found similar results. The results of these studies viewed together will have implications for diagnoses in children.

DISCUSSION OF PRESENTATIONS

Following Dr. Klerman's presentation (Chapter 1), three issues were discussed. The first had to do with the availability of data to validate the concept of melancholia. An overview of a conference conducted in 1982 by Dr. Robert Hirschfeld at the annual meeting of the American College of Neuropsychopharmacology was presented. The purpose of the conference was to review the current status of the validity of the concept "endogenous." The following endogenous subtypes were reviewed: RDC endogenous, which is the broadest concept; *DSM-III* melancholia, which is the most restricted concept and focuses on diurnal variation and guilt; and the Nelson–Charney concept of autonomous, which is also restricted and would include the more psychotic and guilt-ridden patients.

Investigators were asked to reanalyze their data on the basis of these subtypes to determine if the subtypes were sensitive to family aggregation. One problem reported was that the majority of persons in inpatient samples meet the criteria of endogenous. However, the results of the analyses from a number of these studies showed no increased familial aggregation with the various definitions of the endogenous subtypes. Although major depression in a proband increased familial aggregation in first-degree relatives, the specific subtypes did not increase aggregation in relatives over and above that found in the relatives of probands without the subtype. Moreover, treatment data presented at that conference by Robert Prien did not show sensitivity to the subtypes. The only evidence for some sensitivity of the endogenous subtypes was from the sleep data presented by David Kupfer. The conclusion of the conference was that the endogenous subtypes could not be validated by existing methods. However, no one was yet willing to give up these subtypes.

Commenting on the conference, Dr. Kupfer noted that investigators approached the validation of subtypes from two viewpoints: defining biological markers in patients and examining subtypes, and defining patients by clinical subtypes and looking for biological differentiation. He noted that, in general, these studies were not fruitful, because neither the neurochemical nor the neuroendocrine studies showed positive findings. Further, he believed that sleep studies in and of themselves represented an insufficient data base.

The next question raised had to do with the multiple meanings of "atypical affective disorder." There was some dissatisfaction with this term. It can indicate insufficient information, an unusual presentation, or an undiagnosable condition. As such, "atypical" has no communicative value. Some participants believed that there was value in separating out the patients who definitely fit the criteria for various disorders from those who almost fit. The atypical category includes those patients who do not quite make the major category. It is particularly useful to have narrow categories for research studies of causes. Although there was agreement that the atypical category is useful, there was also agreement that it needed further elaboration and that the term was too broad. Only a small number of patients (10%) in studies conducted in St. Louis were in fact undiagnosable. This was confirmed by Dr. Akiskal, who found that only 6% of patients coming to his mood clinic had atypical bipolar disorders, and another 2.5% were considered undiagnosed after six months of follow-up. However, Dr. Weissman pointed out that in epidemiologic or family studies of nonpatients, there are much higher rates of atypical disorders because of insufficient information or the presence of individuals on the milder ends of the clinical spectrum.

The discussion ended with questions as to the utility of the primary–secondary continuum (which does not appear in *DSM-III*) as a presumption of sequence in establishing a hierarchy. There was agreement that attention should be given to the possible value of including the primary–secondary distinction in future versions of *DSM-III*.

Two issues were raised in the discussion of Dr. Kupfer's presentation (Chapter 2). The first concerned the value of the subtypes of depression as currently defined. Although there was general consensus that major depression as a broad group was clinically useful, it was concluded that psychobiological studies will need to focus on the discrete subtypes. The point was made that the subtypes as currently defined may or may not be validated by empirical investigations. One discussant believed that the subtypes of melancholia and delusional depression had the most promise of being validated, but noted that validation solely on the basis of sleep studies would not be sufficient.

From a methodological perspective it was suggested that the approach used by Dr. Buxbaum and associates at NIMH might prove fruitful. The approach begins with patients with biological abnormalities that can be used as markers to determine how the clinical subtypes, as currently defined, aggregate in these patients. Others believed that although the approach has potential, it also has problems: One must determine how to carefully define the biological variables and their measurements and cutoff points. The biological variables will have to be measured carefully, and researchers will need to pay close attention to the clinical and diagnostic variables and develop settings in which such complex studies can be accomplished. The studies will also need to examine family history and genetic loading as well as the clinical descriptive phenomena.

A second question arose concerning the value of the delusional subtype. There was disagreement among the participants as to whether or not delusional depression has been validated as a distinct subtype. Studies at Yale have found that delusional depression predicts higher familial aggregations in relatives for both delusional subtypes and major depression. Furthermore, bipolar disorders may be increased in the relatives of those with delusional depression. To date, however, these findings have not been replicated. It was pointed out that the Swedish adoption-study data indicate that there was no great aggregation of depression among biological parents of adopted-away children who had delusional depression.

The discussion following Dr. Clayton's presentation (Chapter 4) focused on whether schizoaffective disorders should be further defined or dropped from this diagnostic category. Current usage involves retaining the category without diagnostic criteria for those situations in which a clinician is unable to make a differential diagnosis between affective disorder and either schizophreniform disorder or schizophrenia. It was pointed out that the use of bipolar disorders with mood-congruent or mood-incongruent psychotic features captured most of the schizoaffective manics. The schizoaffective depressed patients, however, clearly represent a more heterogeneous group. The syndrome appears to be related to both schizophrenia and depression, but not to bipolar disorder. The issue seemed to be further confounded as the point was made that data from twin and fostering studies on schizoaffective disorders conducted in Germany and Denmark suggest that schizoaffective disorders appear to be in the schizophrenia spectrum. Because the treated course of the disorder remains unclear, some argued that more precise definition of the syndrome is required so that patients meeting specific criteria can be studied in greater detail. There was no agreement, however, as to how one would define such patients. An alternative proposition was to delete the category entirely, thus forcing clinicians to diagnose and treat schizoaffective patients as if they had affective disorders. It was noted that many patients who present with both mood and thought disorders often have family histories that include relatives with both schizophrenia and affective disorders, and their treatment involves the use of medications for both the affective disorders and psychotic disorders. At a more general level, the discussion of schizoaffective disorders highlighted the problems presented by diagnostic entities that either are defined entirely by exclusion or are used as residual categories.

The discussion of Dr. Akiskal's presentation (Chapter 3) centered around the boundaries between axis I and axis II. Two issues were raised: The first concerned how to treat spectrum disorders currently regarded as personality disorders under axis II. The question was posed: Should these disorders continue to be listed as personality disorders, or should they be listed with the major axis I disorder with which they are associated? It was suggested that where there is empirical evidence that an axis II disorder is an attenuated form of the axis I major disorder, it should be classified under axis I. If this principle were followed, schizotypal personality disorder could be brought to axis I as a milder form of schizophrenia, just as psychothymia, hyperthymia, and dysthymia are currently classified with their respective major affective disorders.

In response to the question whether or not axis I implies a biological cause, and axis II a nonbiological cause, there was strong agreement that this is not the case. The point was made that the concept underlying axis I is the existence of a clear break, with the disorder being discontinuous from previous function. On axis II, the disorder represents an unfolding of what is already in the personality. In either instance, the underlying process can be biological or nonbiological or some combination of the two.

REFERENCES

Angst J, Dobler-Mikola A: The Zurich study: III. diagnosis of depression. Eur Arch Psychiatr Neurol Sci 234:30–37, 1984

Leckman JF, Merikangas KR, Pauls DL, et al: Anxiety disorders and depression: contradictions between family study data and DSM-III convention. Am J Psychiatry 140:880–882, 1983a

Leckman JF, Weissman MM, Merikangas KR, et al: Panic disorder and psychiatric illness in families of depressed probands. Arch Gen Psychiatry 40:1055–1060, 1983b

Merikangas KR, Bromet EJ, Spiker DG: Assortative mating, social adjustment, and course of illness in primary affective disorder. Arch Gen Psychiatry 40:795–800, 1983

Myers JK, Weissman MM, Tischler GL, et al: Six-month prevalence of psychiatric disorders in three communities: 1980–82. Arch Gen Psychiatry 41:959–967, 1984

Regier DA, Myers JK, Kramer M, et al: The NIMH Epidemiologic Catchment Area (ECA) program: historical context, major objectives and study population characteristics. Arch Gen Psychiatry 41:934–941, 1984

Weissman MM, Gershon ES, Kidd KK, et al: Psychiatric disorders in the relatives of probands with affective disorders: the Yale–NIMH collaborative study. Arch Gen Psychiatry 41:13–21, 1984a

Weissman MM, Kidd KK, Prusoff BA: Variability in rates of affective disorders in relatives of depressed and normal probands. Arch Gen Psychiatry 39:1397–1403, 1982

Weissman MM, Leckman JF, Merikangas KR, et al: Depression and anxiety disorders in parents and children: results from the Yale family study. Arch Gen Psychiatry 41:845–852, 1984b

Weissman MM, Prusoff BA, Gammon GD, et al: Psychopathology in the children (ages 6–18) of depressed and normal parents. J Am Acad Child Psychiatry 23:78–84, 1984c

PART II

The nonaffective functional psychoses

The focus of Part II is the nonaffective functional psychoses in *DSM-III,* with emphasis on the schizophrenic, schizophreniform, and paranoid disorders. In discussing the schizophrenic and schizophreniform disorders, Nancy Andreasen highlights a number of issues that have been foci of controversy since the introduction of *DSM-III.* These include the duration criterion, the characteristic symptoms, the age criterion, the organic exclusion criterion, and the validity of the subtypes. Noting that there has been relatively little systematic research on the paranoid disorders, in contrast to the situation with schizophrenia and affective illness, Kenneth Kendler examines the recent literature on paranoid disorders as defined by *DSM-III* and suggests possible changes in the diagnostic criteria for paranoid disorders.

The other syndromes among the nonaffective psychoses for which there are specified criteria are brief reactive psychosis, schizoaffective disorder, and atypical psychosis. Atypical psychosis is purely a residual category in *DSM-III* and is not formally covered in this volume. Schizoaffective disorder is discussed in Part I on affective disorders. In the "Overview," I touch on brief reactive psychoses, address a few additional issues relevant in a consideration of schizophrenic and schizophreniform disorders, and provide a summary of the salient issues that arise in Part II.

John E. Helzer

6 Schizophrenia and schizophreniform disorders

NANCY C. ANDREASEN

The definitions of schizophrenia and schizophreniform disorder appearing in *DSM-III* represent a conservative revolution. These definitions, written in the early 1970s, narrowed the concept of schizophrenia with a few swift strokes of the typewriter keys. American psychiatry, which had been using a relatively broad Bleulerian definition of the disorder for many years, was returned to a more conservative conceptualization similar to that of the founding father of modern psychiatric nosology and arch-rival of Bleuler (1950): Emil Kraepelin (1919). Acute and chronic schizophrenias, which had happily resided together as siblings within the schizophrenia family in *DSM-I* and *DSM-II*, were split apart. Indeed, some might even say that acute schizophrenia (renamed schizophreniform disorder) was shuffled off to a foster home among the "psychoses not elsewhere classified." Affective forms of schizophrenia, or schizoaffective disorders, were also removed, as were nonpsychotic forms such as simple schizophrenia. Because many patients who had been called schizophrenic in the older system could no longer be given this diagnosis, the changes seemed revolutionary to many. On the other hand, because these changes represent a return to earlier ideas and perhaps represent a correction of a tendency toward extremism in American psychiatry, some would say they are essentially conservative in spirit.

The decision to return to a more traditional definition of schizophrenia was shaped by a number of recent "life events" that occurred during the years just before *DSM-III* was written. Many of these suggested that the broad American concept of schizophrenia needed rethinking. During the late 1960s and early 1970s, several important cross-national studies of schizophrenia were conducted: the International Pilot Study of Schizophrenia, and the US/UK study (Wing, 1970; Kendell et al., 1971; Wing, Cooper, and Sartorius, 1974; Wing and Nixon, 1975). Both these studies suggested that American psychiatrists, at least as represented by those working in New York City and Washington, D.C., often tended to see schizophrenia in patients whom their international colleagues would view as manic-depressives and in general tended to diagnose schizophrenia more frequently. These large international studies also placed great emphasis on improving the reliability of diagnosis and evaluation of symptoms. Thus, they tended to minimize Bleulerian symptoms, which were considered hard to define reliably, and to focus instead on symptoms that might be more "objective," such as delusions or hallucinations.

Through the influence of John Wing, Frank Fish, and other British psychiatrists, more emphasis was placed on Germanic approaches to phenomenology (Fish, 1962; Wing, 1970; Hamilton, 1974; Wing et al., 1974). The Schneiderian school, which stressed the pathognomonic nature of "first-rank symptoms," assumed great importance (Schneider, 1959; Mellor, 1970; Mellor, Sims, and Cope, 1981; Hoenig, 1982). First-rank symptoms were, at least for a time, seen as the solution to the eternal problem of identifying the "pathognomonic symptom of schizophrenia." Further, they were codified in standard interviewing instruments such as the Present State Examination and the Schedule for Affective Disorders and Schizophrenia (SADS) (Wing, 1970; Wing et al., 1974; Endicott and Spitzer, 1978). Early in the 1970s a few canny American psychiatrists working at Washington University in St. Louis developed another solution to the problem. They wrote a set of diagnostic criteria for schizophrenia, as well as criteria for 12 other major psychiatric disorders, thereby laying the foundation for the diagnostic criteria throughout all of *DSM-III* (Feighner et al., 1972). The Washington University criteria (sometimes also called the Feighner criteria) relied heavily on the duration of symptoms, as well as characteristic patterns of symptoms, in order to isolate relatively homogeneous diagnostic groups. In the case of schizophrenia, the Washington University criteria specified that patients must be ill for at least six months.

These influences all impinged on the *DSM-III* definition of schizophrenia. The new schizophrenia is a disorder lasting at least six months, including both prodromal and residual periods, that is characterized primarily by delusions and hallucinations during the active period of illness. The description of characteristic symptoms places great emphasis on Schneiderian first-rank symptoms, although a deferential nod is made in the direction of such classic Bleulerian symptoms as types of formal thought disorders or affective flattening.

It is now nearly 10 years since the first draft of the criteria and description of schizophrenia were written. Although most clinicians seem generally satisfied with the direction taken in *DSM-III*, a number of issues and problems remain, some more serious than others. Most of the controversy has focused on the following five areas:

1. the duration criterion
2. the characteristic symptoms
3. the age criterion
4. the organic exclusion criterion
5. the validity of the subtypes

THE DURATION CRITERION

The requirement that the illness be present for at least six months was borrowed principally from the Washington University criteria. The reason that the authors of the Washington University criteria specified a relatively long

Table 6.1. *Duration of illness before admission as a predictor of outcome*

Outcome	6 months		>6 months	
	N	%	N	%
Recovered	93	31	28	7
Improved	138	46	93	23
Some deterioration	67	22	287	70
Total	298		408	

Source: Astrup and Noreik (1966).

duration of illness is clear: They wanted to narrow an overbroad concept and to eliminate those patients with brief psychotic episodes, particularly when these episodes might in fact be some type of affective illness. But why choose six months rather than two months, five months, nine months, or one year? Any specific duration seems relatively arbitrary. The principal evidence available at the time for selecting six months rather than some other time period appears in a book on psychotic disorders by Astrup and Noreik (1966) and is summarized in Table 6.1. They looked at the duration of illness before admission as a predictor of outcome. They split the data into a variety of durations and a variety of outcomes, which appear in full form in their book and have been summarized and collapsed in Table 6.1. These data suggest that the six-month-duration criterion can be a useful predictor of outcome in this large sample of over 700 patients. Seventy-seven percent of those who had been ill less than six months either recovered or improved, whereas only 22% showed signs of deterioration. On the other hand, among the patients who had been ill for more than six months, only 30% recovered or improved, whereas 70% showed some deterioration.

More recent data have raised some questions about the value of this criterion. Coryell and Tsuang (1982) examined a subsample of patients from the Iowa 500 and non-500 studies. They identified a subsample of 214 patients who met *DSM-III* criteria for schizophreniform disorder and compared them to similar patients meeting criteria for schizophrenia, unipolar depression, and bipolar disorder. The lengths of follow-up periods varied from 2.2 to 4.3 years on the average. As Table 6.2 indicates, both types of affective illnesses tended to have relatively good outcomes, with 79% of bipolar patients and 74% of unipolar patients either recovered or improved. Alternatively, 24% of schizophrenic patients were recovered or improved, a significantly lower percentage than found in affective illness, although somewhat higher than that noted in the data of Astrup and Noreik. What is surprising, however, is the extremely low recovery or improvement rate among the schizophreniform patients: only 44%, with 57% being unimproved.

Table 6.2. *Outcome of psychotic disorders: Iowa 500 and non-500*

	N	Mean length of follow-up	Outcome (%)		
			Recovered	Improved	Unimproved
Bipolar disorder	86	2.2	55	24	21
Unipolar depression	203	4.3	59	15	26
Schizophreniform disorder	83	2.6	16	28	57
Schizophrenia	214	2.6	8	16	76

Sources: Coryell and Tsuang (1982).

The advantage of this sample is that it describes the natural history of the illness in a period prior to development of the wide range of modern neuroleptic treatments. A disadvantage, however, is that the findings may not be generalizable to samples collected more recently. Coryell and Tsuang did, however, examine recovery rates in a subsample of patients who had received no treatment at all (treatments received by the patients in this study were administered in the preneuroleptic era and consisted principally of insulin-shock therapy and electroconvulsive therapy). When treatment is controlled for by examining only those patients who did not receive somatic therapy, there is little difference in outcome between the schizophrenic and schizophreniform patients. Seven percent of the schizophrenics recovered, and 16% improved, whereas 77% were unimproved; similarly, 17% of the schizophreniform patients recovered, 19% improved, and 65% were unimproved. Thus, the natural histories of these two disorders appear to be quite similar and suggest that dividing patients into two separate groups on the basis of duration of symptoms alone may be of little predictive value.

Coryell and Tsuang also examined another external validator of the six-month-duration criterion. Using family-history data, they found somewhat different patterns of familial rates, as shown in Table 6.3. The highest morbid risk for schizophrenia is found among the relatives of the schizophrenic probands, whereas the rate for patients suffering from schizophreniform disorder is intermediate between the rates for schizophrenia and affective disorder. On the other hand, the morbid risk for affective disorder is much higher among the relatives of probands suffering from affective disorder, and the rates are quite similar among the relatives of patients suffering from schizophrenia and schizophreniform disorder. These results suggest that schizophrenia and schizophreniform disorder resemble one another more than they resemble affective illness, although the relatives of schizophrenics are more frequently affected with schizophrenia than are the relatives of schizophreniform patients. This suggests that schizophrenia may be a somewhat more severe and "familial" illness. Nevertheless, these data must be interpreted quite conservatively. The family-

Table 6.3. *Schizophrenia versus schizophreniform disorder: familial rates of illness*

	Proband N	Relative N	Morbid risk for schizophrenia		Morbid risk for affective disorder	
			$\overline{X}$	SD	$\overline{X}$	SD
Schizophrenia	235	1280	2.78	0.58	5.84	0.87
Schizophreniform disorder	93	513	1.82	0.74	6.49	1.52
Affective disorder	325	1932	0.60	0.19	13.48	0.99

Source: Coryell and Tsuang (1982).

history method has inherent strengths, in that it provides information on all possible relatives, living or dead, but also it is probably less valid than data based on direct interview. Further, Coryell and Tsuang did not attempt to determine the morbid risk for schizophreniform disorder among relatives, which would have been helpful in trying to determine if these two syndromes are genetically independent of one another.

THE CHARACTERISTIC SYMPTOMS

The diagnostic criteria for schizophrenia and those for schizophreniform disorder require that at least one from a set of six characteristic symptoms be present during some phase of the illness. As this listing indicates, delusions and hallucinations are given considerable prominence. At the time *DSM-III* was being written, both clinical and research lore suggested that delusions and hallucinations were easier to define, more objective, and more likely to be reliable than other common symptoms of schizophrenia. The text accompanying the criteria goes into considerable detail in describing other types of symptoms, but these are given little prominence in the criteria. Only criterion 6 focuses on classic Bleulerian symptoms.

Clinical and research lore was changing, however, during the years that *DSM-III* was in progress and has continued to change since *DSM-III* went to press. The bulk of the current evidence suggests that delusions and hallucinations are not necessarily more reliable than other types of symptoms and that they may have been given undue prominence in the criteria for schizophrenia. Table 6.4 contains an up-to-date summary of the reliability of delusions and hallucinations as reported for three different systems (Endicott et al., 1982). The data base consisted of the SADS, supplemented by some additional questions. Patients were interviewed jointly in an interrater reliability design and provided scores for the various criteria after the interview was completed.

Table 6.4. *Characteristic symptoms: reliability of delusions and hallucinations in three different systems*

Item	κ
Research Diagnostic Criteria	
Thought broadcasting, insertion, withdrawal	.45
Delusions of control, bizarre delusions	.85
Nonpersecutory or jealous delusions	.77
Delusions and hallucinations for one week	.87
Auditory hallucinations (specific type)	.71
Nonaffective verbal hallucinations	.76
Hallucinations daily	.62
DSM-III	
Delusions of control	.25
Thought broadcasting	.48
Thought insertion	−.02
Other bizarre delusions	.29
Nonpersecutory or jealous delusions	.59
Persecutory delusions plus hallucinations	.42
Auditory hallucinations (specific type)	.31
Nonaffective auditory hallucinations	.47
Yale system	
Delusions	.81
Auditory hallucinations	.86
Visual hallucinations	.44
Other hallucinations	.90
Paranoid ideation	.74
Widespread delusions	.28
Bizarre delusions	.66

Source: Endicott et al. (1982).

Whereas the RDC and Yale system showed good reliability for delusions and hallucinations generally, the first-rank symptoms of thought broadcasting, insertion, and withdrawal had relatively low κ values, as did visual hallucinations and widespread delusions. Application of the criteria for *DSM-III* fared much less well. Statistical tests of significance are not appropriate for deciding on an appropriate κ, but most investigators consider a κ of .5 or .6 to be acceptable and κ of .7 or greater to be good. Only one of the *DSM-III* criterion symptoms, nonpersecutory or jealous delusions, had a κ of .5 or greater. Other studies have also shed some doubt on the superior reliability of these more "objective" symptoms.

Reliability is but one indicator of the usefulness of criterion symptoms. There are other relevant questions we must ask about symptoms used in diagnostic criteria:

> Are they common enough to be present in enough patients so that the diagnosis can be made accurately?
> Are they specific to a given disorder, or do they occur in many different disorders?

The first issue, base rate, is particularly important. If a symptom or sign (e.g., thought withdrawal) occurs infrequently but is pathognomonic of a disorder (e.g., schizophrenia), then that symptom is useful diagnostically when it occurs, but it probably should not be incorporated as a criterion symptom in a standard nomenclature if its base rate is only 5%–10%. Criteria should be limited to those symptoms that occur relatively frequently.

The second question is even more difficult conceptually. In an ideal medical world, symptoms would occur only in specific disease types and would not cross over from one disease to another. But in the real medical world we have fever in pneumonia, tuberculosis, heat stroke, and alcohol withdrawal, not to mention hallucinations in schizophrenia, affective illness, delirium, and drug intoxica-tion. Searching for specific or pathognomonic symptoms is somewhat like looking for the philosopher's stone or the Holy Grail. Nevertheless, it is useful to ask ourselves how specific typical symptoms really are. This exercise is particularly useful for symptoms that have been argued to be specific to a particular disorder or pathognomonic of it.

Tables 6.5 and 6.6 address the issue of the base rate for first-rank symptoms. Koehler and associates have compared the frequencies with which these symptoms were rated in four different studies: their own study in Germany (Koehler, Guth, and Grimm, 1977), a study in England by Mellor (1970), a study of an American sample by Carpenter, Strauss, and Muleh (1973), and an international sample by Carpenter and Strauss (1974). The base rate for any single Schneiderian symptom was relatively low and tended to vary somewhat unnervingly from one center to another. The British were the most parsimonious in their recognition of first-rank symptoms, whereas the Germans were most lavish. Table 6.5 shows which first-rank symptoms were present in patients who had any type of first-rank symptoms, and Table 6.6 shows the overall base rate for all such symptoms in schizophrenia. Again, the numbers varied significantly, ranging from a low of 34% to a high of 72%. Americans appeared to vary among themselves regarding the frequency with which these symptoms were diagnosed, and the rates varied greatly even within a single method, such as examination of case records.

When first-rank symptoms were originally introduced to English-speaking psychiatrists, they were touted as being highly specific. If they were present, a diagnosis of schizophrenia was virtually certain. This view was widely accepted during the late 1960s and early 1970s, but in the mid-1970s a series of studies began to question the specificity of first-rank symptoms. Table 6.7 summarizes

Table 6.5. *Frequency distributions for 10 first-rank symptoms in Schneider-positive schizophrenic patients*

First-rank symptom	Germany: current study (*N* = 69)	England: Mellor (*N* = 173)	United States: Carpenter et al. (*N* = 53)	International: Carpenter & Strauss (*N* = 354)
Audible thoughts	1.5	11.6	20	28
Voices arguing	7.2	13.3	–	22
Voices commenting	24.6	13.3	–	10
Thought broadcasting	27.5	21.4	33	26
Thought insertion	17.4	19.7	20	23
Thought withdrawal	24.6	9.8	15	25
"Made" affect and "made" impulse	1.5	9.3	11	16
"Made" volition	20.3	9.2	28	29
Somatic passivity	37.7	11.6	17	–
Delusional perception	55.1	6.4	–	–

Source: Koehler et al. (1977).

Table 6.6. *Incidences of first-rank symptoms (FRS) in schizophrenia*

Type of study	Number of schizophrenics	% with FRS
Case record		
Huber (1967)	195	72
Taylor (1972)	78	28
Abrams & Taylor (1973)	71	34
Prospective		
Mellor (1970)	166	72
Carpenter et al. (1973)	103	51
Carpenter & Strauss (1974)	801	57

Source: Koehler et al. (1977).

three such studies, two by Taylor and Abrams (1973, 1975) and a third by Carpenter and associates (1973). These studies suggest that first-rank symptoms do occur in a substantial number of patients suffering from affective illness. Table 6.8 addresses another related issue, the specificity of delusions and hallucinations in general, with particular emphasis on mania. This table shows the rates at which delusions and hallucinations were observed in teams led by British and American investigators. Brockington, Wainwright, and Kendell (1980) found

Table 6.7. *Specificity of first-rank symptoms (FRS)*

	Sample	% with FRS
Taylor & Abrams (1975)	53 manics	8
Taylor & Abrams (1973)	52 manics	12
Carpenter et al. (1973)	66 manics	23
	119 depressives	16

Table 6.8. *Characteristic symptoms: specificity of delusions and hallucinations – percentages of manic patients affected*

	Brockington et al. (1980) (%)	Taylor & Abrams (1975) (%)
Delusions of persecution	47	42
Auditory hallucinations	25	48
Visual hallucinations	3	27
Olfactory hallucinations	6	15
Delusions of reference	50	–
Delusions of control	14	–
Thought broadcasting or insertion	9	–

high frequencies of delusions and hallucinations in mania, as did Taylor and Abrams (1973). These studies confirm what most clinicians know full well: Patients suffering from affective illness may have prominent symptoms of psychosis.

In Bleulerian terminology, delusions and hallucinations are "accessory symptoms," and Bleuler was among the earliest to argue that they should not be considered specific to schizophrenia. Bleuler did believe, however, that there were specific or pathognomonic symptoms that were fundamental to the illness. These are usually summarized in the Bleulerian "four A's," which dominated American thinking about schizophrenia throughout most of this century: association, affect, autism, and ambivalence. In particular, Bleuler believed that some form of the "characteristic disturbance in thinking" was present in each and every case.

As delusions and hallucinations began to return to prominence during the 1960s, the era when structured interviews and diagnostic criteria were being invented, the Bleulerian four A's were looked on with some contempt. Such symptoms were considered "soft" and subjective and therefore highly unrelia-ble. Clinicians could not agree on definitions of "associative loosening," and thought disorder was something that occurred inside the "black box" of the

Table 6.9. *Characteristic symptoms: reliability of types of thought disorder*

	κ
Negative	
Poverty of speech	.81
Poverty of content	.77
Alogia	.88
Positive	
Derailment	.83
Incoherence	.80
Illogicality	.80
Tangentiality	.58
Pressured speech	.89
Others	
Circumstantiality	.74
Perseveration	.74
Distractibility	.78
Clanging	.58
Neologisms	.39
Echolalia	.39
Blocking	.79

Source: Andreasen (1979b).

patient's head. "Affective flattening" was equally unreliable. Nevertheless, because formal thought disorder was a symptom of both historical and clinical significance, investigators eventually made attempts to develop improved definitions. A particularly useful approach was to look at subtypes or subcategories of an inclusive concept like "formal thought disorder" and encourage interviewers and raters to approach the concept through anatomic dissection (Andreasen, 1979a,b,c). One cannot know what a patient is thinking, but one can make inferences about thought by means of the objective behavior that occurs when the patient speaks. Many different kinds of abnormalities in language behavior can be observed. Clinicians can look for these various specific kinds of abnormalities and make a judgment as to whether or not the patient exhibits disorganized speech and, by inference, disorganized thinking.

The reliability of one such approach is summarized in Table 6.9. The definitions of various types of thought disorder in the glossary of *DSM-III* are based principally on this study. As Table 6.9 indicates, this approach to defining thought disorder leads to a high level of reliability. A different perspective on the issue of reliability is given by Table 6.10, which compares the frequencies with which various types of formal thought disorder (FTD) are observed in two different samples of schizophrenic patients. As Table 6.10 indicates, although

Table 6.10. *Comparison of TLC[a] abnormalities in two different samples of schizophrenics*

Variable	1979 sample (N = 45)		1983 sample (N = 50)		χ^2	p
	N	(%)	N	(%)		
I. *Negative FTD*						
Poverty of speech	13	(29)	15	(30)	0.04	.84
Poverty of content	18	(40)	14	(28)	1.53	.22
II. *Positive FTD*						
Pressure of speech	12	(27)	10	(20)	0.59	.56
Tangentiality	16	(36)	10	(20)	2.88	.09
Derailment	25	(56)	31	(62)	0.41	.52
Incoherence	7	(16)	15	(30)	2.78	.10
Illogicality	12	(27)	15	(30)	0.13	.72
III. *Other*						
Circumstantiality	2	(4)	8	(16)	3.36	.93
Loss of goal	20	(44)	15	(30)	2.12	.15
Perseveration	11	(24)	12	(24)	2.41	.12
Distractible speech	1	(2)	3	(6)	—[b]	.35

[a]Thought, language, and communication.
[b]Where no statistic is reported, Fisher's exact test was used.

these two samples were collected at different times and evaluated by different sets of raters, the simple fact that the definitions were standardized has led to nearly identical frequencies in the base rates for most of the symptoms. These findings provide relatively strong evidence that types of thought disorder can be defined reliably and have considerable stability. A similar stability was found for the ratings of types of thought disorder in manic patients.

On the other hand, as Table 6.11 indicates, contrary to conventional Bleulerian wisdom, the various types of formal thought disorder are not highly specific. Some types of thought disorder, such as poverty of speech, poverty of content, derailment, illogicality, tangentiality, pressured speech, and perseveration, occur with great frequency in schizophrenia. A discriminant-function analysis has indicated that a polythetic cluster of "negative" types of formal thought disorder versus "positive" formal thought disorder is quite useful in distinguishing between manic and schizophrenic patients, reliably differentiating them about 80% of the time (Andreasen, 1979c). Thus, although the mere presence or absence of formal thought disorder is not diagnostically useful, the patterning of types of thought disorder may be. Some types of thought disorder often discussed in textbooks of psychopathology, such as neologisms or blocking, tend to have very low base rates, at least in patients seen in relatively acute treatment

Table 6.11. *Characteristic symptoms: specificity of thought disorder*

	Schizophrenia (N = 45) (%)	Mania (N = 32) (%)	Depression (N = 37) (%)
Negative			
Poverty of speech	29	6	22
Poverty of content	40	19	17
Alogia			
Positive			
Derailment	56	56	14
Incoherence	16	16	0
Illogicality	27	25	0
Tangentiality	36	34	25
Pressured speech	27	72	6
Others			
Circumstantiality	4	25	31
Perseveration	24	34	6
Distractibility	2	31	0
Clanging	0	9	0
Neologisms	2	3	0
Echolalia	4	3	0
Blocking	4	3	6

Source: Andreasen (1979b).

Table 6.12. *Reliability and specificity of "negative symptoms"*

	Intraclass R	Depressives (N = 12)	Schizophrenics (N = 11)
Alogia	.877	1.08	2.00
Affective flattening	.696	2.83	3.32
Anhedonia	.731	3.50	3.50
Avolition	.763	3.25	3.55
Attentional impairment	.749	1.83	1.41

Source: Andreasen (1982a).

settings such as university hospitals. It should perhaps be noted that one of the more diagnostically useful types of formal thought disorder, poverty of speech, is omitted from the current criteria for schizophrenia and probably should be included in the future.

Since the writing and publication of *DSM-III,* investigators studying schizophrenia have become increasingly interested in a new grouping of symptoms that are quite similar to the older Bleulerian symptoms. Frequently these are referred to as "negative symptoms." Although investigators do not always agree which symptoms should be included under the heading of negative symptoms, one popular grouping is summarized in Table 6.12. These symptoms appear in a widely used rating scale, the Scale for Assessment of Negative Symptoms (SANS), that provides definitions, rating scales, and anchor points for the components of each of these negative symptoms (Andreasen, 1982a,b). As Table 6.12 indicates, these five negative symptoms are highly reliable. On the other hand, at least in a relatively small sample of depressives and schizophrenics, they are not particularly specific. Nevertheless, as a later discussion of the subtyping of schizophrenia indicates, when they are present in schizophrenic patients, they may have a high degree of predictive validity.

As the foregoing discussion indicates, there is no simple answer to the questions raised earlier:

> Which are the best symptoms to include in the diagnostic criteria for schizophrenia?
>
> How many symptoms should be required in order to yield maximum discrimination?
>
> Have delusions and hallucinations been overemphasized at the expense of other types of symptoms?

Investigators interested in schizophrenia need to do more work with relatively large samples of schizophrenics and affectively ill patients in order to determine which symptoms have the greatest discriminating power. Work completed to date does suggest, however, that delusions and hallucinations may be overemphasized in the present criteria. They appear to be no more reliable than other symptoms common in schizophrenia, such as types of thought disorder, affective flattening, or avolition, and they are also no more specific or pathognomonic. Indeed, the bulk of current evidence suggests that there is no single symptom of schizophrenia that can be considered pathognomonic or specific. Future research must attempt to identify a polythetic clustering of symptoms that have strong predictive validity. As is discussed in a later section in this chapter, much of the current evidence implies that Bleulerian or negative symptoms may actually have more promise in this area than do delusions and hallucinations or other positive symptoms.

THE AGE CRITERION

Kraepelin's dementia praecox was a disorder that occurred principally in young people; hence its name: a dementing illness that begins early in life. Bleuler later argued that schizophrenia might begin at any age, although he conceded that early ages of onset were more common. Later investigators have described a syndrome of involutional paraphrenia, characterized by a relatively late onset of suspiciousness and delusional thinking in individuals who frequently have experienced some sensory loss (Roth, 1955). The authors of *DSM-III,* while recognizing the likely validity of this syndrome, believed that it was probably a disorder different from the schizophrenia observed in younger individuals. Consequently, a criterion requiring onset prior to age 45 was included in order to make the category of schizophrenia more homogeneous.

Although the inclusion of an age criterion has led to considerable discussion, and the merits of this criterion are still not clear, I am not aware of any new evidence supporting or attacking the age criterion since the publication of *DSM-III*. At the moment, the principal argument in favor of this criterion is that it is more likely to isolate a biologically homogeneous group of patients in whom the search for some underlying cause or causes is more likely to be productive. Very likely, those patients who have an onset of psychotic symptoms late in life are developing their symptoms from a somewhat different biological and perhaps genetic substrate. On the other hand, those who criticize this criterion would argue that the null hypothesis has not been disproved. People who develop psychotic symptoms late in life and those who develop them at an early age may be genotypically nearly identical, differing only in their age of onset. Such critics would argue that the burden of proof that such patients are biologically different rests on the authors of *DSM-III*, who chose to write in an age criterion for the first time.

THE ORGANIC EXCLUSION CRITERION

The organic exclusion criterion states simply (and rather laconically and even obscurely): "Not due to any Organic Mental Disorder or Mental Retardation." Presumably this means that the ability to meet the previous five criteria, A–E, is not due to an organic mental disorder or mental retardation, but it might mean that schizophrenia can never be diagnosed in people who meet criteria for an organic mental disorder or mental retardation. Users of *DSM-III* tend to be confused on that issue, and it should be clarified by a clearer statement in the criteria themselves.

Some help is provided in the text, which points out that mentally retarded patients or patients with organic mental disorders may also have schizophrenia, although double diagnoses should be given only with great caution. In providing useful guidelines for distinguishing between organic mental disorders and schizophrenia, the text comes down hard on the absence of memory impairment or disorientation. There is an increasingly large body of evidence suggesting that schizophrenic patients may have significant short-term and long-term impairments in both disorientation and memory (Roth, 1955; Heaton, Baade, and Johnson, 1978; Chapman, 1979). Indeed, these may even be among the core symptoms of the disorder.

The problem with the organic criterion is worsened because of the old tradition of distinguishing between functional and organic disorders in psychiatry and in medicine generally. Although this distinction is not written into *DSM-III*, it is a tradition that is widespread and has been slow to die out. On the one hand there are functional disorders, which have no known organic basis, and on the other there are the organic disorders, which in psychiatry have typically included drug intoxications, deliria, and the various dementias. Although *DSM-*

III generally avoids discussions of etiology, it does state that the organic mental disorders are the only ones for which we know the causes. By implication, schizophrenia, affective illness, and the anxiety disorders have no known organic causes.

Yet, there is a vast amount of evidence in the research literature supporting various types of organic causes for all these disorders, making it difficult to explain the organic exclusion criterion sensibly to residents and medical students well versed in the lore of neurochemistry, neuropharmacology, neurophysiology, neuroendocrinology, and neuropathology. If schizophrenia or affective illness is not due to an organic mental disorder, then how does one explain the dopamine hypothesis, the neuropeptide data, the platelet MAO research, the CT scan research, the mechanisms of drug actions, and all that other stuff? To try to explain that those factors are not used to define organic mental disorders in the psychiatric "Talmud" can leave one feeling very foolish.

I am not sure what the solution is, but somehow in future editions, at least in the case of schizophrenia, we need to face squarely all the evidence that has accumulated to suggest that there is some type of brain abnormality in schizophrenia. This is supported by CT scan studies showing ventricular enlargement, occasional instances of cortical atrophy, and occasional examples of cerebellar atrophy (Johnstone et al., 1976; Weinberger et al., 1979, 1980; Andreasen et al., 1982). Various neuropathological findings have been noted in postmortem brains (Stevens, 1982). Further, repeatedly postmortem brain research has shown an increase in D_2 receptors, even in untreated patients (Crow et al., 1982). Neurophysiological studies point to possible deficits in the subcortical mechanisms monitoring attention, as manifested by abnormalities in eye tracking (Levin, 1982). Large numbers of neuropsychological studies have repeatedly demonstrated deficits in orientation, memory, attention, and language (Roth, 1955; Heaton et al., 1978; Johnstone et al., 1978; Chapman, 1979; Golden et al., 1980; Andreasen et al., 1982). The question is not whether or not there is likely some brain abnormality in schizophrenia, but rather where it is, whether or not different syndromes within schizophrenia are due to different localizations or mechanisms, and what mechanisms are involved.

SUBTYPING OF SCHIZOPHRENIA

After acute, latent, simple, and schizoaffective schizophrenia were removed from the subtypes of schizophrenia, *DSM-III* was left with a stripped-down, modernized (but actually quite traditionally Kraepelinian) approach to subtyping. The subtypes consist of disorganized (equivalent to hebephrenic), catatonic, paranoid, undifferentiated, and residual. This new approach has elicited a number of different criticisms.

One criticism relates to the overall grouping of subtypes of schizophrenia, as compared with the affective disorders. Whereas the affective disorders have been brought together and include both mild and severe forms, ranging from mania with mood-incongruent psychotic features to dysthymic disorder, the schizophrenias have been split asunder. Latent schizophrenia has not really disappeared, but instead has reappeared under the heading of personality disorders as schizotypal personality. On the other hand, among the affective disorders, what used to be a personality disorder has now been moved to the main category of affective disorders and is called cyclothymic disorder. There is a certain inconsistency in this approach. The inconsistency is all the more remarkable because there may be stronger genetic evidence for grouping schizotypal personality with the schizophrenias than for grouping cyclothymic personality with the affective disorders. In any case, symmetry and consistency – so much a feature of *DSM-III* most of the time – are missing in this instance.

Another problem with the subtypes arises because of the disappearance of simple schizophrenia. The critics of this subtype argued that it was rarely used, and others argued that an overdiagnosis of simple schizophrenia was one of the reasons that schizophrenia in general was overdiagnosed in the United States. Whichever of these opposing statements may be the case does not matter, because neither is well supported by research evidence. A more serious matter of concern is the resurgence of interest in mild or less florid types of schizophrenia that are manifested by prominent negative symptoms. The recent research on negative symptoms suggests that patients whose illness is characterized by loss of volition, inattention, poverty of speech, and the other "nonpsychotic" symptoms that characterize simple schizophrenia may have a syndrome with the worst prognosis – a syndrome that is refractory to treatment and sometimes is characterized by an underlying structural brain abnormality. Under the current *DSM-III* system, these patients cannot be diagnosed as having schizophrenia. Many of these patients may in fact have what is referred to as "residual schizophrenia," but this subtype can be diagnosed only when there is a clear past history of delusions and hallucinations. If old records are not available and the patient is too impaired to describe previous symptoms, then the clinician may be confronted with a patient who has a clear case of schizophrenia but cannot be diagnosed as such.

A final problem with the subtypes used in *DSM-III* is that they lack strong predictive value, at least given their current definitions. Once the acute-versus-chronic distinction is eliminated, the strongest data in the older research literature support subdividing schizophrenia simply into paranoid and nonparanoid subtypes. The definitions of the disorganized, catatonic, and undifferentiated types are not well supported by any substantial body of research data and have no clear construct or predictive validity. A fresh approach to the subtyping of schizophrenia should certainly be considered for *DSM-IV*.

One fresh approach that combines face, construct, and predictive validity is the subtyping of schizophrenia into positive, mixed, and negative (Crow, 1980). This approach was not proposed until after the publication of *DSM-III*, although hints of its utility appeared in earlier literature. Simply stated, this approach subdivides schizophrenics into two main groups, with mixed schizophrenia providing a bridge between the two extremes. The defining features of these subtypes appear in Table 6.12. Positive schizophrenia is characterized by a good premorbid adjustment, a relatively more acute onset, and prominent positive or florid symptoms during the active phase of illness. Positive symptoms include delusions, hallucinations, positive formal thought disorder, bizarre behavior, and perhaps catatonic features. Most of these symptoms respond well to treatment with neuroleptics, and consequently the prognosis for positive schizophrenia tends to be relatively good. The underlying abnormality in positive schizophrenia is hypothesized to be in the dopaminergic system, perhaps within the limbic system, or to involve some other type of neurochemical abnormality. This mechanism explains why it is more easily reversed through treatment with neuroleptics. On the other hand, negative schizophrenia is characterized by a poor premorbid adjustment, suggesting an underlying pathological process beginning relatively early in life. Its onset is insidious, and it is often difficult to date the precise time of onset. The most prominent symptoms are negative, including symptoms such as alogia, affective flattening, avolition, and anhedonia. These symptoms tend to respond poorly to treatment with neuroleptics, suggesting that the underlying mechanism may be some structural change in the brain that is irreversible. This possibility is supported by the fact that patients with negative symptoms are more likely to show ventricular enlargement on CT scans, and ventricular enlargement tends to be associated with negative symptoms.

Table 6.13 shows the results of one study that used this new approach to the subtyping of schizophrenia (Andreasen, 1982a,b). Fifty-two patients were subdivided into three groups using predefined criteria for subtyping based on the presence and prominence of positive versus negative symptoms. As that table indicates, patients with negative symptoms tend to have poor premorbid adjustment, poor employment records, ventricular enlargement as measured by CT scanning, and impairment in cognitive performance as measured by the Mini Mental Status examination. They differ from patients with positive schizophrenia on all these major validating variables. Thus, this newer method of subtyping has some initial support, and it is currently a major area of research in schizophrenia.

SUMMARY

Based on this review, one might predict that major changes will be made in the definitions of schizophrenia in *DSM-IV*. Although it is somewhat disheartening to note that the *DSM-III* definitions are already becoming outdated, it also is an observation that can be made with some pride. Our knowledge concerning schizophrenia progressed remarkably between *DSM-II* and *DSM-III*. Even greater strides probably will be taken between *DSM-III* and *DSM-IV*. In fact, the improvements made in *DSM-III*, such as careful attention to its definitions and an attempt to narrow them in a useful way, have probably permitted many of those advances to occur already. They should help to yield

Table 6.13. *Sociodemographic characteristics*

Variable	Type of schizophrenia			$p > F$	Duncan's follow-up test ($\alpha = .05$)
	Negative (N) ($N = 16$)	Mixed (M) ($N = 18$)	Positive (P) ($N = 18$)		
Age (yr, mean ± SD)	34.37 ± 14.49	27.28 ± 7.73	28.72 ± 8.09	.1241	
Education (yr, mean ± SD)	11.06 ± 1.48	12.06 ± 2.44	13.55 ± 2.04	.0032	P > M, N
Premorbid adjustment, Phillips scale (mean ± SD)	8.40 ± 3.58	5.50 ± 3.20	5.05 ± 1.95	.0047	N > M, P
Female (%)	50	44	50	.9336[a]	
Single (%)	63	67	78	.6175[a]	
Employed (%)	6	41	55	.0066[a]	P, M > N
VBR (mean ± SD)	8.48 ± 4.55	5.20 ± 2.93	4.59 ± 3.24	.0063	N > M, P
Mini Mental Status (mean ± SD)	20.60 ± 8.96	26.47 ± 3.00	28.67 ± 1.88	.0011	P, M > N

[a]Some observations are missing for some of the variables.

120

DSM-IV definitions that will be strongly tied to theories and facts concerning etiology and that will possess a stronger ability to predict important clinical variables such as response to treatment or long-term outcome.

REFERENCES

Abrams R, Taylor MA: First-rank symptoms, severity of illness, and treatment response in schizophrenia. Compr Psychiatry 14:353–355, 1973

Andreasen NC: Affective flattening and the criteria for schizophrenia. Am J Psychiatry 136:944–947, 1979a

The clinical assessment of thought, language, and communication disorders, I: the definition of terms and evaluation of their reliability. Arch Gen Psychiatry 36:1315–1321, 1979b

The clinical assessment of thought, language, and communication disorders, II: diagnostic significance. Arch Gen Psychiatry 36:1325–1330, 1979c

Negative symptoms in schizophrenia: definition and reliability. Arch Gen Psychiatry 39:784–788, 1982a

Negative v. positive schizophrenia: definition and validation. Arch Gen Psychiatry 39:789–794, 1982b

Andreasen NC, Smith MR, Jacoby CG, et al: Ventricular enlargement in schizophrenia: definition and prevalence. Am J Psychiatry 139:292–296, 1982

Astrup C, Noreik K: Functional Psychoses: Diagnostic and Prognostic Models. Springfield, Ill, Charles C Thomas, 1966

Bleuler E: Dementia Praecox or the Group of Schizophrenias. Translated by Zinkin J. New York, International Universities Press, 1950

Brockington IF, Wainwright S, Kendell RE: Manic patients with schizophrenic or paranoid symptoms. Psychol Med 10:73–83, 1980

Carpenter WT, Strauss JS: Cross-cultural evaluation of Schneider's first-rank symptoms: a report from the International Pilot Study of Schizophrenia. Am J Psychiatry 131:682–687, 1974

Carpenter WT, Strauss JS, Muleh S: Are there pathognomonic symptoms in schizophrenia? An empiric investigation of Schneider's first-rank symptoms. Arch Gen Psychiatry 28:847–852, 1973

Chapman LJ: Recent advances in the study of schizophrenic cognition. Schizophr Bull 5:568–580, 1979

Coryell W, Tsuang MT: DSM-III schizophreniform disorder: comparisons with schizophrenia and affective disorder. Arch Gen Psychiatry 39:66–69, 1982

Crow TJ: Molecular pathology of schizophrenia: more than one disease process? Br Med J 280:1–9, 1980

Crow TJ, Cross AJ, Johnstone EC, et al: Changes in D2 dopamine receptor numbers in post-mortem brain in schizophrenia in relation to the presence of the type 1 syndrome and movement disorder, in Brain Peptides and Hormones. Edited by Collu R et al. New York, Raven Press, 1982

Endicott J, Nee J, Fleiss J, et al: Diagnostic criteria for schizophrenia: reliabilities and agreement between systems. Arch Gen Psychiatry 39:884–889, 1982

Endicott J, Spitzer RL: A diagnostic interview: the Schedule for Affective Disorders and Schizophrenia (SADS). Arch Gen Psychiatry 35:837–844, 1978

Feighner JP, Robins E, Guze SB, et al: Diagnostic criteria for use in psychiatric research. Arch Gen Psychiatry 26:57–63, 1972

Fish FJ: Schizophrenia. Bristol, England, John Wright & Sons, 1962

Golden CJ, Moses JA, Zelazowski R, et al: Cerebral ventricular size and neuropsychological impairment in young chronic schizophrenics: measurements by the standardized Luria–Nebraska neuropsychological battery. Arch Gen Psychiatry 37:619–623, 1980

Hamilton M (ed): Fish's Clinical Psychopathology: Signs and Symptoms in Psychiatry. Bristol, England, John Wright & Sons, 1974

Heath RG, Franklin DE, Walker CF, et al: Cerebellar vermal atrophy in psychiatric patients. Biol Psychiatry 17:569–583, 1982

Heaton RK, Baade LE, Johnson KL: Neuropsychological test results associated with psychiatric disorders in adults. Psychol Bull 85:141–162, 1978

Hoenig J: Kurt Schneider and anglophone psychiatry. Compr Psychiatry 23:391–400, 1982

Huber G: Symptomwandel der Psychosen und Pharmakopsychiatrie, in Pharmakopsychiatrie und Psychopathologie. Edited by Kranz H, Heirich K. Stuttgart, Thieme, 1967

Johnstone EC, Crow TJ, Frith CD, et al: Cerebral ventricular size and cognitive impairment in chronic schizophrenia. Lancet 2:924–926, 1976

The dementia of dementia praecox. Acta Psychiatr Scand 57:305–324, 1978

Kendell RD, Cooper JR, Gourlay AJ, et al: Diagnostic criteria of American and British psychiatrists. Arch Gen Psychiatry 25:123–130, 1971

Koehler A, Guth W, Grimm G: First-rank symptoms of schizophrenia in Schneider-oriented German centers. Arch Gen Psychiatry 34:810–813, 1977

Kraepelin E: Dementia Praecox and Paraphrenia. Translated by Barkley RM, edited by Robertson GM. Edinburgh, E&S Livingstone, 1919

Levin S, Jones A, Stark L, et al: Identification of abnormal patterns in eye movements of schizophrenic patients. Arch Gen Psychiatry 39:1125–1130, 1982

Mellor CS: First-rank symptoms of schizophrenia, 1: the frequency in schizophrenics on admission to hospital; 2: differences between individual first-rank symptoms. Br J Psychiatry 117:15–23, 1970

Mellor CS, Sims AC, Cope RV: Change of diagnosis in schizophrenia and first-rank symptoms: an eight-year follow-up. Compr Psychiatry 22:184–188, 1981

Roth M: The natural history of mental disorder in old age. J Ment Sci 101:281–301, 1955

Schneider K: Clinical Psychopathology. Translated by Hamilton MW. New York, Grune & Stratton, 1959

Stevens J: Neuropathology of schizophrenia. Arch Gen Psychiatry 39:1131–1139, 1982

Taylor MA: Schneiderian first-rank symptoms and clinical prognostic features in schizophrenia. Arch Gen Psychiatry 26:64–66, 1972

Taylor MA, Abrams R: The phenomenology of mania: a new look at some old patients. Arch Gen Psychiatry 29:520–522, 1973

Acute mania: clinical and genetic study of responders and nonresponders to treatments. Arch Gen Psychiatry 32:863–865, 1975

Weinberger DR, Bigelow LB, Kleinman JE, et al: Cerebral ventricular enlargement in chronic schizophrenia: an association with poor response to treatment. Arch Gen Psychiatry 37:11–13, 1980

Weinberger DR, Torrey EF, Neophytides AN, et al: Structural abnormalities in the cerebral cortex of chronic schizophrenic patients. Arch Gen Psychiatry 36:935–939, 1979

Wing JK: A standard form of psychiatric Present State Examination (PSE) and a method for standardizing the classification of symptoms, in Psychiatric Epidemiology. Edited by Hare EH, Wing JK. London, Oxford University Press, 1970

Wing JK, Cooper JE, Sartorius N: The Measurement and Classification of Psychiatric Symptoms. Cambridge, Cambridge University Press, 1974

Wing JK, Nixon J: Discriminating symptoms in schizophrenia: A report from the International Pilot Study of Schizophrenia. Arch Gen Psychiatry 32:953–959, 1975

7 Paranoid disorders in DSM-III

A critical review

KENNETH S. KENDLER

This review has two major goals. The first is to critically examine the recent literature dealing with the diagnostic entity of paranoid disorder as defined by *DSM-III*. The second goal is to suggest, on the basis of this work, possible changes in the diagnostic criteria for this disorder. Compared with the other two major "functional" psychoses, schizophrenia and affective illness, paranoid disorders have been the focus of relatively little systematic research. Furthermore, most of the work conducted has focused on the validity of the specific diagnostic entities rather than examining the validity of specific diagnostic criteria for paranoid disorders. This focus of research is best understood from a historical perspective (Lewis, 1970; Kendler and Tsuang, 1981).

The major contribution of Emil Kraepelin to psychiatric diagnosis is widely regarded as his division of the functional psychoses into two major entities: dementia praecox (or schizophrenia) and manic-depressive insanity (or affective illness). Although it is less widely recognized, Kraepelin always believed that a third major functional psychotic illness existed that he termed paranoia (Kraepelin, 1904). Whereas the division between schizophrenia and affective illness has achieved wide acceptance, the independence of the diagnosis of paranoia has been more frequently questioned. As Kraepelin (1916) wrote, the diagnostic independence of paranoias

... may be assailed from two different points of view. First, we may ascribe them to chronic mania in the sense used by Specht. [Second] we may conceive of the possibility that paranoia represents a form of schizophrenic delusional system of especially slow and mild course; the paranoid tendency might be conceived as a minor sort of "latent schizophrenia."

In the years since Kraepelin's work, several eminent psychiatrists have indeed suggested that paranoia represents a mild form of schizophrenia (Kolle, 1931; Sakel, 1958; Schneider, 1959). For example, Sakel wrote that

the group paranoia presents an almost unified symptom complex which is so distinct from other schizophrenic pictures that for a long time it has been considered as a separate disease entity. It should be made perfectly clear at this point that paranoia is one manifestation of the schizophrenic disease process.

124

More rarely, it has been suggested that paranoid disorders are subforms of affective illness (Specht, 1901). The uncertainty regarding this group of disorders is reflected in the description of paranoid states in *DSM-II*. After suggesting how paranoid states may be differentiated from schizophrenia and affective illness, *DSM-II* states that "most authorities, however, question whether disorders in this group are distinct clinical entities and not merely variants of schizophrenia or paranoid personality." *DSM-III* contains the following similar statement in the description of paranoid disorders:

The boundaries of this group of disorders and their differentiation from such other disorders as severe Paranoid Personality Disorder and Schizophrenia, Paranoid Type, are unclear.

Given the uncertainty about the validity of the entire diagnostic category, it is understandable that research has focused primarily on the question whether or not the general syndrome of paranoid disorders is a nosologically distinct entity, rather than on finer points of specific diagnostic criteria. Therefore, this chapter initially reviews recent studies that have addressed the question of nosologic validity of paranoid disorders. Specifically, we evaluate three alternative hypotheses regarding the diagnosis of paranoid disorder. These hypotheses are that paranoid disorder should be considered (1) a subtype of schizophrenia, (2) a subtype of affective illness, or (3) an independent diagnostic entity unrelated to schizophrenia or affective illness.

A resolution of the diagnostic controversy over the paranoid disorders has been hindered by the variety of different terms that have been applied to this diagnostic grouping. However, because most investigators defined their study groups in a manner at variance with *DSM-III*, we use the terms originally proposed by each investigator. The general outline of their diagnostic approaches to this disorder is reviewed, but for specific details, the interested reader should consult the primary reports.

REVIEW OF RECENT LITERATURE ON THE NOSOLOGIC VALIDITY OF PARANOID DISORDERS

The most logical starting point for a review of "recent" research on the diagnosis of paranoid disorders is an article published in 1977 by Winokur entitled "Delusional Disorder (Paranoia)." That article described a systematic chart-review study from the records of the University of Iowa Psychopathic Hospital. Applying rigorous criteria that admitted only patients demonstrating any nonbizarre delusion without evidence of hallucinations, affective illness, inappropriate or flat affect, or organic brain syndrome, Winokur identified 29 patients. The following delusional themes were observed in descending order of frequency: persecution, reference, jealousy, somatic (hypochondriacal), and grandiose. Consistent with the previous descriptive literature, he found that the average age at onset for these patients was in the late thirties, considerably later than that found for schizophrenics in the same hospital. In contrast to schizophrenic patients, a substantially higher proportion of patients with delusional disorder had good premorbid work histories, were discharged to the community, and had good occupational outcomes. Of the 19 patients, only 2 had changes in their diagnoses at follow-up: one to schizophrenia and one to affective illness. Using family-history data from the hospital records, Winokur found a risk for "major chronic illness" in their first-degree relatives of 2.4%. From the diagnostic perspective of the Washington University school, "major chronic illness" is usually considered to be schizophrenia. However, of the four relatives of his probands with paranoia with "major chronic illness," two or three of them had paranoia themselves. Therefore, the better estimate for the risk for schizophrenia in these relatives was 0.6%–1.2%. The risk for affective illness (2.4%) in these relatives was also low.

The next significant report relevant to the *DSM-III* concept of paranoid disorder was a review that examined all previous empirical studies that had addressed the question of the nosologic validity of paranoia (Kendler, 1980a). Only 20 such studies were found. The definition used for this literature review was similar to that employed by Winokur and did not imply an insidiously developing chronic disorder. To differentiate this syndrome from cases of paranoid psychosis accompanied by prominent hallucinations, Kendler proposed the alternative term for this entity of "simple delusional disorder."

In addition to the report by Winokur noted earlier, only two other family studies were found that had examined the frequency of psychopathology in the relatives of patients with paranoia. Neither study showed an increased risk for affective illness in these relatives as compared with that expected from studies in the literature. However, both studies found a slightly increased risk for schizophrenia in these relatives over what might be expected in the general population (1.5%–2.4%, as compared with the usual rate in the population of 0.8%–1.0%). Nonetheless, these risks for schizophrenia were much lower than the 6%–15% risk for schizophrenia usually found in the first-degree relatives of schizophrenics.

Three studies were found that suggested that the premorbid personalities of patients with paranoia differed from that found for schizophrenics. Premorbidly, patients with paranoia were more frequently schizoid. When restricting studies to those that specified that hallucinations were absent in the cases of paranoia, only four studies were found that examined the demographic characteristics of patients with paranoia and schizophrenia. None were found that compared demographic factors for paranoia and affective illness. Compared with schizophrenics, the few available studies suggested that patients with paranoia had a later age of onset and more frequently were married. Evidence from one study suggested that immigration increased the risk for paranoia much more than for schizophrenia.

Two studies showed that patients with paranoia and those with schizophrenia performed differently on psychological tests such as the MMPI. Two other studies measuring simple biological variables (amenorrhea and blood pressure) found patients with paranoia to differ from schizophrenics.

In addition to the study by Winokur (1977), three reports examined the diagnostic stability of cases of paranoia. The largest and methodologically soundest of these reports were those of Retterstøl (1966, 1970). These reports found that a small but significant percentage (3%–22%) of patients with delusional disorders are found on follow-up to have developed schizophrenia. Two of the reports noted a few patients (3–6%) who developed affective illness during the follow-up period. Only the studies of Retterstøl provided useful information on other follow-up data. He found that at follow-up, a much higher percentage of patients with paranoid psychosis than those with schizophrenia were self-supporting. Furthermore, during the follow-up period, the percentage of patients with paranoid psychosis who were out of work for any prolonged period or had to be rehospitalized was much less than that for the schizophrenics.

The conclusion of Kendler's review was that relatively little systematic data existed that addressed the question of the nosologic validity of paranoia. Of the published studies, all but a few would not meet current criteria for methodologic rigor. The few studies that addressed the question of the relationship between paranoia and affective illness did not support a strong link between the two disorders. The information regarding the relationship between paranoia and schizophrenia was less clear-cut. Whereas a number of studies supported the independence of the two disorders, other studies were consistent with the hypothesis that at least some cases of paranoia are etiologically related to schizophrenia.

The next important study on paranoid disorders was published in 1980 by Watt and associates, based on the Aberdeen case register in northeast Scotland. The authors searched the case register for all cases diagnosed as paranoid state or paranoid schizophrenia. Of the 905 cases obtained, they randomly chose 300 for a case-record review. Applying criteria for "paranoid states" similar to those of Winokur and Kendler, except that hallucinations were permitted and the age of first presentation was required to be after 35, they found 24 patients meeting these criteria. The delusional themes found in these patients were, in descending order of frequency, persecutory, jealous, somatic (hypochondriacal), and grandiose. The peak ages of onset for their cohort were the late thirties and early forties. In the most important part of the study, the authors searched the case register for the 127 siblings of the 24 patients with paranoid state. Only one case of possible schizophrenia was found. The prevalence of schizophrenia in the siblings of their patients with paranoid state was therefore less than 1.0%, or indistinguishable from that expected in the general population. These authors concluded that in their register, paranoid state did not appear to have a familial relationship to schizophrenia.

Another family study of paranoid disorder was published by Kendler and Hays in 1981. The study was based on a cohort of 147 clinically diagnosed schizophrenics who had been intensively studied by Hays. In addition to detailed clinical evaluations, Hays had completed family histories on all these patients that included a review of available hospital records of relatives. Blind to family-history information, Kendler examined the case notes and symptom checklists for the 147 patients and rediagnosed 12 of them as having what he termed delusional disorder. Because of the manner in which the symptoms were recorded by Hays, the definition of delusional disorder in this report deviated somewhat from those in other publications. Only cases of persecutory delusions were included with or without hallucinations. Cases were excluded if they had any of the following "schizophrenic" symptoms: thought disorder, passivity symptoms, primary delusions, catatonic symptoms, or flattened affect. The blind was then broken, and the frequencies of various psychiatric disorders in the first-degree relatives or first- and second-degree relatives of the probands with delusional disorder and the remaining schizophrenic probands were compared. No significant differences were found between the two groups of relatives for the following disorders: bipolar affective illness, unipolar affective illness, sociopathy, anxiety disorder, or obsessional disorder. However, schizophrenia was much less frequent in the first-degree relatives of the delusional disorder probands (1 of 58 = 1.7%) than in the first-degree relatives of the schizophrenics (47 of 639 = 7.4%) (exact p = .076). When first- and second-degree relatives were considered, the difference became statistically significant (0.6% vs. 3.8%, respectively, exact p = .011). This study incorporated two important methodologic advances over previous family investigations of paranoid disorder. First, the study contained a comparison group of schizophrenic probands, so that the same diagnostic approach was used for the relatives of the schizophrenic and paranoid disorder probands. The interpretation of the study did not have to rely on literature values for the frequency of schizophrenia in the families of schizophrenics. Second, the diagnosis of the probands was made blind to knowledge of the relatives. However, two potential weaknesses of this study are also noteworthy. First, the cases of delusional disorder selected were not representative of all cases of this disorder, because for this study they had initially to have been considered as clinically schizophrenic. Second, the family histories were collected by the same investigator who examined the probands.

In a study published in 1981, Kendler, Gruenberg, and Strauss applied the adoption method in an attempt to clarify the genetic relationship between paranoid disorder and schizophrenia and the related "spectrum" disorders. This study was part of an independent analysis of the interviews with relatives from the Greater Copenhagen sample of the Danish Adoption Study of Kety and associates. For this particular report, the authors applied criteria for delusional disorder to these interviews and found that five cases met the criteria. Of these five patients, two had only somatic delusions, two had both persecutory and grandiose delusions, and one had referential and persecutory delusions. Whereas the schizophrenia spectrum disorders (here defined as schizophrenia plus schizotypal personality disorder as defined by *DSM-III*) were heavily concentrated in the biological relatives of the schizophrenic adoptees, none of the five patients with delusional disorder was biologically related to a schizophrenic. The distributions of the cases of schizophrenia spectrum disorder and delusional disorder in the relatives were significantly different. In this sample, delusional disorder did not appear to be part of the "schizophrenia spectrum."

In 1982, Munro published a monograph that summarized a number of years of work on the diagnostic entity he terms "monosymptomatic hypochondriacal psychosis" (MHP). This syndrome is conceptualized by Munro as clinically similar to classic paranoia, except that the delusions are of a somatic or hypochondriacal nature. Although his observations were uncontrolled, at least two of his conclusions warrant attention. First, the syndrome of MHP is not strikingly rare, although many cases present to nonpsychiatric physicians. Second, in at least some cases, a dramatic clinical response is seen to the antipsychotic drug pimozide. He makes a strong case that MHP is often overlooked as a diagnostic possibility and should best be regarded as a subtype of paranoia.

The last of the recently published studies that addressed the question of the nosologic validity of paranoid disorders is a review of published hospital admission records that compared the demographic characteristics of patients with paranoid disorder, schizophrenia, and affective illness (Kendler, 1982). Unlike the earlier review, this study was not restricted to reports in which the absence of auditory hallucinations in paranoid disorder was specified. Rather, diagnostic categories roughly equivalent to the *DSM-II* disorder of paranoid states were included, such as paranoid condition, paranoid reaction, paranoid psychosis, and so forth. Over 61,000 cases of admissions for paranoid disorder were contained in the 17 major reports or series of reports reviewed. The demographic characteristics of the admissions with paranoid disorder were compared with those found for schizophrenia and affective illness in the same report. A summary of the results is given in Table 7.1. Like affective illness, but unlike schizophrenia, paranoid disorder is predominantly an illness of middle-to-late adult life that usually occurs in individuals who are or have been married. Like schizophrenia, but unlike affective illness, paranoid disorder occurs more frequently in low socioeconomic classes and produces a poor chance for full recovery. Paranoid disorder occurs more frequently in immigrants than either schizophrenia or affective illness. From a demographic perspective, paranoid disorder was found to closely resemble neither schizophrenia nor affective illness.

Before concluding this section, it is important to note what has not been included. Many studies have examined "paranoia" or "the paranoid," which, unfortunately, have no direct relevance to paranoid disorders as defined by *DSM-III*. For example, Oxman, Rosenberg, and Tucker (1982) recently examined "The Language of Paranoia" using speech-content analysis. However, of their 24 "paranoid subjects," only 6 had true paranoia, the remainder having paranoid schizophrenia or delusions in the setting of affective illness or organic brain syndrome. Another author, Magaro, has published extensively on cognitive studies of "the paranoid." However, as he makes clear in a recent review article (Magaro, 1981), he uses this term to include (and consist mainly of) paranoid schizophrenics.

What can be concluded from the studies reviewed regarding the diagnostic validity of paranoid disorder? Little support is provided for the hypothesis that a substantial proportion of patients with paranoid disorder really suffer from a form of affective illness. There is no evidence that the risk for affective disorder

Table 7.1. *Demographic characteristics of delusional disorder (DD) compared with schizophrenia (S) and affective illness (AI)*[a]

Demographic variable	DD compared with S	DD compared with AI
Age at first admission	Much older	Similar
Sex	More likely female	More likely male
Marital status	More likely to be or have been married	Similar
Social background	Similar	More likely disadvantaged
Place of birth	More likely immigrant	More likely immigrant
Condition at discharge	Similar	Less likely recovered
Length of hospitalization	Somewhat shorter	Longer

[a] Based on information reviewed by Kendler (1982).

in the relatives of patients with paranoid disorder differs from that expected in the general population and is therefore much lower than that found in the relatives of patients with affective illness. Very few patients with paranoid disorder followed for long periods of time develop classic affective illness. Demographic data suggest that, compared with affective illness, paranoid disorder more frequently occurs in people from low socioeconomic groups and produces a much lower chance for full recovery.

Overall, the evidence is less conclusive regarding the relationship between paranoid disorder and schizophrenia. The majority of studies do not support the hypothesis that paranoid disorder is a subtype of schizophrenia. Although in several of the early family studies relatives of patients with paranoid disorder had an increased risk for schizophrenia, in no study did it begin to approach the increased risk commonly seen in relatives of schizophrenics. Furthermore, more recent family studies have shown no evidence of increased risk for schizophrenia in relatives of paranoid disorder patients. At least one earlier uncontrolled study suggested an increased frequency of paranoid disorder in the relatives of schizophrenics (Fisher, 1973); however, this result was not replicated in a more recent controlled investigation (Kendler et al., 1981). Compared with schizophrenics, patients with paranoid disorder tend to have a different premorbid personality and to have a substantially better prognosis. Unlike schizophrenia, paranoid disorder is predominantly a disorder of middle-to-late adult life, usually occurring in people who are or have been married. The evidence that supports most strongly a link between paranoid disorder and schizophrenia is the finding from several follow-up studies that 5%–20% of patients with paranoid disorder will eventually develop schizophrenia.

The most parsimonious explanation for these findings is that a small but nontrivial minority of cases of paranoid disorder are etiologically related to schizophrenia. It is in these cases that the paranoid disorder "syndrome" may represent a prodromal manifestation of a schizophrenic disorder. However, the evidence suggests that a substantial majority of cases of paranoid disorder have no close etiologic relationship to schizophrenia.

Although the evidence gathered to date can hardly be regarded as conclusive, the available data do support the hypothesis that the majority of patients suffering from paranoid disorder have a condition unrelated to either schizophrenia or affective illness. Therefore, it is worthwhile inquiring if information is available to evaluate any of the specific criteria for paranoid disorder contained in *DSM-III.*

EVALUATION OF SPECIFIC CRITERIA FOR PARANOID DISORDER IN *DSM-III*

Of the seven criteria for paranoid disorder in *DSM-III,* sufficient empirical evidence exists to evaluate only one of them. Four of the criteria (B, D, F, and G) contain the core exclusion criterion that has been implicit in diagnostic perspectives on this disorder since Kraepelin. If the delusion occurs in the setting of specific schizophrenic symptoms (criterion D), bizarre behavior or affect (criterion B), an affective syndrome (criterion F), or an organic brain disorder (criterion G), then paranoid disorder cannot be diagnosed. Few or no data exist specifically evaluating these exclusion criteria, because implicitly or explicitly they have been used in all studies of paranoid disorder or related diagnostic categories.

DSM-III provides two major inclusion criteria for paranoid disorder: "persistent persecutory delusions or delusional jealousy" (criterion A) and "duration of illness of at least one week" (criterion C). No specific information is available to evaluate the required duration of illness for paranoid disorder in *DSM-III,* although most studies of this group of disorders have required patients to be ill for longer periods of time. However, both historical precedent and some empirical data are available to evaluate the restriction of cases of paranoid disorder to individuals demonstrating only delusions of persecution or jealousy.

Since the time of Kraepelin, patients with erotic, grandiose, and referential delusions have been included within the category of paranoid disorder. Although Kraepelin was uncertain whether or not cases of paranoia with somatic delusions existed, the observations of Munro (1982) and others such as Retterstøl (1968) clearly establish the existence of such a syndrome. A small amount of empirical evidence is available to evaluate this criterion. First, Retterstøl (1968), Winokur (1977), Watt and associates (1980), and Kendler and associates (1982), in their studies of paranoid psychotic disorders, noted patients with somatic, referential, erotic, and/or grandiose delusions. None of these authors noted that such patients were fundamentally different from the more common patients displaying persecutory delusions. Second, data are available from three Scandinavian studies of paranoid psychotics and schizophrenics in which both the type of delusion at index admission and the long-term outcome were reported (Kendler, 1980b). If certain delusions are specific for paranoid disorders, then the presence of these delusions on admission ought to predict a nonschizophrenic outcome. Furthermore, if certain delusions are specific for schizophrenia, their presence on admission ought to predict a schizophrenic outcome. Across the three studies, there was no agreement that a given type of delusion could predict a schizophrenic or nonschizophrenic outcome. In fact, of the 17 comparisons, only one was significant at the .05 level. This difference, which could have occurred by chance, was opposite to that predicted by the *DSM-III* (i.e., that hypochondriacal delusions predicted a nonschizophrenic outcome). The available empirical evidence, albeit not extensive, does not support the criterion of *DSM-III* to include in paranoid disorders only those cases with delusions of persecution or jealousy.

POTENTIAL FUTURE DIRECTIONS

From a nosologic perspective, a number of important questions concerning paranoid disorders remain unanswered. We lack any good information about the relationship between chronic and acute paranoid disorders. Are they subforms of the same disorder, or do they represent fundamentally different syndromes? If the patients in a subgrouping of paranoid disorder go on to develop schizophrenia, is there any way such patients can be identified early in their courses? I have seen two such patients, and both were atypical in that the onset of their "paranoid disorder" was before age 25. Both progressed to a full schizophrenic syndrome within two years. Perhaps patients with an early age of onset of the "paranoid disorder" (i.e., before age 25) are particularly prone to develop schizophrenia. No mention has been made of criterion E for paranoid disorder in *DSM-III* (absence of prominent hallucinations). Clinically, cases occur with a syndrome indistinguishable from paranoid disorder, except for the presence of auditory hallucinations. Should these patients be considered cases of paranoid disorder? Two family studies of paranoid disorder had subgroups with auditory hallucinations (Watt et al., 1980; Kendler and Hays, 1981), and in neither did that subgroup differ from the patients without hallucinations. Such cases illuminate our lack of knowledge of the precise phenomenological boundary between paranoid disorder and paranoid schizophrenia. Lastly, we know little about the relationships among the different delusional syndromes seen in paranoia. Are there any fundamental differences between cases of paranoia with somatic delusions versus those with erotic or persecutory delusions?

Although this is not precisely in the purview of *DSM-III*, it is worth noting that whereas a great deal remains unknown about the diagnosis of paranoid disorder, even less is known about the treatment of the disorder. No controlled, double-blind study of any treatment modality for this disorder is currently available in the literature. Given that evidence is accumulating that Kraepelin was correct in regarding paranoid disorder as a distinct psychotic syndrome, our ignorance regarding the treatment of this disorder is increasingly difficult to justify.

SUMMARY

As compared with schizophrenia or affective illness, little systematic research has been conducted on paranoid disorder. Most of the available studies address the question of the nosologic validity of this condition. The evidence to date suggests that the majority of patients with paranoid disorder are best regarded as suffering from a separate psychotic disorder closely related to neither schizophrenia nor affective illness. A small subgroup of patients with paranoid disorder probably have a disorder etiologically related to schizophrenia. Of the seven criteria for paranoid disorder in *DSM-III,* empirical evidence is available to evaluate only one. Neither historical precedent nor the available data support the restriction of paranoid disorder in *DSM-III* to only patients displaying delusions of persecution or jealousy.

REFERENCES

Fisher M: Genetic and environmental factors in schizophrenia. Acta Psychiatr Scand [Suppl] 238:1–152, 1973

Kendler KS: The nosologic validity of paranoia (simple delusional disorder): a review. Arch Gen Psychiatry 37:699–706, 1980a

Are there delusions specific for paranoid disorders vs. schizophrenia? Schizophr Bull 6:1–3, 1980b

Demography of paranoid psychosis (delusional disorder): a review and comparison with schizophrenia and affective illness. Arch Gen Psychiatry 39:890–902, 1982

Kendler KS, Gruenberg AM, Strauss JS: An independent analysis of the Copenhagen sample of the Danish adoption study of schizophrenia, III: the relationship between paranoid psychosis (delusional disorder) and the schizophrenia spectrum disorders. Arch Gen Psychiatry 38:985–987, 1981

Kendler KS, Hays P: Paranoid psychosis (delusional disorder) and schizophrenia: a family history study. Arch Gen Psychiatry 38:547–551, 1981

Kendler KS, Tsuang MT: Nosology of paranoid schizophrenia and other paranoid psychoses. Schizophr Bull 7:594–610, 1981

Kolle K: Die Primare Verruckheit. Leipzig, Thieme, 1931

Kraepelin E: Clinical Psychiatry: A Textbook for Students and Physicians. Edited and translated by Diefendorf AR. New York, Macmillan, 1904

Kraepelin on "paranoid conditions." Translated by Gosline HI. Alienist and Neurologist 37:184–210, 1916

Lewis A: Paranoia and paranoid: an historical perspective. Psychol Med 1:2–12, 1970

Magaro P: The paranoid and the schizophrenic: the case for distinct cognitive style. Schizophr Bull 7:632–661, 1981

Munro A: Delusional hypochondriasis: a description of monosymptomatic hypochondriacal psychosis (MHP). Clarke Institute of Psychiatry Monograph Series, 5, 1982

Oxman TE, Rosenberg SD, Tucker, GJ: The language of paranoia. Am J Psychiatry 139:275–282, 1982

Retterstøl N: Paranoid and Paranoiac Psychoses. Springfield, Ill, Charles C Thomas, 1966

Paranoid psychoses with hypochondriac delusions as the main delusion: a personal follow-up investigation. Acta Psychiatr Scand 44:334–353, 1968

Prognosis in Paranoid Psychoses. Springfield, Ill, Charles C Thomas, 1970

Sakel M: Schizophrenia. New York, Philosophical Library, 1958

Schneider K: Clinical Psychopathology. New York, Grune & Stratton, 1959

Specht G: Ueber den pathologischen Affect in der chronischen Paranoia. Leipzig, Bohme, 1901

Watt JAG, Hall DJ, Olley PC, et al: Paranoid states of middle life: familial occurrence and relationship to schizophrenia. Acta Psychiatr Scand 61:413–426, 1980

Winokur G: Delusional disorder (paranoia). Compr Psychiatry 18:511–521, 1977

8 *Overview*

JOHN E. HELZER

Before summarizing the discussion generated by the chapters of Drs. Andreasen and Kendler, I would like to touch on a few additional issues relevant to schizophrenia and include a few remarks about schizophreniform disorder and brief reactive psychosis.

OUTCOMES IN VARIOUS PSYCHOTIC STATES

Table 8.1 shows data from Coryell, Tsuang, and McDaniel (1982) regarding outcomes in various psychotic states. As noted by Dr. Andreasen, the unimproved rate among schizophreniform cases after two to four years seems high at 56%. However, the recovery rates for schizophreniform disorder, in both Table 8.1 and Andreasen's Table 6.2, are about twice as high as those for schizophrenia, and in the latter table the proportion improved is nearly twice as great. This finding of a better outcome for *DSM-III* schizophreniform illness is consistent with findings in a sample of 125 consecutive admissions with functional psychosis from Netherne Hospital, first collected as part of the U.S./U.K. study and followed up an average of approximately six years later by Ian Brockington. Unlike the patients of Coryell and associates, these patients were selected after the advent of psychotropic drugs. Table 8.2 shows that although there is considerable similarity in the types of symptoms seen during the follow-up period, outcome for the schizophreniform patients is much better in terms of the proportion of the follow-up period spent in the hospital (12% versus 45% for the schizophrenics). Outcome is also better in terms of social functioning (a lower score on the social status scale indicates better adjustment) and in terms of the general outcome regression score, which takes into account various types of nonsymptom outcomes (Helzer, Brockington, and Kendell, 1981).

Another finding in both the study of Coryell and associates and the Netherne Hospital sample is relevant to a point made by Dr. Clayton in her discussion of the affective disorders concerning the occurrence of mood-congruent and mood-incongruent psychotic features in affective illness. In the Netherne series, we compared outcomes for patients diagnosed as having schizophrenia and schizophreniform disorder to outcomes for those diagnosed as having nonpsychotic depression, as well as depressives with mood-congruent and mood-

135

Table 8.1. *Short-term outcome by diagnosis: patients without somatic therapy*

		N	Outcome (%)		
			Recovered	Improved	Unimproved
A.	Nonpsychotic major depression	78	69.2	10.3	21.8
B.	Major depression with mood-congruent psychotic features	71	43.7	21.1	35.2
C.	Major depression with mood-incongruent psychotic features	43	32.6	32.6	34.9
D.	Schizophreniform disorder	48	16.6	18.8	64.6
E.	Schizophrenia	171	7.0	15.8	77.2

Source: Coryell et al. (1982).

incongruent psychotic phenomena. Table 8.3 shows the results, which are in fact similar to those of Coryell and associates shown in Table 8.1. Nonpsychotic depressives tend to have more affective symptoms and to have better (i.e., lower) general outcome regression scores. Those with mood-congruent psychotic symptoms tend to fall in an intermediate position (Brockington et al., 1982).

THE DURATION CRITERION IN THE *DSM-III* DEFINITION OF SCHIZOPHRENIA

It has been suggested that the six-months-of-illness criterion is inappropriate, that this is evidence of established chronicity and does not contribute to differentiation between the functional psychoses, because having been ill for six or more months is likely to predict poor outcomes for all psychotic patients. This issue has been examined elsewhere (Helzer, Kendell, and Brockington, 1983).

In the sample of 125 consecutive admissions for functional psychosis noted earlier, there were 69 patients who had been ill for six months or longer at index and 18 who met the full *DSM-III* criteria for schizophrenia. In Table 8.4 we show how these compare in predicting an outcome diagnosis of schizophrenia. It can be seen that the six-month criterion alone is quite overinclusive for predicting this outcome; the κ value and the specificity are low, and the false-positive rate is high. This same pattern was observed when a non-*DSM-III* diagnosis of schizophrenia was used as the outcome criterion. In addition, outcomes were significantly worse for those meeting the full criteria when we examined such follow-up measures as social functioning, employment, and the occurrence of psychotic versus affective symptoms during the follow-up period (Helzer et al., 1983). Because many of those who met the six-month-illness criterion went on to have good outcomes, it does not seem inherently tautological to include the duration of illness as part of the definition of schizophrenia (i.e.,

Table 8.2. *Comparison of DSM-III schizophrenia and schizophreniform disorder*

	Pathologic symptom scale scores							General outcome measures		
	N	Manic	Passivity	Auditory hallucination	Delusion	Persecution	Defect	Time in hospital (%)	Combined social status score	Outcome regression score
Schizophrenia	19	3.4	18.0	15.8	38.7	26.0	26.1	46	54	2.53
Schizophreniform disorder	7	13.0	20.4	13.4	34.0	20.9	8.1	12	34	1.46
p	–	.04	NS	NS	NS	NS	NS	.02	.03	.02

Source: Helzer et al. (1981).

Table 8.3. Outcome during six-year follow-up for Netherne series patients with depression diagnosed according to DSM-III

Outcome variable[a]	DSM-III diagnosis		
	Major depression (nonpsychotic) (N = 45)	Depression with mood-congruent psychotic features (N = 11)	Depression with mood-incongruent psychotic features (N = 14)
Psychopathology scale scores (mean)			
Passivity experience	1.4	1.8	10.2[b]
Auditory hallucinations	0.6	7.6[c]	25.0[b]
Delusion formation	8.2	26.2[d]	37.8[e]
Ideas of persecution	7.2	22.4[d]	36.4[e]
Defect state	1.6	0.5	5.2[c]
Depression	28.4	43.9[c]	27.1
Manic symptoms	14.7	24.6	3.4[c]
Psychopathology discriminant score	+1.58	+1.51	−0.09[e]
Diagnosis (number of patients)			
At least one schizoaffective episode	2	7[e]	8[e]
Final diagnosis of schizophrenia	4	1	10[e]
Final diagnosis of bipolar affective disorder	13	6	1
General outcome			
Number of patients who failed to recover from index episode	4	2	7[d]
Mean percentage of follow-up period spent in hospital	17.1	15.3	11.4[d]
Mean general outcome regression score	1.38	1.49	1.60

[a]The statistical comparisons between patients in each of the two categories of psychotic depression and the 45 patients with nonpsychotic depression are shown here.

[b]$p < .001$.

[c]$p < .05$.

[d]$p < .01$.

[e]$p < .0001$.

Source: Brockington et al. (1982). Am J Psychiatry 139:1022–1027, 1982. Copyright 1982, The American Psychiatric Association. Reprinted

Table 8.4. *Values of DSM-III schizophrenia criteria (N = 18) versus six or more months of illness (N = 69) in predicting diagnostic outcome*

Index condition	Raw agreement (%)	κ	Sensitivity (%)	Specificity (%)	No. (%) of false-negative cases	No. (%) of false-positive cases
Predicting outcome diagnosis of schizophrenia						
Index DSM-III schizophrenia	75	0.24	31	91	22 (21)	8 (44)
Ill ≥ 6 months at index	59	0.15	78	52	7 (13)	43 (62)
Predicting final diagnosis of schizophrenia						
Index DSM-III schizophrenia	75	0.36	37	99	29 (28)	1 (6)
Ill ≥ 6 months at index	62	0.24	74	55	12 (23)	34 (49)
Predicting outcome DSM-III diagnosis of schizophrenia						
Index DSM-III schizophrenia	92	0.69	70	96	6 (6)	4 (22)
Ill ≥ 6 months at index	57	0.07	90	50	2 (4)	50 (72)

Source: Helzer et al. (1983).

139

this does not appear to be prima facie evidence of established chronicity). We saw from the earlier analysis of schizophreniform cases that the cross-sectional schizophrenic symptoms, as required by *DSM-III*, do not necessarily predict a schizophrenic outcome, and we see from this latter analysis that psychotic illness for six months is not a strong predictor. It seems to be the combination of symptoms and duration that is predictive of long-term schizophrenic illness.

BRIEF REACTIVE PSYCHOSIS

There does not seem to have been much research done yet regarding this specific category. Scandinavian investigators have perhaps written the most about the "reactive psychoses," but this has not necessarily been the *DSM-III* definition. Some Scandinavian investigators believe that the *DSM-III* definition of brief reactive psychosis is too narrow because it relies so heavily on duration (i.e., if the psychosis lasts more than two weeks, the diagnosis has to be changed). The feeling is that there are many cases that meet the intent of the *DSM-III* definition and would otherwise be classified as brief reactive psychosis but for the duration of illness. In these cases, the illness persists for several weeks, sometimes several months, but does completely and permanently remit (N. Retterstøl, pers. commun.). Conceptually it is awkward to have to think of changing the diagnosis as an illness persists from two weeks to three. However, as already discussed for schizophreniform and schizophrenic illnesses, adding some duration criterion may greatly enhance prediction of long-term outcome. Any duration criterion is to a degree arbitrary, and the two-week criterion for brief reactive psychosis may be too short, but it would appear at this time that the necessary studies to answer this particular question have yet to be done.

SUMMARY OF THE DISCUSSION OF ANDREASEN'S AND KENDLER'S CHAPTERS

In her formal presentation, Dr. Andreasen discussed the appropriateness of the exclusionary age criterion for *DSM-III* schizophrenia. During the discussion there was a focus on the opposite end of the age spectrum, namely, persons who are very young at onset of the illness. It was asked if early-onset schizophrenia should be conceptualized as a separate illness, an atypical form, or the same illness modified by developmental factors. It was pointed out that the Isle of Wight studies had shown a correlation between early onset of schizophrenia and poor outcome. However, this is true in other illnesses as well and would not necessarily be a compelling reason to classify early-onset cases differently.

Two points were raised concerning the duration criterion for schizophrenia. The rationale for a duration of six months was discussed by Dr. Andreasen, but it was pointed out that duration is obviously a continuous variable. It would be interesting to know if some lesser duration would be just as predictive of poor outcome as six months seems to be. For example, it would be useful to follow first-admission patients who have had index episodes of various lengths to see how this variable is related to outcome, a replication of Astrup and Noreik's work. There seems to be an impression that a duration of less than six months might be as predictive of poor outcome, but few specific data are available as yet. One methodological point was raised concerning the use of the *DSM-III* criteria to define study samples. In selecting patients for study, it is important to make a distinction between those who have not yet been ill for six months but are still symptomatic and those who have recovered from illness within a six-month period. Lastly, the point was made that the duration criterion also has utility in the differentiation of mania and schizophrenia. Cross-sectionally, manic patients can be quite psychotic, but a six-month continuous duration of active psychotic symptoms is unusual in mania, and this criterion helps prevent a misdiagnosis of schizophrenia in manic patients.

One additional point was made concerning the change in scope of the diagnosis of schizophrenia from a relatively broad definition in *DSM-II* to a more restrictive definition in *DSM-III*, the latter implying chronic illness and poor outcome. It was pointed out that according to *DSM-III*, schizophrenia is an illness from which, by definition, one cannot recover. This is true because criterion C specifies that some sign of the illness must be present at the time of evaluation. If the subject is completely free of all sign of illness, the diagnosis cannot be given regardless of having met the full criteria at some earlier time.

One discussant supported the suggestion mentioned by Helzer that two weeks of illness may be too restrictive a criterion for brief reactive psychosis. Some data from a study in progress were mentioned in which a few cases had been found of a psychotic illness that appeared to be reactive to precipitating circumstances, but that lasted up to three to four months. However, several of these patients seemed to have had relapses of illness some years later, suggesting an underlying illness diathesis rather than a purely "reactive" illness. Furthermore, it was not clear if the "precipitating circumstances" in these cases were of the same order of severity as those specified by *DSM-III* (i.e., serious enough to "evoke significant symptoms of distress in almost anyone!").

During the discussion, the question arose again whether paranoid disorders should be classified with the schizophrenias rather than separately. In addition to Dr. Kendler's formal review of this issue, it was noted in the discussion that in at least one more study, the morbid risk of schizophrenia in family members of paranoid schizophrenics was in the same range as (or perhaps even higher than) that in the family members of other schizophrenics, but the morbid risk for schizophrenia in the family members of probands with paranoid illness was much lower. This would argue in favor of continued separation of these two diagnostic groups. One confounding problem here that was pointed out is the differential in the ages of onset for paranoid illness versus schizophrenia, but this is hard to control for, because late-onset cases of schizophrenia are relatively rare. It was noted in the discussion that paranoid disorder might be an attenuated form of schizophrenia, but this is not the most plausible hypothesis, and current evidence seems to favor maintaining the diagnostic distinction between these two categories as *DSM-III* has done.

CONCLUSION

For the most part, recommendations from this segment of the conference were in the form of suggestions for future investigations rather than for specific changes in the *DSM-III* criteria. What little data are available suggest that schizophrenia and schizophreniform disorder, together with nonpsychotic, mood-congruent, and mood-incongruent psychotic depressions, may form a useful continuum in terms of outcome. This must be considered only tentative because of the scarcity of appropriate follow-up data, but this preliminary lead should be pursued, and one practical issue should be examined: the interrater reliability of the judgment about mood congruence. Other areas in which more research is needed are the six-month criterion for schizophrenia and the two-week criterion for brief reactive psychosis. Are these two duration criteria too restrictive? Should the former be shortened and the latter lengthened? There seems to be more evidence at present that the two-week criterion may be too short, but these are both areas for critical review and future study.

More work is needed regarding interrater reliability and the predictive utility of negative versus positive symptoms in schizophrenia and how these might be optimally combined in a subtyping scheme. The limitations of the current subtype concept were pointed out, and observations about negative and positive symptoms might form the basis of a useful replacement.

Another suggestion, arising in Dr. Kendler's review, is to consider including more delusions, such as somatic and certain types of referential delusions, in the definition of the paranoid disorders. There is somewhat more current evidence in favor of this change, and it is something that might be contemplated in a revision of *DSM-III*.

The one item that does seem to be in need of change in the next *DSM-III* revision is the organic exclusion criterion for psychoses. The accumulating evidence that patients with "functional" psychoses may have certain consistent types of brain abnormalities renders this exclusion difficult at the present time and may render it obsolete in the near future. This is a problem not only in the nonaffective psychoses but also in the affective disorders and even the anxiety disorders. No specific suggestion for how these changes might be made was forthcoming, but the wording of this exclusion item should be altered so that the possibility of an organic basis for these illnesses is recognized in the specified criteria.

REFERENCES

Brockington IF, Helzer JE, Hillier VF, et al: Definitions of depression: concordance and prediction of outcome. Am J Psychiatry 139:1022–1027, 1982

Coryell W, Tsuang MT, McDaniel J: Psychotic features in major depression: is mood congruence important? J Affect Dis 4:227–236, 1982

Helzer JE, Brockington IF, Kendell RE: Predictive validity of DSM-III and Feighner definitions of schizophrenia: a comparison with Research Diagnostic Criteria and CATEGO. Arch Gen Psychiatry 38:791–797, 1981

Helzer JE, Kendell RE, Brockington IF: Contribution of the six-month criterion to the predictive validity of the DSM-III definition of schizophrenia. Arch Gen Psychiatry 40:1277–1280, 1983

PART III

Organic mental disorders, substance-use disorders, and psychosexual disorders

Part III encompasses three rather disparate entities: organic mental disorders, substance-abuse disorders, and psychosexual disorders. Perhaps the only common element these three topics have is that they bring the psychiatrist in contact with other physicians, agencies, and society more than do most psychiatric conditions. Although these diagnostic entities represent common clinical problems, except in specific portions of the psychiatric community, they do not seem to attract as much psychiatric intellectual enthusiasm as do the affective disorders and schizophrenia. Whether or not this is due to the fact that the conditions included in these diagnostic groups have clear-cut symptoms and specific causes and allow little room for speculation remains to be seen.

The contributors to Part III were selected primarily because they are experts on these topics, and most were not members of the original *DSM-III* task force. The latter factor was deemed important because it was believed that they might give a more objective view than would authors with a more proprietary interest. However, two of the authors surveyed many of the people who were on the *DSM-III* committee and also other "experts" in the field. Basically, with some minor changes, almost all "experts" found *DSM-III* usable and in fact quite good, but even so the suggestions for improvements in *DSM-III* and the conceptualizations presented raise serious questions for those immersed in the process of nosology and classification.

Gary Tucker

9 *DSM-III organic mental disorders*

MICHAEL ALAN TAYLOR

DSM-III (American Psychiatric Association, 1980) is praised primarily for its use of explicit, operationally defined diagnostic criteria. Often overlooked, but of more fundamental and long-lasting importance, is *DSM-III*'s reorganization of a nosology of mental illness that had been in existence since the nineteenth century. Neuroses and psychophysiologic (or psychosomatic) disorders have been discarded as unacceptably biased concepts, and organic brain syndromes and affective disorder are no longer, by definition, psychoses. These nosologic changes are supported by a broad literature and further justified by the need to produce a classification system of acceptable reliability based on diagnosis according to shared descriptive clinical features. The goal: reducing idiosyncratic decision making by individual practitioners, a major source of past diagnostic unreliability in psychiatry (Skodol and Spitzer, 1982).

The *DSM-II* category of organic brain syndromes (OBS) (American Psychiatric Association, 1968) has also undergone significant internal alteration, although conceptually its relationship to other clinical categories remains unchanged. This chapter briefly reviews these intracategory alterations, discusses the conceptual difficulties of the OBS category, now termed organic mental disorders (OMD), and suggests changes in the concept and its definitions.

DSM-II

DSM-II categorized OBS as mental disorders caused by diffuse brain dysfunction that leads to deficits in orientation and intellectual functioning (e.g., memory, judgment, comprehension) and to changes in affective modulation (lability or shallowness). Despite evidence to the contrary (Slaby and Wyatt, 1974; Torack, 1978; Benson, 1982), acute onset and reversibility were considered synonymous with delirium, and insidious onset and irreversibility were considered synonymous with dementia. Regional hemispheric syndromes (e.g., frontal, temporal, parietal) and focal dysfunction were ignored. Severity and psychosis were linked by the definition that OBS with psychosis was characterized by dysfunction of sufficient severity to interfere grossly with the ability to perform activities of daily living. Thus, patients with mild cerebral dysfunction, hallucinations, and delusions could be classified nonpsychotic, and patients with severe cerebral dysfunction and no signs of hallucinations or delusions were classified psychotic.

DSM-III OMD

Based on a large body of data, the linkage between psychosis and severity of illness is eliminated in *DSM-III*. Acute onset and reversibility are no longer considered synonymous with delirium, and insidious onset and irreversibility are no longer considered synonymous with dementia. The inclusion of the amnestic syndrome recognizes for the first time circumscribed symptom clusters, and categories such as organic personality disorder can be used to label patients who have behavioral changes secondary to focal brain disease. In total, 10 subcategories are subsumed under the heading OMD. These include dementia and delirium; organic amnestic syndrome; hallucinosis; delusional, affective, and personality syndromes; intoxications and withdrawal states; and a residual/atypical syndrome.

DSM-III further makes a fundamental distinction between OBS and OMD. It states:

"Organic brain syndrome" is used to refer to a constellation of psychological or behavioral signs and symptoms without reference to etiology (e.g., Delirium, Dementia); "organic mental disorder" designates a particular organic brain syndrome in which the etiology is known or presumed (e.g., Alcohol Withdrawal Delirium, Multi-infarct Dementia). [p. 101]

An OMD is diagnosed by first "recognizing the presence of one of the Organic Brain Syndromes" and then "by demonstrating, by means of the history, physical examination, or laboratory tests, the presence of a specific organic factor judged to be etiologically related to the abnormal mental state." An escape clause, however, permits "under certain circumstances . . . a reasonable inference of an organic factor . . . from the clinical features alone, in which case only step [one is] necessary for diagnosis" (p. 101).

The definition and conceptualization of OMD are of particular importance because their application transcends the boundary of the category. The diagnostic criteria for *DSM-III* schizophrenia, affective disorder, paranoid disorder, and other psychotic disorders include in each case the injunction "not due to any organic mental disorder." To be able to diagnose these conditions, the clinician must first exclude OMD, and this cannot be done unless OMD is clearly defined. In its present form, the OMD category has significant intracategory and intercategory defects, which makes its application problematic and will require remediation if OMD is to be an optimally useful part of psychiatric nosology.

INTRACATEGORY PROBLEMS WITH *DSM-III* OMD

Although patients with mental disorders secondary to circumscribed lesions can be included in several *DSM-III* OMD subcategories, these are limited to either an amnestic syndrome or the traditional "functional" syndromes (e.g., schizophrenia, affective disorder, personality disorder) secondary to identifiable brain disease. There are, however, other clearly delineated conditions observed in psychiatric settings that can now only be classified as atypical or mixed OBS. These include a variety of psychomotor states and syndromes associated with circumscribed regional cortical lesions. It is important for the clinician to be able to identify these conditions, because there are specific treatments for the psychomotor states (Delgado-Escueta, Treiman, and Walsh, 1983), and regional cortical syndromes reflect a wide variety of pathological conditions, some life-threatening (e.g., tumors) and some remedial (e.g., tumors, arteriovenous malformations, stroke) (Scheinberg, 1981).

PSYCHOMOTOR STATES

Behavioral changes associated with epilepsy are common and can directly relate to the seizure itself (i.e., the ictal state), to the prodromal (hours to weeks preceding the seizure) or postictal (hours to days subsequent to the seizure) periods, or to the interictal period. Because the seizure itself rarely lasts more than 15 minutes and is most often less than a minute, the behaviors that lead to psychiatric hospitalization or treatment are typically nonictal (Fenton, 1981b; Strub and Black, 1981; Benson and Blumer, 1982).

Prodromal symptoms usually develop a few hours or days prior to the seizure. Irritability and dysphoria are most common, although psychosis can occur. Prodromal syndromes usually improve following the seizure. Observation of this relationship contributed to the development of induced seizures for treatment of psychiatric disorders (Meduna, 1938; Trimble, 1982).

Ictal phenomena requiring psychiatric treatment are most commonly seen in patients with complex partial seizures. Another term used to identify these syndromes is psychomotor epilepsy. Temporal-lobe epilepsy (TLE) is the most common type of psychomotor epilepsy. Epilepsy arising in other cortical areas, particularly the frontal lobes, can also produce complex psychomotor phenomena. Petit mal status has also been reported to produce a confusional psychosis that can last for days or weeks. However, any chronic generalized seizure disorder can eventually result in psychosis (Beard and Slater, 1962; Davidson and Bagley, 1969; Toone, 1981; Trimble, 1982).

Psychomotor, or complex partial seizure, syndromes are associated with some alteration in consciousness. The alteration can be extremely subtle, during which patients may appear only slightly hesitant or somewhat distracted in their responses. Perplexity, oneiroid states, syndromes characterized by disorientation and agitation, and complex behavior patterns during which the patient is unresponsive to all but the most intense stimulation (e.g., shouting, physical restraints) can also occur. Absence phenomena are also observed, but these tend to be longer and less frequent than those of petit mal and more gradual in onset and termination. Psychomotor episodes tend to be short in duration, frequent, and, for a given patient, similar in form and content from one episode to another (Beard and Slater, 1962; Davidson and Bagley, 1969; Fenton, 1981b;

Toone, 1981; Benson and Blumer, 1982; Koella and Trimble, 1982; Trimble, 1982).

Virtually every psychopathological feature has been reported during psychomotor states. The classic psychomotor ictal presentation is that of temporal-lobe epilepsy and is characterized by automatic, repetitive behaviors termed automatisms that can take the form of complicated acts. Some reported automatisms are laughing, weeping, sobbing, raging, screaming, lip smacking, chewing, swallowing, rubbing, scratching, grimacing, assuming odd postures, dressing and undressing, continual repetition of the same phrases, getting something to eat or drink, fugue states, and violent behavior. Other repetitive ictal behaviors are coughing, sneezing, yawning, hiccupping, gagging, vomiting, and belching. During the seizure, the patient may appear unblinking, wide-eyed, expressionless, or staring ahead or to one side. Partial or complete loss of posture may occur, as well as pupillary dilation, pallor or flushing, perioral cyanosis, salivation, sweating, tachycardia, hypertension, gastrointestinal motility changes, incontinence of urine (rarely of feces), respiratory rate changes, gasping, or even apnea.

Associated experiences include alteration in mood, forced thinking, feelings of impending doom and anxiety, sensations of false familiarity (déjà vu) or unfamiliarity (jamais vu), depersonalization and derealization, oneiroid states, visual distortions (macropsia, micropsia), hallucinations (pleasant and unpleasant) in any sensory modality (particularly visual, olfactory, and gustatory), autoscopic phenomena (hallucinating oneself), and abdominal pains or a feeling of abdominal emptiness (hollowness) that "rushes" up into the subcostal area (sometimes through the chest and into the head). These episodes usually are short in duration and always are followed by some degree of amnesia for the event and some postictal fatigue, sleepiness, confusion, or depression (Beard and Slater, 1962; Davidson and Bagley, 1969; Fenton, 1981b; Toone, 1981; Benson and Blumer, 1982; Koella and Trimble, 1982; Trimble, 1982). Although most ictal phenomena are not lateralizable to the side of the seizure focus, several studies (Hecaen, 1962; Gainotti, 1972; Ahern and Schwartz, 1979; Sackeim et al., 1982) have demonstrated that sudden, transient, shallow expressions of sadness or tearfulness are associated with nondominant-hemisphere lesions, whereas sudden, transient, shallow expressions of euphoria or laughter are associated with dominant-hemisphere lesions.

Other ictal syndromes include the following: There is a parietal-lobe syndrome characterized by feelings that body parts are unusually heavy, dead, as if made of metal, with painful tingling similar to electrical shocks, unpleasant coldness, burning feelings, feelings that an arm or leg is moving on its own, experiences of body parts in new locations (e.g., a hand in one's abdomen), and/ or altered attitude toward pain (painful stimuli become pleasant, so that self-inflicted painful injuries may result). These experiences may lead to secondary delusional ideas of being possessed, being controlled by an outside force, or being dead (Critchley, 1953). There is a frontal-lobe syndrome characterized by speech arrest, periods of shallow euphoria and depression, irritable outbursts, dysphoria, posturing, diminished wakefulness, hyperactivity, disorientation, uncontrollable confabulations, and lack of self-control (Teuber, 1964; Luria, 1969; Hecaen and Albert, 1975; Lishman, 1978; Dammasio, 1979).

Postictal behaviors usually last only a few minutes, but can extend to several hours or days. These behaviors are more variable and complex than most ictal phenomena and include confusion, orienting behaviors (looking about, walking around, absent-minded talking, straightening up one's clothes), sleepiness, irritability (including violent rage behavior), sexual arousal, sexual behaviors that usually are socially inappropriate, and undressing. Confusional or delirious states lasting hours or days can occur, usually after grand mal seizures. Hallucinations and delusions can also occur. These postictal psychoses characteristically fluctuate in severity from day to day or from hour to hour. They are occasionally mistaken for schizophrenic psychoses, but a history of seizurelike phenomena or episodes, an alteration in consciousness, or fluctuation in symptom severity should alert the clinician. The postictal-period EEG findings in these patients usually will be abnormal, characterized by diffuse slow activity (Beard and Slater, 1962; Davidson and Bagley, 1969; Fenton, 1981b; Toone, 1981; Benson and Blumer, 1982; Koella and Trimble, 1982; Trimble, 1982).

Patients with petit mal epilepsy may also experience a prolonged subacute delirious state with altered consciousness, termed petit mal status. These episodes, lasting from hours to several weeks, are characterized by confusion or perplexity, hallucinations, vague delusional ideas, rambling speech, and agitation. The EEG characteristically shows a spike-wave pattern (Roger, Lob, and Tassinari, 1974; Ellis and Lee, 1978; Marsden and Reynolds, 1982).

Interictal behavioral changes are varied (Davidson and Bagley, 1969; Fenton, 1981a,b; Benson and Blumer, 1982; Koella and Trimble, 1982; Trimble, 1982), occur in 40% to 60% of epileptics, and do not predict location of lesion or type of seizure disorder. Many nonepileptic psychiatric patients also exhibit these behaviors. Excluding behaviors associated with mental retardation or developmental lag, the most common behavioral changes are those in personality. These personality changes associated with chronic epilepsy usually take a decade or more to develop. Although *DSM-III* includes the category organic personality syndrome, the required diagnostic criteria do not reflect the behaviors generally described in the personalities of chronic epileptics.

The most common personality syndrome associated with epilepsy has been termed "adhesive" or "viscious." Patients with an adhesive personality are verbose, circumstantial, and perseverative. They are slow in thinking and speak in a pedantic manner. They lose sight of basic concepts and themes and focus on minutiae. Nothing is trivial; every detail must be considered ad nauseam, mulled over, and digested in a humorless fashion. These patients lack spontaneity and use common expressions of speech and trite sayings almost to the exclusion of original word sequencing.

A second interictal personality is characterized by a profound deepening of the patient's emotional responses. These patients tend to overrespond to provocative stimuli. They have explosive rages, followed by hearty good-naturedness. They are emotionally labile, rash, suggestible, and excitable. They may develop a heightened sense of justice, morality, or religious conviction. For these patients, mundane, petty events assume cosmic significance. Detailed, perseverative, and trite written records may be kept, filling page after page of notebooks and scraps of paper with "universal truth." On occasion, these patients become suspicious and develop vague delusional ideas. An interictal personality syndrome has been specifically described in temporal-lobe epileptics (Bear and Fedio, 1977). It is unlikely that these behaviors (hypergraphia, global hyposexuality, circumstantiality, and pseudoabstractness) are specific (Mungas, 1982). Other interictal syndromes, in order of decreasing incidences, are anxiety states, depression, and neurasthenia. Deviant sexual behavior can also occur, and all late-onset (35 years of age or older) major changes in sexual behavior (e.g., transvestism, fetishism, homosexuality) should be suspect as manifestations of a seizure disorder (Davidson and Bagley, 1969; Fenton, 1981a,b; Benson and Blumer, 1982; Koella and Trimble, 1982; Trimble, 1982).

REGIONAL CORTICAL SYNDROMES

Two major frontal-lobe syndromes have been described in association with massive frontal-lobe injury: the convexity syndrome and the medial-orbital syndrome (Luria, 1966, 1973; Milner, 1969, 1971; Lishman, 1973; Black, 1974; Levin, 1978; Pincus and Tucker, 1978; Heilman and Valenstein, 1979; Miller, 1979).

The *convexity syndrome,* related to lesions within or near the lateral surface of the frontal lobes, is characterized by "negative symptoms." These patients are apathetic, indifferent to their surroundings, and emotionally unresponsive. They appear to have lost all drive and ambition. Loss of social graces is common, and they frequently appear disheveled and dirty. Their movements are slow and reduced in frequency (motor inertia). Occasionally they may remain in positions for prolonged periods (catalepsy) and may posture. Slight flexion at the waist, knees, and elbows is a typical body position for these patients. They occasionally move with a floppy shuffling gait, progressively picking up steam only to then gradually slow down to a stop (glissando/deglissando gait). Unlike patients with Parkinson's disease, their muscle tone is decreased, and "pill rolling" is not present. These patients have difficulty attending to tasks, but do respond to irrelevant, particularly intense stimuli. They will tend to walk next to walls (just touching them), rather than in the middle of the hallway, and may even follow architectural contours rather than take a direct route across open space.

If the convexity syndrome is due to dominant-hemisphere pathology, it may also be associated with deficits in language and in verbal thinking. Impoverished thinking (vague and without detail) is almost always present; verbal fluency is significantly impaired; speech is often stereotyped, with perseverative and verbigerated utterances; and Broca's aphasia or transcortical aphasia may be present. Most frontal-lobe cognitive and "soft" neurologic signs can be observed in these patients, who may also be dyspraxic (gait, buccolinguofacial, ideomotor) and incontinent of urine. There is no *DSM-III* category for these patients other than "atypical organic brain syndrome."

A second frontal-lobe syndrome is associated with dysfunction in the orbito-medial areas of the frontal lobes. Some patients may be asthenic and easily fatigued, bland akinetic, aphonic, withdrawn, and fearful. They may show diminished wakefulness and be in an oneiroid state or even stuporous. Other patients may have an intense affect, expressing euphoria, irritability, or extreme lability of affect, with rapid mood shifts and mixed and cycling mood states. Witzelsucht is common. These affectively intense patients are hyperactive and overresponsive to stimuli. They rapidly terminate one incomplete goal-directed behavior only to start another and may appear frenetic as they run about from one activity to another, never completing a task. These patients lose their inhibitions and become reckless. They are impulsive and may engage in buying sprees or other high-risk behaviors. They lack foresight, cannot make decisions, are unable to persevere, and have uncontrollable associations. They are strongly stimulus-bound, distractable, intrusive, and importunate. They will interrupt conversations and will mimic an examiner's movements and comments. These are the patients who, despite repeated injunctions, will repeat behaviors such as entering a room in which a group of people are in conference or pulling fire alarms or changing channels continually on television sets, simply because they see them. These patients may have uncontrollable, often fantastic confabulations, and when prevented from doing as they please, they may have violent outbursts.

The obvious similarity in behavior between these patients and patients with bipolar affective disorder requires particularly careful diagnostic evaluation. Localized CT scan and EEG abnormalities, focal neurologic signs, the shallowness of affect, a prolonged and insidious onset, a chronic nonepisodic course, and a negative family history for affective disorder would suggest coarse disease. Using *DSM-III* terminology, these patients would be labeled as having organic affective disorder.

PARIETAL-LOBE SYNDROMES

Coarse lesions of the parietal lobes can be associated with significant psychopathology (e.g., delusional ideas, experiences of alienation), which can lead to misdiagnosis and inappropriate treatment for a "functional" disorder (Critchley, 1953; Luria, 1973; Pincus and Tucker, 1978; Heilman and Valenstein, 1979; Strub and Black, 1981). Two general patterns of symptoms have been observed in patients with parietal-lobe lesions. Lesions of the *dominant parietal lobe* usually are associated with disorders of language (dyslexia, word-finding problems, conduction aphasia), problems with calculation, dyspraxias (ideomotor, kinesthetic), difficulties in abstraction, and contralateral sensory deficits (agraphasthesia, astereognosis) and motor deficits (hypotonia, posturing, paucity of movement). The best-known dominant-parietal-lobe syndrome is the controversial Gerstmann's syndrome (dysgraphia, dyscalculia, right–left disorientation, finger agnosia) putatively involving a lesion in the posterior-inferior aspect (angular gyrus) of the dominant parietal lobe. Although the validity of the syndrome has been questioned by some authors, it has been reported (Birkett, 1967) in over 20% of chronic psychiatric patients.

Lesions of the *nondominant parietal lobe* are associated with profound (occasionally delusional) denial of illness (anosognosia), left-sided spatial neglect, constructional difficulties, problems getting dressed, and contralateral sensory and motor deficits. Capgras's syndrome (delusional ideas that close friends or relatives are impostors) and the first-rank symptom of experience of alienation (body parts or thoughts not belonging to one) have been described in patients with nondominant-parietal-lobe lesions. These patients may also have difficulties orienting themselves in their environments. They complain that "things look confused" or "jumbled." They say they cannot find their way along previously familiar routes and that they can no longer drive because they lose track of the other vehicles around them. They may complain that their bodies are somehow different – that an arm or leg feels heavy, bigger than usual, or not always being sure of the location of an arm or leg.

TEMPORAL-LOBE SYNDROMES

Some patients without temporal-lobe epilepsy will nevertheless have temporal-lobe lesions. Patients with stroke, head injury, viral disease (particularly herpes), vascular malformations, and degenerative diseases involving the temporal lobes can present with delusions, hallucinations (particularly auditory and visual), and mood disturbances. Patients with posterior (temporoparietal) aphasia and patients with formal thought disorders share many of the same elements of language dysfunction. There is a strong association between temporal-lobe dysfunction and psychopathology, and the absence of a classic epileptic picture and course is not sufficient to eliminate a temporal-lobe cause from the differential diagnosis of a psychotic patient (Luria, 1973; Heilman and Valenstein, 1979; Koella and Trimble, 1982; Trimble, 1982).

Disturbances in language and memory are most commonly observed in psychiatric patients with temporal-lobe dysfunction. When the dysfunction is in the dominant temporal lobe, euphoria, auditory hallucinations (often "complete" voices), formal thought disorder and primary delusional ideas will be the likely psychopathology. These clinical phenomena will be associated with such cognitive deficits as decreased learning and retention of verbal material (read or heard), poor speech comprehension, and poor reading comprehension. When the dysfunction is in the nondominant temporal lobe, dysphoria, irritability, depression, and loss of emotional expression (aprosodia) will be the likely psychopathology. These clinical phenomena will be associated with such cognitive deficits as decreased recognition and recall of visual and auditory nonverbal material, amusia (loss of ability to repeat musical sounds), poor visual memory, decreased auditory discrimination and comprehension of tonal patterns, and decreased ability to learn and recognize nonsense figures and geometric shapes. Bilateral temporal-lobe involvement is usually associated with dementia (Slaby and Wyatt, 1974; Torack, 1978; Benson, 1982).

OTHER OMISSIONS IN *DSM-III*

A particularly striking omission in the *DSM-III* OMD category is the absence of an organic anxiety syndrome. This is mirrored by the failure to include "no evidence of OMD" as an exclusion criterion for *DSM-III* anxiety disorders. MacKenzie and Popkin (1983) have suggested criteria for this syndrome, which is essentially indistinguishable from primary anxiety states. An illness onset after age 35 should alert the clinician to the possibility of such a disorder (Lader and Marks, 1971), which has been reported in association with a wide variety of neurologic, endocrine, infectious, collagen, circulatory, and other disorders (Table 9.1) (Weil, 1959; Harper and Roth, 1962; Lader and Marks, 1971; Fajans, 1977; Hickler and Thorn, 1977; Ingbar and Woeber, 1977; Hall, 1980a; Nemiah, 1980; Trimble and Grant, 1982).

Another omission from the OMD category is postconcussion syndrome, which now must be subsumed under the atypical OMD subcategory. A common sequela of mild-to-moderate head trauma, this syndrome is characterized by headache, dizziness or vertigo, impaired concentration, anterograde memory problems, irritability, and lack of energy. Mild depressive features are commonly observed. These patients often are dysphoric, experience a variety of physiologic signs associated with anxiety states (e.g., tachycardia, palpitations), and have reduced work capacities (Merskey and Woodforde, 1972; Sisler, 1978; Strub and Black, 1981; Alexander, 1982). These patients may exhibit abnormal caloric testing (Harrison, 1956), and many exhibit unequivocal vestibular dysfunction by electronystagmography and abnormal brain-stem auditory-evoked potentials (Rowe and Carlson, 1980). In one study (Rowe and Carlson, 1980), only 21% of patients were normal on both measures.

In addition, there are no *DSM-III* OMD categories and no OMD exclusion criterion for "organic" anorexia nervosa, obsessive–compulsive disorder, or multiple personalities, although each of these has been associated with coarse neurologic disease (Schenk and Bear, 1981; Pitman, 1982; Weller and Weller, 1982).

OPERATIONAL-DEFINITION PROBLEMS

Among the criteria for each OMD syndrome, disorientation, loss of intellectual abilities, memory impairment, and impaired thinking are most frequently required for a positive diagnosis. The amnestic syndrome specifically requires impairment in short- and long-term memory. Unfortunately, the choice of a method of assessment for these functions is left to the individual clinician, with only rudimentary suggestions about how to evaluate them and what constitutes an abnormal response. This is particularly disturbing because

Table 9.1. *Known causes of anxiety*

Neurological – 25%
1. Cerebral vascular disorders
2. Sequelae to head injury
3. Postencephalitic disorders
4. Cerebral syphilis
5. Multiple sclerosis
6. Brain tumor (general)
7. Tumors of third ventricle (specifically)
8. Diencephalic autonomic epilepsy
9. Posterolateral sclerosis
10. Postconcussive syndrome
11. Wilson's disease
12. Huntington's chorea
13. Combined systemic disease
14. Polyneuritis
15. Myasthenia gravis
16. Dementia

Endocrine – 25%
1. Thyroid disorders
    a. Hyperthyroidism
    b. Hypothyroidism
2. Pituitary disorders
    a. Hypopituitarism
    b. Hyperpituitarism
3. Parathyroidism
    a. Hypoparathyroidism
    b. Hyperparathyroidism
4. Ovarian dysfunction
5. Testicular deficiency
6. Pancreatic disorders
    a. Hypoglycemia
    b. Diabetes mellitus
    c. Pancreatic carcinoma
    d. Hyperglycemia
7. Adrenal cortical disorders
    a. Adrenal cortical insufficiency (Addison's disease)
    b. Adrenal cortical hyperplasia (Cushing's disease)
    c. Adrenal tumors

Chronic infections – 12%
1. Tuberculosis
2. Brucellosis
3. Malaria
4. Atypical viral pneumonia
5. Viral hepatitis
6. Mononucleosis

Rheumatic–collagen vascular disorders – 12%
1. Rheumatoid arthritis
2. Lupus (systemic lupus erythematosus)
3. Polyarteritis nodosa
4. Temporal arteritis

Circulatory disorders – 12%
1. Anemia (various causes)
2. Cerebral anoxia
3. Cerebral insufficiency
4. Paroxysmal atrial tachycardia
5. Coronary insufficiency

Other – 14%
1. Nephritis
2. Other malignancies (e.g., oat-cell carcinoma of the lung)
3. Nutritional disorders
4. Drug-induced, particularly in the elderly
5. Meniere's disease (early)
6. Drug abuse
7. Fasting hypoglycemia
8. Caffeine sensitivity

Source: Adapted from Hall (1980a).

the *DSM-III* "escape clause" permits the diagnosis of OMD without historical or physical examination or laboratory verification, and the interrater-reliability figures for the OMD category have been marginal in initial field trials (Spitzer, Forman, and Nee, 1979; Hyler, Williams, and Spitzer, 1982). The terminology for these cognitive criteria was severely criticized by Lipowski (1978) in his critique of *DSM-II*. They remain virtually unchanged in *DSM-III*.

There are, however, many cognitive tasks of known reliability and validity that are adaptable to the clinical examination and could provide more standardized and meaningful information for diagnosis. For example, Benton and associates (1983) have standardized a test of orientation (Table 9.2) that can be scored reliably. Normative data and the performances of patients with brain damage and psychiatric disorders provide evidence that the test can discriminate these different patient groups. A six-item orientation-memory-concentration test of cognitive impairment (Katzman et al., 1983) (Table 9.3) based on an assessment instrument developed by Blessed, Tomlinson, and Roth (1968) also shows promise as a brief measure of cognitive function that could be included as part of a standard clinical evaluation of patients. The Mini-Mental State (Folstein, Folstein, and McHugh, 1975) also includes a scored orientation item, as well as items testing registration, attention, calculation, recall, language, and constructional abilities. This quick, easily administered paper-and-pencil battery is also helpful in identifying patients with diffuse intellectual impairment (dementia or delirium) and correlates well with CT scan evidence of diffuse cortical atrophy (Tsai and Tsuang, 1979). Taylor and associates (1980a) have also developed a brief, reliable battery of cognitive tasks for use during the mental-status examination. This battery (Table 9.4) tests for specific items (e.g., apraxia, constructional ability, aphasia) required by *DSM-III* for the diagnosis of dementia.

There are also numerous tests of memory function available to the clinician. Memory assessment should include an evaluation of span of immediate retention, learning, and retrieval of recently learned and long-stored information. Specific verbal- and visual-memory testing should be done. Questioning patients about their past life events and the sequence of events and details of the recent illnesses can provide an impression of their memory functions. If the OMD categories are to prove valid, however, more standardized and more specific memory assessment will be required, because there have been numerous studies (Sternberg and Jarvik, 1976; Abrams, Redfield, and Taylor, 1981; Caine, 1981; McAllister, 1981) demonstrating that many psychiatric patients with "functional" diagnoses do poorly on the more global memory items used in the typical clinical examination. Table 9.5 displays several memory tests that are brief, reliable, and sensitive to brain damage (Lezak, 1983, pp. 414–74; Benton et al., 1983).

Impairment in abstract thinking is one criterion for the diagnosis of dementia. *DSM-III* characterizes this impairment as "concrete interpretation of proverbs, inability to find similarities and differences between related words, difficulty in defining words and concepts, and other similar tasks." Unfortunately,

Table 9.2. *Test of orientation*

Administration

What is today's date? (The patient is required to give month, day, and year.)

What day of the week is it?

What time is it now? (Examiner makes sure that the patient cannot look at a watch or clock.)

Scoring

Day of week: 1 error point for each day removed from the correct day to a maximum of 3 points.

Day of month: 1 error point for each day removed from the correct day to a maximum of 15 points.

Month: 5 error points for each month removed from the correct month, with the qualification that if the stated date is within 15 days of the correct date, no error points are scored for the incorrect month (for example, May 29 for June 2 = 4 error points).

Year: 10 error points for each year removed from the correct year to a maximum of 60 points, with the qualification that if the stated date is within 15 days of the correct date, no error points are scored for the incorrect year (for example, December 26, 1982, for January 2, 1983 = 7 error points).

Time of day: 1 error point for each 30 minutes removed from the correct time to a maximum of 5 points.

The total number of points constitutes the patient's obtained score.

Source: Adapted from Benton et al. (1983): *Contributions of Neuropsychological Assessment.* ©1983, Oxford University Press.

Table 9.3. *Six-item orientation–memory–concentration test*

Items	Maximum error	Score[a]	Weight	
1 What year is it now?	1	——	× 4	=
2 What month is it now?	1	——	× 3	=
Memory phrase				
Repeat this phrase after me: "John Brown, 42 Market Street, Chicago"				
3 About what time is it? (within 1 hour)	1	——	× 3	=
4 Count backward 20 to 1	2	——	× 2	=
5 Say the months in reverse order	2	——	× 2	=
6 Repeat the memory phrase	5	——	× 2	=

[a]Score of 1 for each incorrect response; maximum weighted error score = 24. Normal or minimal impairment ≤ 8; moderate impairment 9–19; severe impairment ≥ 20.

Source: Katzman et al. (1983), *American Journal of Psychiatry* 140(6):734–739. Copyright 1983 The American Psychiatric Association. Reprinted by permission.

proverb interpretation is the most widely used of these suggestions, despite evidence that responses to proverbs do not correlate well with deficits in abstract thinking (Reed, 1968; Andreasen, 1977; Reich, 1981) and that fewer than 22% of non-brain-damaged adults fully understand them (Matarozzo, 1972). Difficulty in defining words is also unrelated to abstract thinking, and all the suggested tasks have large language components that might lead to an erroneous diagnosis of dementia in a schizophrenic with thought disorder or in a patient with a fluent aphasia and a deficit in auditory comprehension.

Likewise, thinking is not a monolithic function, and no single test spans the various cognitive processes subsumed under that rubric. A more meaningful approach would be assessment of the several areas of thinking that would lead to a reliable and valid conclusion about a patient's abstract thinking. The non-proverb parts of the comprehension subtest of the WAIS (Lezak, 1983, pp. 259–62), the WAIS subtest on verbal concept formation (similarities) (Lezak, 1983, pp. 265–6), and tests of reasoning (verbal and pictorial absurdities) from the Stanford–Binet (Lezak, 1983, pp. 494–5) are each readily adapted to the clinical examination and as a group should provide an adequate assessment of a patient's thinking.

In addition, the criteria for delirium include "clouding of consciousness," defined as "reduced clarity of awareness of the environment [with] reduced capacity to shift, focus, and sustain attention to environmental stimuli." It is, however, well known that several "functional" disorders (e.g., catatonia, depression, mania, hysteria) are associated with stuporous stages in which patients have reduced responsivity to stimuli and apparent fluctuations of awareness. Oneiroid or dreamlike states of perplexity and altered awareness have also been described in these disorders (Berrios, 1981). Although often clinically indistinguishable from the stupor described in neurologic syndromes, "psychiatric stupor" is rarely associated with abnormal clinical EEG findings. The stupor of delirium and other forms of OMD, on the other hand, is invariably associated with diffuse high-voltage slow activity (Fishgold and Mathis, 1959; Lipowski, 1967; Plum and Posner, 1972; Posner, 1978).

Finally, the OMD subcategories of organic delusional syndrome, organic hallucinosis, organic affective disorder, and organic personality syndrome present the additional problem of each diagnosis being based on a known or presumed cause. Causes for each syndrome are being identified at an extraordinary rate, and supplemental lists of systemic and neurologic causes of mental syndromes would be helpful.

INTERCATEGORY PROBLEMS WITH *DSM-III* OMD

There are two basic *DSM-III* OMD intercategory problems. The first, the term "organic mental disorder," on cursory examination, may appear a semantic issue, but is in fact an issue fundamental to our nosology and conceptualization of mental illness. The second problem concerns the criterion used

Table 9.4. *Some mental-status cognitive tasks*

Task	Dysfunction	Abnormal response	Suggested localization
Spell "earth" backward	Concentration	Any improper letter sequence	Frontal lobes
Serial sevens	Concentration	One or more errors or longer than 90 seconds	Frontal lobes
Name the day of the week, month, year, location	Global disorientation	Any error	Frontal lobes (if memory intact)
Repeat: "No ifs, ands, or buts," "The President lives in Washington," "Methodist Episcopal," "Massachusetts"	Expressive language	Missed words or syllables; repetition of internal syllables; dropping of word endings	Dominant frontal lobe
Name common objects (key, watch, button, etc.)	Anomia	Cannot name; word approximations; describes functions rather than word	Dominant temporal lobe, angular gyrus
Conversation during examination	Receptive language	Word approximations, neologisms, word salad, stock words, tangential speech	Dominant temporal lobe
a. Repeat four words or items (e.g. blue, chair, swim, glove)	Immediate recall	One or more errors	Temporal lobes/frontal lobes (hippocampus)
b. Remember them after 10 minutes with interposed tasks	Recent memory	One or more errors	Temporal lobes (hippocampus, thalamus, fornix, mammillothalamic tract)
c. Provide accurate detail and sequence of past events	Long-term memory	Significant loss of detail; confused sequence	Temporal lobes (hippocampus)
Copy examiner's hand and arm movements (each hand/arm)	Dyspraxia	Any error, mirror movements	Contralateral parietal lobe

160

Instruction	Deficit	Description	Localization
Demonstrate use of key, hammer, flipping a coin a. Left hand only plus some expressive language difficulty b. Both hands	Ideomotor apraxia	Use of hand as object; failure to use fine hand and wrist movements; verbal overflow	Dominant parietal lobe, disconnected from nondominant frontal lobe Dominant frontal lobe or anterior corpus callosum Dominant parietal lobe, arcuate fasciculus
Name fingers	Finger agnosia	Two or more errors; cannot identify after examiner numbers each	Dominant parietal lobe
Calculations	Dyscalculia	Errors in borrowing or carrying over when concentration is intact	Dominant parietal lobe
Write a sentence	Dysgraphia	No longer able to write cursively; loss of word structure; abnormally formed letters	Dominant parietal lobe
In individual steps, copy sentence, read it, and do what it says ("Put the paper in your pocket")	Dysgraphia, dyslexia, comprehension	No longer able to write cursively; loss of sentence structure; loss of word structure; abnormally formed letters	Dominant temporoparietal lobe
Place left hand to right ear, right elbow, right knee; same for right hand	Right/left disorientation	Two or more errors or two or more 7-second delays in carrying out tasks	Dominant parietal lobe
Copy the outline of simple objects (e.g., Greek cross, key)	Construction apraxia	Loss of gestalt, loss of symmetry, distortion of figures	Nondominant parietal lobe
Camouflaged object(s)	Visual-perception deficit	Cannot name when camouflaged, can name when clear	Occipital lobes

Source: Adapted from Taylor et al. (1980a), *Journal of Nervous and Mental Disease* 168(3):167–170. Copyright 1980 The Williams & Wilkins Co., Baltimore.

Table 9.5. *Clinical tests of memory*

Test	Tasks	Abnormal response	Dysfunction
Verbal Automatism (long-term memory)	Recitation of information learned by rote in early childhood (e.g., alphabet, number series, simple multiplication tables, days of week, months of year, the Pledge of Allegiance, childhood rhymes & prayers)	Any error Unable to start or complete sequence	Mild, diffuse Severe, diffuse If acute condition, attentional or altered consciousness
Serial Digit Learning (span of immediate retention)	Learning of 8- or 9-digit series; maximum of 12 trials; two consecutive correct repetitions are required; points are awarded for correct digits and sequencing	Unable to learn sequence in 12 trials Score < 8	Severe brain dysfunction Mild to moderate dysfunction
Paired Associate Learning (short-term learning)	Ten word pairs (6 easy & 4 hard); read three times, with memory trial following each reading; total score is ½ sum of all correct associations of easy pairs plus sum of all correct associations of hard pairs	*Maximum score is 21* Ages: 20–39, score ≤ 13 40–54, score ≤ 10 55–69, score ≤ 7 ≥ 70, score ≤ 6	Severe impairment if patient alert and attentive
Babcock Story Recall (immediate retention & retrieval)	A 21-unit paragraph is read; patient immediately tries to recall; paragraph read second time, and patient tries to recall 20 minutes later; each unit correct earns 1 point; immediate-recall score adjusted by adding 4 points	*Maximum score is 25* Immediate recall Score 11 *Maximum score is 21* Delayed recall after second reading Score 11	Moderate to severe dysfunction if patient alert and attentive
Memory for Designs	Fifteen geometric designs each presented for 5 seconds; patient immediately tries to reproduce designs	1 point for two or more errors when gestalt of design preserved 2 points when configuration lost or major element missing 3 points for rotations and reversals, failure to draw anything	Normal (0–4) Borderline (5–11) Brain damage (12)

to categorize an OBS as an OMD and the functional syndromes as non-OMD disorders. I discuss this criterion first.

To diagnose an OBS as an OMD and to rule out an OMD when considering a functional illness, *DSM-III* requires assessment of historical, physical-examination, or laboratory-test variables designed to discriminate OMD syndromes from non-OMD syndromes. During the past two decades, however, a large body of data has accumulated that makes this discrimination difficult if the traditional neurologic versus nonneurologic variables are used without qualification. For example, to automatically label a patient as having OMD rather than schizophrenia on the basis of that patient having abnormal EEG findings would be to ignore the literature that demonstrates that 40% or more of schizophrenics have abnormal EEG findings (Tucker et al., 1965; Vianna, 1975; Abrams and Taylor, 1979). The criterion needs to be more specific and reflective of research on the biology of mental disorders.

HISTORICAL ANTECEDENTS OF OMD

Although virtually any neurologic disease can lead to behavioral changes (Table 9.6), head trauma is the most common antecedent of brain syndromes. To be of sufficient magnitude to result in subsequent behavioral changes, a closed head injury will likely be associated with a skull fracture, unconsciousness of 30 minutes or longer, anterograde amnesia of several hours or longer, focal neurologic signs (even if transient), or blood in the spinal fluid. "Bumps on the head," even when suturing is required, do not correlate highly with most brain syndromes (Luria, 1969; Lishman, 1973, 1978; Hendrie, 1978; Levin, 1978; Sisler, 1978; Miller, 1979; Strub and Black, 1981; Alexander, 1982). Mild-to-moderate trauma, however, is a typical antecedent of the postconcussion syndrome (Harrison, 1956; Merskey and Woodforde, 1972; Rowe and Carlson, 1980).

A history of documented epilepsy is also commonly associated with behavior syndromes (Beard and Slater, 1962; Davidson and Bagley, 1969; Roger et al., 1974; Bear and Fedio, 1977; Ellis and Lee, 1978; Lishman, 1978; Fenton, 1981a,b; Toone, 1981; Benson and Blumer, 1982; Koella and Trimble, 1982; Marsden and Reynolds, 1982; Trimble, 1982), as is a history of major systemic disease. Of these, those most frequently associated with behavioral change include: endocrinopathies, lupus erythematosus, diabetes, extensive cardiovascular disease (particularly arrhythmias, heart failure, myocardial infarction, endocarditis, vasculitis), cancer, nutritional deficiencies, metabolic acidosis, chronic infection, and blood dyscrasias. Exposure to toxic substances (organic solvents, carbon monoxide, heavy metals) and chronic substance abuse may also result in a brain syndrome (Hall, 1980c; Speidel and Rodewald, 1980).

PHYSICAL SIGNS OF OMD

Physical-examination findings consistent with OMD include focal neurologic features (e.g., abnormal cranial nerve signs, abnormal reflexes, paralysis)

Table 9.6. *Neurologic conditions often associated with behavioral syndromes*

Intracranial hemorrhage	Brain abscess	Multiple sclerosis
Epilepsy	Syphilis	Parkinson's disease
A–V malformation	Toxoplasmosis	Huntington's chorea
Aneurysm	Hypoxia	Wilson's disease
Acute vascular occlusion	Transient ischemia	Alzheimer's disease
Cerebral infarct(s)	Hydrocephalus	Pick's disease
Intracranial neoplasm	Cerebral abscess	
Meningitis	Viral encephalitis	

and sufficient signs of a systemic illness known to produce behavioral change (Slaby and Wyatt, 1974; Hendrie, 1978; Lishman, 1978; Pincus and Tucker, 1978; Torack, 1978; Hall, 1980c; Speidel and Rodewald, 1980; Strub and Black, 1981; Benson, 1982). "Soft" neurologic signs (e.g., motor impersistence, adventitious motor-overflow, gegenhalten, palmomental reflex, poor double simultaneous discrimination) have been reported in 40% to 70% of functional psychotics and are not useful in discriminating OMD from other psychiatric conditions (Rochford et al., 1970; Cox and Ludwig, 1979; Quitkin, Rifkin, and Klein, 1979; Taylor et al., 1980a; Nasrallah et al., 1983).

LABORATORY FEATURES OF OMD

The use of laboratory studies to identify OMD has been complicated by recent studies demonstrating that schizophrenics and patients with affective disorders have abnormalities on a variety of such measures. Nevertheless, there are specific differences in the laboratory findings for functional patients and patients with OMD that can be useful in operationally defining the *DSM-III* discriminating criterion.

Numerous computer-enhanced tomographic studies (Luchins, Weinberger, and Wyatt, 1979, 1982; Weinberger et al., 1979, 1982; Golden et al., 1981; Moriguchi, 1981; Tanaka et al., 1981; Frangos and Athanassenas, 1982; Nasrallah et al., 1982a; Nyback et al., 1982) have found that, compared with normal controls, schizophrenics have enlarged lateral ventricles, reduced cortical thickness, decreased gray-matter density, greater or reversed cerebral asymmetry, and reduced cerebellar mass. Several investigators have reported similar findings in patients with affective disorder (Nasrallah, McCalley-Whitters, and Jacoby, 1982b; Tanaka et al., 1982) and in psychiatrically ill children (Reiss et al., 1983), whereas others have failed to confirm differences between patients and controls (Andreasen et al., 1982; Benes et al., 1982; Jernigan et al., 1982a,b). Although theoretically interesting, these findings are primarily based on group-mean comparisons, and few individual subjects have CT scan images that would be reported as clinically abnormal. An individual scan characterized as clinically abnormal (e.g., circumscribed lesion, significant cortical atrophy) is consistent with the diagnosis of OMD (Torack, 1978; Tsai and Tsuang, 1979; Strub and Black, 1981; Benson, 1982; Cummings, 1982).

Similarly, numerous studies have reported that 40% to 50% of schizophrenics have clinically abnormal resting EEG findings (Tucker et al., 1965; Vianna, 1975; Abrams and Taylor, 1979), usually nonspecific slowing. None of these studies, however, has been able to demonstrate a characteristic schizophrenic EEG pattern. Although less numerous, EEG studies in affective disorder (Abrams and Taylor, 1979; Kadrmas and Winokur, 1979) and other non-OMD conditions (Kiloh, McComas, and Osselton, 1974) have also failed to identify specific abnormalities. A resting EEG showing a specific clinical abnormality (e.g., spike-and-low-wave complexes, paroxysmal bursts of slow waves, circumscribed abnormalities) is inconsistent with a functional diagnosis and indicates the patient may have an OMD. Power-spectrum studies (Itil, Saletu, and Davis, 1972; Flor-Henry, 1976; Volavka et al., 1981) and evoked-response studies (Rockstroh et al., 1982), each suggesting differences between psychotic patients and normal controls, have not yet proved useful diagnostically. Evoked-response studies, however, can be helpful in determining the presence of demyelinating disease (Green and Walcoff, 1982; Haldeman et al., 1982).

Neuropsychological testing of affective-disorder patients and schizophrenics has captured the imagination of many investigators. Despite a common notion that schizophrenics exhibit dominant-hemisphere dysfunction, whereas affectives exhibit nondominant-hemisphere dysfunction, the data overwhelmingly demonstrate most schizophrenics to have bilateral and diffuse cognitive impairment (perhaps more profound in the anterior dominant regions), whereas a smaller proportion of affectives have evidence of bilateral anterior impairment and general nondominant-hemisphere dysfunction (Marin and Tucker, 1981; Silverstein and Meltzer, 1983; Taylor and Abrams, 1984). A circumscribed neuropsychological deficit is inconsistent with the major functional psychoses and suggests an OMD (Golden, 1978; Heilman and Valenstein, 1979). There have been few neuropsychological studies of other functional disorders, and clearcut patterns of dysfunction have not been reported. None of these disorders, however, appears to be associated with severe or focal cognitive impairment (Marin and Tucker, 1981).

Any cerebrospinal fluid abnormality, any abnormal blood finding associated with causes of dementia (e.g., low serum B_{12}, low serum T_3), or other laboratory finding consistent with a systemic illness known to produce behavioral change (e.g., x-ray evidence of pneumonia, EKG evidence of recent myocardial infarction) should strongly influence the clinician toward a diagnosis of OMD, as these abnormalities are rarely reported in the primary functional states (Slaby and Wyatt, 1974; Pincus and Tucker, 1978; Torack, 1978; Scheinberg, 1981; Strub and Black, 1981; Benson, 1982). On the other hand, in some samples of psychotic patients, nearly 40% had systemic illness (Hall, 1980b), which appeared to be the most likely cause of the behavioral syndrome. Investigative techniques such as topographic brain electrical mapping (Morihisa, Duffy, and

Wyatt, 1983) and studies of cerebral blood flow (Mathew et al., 1982; Ariel et al., 1983; Uytdenhoef et al., 1983) show promise as discriminating measures for different behavioral syndromes. Many more patients, however, will have to be studied by these techniques before consistent and clear-cut differences will emerge.

OMD: A CONCEPTUAL PROBLEM

The second basic *DSM-III* OMD intercategory problem is conceptual. *DSM-III* explicitly states the following:

Differentiation of Organic Mental Disorders as a separate class does not imply that non-organic ("functional") mental disorders are somehow independent of brain processes. On the contrary, it is assumed that all psychological processes, normal and abnormal, depend on brain function. Limitations in our knowledge, however, sometimes make it impossible to determine whether a given mental disorder in a given individual should be considered an organic mental disorder (because it is due to brain dysfunction of *known* organic etiology) or whether it should be diagnosed as other than an Organic Mental Disorder (because it is more adequately accounted for as a response to psychological or social factors [as in Adjustment Disorder] or because the presence of a specific organic factor has not been established [as in Schizophrenia]). [pp. 101–2]

However, the idea that failure to establish a specific organic factor in schizophrenia is what separates it from OMD cannot be reconciled with the fact that we do not know the specific organic factors for so many disorders traditionally included in the OMD category. Alzheimer's disease, Huntington's chorea, Pick's disease, and multiple sclerosis are but a few examples. To redefine "specific organic factor" to mean evidence of brain dysfunction rather than to mean "cause" is also inconsistent, because EEG (Tucker et al., 1965; Itil et al., 1972; Kiloh et al., 1974; Vianna, 1975; Flor-Henry, 1976; Abrams and Taylor, 1979; Kadrmas and Winokur, 1979; Volavka et al., 1981; Rockstroh et al., 1982), CT scan (Luchins et al., 1979, 1982; Weinberger et al., 1979, 1982; Golden et al., 1981; Moriguchi, 1981; Tanaka et al., 1981, 1982; Frangos and Athanassenas, 1982; Nasrallah et al., 1982a,b; Nyback et al., 1982; Reiss et al., 1983), neuropsychological (Flor-Henry, 1976; Marin and Tucker, 1981; Silverstein and Meltzer, 1983; Taylor and Abrams, 1984), and neurotransmitter and neuroendocrine studies (Van Praag et al., 1981; Henn and Nasrallah, 1982; Potkin et al., 1983; Rosenbaum et al., 1983; Schatzberg et al., 1983; Stahl et al., 1983; Swann et al., 1983; Targum, 1983), in schizophrenia and affective disorder clearly indicate that these patients have brain dysfunctions of some kind. The genetic data in affective disorders (Taylor and Abrams, 1980; Taylor, Abrams, and Hayman, 1980b) are particularly compelling evidence that these patients suffer from a condition whose major determinant is biological. Finally, to redefine "specific organic factor" to mean "neuropathological abnormality" is at best a short-term evasion of the problem, because the biological data in the major psychoses certainly imply neuropathologic abnormality at some level, and several forms of epilepsy, an accepted neurologic disorder, have no distinguishable neuropathologic abnormality (Mathieson, 1982; Young et al., 1982).

The term "functional" was originally employed to mean biochemical or physiological. Only with the ascendancy of psychoanalytic thinking in the 1930s and 1940s did "functional" become synonymous with "psychological." Schizophrenia, for example, became a "reaction" rather than a subtle form of brain disease. The term "OMD" is a vestige of the notion that there are behavioral syndromes divorced from brain function. Its meaning literally implies that the rest of our nosology is inorganic or nonorganic. Both ideas (rejected in the text of *DSM-III*) are clearly untenable in an era of modern biological science.

Although this chapter highlights the differences between functional syndromes and OMD to better operationally define the present *DSM-III* criteria discriminating the two categories, in fact there is much evidence that at least schizophrenia and affective disorder are syndromes of brain disorder. The disorder is subtle and not clearly measurable, but its presence is inescapable. The terms "neuroses," "psychosomatic," and "psychophysiological" were abandoned and the term "hysteria" virtually abandoned because each reflected concepts no longer consistent with modern ideas of mental illness. OMD is also such a term. The syndromes subsumed under that heading might be neurological, clearly measurable or coarse brain disorders, but they are surely no more organic than other mental disorders.

SUGGESTED CHANGES IN THE *DSM-III* OMD CATEGORY

1. Eliminate the distinction between OBS and OMD. Eliminate the "escape clause" permitting the diagnosis OMD without evidence of coarse brain disease.
2. Include the following additional subcategories:
   a. Psychomotor states
   b. Regional cortical syndromes (e.g., frontal lobe, parietal lobe, temporal lobe)
   c. Anxiety states secondary to coarse brain disease or systemic illness
   d. Postconcussion syndrome
   In addition, the criteria for each anxiety disorder, obsessive–compulsive disorder, and anorexia nervosa should each include the criterion "no evidence of neurologic illness or systemic disease known to produce this behavioral syndrome."
3. Operationally redefine the terms "disorientation," "memory impairment," "loss of intellectual abilities," and "defect in abstract thinking." This redefinition should be based on standardized, reliable, valid, and clinically practical tests of cognition. Some suggested tests:
   a. *For orientation:* Benton's Orientation Test
   b. *For general intellectual abilities:* Mini-Mental State
   c. *For various aspects of memory function:* Verbal Automatism Tests, Serial Digit Learning, Paired Associate Learning, Babcock Story Recall, Memory for Designs
   d. *For various aspects of abstract thinking:* Nonproverb parts of the WAIS comprehension subtest, WAIS Verbal Concept Formation (similarities),

tests of reasoning (Verbal and Pictorial Absurdities Tests of the Stanford–Binet)

4. Operationally redefine "neurologic stupor" to require the presence of an abnormal EEG.
5. Provide a list of CNS and systemic conditions known to cause behavioral syndromes.
6. Put into operation the criterion requiring historical, physical-examination, or laboratory evidence of brain dysfunction.
7. Replace the term "organic mental syndrome" (some suggested terms: behavioral neurologic disorder, behavioral coarse brain disorders).

REFERENCES

Abrams R, Redfield J, Taylor MA: Cognitive dysfunction compared in schizophrenia and affective disorder. Br J Psychiatry 139:190–194, 1981

Abrams R, Taylor MA: Differential EEG patterns in affective disorder and schizophrenia. Arch Gen Psychiatry 36:1355–1358, 1979

Ahern GL, Schwartz GE: Differential lateralization for positive versus negative emotion. Neuropsychologia 17:693–698, 1979

Alexander MP: Traumatic brain injury, in Psychiatric Aspects of Neurologic Disease, Vol II. Edited by Benson DF, Blumer D. New York, Grune & Stratton, 1982, pp 219–248

American Psychiatric Association: Diagnostic and Statistical Manual of Mental Disorders, third edition. Washington, DC, APA, 1980

Diagnostic and Statistical Manual of Mental Disorders, second edition. Washington, DC, 1968

Andreasen NC: Reliability and validity of proverb interpretation to assess mental status. Compr Psychiatry 18:465–472, 1977

Andreasen NC, Smith MR, Jacoby CG, et al: Ventricular enlargement in schizophrenia: definition and prevalence. Am J Psychiatry 139:292–296, 1982

Ariel RN, Golden CJ, Berg RA, et al: Regional cerebral blood flow in schizophrenics. Arch Gen Psychiatry 40:258–263, 1983

Bear DM, Fedio P: Quantitative analysis of interictal behavior in temporal lobe epilepsy. Arch Neurol 34:454–467, 1977

Beard AW, Slater E: The schizophrenic-like psychoses of epilepsy. Proc R Soc Med 55:311–316, 1962

Benes F, Sunderland P, Jones BD, et al: Normal ventricles in young schizophrenics. Br J Psychiatry 141:90–93, 1982

Benson DF: The treatable dementias, in Neurologic Disease, Vol II. Edited by Benson DF, Blumer D. New York, Grune & Stratton, 1982, pp 123–148

Benson DF, Blumer D: Psychiatric manifestation of epilepsy, in Psychiatric Aspects of Neurologic Disease, Vol II. Edited by Benson DF, Blumer D. New York, Grune & Stratton, 1982, pp 25–47

Benton AL, Hamsher des K, Varney NR, et al: Contributions of Neuropsychological Assessment. A Clinical Manual. Oxford University Press, 1983, pp 3–9, 23–29

Berrios GE: Stupor revisited. Compr Psychiatry 22:466–478, 1981

Birkett DP: Gerstmann's Syndrome. Br J Psychiatry 113:801, 1967

Black WF: Use of the MMPI with patients with recent war-related head injury. J Clin Psychol 30:571–573, 1974

Blessed G, Tomlinson BE, Roth M: The association between quantitative measures of dementia and of senile change in the cerebral grey matter of elderly subjects. Br J Psychiatry 114:797–811, 1968

Caine ED: Pseudodementia, current concepts and future directions. Arch Gen Psychiatry 38:1359–1364, 1981

Cox SM, Ludwig AM: Neurological soft signs and psychopathology, I: findings in schizophrenia. J Nerv Ment Dis 167:161–165, 1979

Critchley M: The Parietal Lobes. New York, Hafner, 1953

Cummings JL: Cortical dementias, in Psychiatric Aspects of Neurologic Disease, Vol II. Edited by Benson DF, Blumer D. New York, Grune & Stratton, 1982, pp 93–120

Dammasio A: The frontal lobes, in Clinical Neuropsychology. Edited by Heilman KM, Valenstein E. Oxford University Press, 1979, pp 360–412

Davidson K, Bagley CR: Schizophrenia-like psychoses associated with organic disorders of the central nervous system: a review of the literature, in Current Problems in Neuropsychiatry, Br J Psychiatry special publication 4, 1969, pp 113–184

Delgado-Escueta AV, Treiman DM, Walsh GO: The treatable epilepsies. N Engl J Med 308:1576–1584, 1983

Ellis JM, Lee SI: Acute prolonged confusion in later life as an ictal state. Epilepsia 19:119–128, 1978

Fajans SS: Hyperinsulinism, hypoglycemia, and glucagon secretion, in Harrison's Principles of Internal Medicine, eighth edition. Edited by Thorn GW, Adams RD, Braunwald E, et al. New York, McGraw-Hill, 1977, pp 586–595

Fenton GW: Personality and behavioral disorders in adults with epilepsy, in Epilepsy and Psychiatry. Edited by Reynolds EH, Trimble MR. Edinburgh, Churchill Livingstone, 1981a, pp 77–91

Psychiatric disorders of epilepsy: classification and phenomenology, in Epilepsy and Psychiatry. Edited by Reynolds EH, Trimble MR. Edinburgh, Churchill Livingstone, 1981b, pp 12–26

Fishgold H, Mathis P: Obnubilations comas et stupeurs. Etudes electroencephaliques. Electroencephalogr Clin Neurophysiol [Suppl 2] 1959

Flor-Henry P: Lateralized temporal-limbic dysfunction and pathology. Ann NY Acad Sci 280:777–797, 1976

Folstein MJ, Folstein SW, McHugh PR: "Mini-mental state": a practical method of grading the cognitive state of patients for the clinician. J Psychiatr Res 12:189–198, 1975

Frangos E, Athanassenas G: Differences in lateral brain ventricular size among various types of chronic schizophrenics: evidence based on a CT study. Acta Psychiatr Scand 66:459–463, 1982

Gainotti G: Emotional behavior and hemispheric side of the lesion. Cortex 8:41–55, 1972

Golden CJ: Diagnosis and Rehabilitation in Clinical Neuropsychology. Springfield, Ill, Charles C Thomas, 1978

Golden CJ, Graber B, Coffman J, et al: Structural brain deficits in schizophrenia: identification by computed tomographic scan density measurements. Arch Gen Psychiatry 38:1014–1017, 1981

Green JB, Walcoff MR: Evoked potentials in multiple sclerosis. Arch Neurol 39:696–697, 1982

Haldeman S, Glick M, Bhatia NN, et al: Colonometry, cystometry, and evoked potentials in multiple sclerosis. Arch Neurol 39:698–701, 1982

Hall RCW: Anxiety, in Psychiatric Presentations of Medical Illness: Somatopsychic Disorders. Edited by Hall RCW. New York, SP Medical and Scientific Books, 1980a, pp 13–35

Medically induced psychiatric disease: an overview, in Psychiatric Presentations of Medical Illness: Somatopsychic Disorders. Edited by Hall RCW. New York, SP Medical and Scientific Books, 1980b, pp 3–9

(ed): Psychiatric Presentations of Medical Illness: Somatopsychic Disorders. New York, SP Medical and Scientific Books, 1980c

Harper M, Roth M: Temporal lobe epilepsy and the phobic-anxiety-depersonalization syndrome. Compr Psychiatry 3:129–151, 1962

Harrison MS: Notes on the clinical features and pathology of postconcussional vertigo with special reference to positional nystagmus. Brain 79:474–482, 1956

Hecaen H: Clinical symptomatology in right and left hemispheric lesions, in Interhemispheric Relations and Cerebral Dominance. Edited by Mountcastle VB. Baltimore, Johns Hopkins Press, 1962, pp 215–243

Hecaen H, Albert ML: Disorders of mental functioning related to frontal lobe pathology, in Psychiatric Aspects of Neurologic Disease, Vol I. Edited by Benson DF, Blumer D. New York, Grune & Stratton, 1975, pp 137–169

Heilman KM, Valenstein E (eds): Clinical Neuropsychology. Oxford University Press, 1979

Hendrie HC (ed): The Psychiatric Clinics of North America, Vol I, Brain Disorders: Clinical Diagnosis and Management. Philadelphia, WB Saunders, 1978

Henn FA, Nasrallah HA: Schizophrenia as a Brain Disease. Oxford University Press, 1982

Hickler RB, Thorn GW: Pheochromocytoma, in Harrison's Principles of Internal Medicine, eighth edition. Edited by Thorn GW, Adams RD, Braunwald E, et al. New York, McGraw-Hill, 1977, pp 557–563

Hyler SE, Williams, JBW, Spitzer RL: Reliability in the DSM-III field trials, interview v. case summary. Arch Gen Psychiatry 39:1275–1278, 1982

Ingbar SH, Woeber KA: Diseases of the thyroid, in Harrison's Principles of Internal Medicine, eighth edition. Edited by Thorn GW, Adams RD, Braunwald E, et al. New York, McGraw-Hill, 1977, pp 501–519

Itil TM, Saletu B, Davis S: EEG findings in chronic schizophrenics based on digital computer period analysis and analog power spectra. Biol Psychiatry 5:1–13, 1972

Jernigan TL, Zatz LM, Moses JA Jr, et al: Computed tomography in schizophrenics and normal volunteers, I: fluid volume. Arch Gen Psychiatry 39:765–770, 1982a

Computed tomography in schizophrenics and normal volunteers, II: cranial asymmetry. Arch Gen Psychiatry 39:771–773, 1982b

Kadrmas A, Winokur G: Manic-depressive illness and EEG abnormalities. J Clin Psychiatry 40:306–307, 1979

Katzman R, Brown T, Fuld P, et al: Validation of a short orientation-memory-concentration test of cognitive impairment. Am J Psychiatry 140:734–739, 1983

Kiloh LG, McComas AJ, Osselton JW: Clinical Electroencephalography, second edition. London, Butterworth, 1974, pp 168–200

Koella WP, Trimble MR (eds): Temporal Lobe Epilepsy, Mania and Schizophrenia and the Limbic System, Advances in Biological Psychiatry, Vol 8. Basel, S Karger, 1982

Lader M, Marks I: Clinical Anxiety. New York, Grune & Stratton, 1971

Levin HS, Grossman RG: Behavioral sequelae of closed head injury: a qualitative study. Arch Neurol 35:720–727, 1978

Lezak MD: Neuropsychological Assessment, second edition. Oxford University Press, 1983

Lipowski ZJ: Delirium, clouding of consciousness and confusion. J Nerv Ment Dis 145:227–255, 1967

  Organic brain syndromes: a reformulation. Compr Psychiatry 19:309–322, 1978

Lishman WA: The psychiatric sequelae of head injury: a review. Psychol Med 3:304–318, 1973

  Organic Psychiatry. London, Blackwell Scientific, 1978

Luchins DJ, Weinberger DR, Wyatt RJ: Schizophrenia, evidence of a subgroup with reversed cerebral asymmetry. Arch Gen Psychiatry 36:1309–1311, 1979

  Schizophrenia and cerebral asymmetry detected by computed tomography. Am J Psychiatry 139:753–757, 1982

Luria AR: Higher Cortical Functions in Man. New York, Basic Science Books, 1966

  Frontal lobe syndromes, in Handbook of Clinical Neurology, Vol II, Localization in Clinical Neurology. Edited by Vinken PJ, Bruyn GW. New York, Elsevier/North Holland, 1969, pp 725–775

  The Working Brain, An Introduction to Neuropsychology. New York, Basic Books, 1973, pp 147–168

McAllister TW: Cognitive functioning in the affective disorders. Compr Psychiatry 22:572–586, 1981

MacKenzie TB, Popkin MK: Organic anxiety syndrome. Am J Psychiatry 140:342–344, 1983

Marin RS, Tucker GJ: Psychopathology and hemispheric dysfunction: a review. J Nerv Ment Dis 169:546–557, 1981

Marsden CD, Reynolds EH: Neurology, in A Textbook of Epilepsy, second edition. Edited by Laidlaw J, Richens A. Edinburgh, Churchill Livingstone, 1982, pp 97–146

Matarozzo JD: Wechsler's Measurement and Appraisal of Adult Intelligence, fifth edition. Oxford University Press, 1972

Mathew RJ, Duncan GC, Weinman ML, et al: Regional cerebral blood flow in schizophrenia. Arch Gen Psychiatry 39:1121–1124, 1982

Mathieson G: Pathology, in A Textbook of Epilepsy, second edition. Edited by Laidlaw J, Richens A. Edinburgh, Churchill Livingstone, 1982, pp 437–456

Meduna LZ: General discussion of the cardiazol therapy. Am J Psychiatry [Suppl] 94:40–50, 1938

Merskey H, Woodforde JM: Psychiatric sequelae of minor head injury. Brain 95:521–528, 1972

Miller E: The long-term consequences of head injury: a discussion of the evidence with special reference to the preparation of legal reports. Br J Soc Clin Psychol 18:87–98, 1979

Milner B: Residual intellectual and memory deficits after head injury, in The Late Effects of Head Injury. Edited by Walker AE, Caveness WF, Critchley M. Springfield, Ill, Charles C Thomas, 1969, pp 84–89

  Interhemispheric differences in the localization of psychological processes in man. Br Med Bull 27:272–277, 1971

Moriguchi I: A study of schizophrenic brains by computerized tomography scans. Folia Psychiatr Neurol Jpn 35:55–72, 1981

Morihisa JM, Duffy FH, Wyatt RJ: Brain electrical activity mapping (BEAM) in schizophrenic patients. Arch Gen Psychiatry 40:719–728, 1983

Mungas D: Interictal behavior abnormality in temporal lobe epilepsy, a specific syndrome or non-specific psychopathology? Arch Gen Psychiatry 39:108–111, 1982

Nasrallah HA, Jacoby CG, McCalley-Whitters M, et al: Cerebral ventricular enlargement in subtypes of chronic schizophrenia. Arch Gen Psychiatry 39:774–777, 1982a

Nasrallah HA, McCalley-Whitters M, Jacoby CG: Cerebral ventricular enlargement in young manic males: a controlled CT study. J Affect Dis 4:15–19, 1982b

Nasrallah HA, Tippin J, McCalley-Whitters M: Neurological soft signs in manic patients, a comparison with schizophrenic and control groups. J Affect Dis 5:45–50, 1983

Nemiah JC: Anxiety state (anxiety neurosis), in The Comprehensive Textbook of Psychiatry, third edition. Edited by Kaplan HI, Freedman AM, Sadock BJ. Baltimore, Williams & Wilkins, 1980, pp 1483–1493

Nyback H, Wiesel FA, Berggren BM, et al: Computed tomography of the brain in patients with acute psychosis and in healthy volunteers. Acta Psychiatr Scand 65:403–414, 1982

Pincus JH, Tucker GJ: Behavioral Neurology, second edition. Oxford University Press, 1978, pp 135–137

Pitman RK: Neurological etiology of obsessive-compulsive disorders? Am J Psychiatry 139:139–140, 1982

Plum P, Posner JB: Diagnosis of Stupor and Coma, second edition. Philadelphia, FA Davis, 1972

Posner JB: Coma and other states of consciousness, in Brain Death. Edited by Korein J. Ann NY Acad Sci 315:215–224, 1978

Potkin SG, Weinberger DR, Linnoila M, et al: 5-Hydroxy-indoleacetic acid in schizophrenic patients with enlarged cerebral ventricles. Am J Psychiatry 140:21–25, 1983

Quitkin F, Rifkin A, Klein DF: Neurologic soft signs in schizophrenia and character disorders. Arch Gen Psychiatry 33:845–853, 1979

Reed JL: The proverbs test in schizophrenia. Br J Psychiatry 114:317–321, 1968

Reich JH: Proverbs and the modern mental status exam. Compr Psychiatry 22:528–531, 1981

Reiss D, Feinstein C, Weinberger DR, et al: Ventricular enlargement in child psychiatric patients. A controlled study with planimetric measurements. Am J Psychiatry 140:453–456, 1983

Rochford JM, Detre T, Tucker GJ, et al: Neuropsychological impairment in functional psychiatric diseases. Arch Gen Psychiatry 22:114–119, 1970

Rockstroh B, Elbert T, Berbaumer N, et al: Slow Brain Potentials and Behavior. Baltimore, Urban and Schwarzenberg, 1982, pp 199–210

Roger J, Lob H, Tassinari CA: Generalized status epilepticus as a confusional state (petit mal status or absence status epilepticus), in Handbook of Clinical Neurology, Vol 15. Edited by Vinken PJ, Bruyn GW. Amsterdam, North Holland, 1974, pp 145–182

Rosenbaum AH, Maruta T, Schatzberg AF, et al: Toward a biochemical classification of depressive disorders, VII: urinary free cortisol and urinary MHPG in depressions. Am J Psychiatry 140:314–317, 1983

Rowe MJ, Carlson C: Brainstem auditory evoked potentials in postconcussion dizziness. Arch Neurol 37:679–683, 1980

Sackeim HA, Greenberg MS, Weiman AL, et al: Hemispheric asymmetry in the expression of positive and negative emotions, neurologic evidence. Arch Gen Psychiatry 39:210–218, 1982

Schatzberg AF, Rothschild AJ, Stahl JB, et al: The dexamethasone suppression test: identification of subtypes of depression. Am J Psychiatry 140:88–91, 1983

Scheinberg P: Modern Practical Neurology, An Introduction to Diagnosis and Management of Common Neurologic Disorders, second edition. New York, Raven, 1981

Schenk L, Bear D: Multiple personality and related dissociative phenomena in patients with temporal lobe epilepsy. Am J Psychiatry 138:1311–1316, 1981

Silverstein M, Meltzer HY: Neuropsychological dysfunction in the major psychoses, in Laterality and Psychopathology. Edited by Flor-Henry F, Gruzelier J. Amsterdam, Elsevier/North Holland, 1983, pp 143–162

Sisler GC: Psychiatric disorder associated with head injury, in The Psychiatric Clinics of North America, Vol I, Brain Disorders: Clinical Diagnosis and Management. Edited by Hendrie HC. Philadelphia, WB Saunders, 1978, pp 137–152

Skodol AE, Spitzer RL: DSM-III: rationale, basic concepts, and some differences from ICD-9. Acta Psychiatr Scand 66:271–281, 1982

Slaby AE, Wyatt RJ: Dementia in the Presenium. Springfield, Ill, Charles C Thomas, 1974

Speidel H, Rodewald G: Psychic and Neurological Dysfunctions after Open-Heart Surgery, First International Symposium, Hamburg, Band 19, Intensivmedizin Notfallmedizin Anasthesiologie. Stuttgart, Georg Thieme, 1980

Spitzer RL, Forman JBW, Nee J: DSM-III field trials, I: initial interrater diagnostic reliability. Am J Psychiatry 136:815–817, 1979

Stahl SM, Woo DJ, Mefford IN, et al: Hyperserotonemia and platelet serotonin uptake and release in schizophrenia and affective disorder. Am J Psychiatry 140:27–30, 1983

Sternberg ED, Jarvik MD: Memory functions in depression. Arch Gen Psychiatry 33:219–224, 1976

Strub RL, Black FW: Organic Brain Syndromes, An Introduction to Neurobehavioral Disorders. Philadelphia, FA Davis, 1981, pp 335–368

Swann AC, Secunda S, Davis JM, et al: CSF monoamine metabolites in mania. Am J Psychiatry 140:396–397, 1983

Tanaka Y, Hazama H, Fukuhara T, et al: Computerized tomography of the brain in manic-depressive patients. A controlled study. Folia Psychiatr Neurol Jpn 36:137–143, 1982

Tanaka Y, Hazama H, Kawahara R, et al: Computerized tomography of the brain in schizophrenic patients: a controlled study. Acta Pychiatr Scand 63:191–197, 1981

Targum SD: Neuroendocrine dysfunction in schizophreniform disorder: correlation with six-month clinical outcome. Am J Psychiatry 140:309–313, 1983

Taylor MA, Abrams R: Reassessing the bipolar-unipolar dichotomy. J Affect Dis 3:195–217, 1980

Cognitive dysfunction in schizophrenia. Am J Psychiatry 141:196–201, 1984

Taylor MA, Abrams R, Faber R, et al: Cognitive tasks in the mental status examination. J Nerv Ment Dis 168:167–170, 1980a

Taylor MA, Abrams R, Hayman M: The classification of affective disorder: a reassessment of the bipolar-unipolar dichotomy, part I: a clinical, laboratory and family study. J Affect Dis 2:95–109, 1980b

Teuber HL: The riddle of frontal lobe function in man, in The Frontal Granular Cortex and Behavior. Edited by Warren JM, Akert K. New York, McGraw-Hill, 1964, pp 410–444

Toone B: Psychoses of epilepsy, in Epilepsy and Psychiatry. Edited by Reynolds EH, Trimble MR. Edinburgh, Churchill Livingstone, 1981, pp 113–137

Torack RM: The Pathologic Physiology of Dementia, with Indications for Diagnosis and Treatment. Berlin, Springer-Verlag, 1978

Trimble MR: The interictal psychoses of epilepsy, in Psychiatric Aspects of Neurologic Disease, Vol II. Edited by Benson DF, Blumer D. New York, Grune & Stratton, 1982, pp 75–88

Trimble MR, Grant I: Psychiatric aspects of multiple sclerosis, in Psychiatric Aspects of Neurologic Disease, Vol II. Edited by Benson DF, Blumer D. New York, Grune & Stratton, 1982, pp 279–298

Tsai L, Tsuang MT: The Mini-Mental State Test and computerized tomography. Am J Psychiatry 136:436–439, 1979

Tucker GJ, Detre T, Harrow M, et al: Behavior and symptoms of psychiatric patients and the electroencephalogram. Arch Gen Psychiatry 12:278–286, 1965

Uytdenhoef P, Portelange P, Jacquy J, et al: Regional cerebral blood flow and lateralized hemispheric dysfunction in depression. Br J Psychiatry 143:128–132, 1983

Van Praag HM, Lader MH, Rafaelsen OJ, et al: Handbook of Biological Psychiatry, Part IV, Brain Mechanisms and Abnormal Behavior Chemistry. New York, Marcel Dekker, 1981

Vianna U: The electroencephalogram in schizophrenia, in Studies of Schizophrenia. Edited by Lader MH. Kent, England, Headley Bros, 1975, pp 54–58

Volavka J, Abrams R, Taylor MA, et al: Hemispheric lateralization of fast EEG activity in schizophrenia and endogenous depression, in Electroneurophysiology and Psychopathology, Advances in Biological Psychiatry, Vol 6. Edited by Mendlewicz J, Van Praag HM (series editors), Perris C, Kemali D, Vacca L (volume editors). Basel, Karger, 1981, pp 72–75

Weil AA: Ictal emotions occurring in temporal lobe dysfunction. Arch Neurol 1:101–111, 1959

Weinberger DR, DeLisi LE, Perman GP, et al: Computed tomography in schizophreniform disorder and other acute psychiatric disorders. Arch Gen Psychiatry 39:778–783, 1982

Weinberger DR, Fuller-Torrey E, Neophytides AN, et al: Lateralized cerebral ventricular enlargement in chronic schizophrenia. Arch Gen Psychiatry 36:735–739, 1979

Weller RA, Weller EB: Anorexia nervosa in a patient with an infiltrating tumor of the hypothalamus. Am J Psychiatry 139:824–825, 1982

Young AC, Costanzi JB, Mohr PD, et al: Is routine computerized axial tomography in epilepsy worthwhile? Lancet 2:1446–1447, 1982

10 An evaluation of the DSM-III substance-use disorders

BRUCE J. ROUNSAVILLE

ABSENCE OF VALIDATING DATA SPECIFIC TO *DSM-III*

Is the *DSM-III* section on substance-use disorders working? A definitive answer to this question would require data collected along the lines described by Robins and Guze (1970) for validating diagnostic entities, such as the following:

1. data regarding the boundaries of the diagnosis, such that the inclusion criteria positively classify those who are judged to have the syndrome by some external standard, and the exclusion criteria rule out those with similar but distinctly different disorders;
2. data on biochemical mechanisms and biological markers that might distinguish the substance-abuse syndromes from each other and from other types of disorders (to some extent, serum and urine tests for presence of the substance being used represent the most nearly definitive such tests in the entire diagnostic system, although a positive test does not establish the diagnosis, and a negative test does not exclude it);
3. family-history data that suggest a coherent pattern of familially transmitted traits or symptoms;
4. follow-up data suggesting a coherent course for the disorder as defined by the current nomenclature, with particular emphasis on the extent to which the disorder is found to be stable (i.e., does not become another disorder).

In the three years following the publication of the *DSM-III*, data of this kind have not been forthcoming, especially in regard to substance-use disorders specifically defined according to *DSM-III* criteria, as opposed to earlier systems such as the Feighner system (Feighner et al., 1972) and the RDC (Spitzer, Endicott, and Robins, 1978). In fact, a literature search in this area produced only two articles pertaining to the utility of *DSM-III* criteria for substance-use disorders. In the first, Craig, Goodman, and Haugland (1982) rediagnosed 102 psychiatric inpatients according to *DSM-III* criteria on the basis of clinical-chart information and compared the diagnoses thus derived with those listed in

This work was supported in part by Grant Ko2 DA 00089-01 MH from the National Institute on Drug Abuse.

the charts, which had been based on *DSM-II* criteria. The only substance-use disorder diagnosed in the study was alcohol abuse or dependence (305.0 and 303.9), and the use of the new diagnostic system did not result in any changes in this category, although changes were noted in the schizophrenia and affective-disorder categories. In a second study comparing diagnoses arrived at using the *DSM-III*, Feighner, and RDC criteria derived on the basis of information gathered with the structured Diagnostic Interview Schedule (1980), Singerman and associates (1981) found the concordance rates among the three systems to be quite high in pairwise comparisons of the diagnostic systems (κ ranging from .84 to .95). Used with 216 individuals in psychiatric and other settings, the level of concordance was higher than those for all other categories except mania. This high concordance was achieved despite numerous small differences in criteria in the three systems, as enumerated by Stoltzman and associates (1981). Thus, the scant amount of information available on the results of using *DSM-III* alcohol-abuse and -dependence criteria in practice suggests that the alterations in criteria result in diagnostic decisions that are largely indistinguishable from those made using earlier systems.

Although these findings may be reassuring to those who were comfortable with the previous systems, the small amount of empirical data thus far published specifically pertaining to *DSM-III* criteria for substance-use disorders is of little help in the process of reevaluating and revising the current system. Despite the lack of investigations that have been completed to date, there is a rich source of data for evaluating the validity of *DSM-III* substance-use criteria in the form of survey material collected as part of the multicenter Epidemiologic Catchment Area (ECA) program sponsored by the National Institute of Mental Health. In this large-scale study, data pertaining to psychiatric disorders have been collected in probability samples in catchment areas in five U.S. cities. The surveys consist of two repeat interviews conducted over the course of one year. The method of obtaining data is the Diagnostic Interview Schedule (1980), which provides sufficient information from which *DSM-III*, Feighner, and RDC diagnoses can be determined. From this data set, a range of studies related to validity of criteria for substance-use disorders can be performed. The following represents a partial list of criterion-related topics that can be investigated using ECA data:

1. Course of illness. One-year follow-up information can be used to determine the stability, test–retest reliability, and prognostic significance of the different substance-use disorders.

2. Symptom groupings. The individual symptoms that are used to determine the diagnoses of the different substance-use disorders can be analyzed using factor analysis and cluster techniques to evaluate dimensions of substance-use disorders. As described later, the current *DSM-III* criteria utilize three dimensions: pathological use, substance-use-associated social impairment, and physiological tolerance and withdrawal. Analysis of items making up the different dimensions may suggest the validity of the current system or suggest different ways for symptoms to be brought together into syndromes. Related to the follow-up portion of the ECA study, the prognostic significance and stability for different aspects of the substance-use syndromes may vary widely, such that, to give a hypothetical example, tolerance may be of little prognostic significance, whereas withdrawal symptoms and medical complications may be comparatively more powerful determinants of subsequent course.

3. Interrelations among substance-use syndromes. The extent to which substance-use disorders coexist may help to better define the syndromes and their courses. Moreover, an evaluation can be made of the concept of "poly–drug abuse" which is believed to be widely seen in practice, but is not included in the *DSM-III* system.

4. Interrelations among substance-use disorders and other categories of psychiatric diagnoses. Knowledge of rates and patterns for other psychiatric disorders in those who meet the criteria for substance-use disorders may provide clues about potential antecedents or consequences of the substance-use disorders and also may be useful in suggesting criteria that can be used to discriminate between coexistent disorders and a disorder that may be diagnosed as an artifact of characteristics of substance-use disorders. For example, an opiate addict or alcoholic may transiently meet many criteria for an affective disorder simply as a result of going through a withdrawal syndrome and may not experience these symptoms in any other context. It would be useful to know which criteria might distinguish between patients with this withdrawal syndrome and those in whom depressive symptoms occur more pervasively.

5. Sensitivity and specificity of criteria for substance-use disorders. An analysis of the sensitivity and specificity of diagnostic criteria requires that agreed-upon external validating criteria be available, and this is unlikely to be the case in the ECA or any other study. However, an approach to this kind of analysis can be made by evaluating those individuals who are currently in alcohol treatment programs. Different diagnostic criteria can be used to establish alcohol-abuse and -dependence diagnoses for these individuals to evaluate the utility of different systems in categorizing treated alcoholics. In a broader analysis, different substance-use disorders in the general population can be evaluated to determine if inclusion or omission of various diagnostic criteria has a marked influence on rates. This kind of analysis can be used to remove redundant criteria and to highlight highly discriminating or important criteria.

Although the ECA program has the potential to provide a wealth of data regarding the validity of diagnostic criteria for substance-use disorders, little empirical work has been accomplished to date since the development of *DSM-III* criteria that might help us to evaluate their utility.

CRITIQUES OF CRITERIA FOR *DSM-III* SUBSTANCE-USE DISORDERS

In the absence of data specifically relevant to *DSM-III* substance-use diagnoses, I attempted to seek out critiques of the current criteria. To do this, I performed a selected survey of literature on trends in the diagnosis of substance-use disorders and obtained verbal critiques from a group of experts in the drug-abuse field, most of whom were listed as having contributed to the sections on substance-use disorders in *DSM-III*. Using this method, I obtained a wide range of critiques, from the general and far-reaching to the highly specific. In the remainder of this chapter, I list the issues raised, examine them critically, and suggest possible responses to the problems.

Characteristics of criteria for DSM-III substance-use disorders

To help the reader understand the critiques that follow, an overview of this section is quoted from Spitzer, Williams, and Skodol (1980):

This section of DSM-III includes disorders in which there are behavioral changes associated with more or less regular use of substances that affect the central nervous system and that in almost all subcultures would be viewed as undesirable. This category combines the DSM-II categories of Drug Dependence and Alcoholism to emphasize that the effects of the maladaptive uses of all substances of potential abuse and dependence are similar.

The Substance Use Disorders are divided into two major types: Abuse and Dependence. In general, Substance Abuse is defined by a pattern of pathological use for at least one month that causes impairment in social or occupational functioning. Examples of pathological use include inability to reduce or discontinue use or remaining intoxicated throughout the day. Substance Dependence is defined by the presence of either tolerance or withdrawal. For Alcohol and Cannabis Dependence, impairment in social or occupational functioning is also required. In the case of tobacco, the presence of a serious physical disorder that the individual knows is exacerbated by tobacco use is also considered evidence of Dependence. . . .

Many substances are associated with both abuse and dependence, including alcohol, barbiturates or similarly acting sedatives or hypnotics, opioids, amphetamines or similarly acting sympathomimetics, and cannabis. . . . Substances for which abuse but not dependence has been demonstrated include cocaine, phencyclidine (PCP) or similarly acting arylcyclohexylamines, and hallucinogens. (Phencyclidine is distinguished from hallucinogens despite some similarities in their effects.) There is also a category of Tobacco Dependence, justifiably included in this section by the potentially serious medical complications of long term use and its inclusion in ICD-9. . . . Poly-substance Use may be classified as such when it is not possible to identify each of the substances involved.

For each Substance Use Disorder in DSM-III, the pattern of use or course of the disorder is coded in the fifth digit as continuous, episodic, or in remission.

General problems with the DSM-III substance-use section

Problem 1: The DSM-III system is not adequate for conceptualizing or denoting coexistent features of substance-use disorders. It is almost universally accepted that there is more to substance-use disorders than simply using a lot of psychoactive drugs. Indeed, the *DSM-III* criteria for substance-use disorders are not intended to denote substance use per se, but behavioral changes associated with more or less regular use of these substances. Individuals with substance-use disorders, in addition to a pattern of pathological use of the substances, have been shown to have problems with social and occupational functioning, medical problems that may be caused or exacerbated by the substance use, and psychopathology, including personality disorders and episodic symptomatic disorders (McLellan et al., 1981; Kosten, Rounsaville, and Kleber, 1982; Rounsaville et al., 1982a,b). There are several areas in which problems may arise in denoting coexistent features of substance-use disorders and in taking them into consideration in treatment:

a. *In treatment planning,* clinicians may need to determine the relationships among substance abuse and coexistent problems and to communicate this to others. For example, is a patient's major depression secondary to his current episode of alcohol abuse, or did the depression long antedate the abuse of alcohol and provide the motivation for it? The approach to treatment may include efforts to curb alcohol abuse and efforts to alleviate depression, which can be offered simultaneously or sequentially. In making the clinical decisions for a treatment approach it may be useful to have a nosologic system that can denote primary and secondary problems. Of course, providing such a system implies that it is possible to determine which disorders are primary and which are secondary, and that may not be possible.

b. *In determining the diagnosis in a substance-use disorder* there is an implication that it is possible to distinguish between antecedents and consequences of substance-use patterns and to determine that the coexisting signs and symptoms are indeed associated with the substance use rather than simply coexisting with it. For example, in the diagnosis of alcohol dependence and alcohol abuse, the criteria include "absence from work, loss of job, . . . arguments or difficulties with family or friends because of excessive alcohol use." In a clinical setting it may be comparatively straightforward to infer consequences of substance use in those coming to treatment. However, in community surveys or in nonpsychiatric settings it may be more difficult to determine if alcohol use caused the social problems or if the social problems caused the alcohol abuse, or if they were both caused by a third factor.

Difficulty in inferring antecedents of drug use from consequences not only is a practical problem for the diagnosis but also points to a general issue regarding the nosologic system, namely, What is the disorder, and how is it distinguished from the consequences of it? This is a fundamental issue in the diagnosis of mental disorders in all categories of the *DSM-III.* For all psychiatric disorders, and specifically for substance-abuse disorders, having adverse consequences from the disorder is seen as part of the disorder itself, or at least as essential in order for the rater to determine that the disorder exists. This decision presumably has been made because there is no consensus regarding the disease processes that underlie most psychiatric disorders. Hence, unless this can be defined and detected in a reliable way, then as a practical matter it is essential to detect consequences of the disorder before one can be sure that the disorder exists. This definition of psychiatric disorders by their consequences may be seen as emblematic of the relatively early stages of our understanding of psychopathology. Because we do not have a clear understanding of underlying disease mechanisms, usually it is not possible to diagnose disorders at an early stage before adverse consequences exist. Moreover, given the potentially stigmatizing consequences of receiving a psychiatric diagnosis, it is potentially harmful to give a diagnostic label unless the disorder is sufficiently severe to lead to adverse consequences. In contrast, for many disorders in general medicine, diagnosis of a disorder can and should precede the onset of serious adverse consequences, as in the case of diagnosing hypertension before organ damage has occurred or detecting cancer at an early stage.

c. *In specialized settings,* such as mental health facilities that do not include services for substance abusers or in substance-abuse treatment units, there is the practical need to be alert to disorders that may not be presented by the patient as the primary reason for seeking treatment. Several investigations have demonstrated that a high percentage of those seeking treatment at substance-abuse treatment units have psychiatric disorders in non-substance-use categories, and, conversely, in general psychiatric clinics, a substantial number of patients have clinically significant substance-use disorders accompanying the problems that are receiving primary treatment emphasis. As a practical matter, detecting disorders that are not the focus of the specialized treatment setting may be haphazard, and omission of a complete diagnosis may undermine the efficiency of the treatment plan. In *DSM-III,* the system allows for a listing of all disorders for which the patient meets the criteria. However, there is no system that will lead to inquiry into diverse areas.

CURRENT *DSM-III* HANDLING OF COEXISTENT FEATURES OF SUBSTANCE-USE DISORDERS. To handle the issue of the multidimensionality of a substance abuser's problems, the *DSM-III* allows documentation of two kinds:

1. Multiple psychiatric disorders can be listed on axis I, and personality disorders can be diagnosed on axis II.
2. Medical disorders, life stress, and social adaptation can be rated on axes III–V.

To handle the issue of the priorities of the diagnoses, *DSM-III* allows the clinician to list the principal diagnosis first on both axis I and axis II.

Regarding the difficulty in determining the consequences of the substance-abuse disorders, *DSM-III* seems to assume that this can be done and/or that the disorders cannot be detected unless consequences are noted.

Regarding the need for clinicians to be alert to disorders that are not the focus of a clinic's specialized interests, a wide-ranging and readily usable structured interview schedule is available in the form of the Diagnostic Interview Schedule (1980), from which a wide range of *DSM-III* disorders can be diagnosed in adults.

POSSIBLE CHANGES IN *DSM-III*

1. Include a primary–secondary distinction. By this scheme, clinicians would make multiple diagnoses to specify within the diagnostic system whether various axis I disorders are primary or secondary. The implication of this denotation would be, at minimum, that the primary diagnosis preceded the secondary diagnosis in time and/or that the development of the secondary disorder was at least partially facilitated or caused by the primary disorder. In this scheme it would be essential to be allowed to omit the primary–secondary distinction if it were not possible to determine priority.

Advantages. The chief advantage of this alteration in the current system would be to allow clinicians to communicate, via the form of their diagnoses, their assessment of the underlying processes of the patient's condition. Moreover, in some disorders, with particular emphasis on depression, it has been argued that the primary–secondary distinction is highly meaningful (Akiskal, 1983) and can be of great significance regarding clinical features, course of illness, and treatment response.

Disadvantages. Inclusion of the primary–secondary distinction in the diagnosis itself, rather than in a clinical summary, may be premature at this time. To start with, this would be somewhat cumbersome to do, involving yet another digit or many more separate diagnostic numbers. More important, it goes against the more modest general principle of the *DSM-III* to describe disorders phenomenologically and without heavy reliance on etiological theories. Making a primary–secondary distinction presupposes that it is truly possible to know which disorder is primary, and it implies that this distinction is of clinical or theoretical significance. Neither of these assumptions is adequately supported by evidence, even in the case of the primary–secondary distinction for affective disorders, the category in which this distinction has received the most attention.

2. Remove the consequences of the substance-use disorders from the diagnostic criteria for the disorders. To handle the practical and theoretical difficulties inherent in using the consequences of the disorder to define and diagnose the disorder, it may be conceptually more sound to define substance abuse and dependence without reference to social consequences. Hence, the disorders would be defined by a pattern of pathological use and evidence of tolerance and/ or withdrawal. By this scheme, the degrees of disability and/or social problems associated with the substance-use disorder could be rated by an extra digit, from "none" to "completely disabling."

Advantages. The advantages of this system would be twofold: (a) It would relieve the diagnostician of the difficult task of having to determine whether various social problems are consequences or causes of the substance-use disorder. (b) It would reflect a theoretical understanding of substance-use disorders that suggests that a pathological pattern of use is the core pattern underlying the abuse of all classes of psychoactive substances. This view, articulated in the proposed World Health Organization model (WHO, 1981), has stirred considerable interest and shows promise, as is discussed later.

Disadvantages. The major disadvantage of eliminating the consequences of substance-use disorders from the diagnostic criteria would be that not enough is known about what constitutes a substance-use disorder in the absence of the consequences of it. This is true not only for the substance-use disorders but also for nearly all the disorders listed in *DSM-III*. For this reason, for most diagnoses, evidence of impairment associated with the disorder is required to make the diagnosis. Thus, for example, for a diagnosis of affective disorder, evidence of impairment associated with symptoms is required for the diagnosis. This is not a trivial matter, in that the ideas of "distress" and "disability" are inherent in the disease concept of psychiatric disorders in *DSM-III* (American Psychiatric Association, 1980), and it is incumbent on a medical model system with diagnostic categories to include strategies for distinguishing manifestations that are within normal limits from those that are abnormal. At present, the rule of thumb governing this decision in making psychiatric diagnoses is to avoid making a diagnosis unless evidence of significant distress or disability is present. To leave this out could undermine the credibility of the diagnostic system. However, if evidence could be brought to bear that compellingly demonstrates an underlying disease process that can be reliably detected in the absence of consequences of the disease (as in the case of hypertension), then this advance could readily be incorporated into the diagnostic system. At present, no adequate body of evidence exists to allow the underlying disease process in substance-use disorders to be detected.

3. Introduce a substance-use axis. By this scheme, the diagnostician would rate every patient for degree of substance use/misuse according to a global rating system.

Advantages. The primary advantage of this system would be that it would force clinicians to consider the importance of substance use in the lives of their patients. Because many patients in general psychiatric settings have clinically significant problems with substance use, an awareness of this issue could profitably be incorporated into the diagnosis and treatment planning for all patients.

Disadvantages. The major disadvantage of handling the multiple-diagnosis problem by adding axes would be that the utility of the multiaxis system would surely decrease if too many axes were included. The ideas for additional axes are numerous, and these must be weighed against the small chance that more than a limited number could actually be used in practice. The current system of allowing for multiple diagnoses and the availability of a diagnostic interview that covers substance-use disorders along with other types of psychiatric disorders may be the most practical system for ensuring that the range of patients' problems is adequately assessed.

Problem 2: The DSM-III system is atheoretical. In common with other diagnoses in *DSM-III*, drug-use disorders are distinguished by phenomenological features that have been shown to occur together in more than a chance fashion to a degree that justifies their being seen as a syndrome. In a field in which there are widely varying and frequently contradictory theoretical explanations for the phenomena observed, the atheoretical *DSM-III* approach may be appropriate given the current state of our knowledge.

DESCRIPTION OF WHO MODEL. Specifically pertaining to the substance-use disorders, the atheoretical nature of the criteria has been criticized because of failure to note the existence of "addictive processes" (Milkman and Sundenwerth, 1982) or of a core "dependence syndrome" (WHO, 1981). The source of the most cogent and convincing statement of the need for a more coherent conceptualization of substance-use disorders is the consensus statement of the World Health Organization Working Group 4, which has been in the process of recommending changes in the substance-use sections of that organization's nomenclature, the *ICD-9* (WHO, 1981). Although the deliberations of this group have not yet yielded recommendations for specific criteria that can be used for diagnosing substance-use disorders, a model for substance-use disorders has been proposed that is believed to have implications for a nosologic system. The WHO model that has been proposed is a complex, dynamic scheme based on behavioral principles that puts forward a "system of reinforcement which initiates and perpetuates substance taking and dependence." Most relevant to possible methods for making diagnoses is a core "dependence syndrome" that is seen as multidimensional, with "various biologic, social and behavioral components," and "exists in degrees." Through the operation of learning-theory principles regarding the operation of stimuli and reinforcement related to learned behavior, the individual develops a core dependence syndrome, the cardinal feature of which is impaired control over substance use. Proposed key elements of the syndrome include the following features (WHO, 1981):

1. *Narrowing of repertoire* – a tendency for the substance-use pattern to become stereotyped around a regular schedule of almost continuous or daily consumption
2. *Salience of substance-taking behavior* – despite negative consequences, substance use is given higher priority than other activities that had previously been important to the subject
3. *Increased tolerance* – more and more of the substance is required to produce behavioral, subjective, and metabolic changes; large amounts of substance can be tolerated
4. *Repeated withdrawal symptoms* – mild to major symptoms characteristic of the particular substance are noted after a period of abstinence characteristic for each substance
5. *Use to avoid withdrawal* – relief or avoidance of withdrawal symptoms by further substance use, as in the case of morning drinking by alcohol-dependent individuals

6. *Compulsion to use substance* – subjective awareness of craving for substance, as well as impaired control over quantity and frequency of intake

7. *Readdiction liability* – a tendency for the syndrome to be rapidly reinstated when substance use is recommenced after a period of abstinence

The WHO model suggests that the dependence syndrome and any disabilities associated with it exist in degrees rather than in an all-or-none fashion. In addition, it is seen as multidimensional, with physical, social, and psychological determinants and consequences being understood as existing in degrees.

Work with the dependence-syndrome construct suggests that it is promising. In the brief period since it was first introduced, the dependence-syndrome construct has received considerable attention from researchers and clinicians working primarily in the alcoholism treatment field. A number of instruments have been developed to assess its usefulness (Hodgson et al., 1978; Stockwell et al., 1979; Chick, 1980; Skinner, 1981; Hesselbrock et al., 1983). Research in both experimental and clinical settings suggests that the severity of dependence predicts attendance at a treatment clinic (Skinner and Allen, 1982), cravings for alcohol after a "priming" drink (Hodgson, Rankin, and Stockwell, 1979), and failure to control drinking following relapse (Hodgson, 1980; Polich and Armor, 1981; Hesselbrock et al., 1983). Although further research is called for, it appears that the dependence-syndrome construct has considerable promise for diagnosis, early detection, and treatment planning (Hodgson, 1980).

Moreover, research is taking place to further validate the dependence-syndrome construct, to refine techniques for detecting and measuring it, and for determining core features that will be characteristic across the use of different classes of substances and in different cultures (Kleber, 1984).

IMPLICATIONS OF THE WHO MODEL FOR CHANGES IN *DSM-III*. Although numerous specific recommendations were made in the WHO memorandum (WHO, 1981), some of which are taken up later, the most important implications of the proposed model for revising the *DSM-III* system would involve two changes:

1. Separate dependence-syndrome elements from "adverse consequences" in diagnosing substance-use disorders. The *DSM-III* currently includes four major elements in the criteria for the substance-use disorders: (a) a pattern of pathological use, (b) evidence of substance-use-associated impairment, (c) evidence for tolerance and withdrawal, and (d) a minimum duration for the "abuse" diagnoses. The core dependence construct proposed in the WHO memorandum involved the first two of these elements, which would thus be the essential features required for substance-use disorders. Drug-related disabilities would be rated as a separate digit, or in some comparable fashion, but would not be considered criteria for the disorder.

Advantages. The primary advantage of distinguishing a core dependence syndrome from other elements of substance-use disorders would be to conform with theoretical ideas about the underlying nature of the disorders that cut across the different substance categories.

Disadvantages. The main disadvantage of organizing *DSM-III* substance-use disorders around the dependence-syndrome construct would be that there is insufficient evidence to date to suggest the validity of the construct or to help in determining what the specific criteria might be to detect its presence or to denote the degrees of its severity. Thus, although several investigators have developed instruments for rating the dependence syndrome, these are insufficiently developed at this point to yield specific criteria by which to determine the degree of dependence on alcohol, and even less evidence is available regarding the use of other categories of substances. In order to displace the current system, which includes disabilities in the diagnostic criteria in accordance with a medical "disease" model, it would be essential that studies from numerous settings be accomplished to demonstrate that the dependence elements are separable from consequences and that the dependence-factor elements are of comparatively great utility for such purposes as predicting the course of the disease. In the absence of such data, the atheoretical model may be a first step preferable to premature adoption of a model based on an underlying theory.

2. Include a rating of degrees of dependence and of drug-related disabilities. A rating system could be devised in the substance-use disorders to denote degrees of the substance-dependence syndrome and of drug-related disabilities with specific anchor points. At present, the way that degrees of substance-use disorders can be rated includes distinguishing between "abuse" and "dependence" and denoting the pattern of abuse or dependence according to time course as episodic, continuous, in remission, or unspecified. In the current system, the key distinguishing element between abuse and dependence is evidence of physiological adaptation to the substance evinced by tolerance or withdrawal symptoms. This difference may involve a difference in the WHO concept of degree of dependence, although only physiological, not behavioral, elements are considered. The denotation of the time course of the disorder is related to the WHO concept of degree of dependence, but only tangentially so.

Advantages. The advantage of rating degrees of substance dependence and disability would result in a greater ability to predict the treatment response or the course of the disorder, superior to that allowed with a categorical, all-or-none system. The best evidence of this would take the form of follow-up studies or experimental studies of patient/treatment matching, which would demonstrate differential outcomes when rating degrees of dependence or substance problems, but which would not yield significant predictions from simply noting the presence or absence of the disorder or the presence of abuse or dependence.

Disadvantages. The main disadvantage of this proposal would be that there is insufficient empirical evidence for its superiority over a categorical approach. Although there is evidence for the multidimensionality of substance-use disorders, particularly as related to treatment outcome (McLellan et al., 1981; Rounsaville et al., 1982), this work has not sufficiently evolved to allow a rating system to be developed that could provide a specific method for rating degrees of dependence or substance-related disability.

SUMMARY OF WHO ALTERNATIVE. Although the WHO conceptualization of substance-use disorders is promising, and developments in assessing it and determining its validity should be taken into consideration when *DSM-III* is revised, it would be premature to recommend specific revisions in *DSM-III* on the basis of this model until more definitive research evidence is available.

Problem 3: Tolerance is a poor criterion for determining dependence. This criticism is pertinent on many levels:

First, there is the theoretical problem that tolerance in *DSM-III* is not complexly specified, whereas the tolerance phenomena are complex and varied. Tolerance may take place through different mechanisms.

Pharmacodynamic tolerance is present when, after exposure to a drug, higher levels of the drug are required at its site of action to produce a given response. Metabolic tolerance is the increased capacity to metabolize a drug: it can be induced by the substance itself or by some other agent. (WHO, 1981)

In addition to different mechanisms of tolerance, different aspects of a given drug's effect may be susceptible to tolerance, whereas others are not. For example, in the case of barbiturates, the euphoric effect is susceptible to tolerance, whereas the respiratory-depression effect is not, making this class of drugs particularly prone to overdose (Jaffee, 1980). Because of the complexity of tolerance phenomena, it is possible that an individual may be incorrectly rated as having developed tolerance to alcohol, when in fact the individual's liver enzymes were induced by another drug. Alternatively, the extent to which one may be able to accurately monitor one's tolerance may be limited, given its complexity. *DSM-III* does specify that the tolerance is to the "desired effect," but this may not really simplify matters.

Second, there are wide individual differences in initial levels of tolerance to drugs. Although *DSM-III* does specify that there need to be "markedly increased amounts" of the substance, and "tolerance" refers to a change in drug effect rather than to an absolute level of drug that can be taken, this is confusing in practice. What does "markedly" mean in an individual case? In order to make the term more precise, a percentage of increase could be specified, or given quantity-frequency numbers could be supplied. However, for the most part, specific amounts of drug are wisely omitted from *DSM-III* criteria because of the large range of individual differences in amounts that can be used without problems.

Third, it is simply too easy to meet the tolerance criteria the way they are currently written. To start with, the phenomenon of tolerance to opiates has been shown to begin with the first use of the drug (Jaffee, 1980). Although "marked" changes are required, the rater is given the option of noting that the subject is using much more of the drug or that the subject uses the same amount of drug but gets much less out of it. Getting much less out of using a drug may be more related to loss of novelty or learning the rituals for using the drug than to development of physiological tolerance. Thus, it is not hard to imagine that many individuals with comparatively weak changes in tolerance may provide a rater with a falsely positive answer to questions about tolerance.

Fourth, in the case of alcoholism, individuals who are at comparatively advanced stages of the disorder have the phenomenon of reversed tolerance, such that less of the drug is required to achieve the desired effect (Segal, 1981).

Fifth, given the specification that tolerance relates to the "desired effect," this is a highly subjective criterion that may be difficult to answer reliably. For example, a heavy drinker may drink pretty much the same amount for many years, although that amount is far greater than the amount he initially used. However, he may simply be unable to remember the earlier, smaller amount of alcohol consumed.

POSSIBLE CHANGES IN *DSM-III*

1. Qualify the term more specifically. Take into consideration the properties of each class of drugs, and try to specify more precisely what "markedly" means.

2. Remove "tolerance" from the criteria for dependence. Though more radical, this move may be more expeditious, with little loss of utility. The remaining criterion to distinguish between abuse and dependence would be the presence of withdrawal symptoms. The main problem with omitting tolerance from the dependence criteria would be that one might miss the individual who uses large amounts of a drug on a daily basis but who has such a steady supply that withdrawal symptoms never occur. In practice, few such individuals exist. Even for readily available, legally obtained substances such as tobacco and alcohol, few heavy users have not at some time found themselves separated from the drug long enough to begin to experience withdrawal symptoms. In the case of substances more difficult to obtain, heavy users typically have difficulties in maintaining their supplies of the drug, such that withdrawal symptoms are a constant threat. Thus, it is not likely that many individuals would be incorrectly labeled as "not dependent" if tolerance were withdrawn from the criteria for substance dependence.

Problem 4: The relationship between substance abuse and substance dependence is inconsistent and illogical in several substance categories. As currently written, because of variations in the criteria for substance dependence across the different categories of drugs, dependence includes and sometimes mixes two different concepts: a "psychological" dependence characterized by a pathological pattern of use and a "physiological" dependence characterized by a substance-specific withdrawal syndrome. This approach may lead to difficulties in practice because it fails to distinguish between two rather different classes of patients:

1. *Iatrogenically addicted individuals* experience tolerance and withdrawal induced by a postoperative medical regimen, but do not exhibit drug-seeking behavior or a pathological pattern of use. It may be useful to have a diagnostic label for these individuals, in that physicians are often called in to aid in with-

drawing them from the substances on which they have become dependent. However, because they have never exhibited a pathological pattern of use, their prognosis is quite different from the prognosis for those whose drug-seeking behavior has come to dominate their lives.

2. *Substance-dependent individuals* have a pattern of pathological use. They are substance-dependent, but typically use illicitly obtained substances and exhibit a pathological pattern of use. They are far more likely to resume substance use following detoxification than are iatrogenically addicted individuals.

It is primarily the second group of individuals who typically come to psychiatric attention, and given the potentially stigmatizing aspects of a substance-dependence diagnosis, it could be argued that the diagnosis should be reserved for them. In fact, for two categories of drugs, cannabis and alcohol, the dependence diagnosis is made only if abuse is also present. However, for the other categories, abuse is not required in order to qualify for a diagnosis of dependence. Hence, for those categories of substances, "abuse" may be a more severe diagnosis and more difficult to achieve, and the implication is that dependence is a more severe condition than abuse. In fact, the terms "dependence" and "abuse" were substitutes for "definite" and "probable" labels that were used in the RDC, on which the *DSM-III* is based (Robins, 1981).

To further complicate the issue, even though "abuse" is intended to be required for a diagnosis of alcohol dependence, it is still possible to make the diagnosis without evidence of a pattern of pathological use. The criteria for alcohol dependence require a "pattern of pathological alcohol use" or "impairment in social or occupational functioning." Hence, it may be possible to make the diagnosis of alcohol dependence too readily – through having family members object to the subject's drinking, and the subject having tolerance to alcohol but not having a pattern of pathological use. A further inconsistency with the alcohol-abuse and -dependence section is that several of the criteria listed under "pattern of pathological alcohol use" are more accurately conceptualized as criteria for "dependence," most notably the "need for daily use of alcohol for adequate functioning." The "need for daily use of alcohol for adequate functioning," though vague, may refer to the need to bolster self-esteem or to the need for daily alcohol use to prevent disabling withdrawal symptoms (Segal, 1981).

POSSIBLE CHANGE IN *DSM-III*

Include "abuse" as a prerequisite for the diagnosis of substance dependence in all categories. This solution would have the advantage of reserving the substance-dependence diagnosis for those who are the patients most typically seen. It would avoid pejorative and clinically misleading labeling of iatrogenically addicted individuals and opiate-dependent newborn children of opiate-dependent mothers.

For such individuals, when a diagnosis is needed at all, a separate set of terms could be used, such as "neuroadaptation" (WHO, 1981) or "dependence without abuse." This solution would make the distinction between abuse and dependence consistent and hierarchical across all classes of substances.

The principal disadvantage of this change would be that a new set of diagnostic labels would be needed to denote medically addicted individuals. In addition, there is the potential problem of not being able to diagnose an individual who is dependent on a substance but who does not quite meet criteria for a "pathological pattern of use" or substance-related social impairment. This might include physicians who are regular users of narcotics but whose substance use has gone undetected and has not yet led to social impairment. To handle this issue, revisions in the criteria for "pattern of pathological use" could be considered.

Specific problems with the DSM-III substance-use section

Problem 1: Attempts to achieve consistency of diagnostic criteria across different categories of drugs have led to meaningless criteria in specific instances

a. *"One-month duration."* A duration of one month is generally required for a diagnosis of substance abuse to be made. The quite reasonable intention of this requirement is to avoid diagnosing individuals who have a single episode of problematic drug use as "abusers" and thereby denoting that more enduring problems exist. However, in many instances, the idea of one month of abuse is not consistent with the way in which the drug is used. For example, in the case of hallucinogens, the typical pattern of even problematic use is episodic, such that even in a period of maximum use the drug may be used only once or twice per month. In the case of alcohol abusers, there are those individuals who are binge drinkers who may have two or three one-week episodes of problem drinking per year. In each episode the disturbance may last less than one month. Clearly the spirit of the one-month-duration criterion is met, if not the letter of the criterion.

b. *"Intoxicated throughout the day."* This criterion for a "pattern of pathological use" is included in several substance-abuse criteria, including those for cocaine abuse, amphetamine abuse, phencyclidine abuse, and so forth. The major problem with this criterion is that it is difficult to apply and may not be relevant to the patterns of use for different classes of substances. For long-acting substances, intoxication throughout the day or even into the next day is an unavoidable aspect of using the drug. For brief-acting substances such as cocaine, the expense of the substance ensures that few individuals stay intoxicated throughout any given day, even if the drug is used several times daily. In addition, the precise meaning of "throughout the day" may be difficult to ascertain in particular individuals, depending on their schedules of work and other social obligations.

POSSIBLE CHANGES IN *DSM-III*

1. Remove the one-month-duration criterion. This solution would solve the inconsistency problems but would then allow single episodes to qualify an individual as an "abuser" of a drug.

2. Tailor the one-month-duration criterion more specifically for each drug. This solution would take into consideration the typical pattern of use for each substance and determine the minimum duration of use or use-related problems accordingly.

3. Apply the phrase "intoxication throughout the day" more specifically for each class of drug or for subgroups in each class of drug. This would have the disadvantage of making the criteria for substance-use diagnoses highly complicated and more difficult to use.

4. Change the general concept of "intoxicated throughout the day" to the more socially relevant concept of "frequently intoxicated when social obligations make drug use inappropriate." This would then include those who drink too heavily at lunch and then return to work, those who have night jobs, and housewives who are intoxicated when they are expected to carry out child-care duties.

Problem 2: "Blackouts" are incorrectly defined in the alcohol-abuse and -dependence criteria. "Blackout" usually is meant to connote amnestic periods in which the individual does not lose consciousness and appears to others to be alert (Segal, 1981). The *DSM-III* criterion does not specify the absence of loss of consciousness and could include individuals who have "passed out." This could be revised by simply noting that amnesia takes place without loss of consciousness.

Problem 3: The quantity and frequency of drug use generally are not specified in the criteria for substance-use disorders, though this is inconsistent. Generally, the absolute quantity and frequency of drug use are not listed as considerations in diagnosing substance-use disorders in the *DSM-III*. This decision probably was made because of the wide variation among the unlearned ability of individuals to tolerate given amounts of different substances. Although age and weight could be used to qualify the amount of drug that can be safely used, this still would not be sufficient to account for variations among individuals. In addition to variations across individuals, there are variations in toxicities of different substances within the same class (e.g., phenobarbital vs. secobarbital), as well as variations for different routes of administration of a given substance. Hence, for a nosologic system, is is probably best to base diagnoses on patterns of use and consequences of use rather than on the amount used.

However, in two specific instances, the *DSM-III* departs from this policy. For alcohol abuse, "occasional consumption of a fifth of spirits" is seen as a criterion for a pattern of pathological use. In the criteria for barbiturate or sedative abuse, the amounts of 600 mg of secobarbital and 60 mg of diazepam are specifically listed. Although it is reasonable to suppose that these relatively large amounts probably would constitute "excessive use" in nearly everyone, it is conceivable that some individuals may be tolerant to these amounts without having a previous pattern of heavy use. In addition, as a practical matter, individuals who abuse barbiturates and sedatives may be taking illicitly obtained and manufactured substances and may not know how much they are using.

POSSIBLE CHANGES IN *DSM-III*. Omit specification of amounts of substances used from all categories of substance-use disorders.

Problem 4: "Cocaine dependence" is not included as a diagnosis. The major point behind this criticism is that a stereotypic pattern of withdrawal phenomena is noted after cessation of heavy cocaine use. These withdrawal phenomena are similar to those noted for withdrawal from amphetamine, but are of briefer duration (Smith and Wesson, 1980; Siegel, 1982; Gawin and Kleber, 1986). However, they can be clinically significant, although the relationship between the onset of withdrawal symptoms in cocaine use may be less strongly linked to repeated use than has been noted with opiates. However, if a syndrome of amphetamine dependence is recognized, then allowing for a diagnosis of cocaine dependence would be most consistent.

POSSIBLE CHANGE IN *DSM-III*. Include the diagnosis of cocaine dependence. The main difficulty with this change relates to one's interpretation of the shorter duration of abstinence phenomena in cocaine users.

Problem 5: The term "substance abuse" is objectionable. The main reasons for objection to the term "abuse" are that it is stigmatizing and imprecise. "Abuse" is an inherently social term and may vary widely across cultures, such that, for example, relatively nondestructive use of alcohol may be considered abuse by subgroups who adhere to religiously prescribed prohibitions of any use whereas in other subcultures the use of alcohol to the point of dependence may be condoned. Moreover, abuse may have many diverse implications.

POSSIBLE CHANGE IN *DSM-III*. The WHO Working Group (WHO, 1981) suggests that the term "abuse" be omitted from public use, with several alternative, more specific terms being substituted to handle the diverse meanings of the word:

1. "Unsanctioned use" would refer to "use of a drug that is not approved by a society or a group within that society."
2. "Hazardous use" would denote "use of a drug that will probably lead to harmful consequences for the users."
3. "Dysfunctional use" would denote "use of a drug that is leading to impaired psychological or social functioning."
4. "Harmful use" would be defined as "use of a drug that is known to have caused tissue damage or mental illness in the particular person."

The advantage of removing "abuse" from our diagnostic systems would be to avoid pejorative labeling and to improve the specificity in the meanings of the terms used. The main disadvantage of adding four terms to substitute for one would be a marked increase in the complexity of the nosologic system. Moreover, the issue of stigmatization and imprecision would be somewhat handled by including specific operational diagnostic criteria for the term "abuse."

Problem 6: The specific items used to diagnose alcohol abuse and dependence may be poorly chosen. The most empirically developed criticism of the validity of the diagnostic criteria for alcohol-use disorders was put forward by Mulford and Fitzgerald (1981). They suggested that the criteria for alcohol-related social problems might be too narrowly defined to allow diagnosis of alcoholics, particularly those who have not sought treatment. They pointed out that little validation work has been done with the Feighner, RDC, and *DSM-III* alcohol-related-problems criteria. Moreover, they provided data from the use of a 10-item Trouble-Due-to-Drinking Scale suggesting that this scale correctly classified as positive only 77% of a group of individuals seeking alcohol treatment or evaluation and 27% of a group of "designated" alcoholics in the community. Because having an alcohol-related problem is required for a *DSM-III* diagnosis of alcohol abuse and is a potential requirement for a *DSM-III* diagnosis of alcohol dependence, the *DSM-III* criteria were criticized as being inadequately sensitive to diagnose a sizable portion of "alcoholics."

There are several problems with the Mulford and Fitzgerald investigation that reduce the impact of their criticism. First, the 10-item Trouble-Due-to-Drinking Scale is similar to but not really equal to the *DSM-III* criteria, which differ in several specific respects. As an example, "Did you ever think you drank too much in general?" is not included as a criterion in the *DSM-III*. Second, the *DSM-III* criteria require other aspects of alcohol use that are not at all covered by the Mulford scale. These include the *DSM-III* alcohol-abuse criterion A requiring a pattern of pathological use and criterion C requiring a minimum duration of one month. Presumably this requirement would make the *DSM-III* even less sensitive than the Mulford scale. However, for the alcohol-dependence diagnosis, "a pattern of pathological use" or "impairment of social or occupational functioning" is required, potentially making *DSM-III* criteria easier to satisfy than the Mulford scale. Thus, the data presented by Mulford and Fitzgerald are not really pertinent to the issue of the sensitivity of the *DSM-III* criteria.

POSSIBLE CHANGE IN *DSM-III*. Despite the aforementioned reservations, the Mulford and Fitzgerald critique of the inadequate level of validation of *DSM-III* criteria is most pertinent and is consistent with that of others (WHO, 1981). A careful investigation of the consistency and discriminatory and predictive powers of the diverse diagnostic criteria used in the *DSM-III* substance-use section is much needed to aid in their refinement.

Problem 7: The term "dependence" is multidimensional
POSSIBLE CHANGE IN *DSM-III*. Divide the term "dependence" into a behavioral/psychological component and a neurophysiological component. This suggestion is also derived from the WHO memorandum (1981) and

reflects the general strategy of separately rating the substantially different dimensions of substance-use disorders. At present, some *DSM-III* diagnoses include the notion of "abuse" with a "pathological pattern of use" as being a part of "dependence," whereas other categories include only evidence of tolerance or withdrawal as sufficient to determine dependence. The most important clinical situation in which this distinction arises is iatrogenically induced dependence to narcotics, in which tolerance and withdrawal can be noted, but there is no drug-seeking behavior or pattern of pathological use. To help in making this distinction, the term "neuroadaptation" is proposed for denoting the physiological changes that underlie the physical component of dependence.

The primary advantage of this change in terminology would be to separate those with iatrogenically induced substance dependence from those whose dependence is coupled with a pattern of pathological use. In practice, in most substance-resistant individuals, the "neuroadaptation" and the "pathological pattern of use" almost invariably coexist. This principle is even recognized in the WHO-model "dependence-syndrome" construct, which includes items that are related to "neuroadaptation" with those related to a "pathological pattern of use" in the same factor. The disadvantage of dividing the terms would be to complicate the way of naming all substance disorders, whereas simply to create a separate category for "iatrogenically induced disorder" or for "dependence without abuse" might be more expeditious.

REFERENCES

Akiskal HS: Diagnosis and classification of affective disorders: new insights from clinical and laboratory approaches. Psychiatr Dev 2:123–160, 1983

American Psychiatric Association: Diagnostic and Statistical Manual of Mental Disorders, third edition. Washington, DC, APA, 1980

Chick J: Alcohol dependence: methodological issues in its measurement: reliability of the criteria. Br J Addict 75:175–186, 1980

Craig TJ, Goodman AB, Hauglan G: Impact of DSM-III on clinical practice. Am J Psychiatry 139:922–925, 1982

Diagnostic Interview Schedule, version two. Rockville Md, National Institute of Mental Health, 1980

Feighner JP, Robins E, Guze SB, et al: Diagnostic criteria for use in psychiatric research. Arch Gen Psychiatry 26:57–63, 1972

Gawin FH, Kleber HD: Cocaine abusers: abstinence symptomatology and psychiatric diagnosis. Arch Gen Psychiatry 43:107–113, 1986

Hesselbrock M, Babor TF, Hesselbrock V, et al: Never believe an alcoholic? On the validity of self report measures of alcohol dependence and related constructs. Int J Addict 18:593–609, 1983

Hodgson RJ: Treatment strategies for the early problem drinker, in Alcoholism Treatment in Transition. Edited by Edwards G, Grant M. Baltimore, University Park Press, 1980, pp 162–177

Hodgson RJ, Rankin JJ, Stockwell TR: Alcohol dependence and the priming effect. Behav Res Ther 17:379–387, 1979

Hodgson R, Stockwell T, Rankin H, et al: Alcohol dependence: the concept, its utility and measurement. Br J Addict 73:339–342, 1978

Jaffee JH: Drug addiction and drug abuse, in The Pharmacological Basis of Therapeutics, sixth edition. Edited by Goodman LS, Gilman L. New York, Macmillan, 1980

Kleber HD: Principal investigator, ADAMHA/WHO project on drug dependence syndromes. Grant R 01 DA03814 from The National Institute of Drug Abuse, 1984

Kosten TR, Rounsaville BJ, Kleber HD: DSM-III personality disorders in opiate addicts. Compr Psychiatry 23:572–581, 1982

McLellan AT, Luborsky L, Woody GE, et al: Are the "addiction-related" problems of substance abusers really related? J Nerv Ment Dis 169:232–239, 1981

Milkman H, Sundenwerth S: Addictive processes. J Psychoact Drugs 14:177–192, 1982

Mulford HA, Fitzgerald JL: On the validity of the Research Diagnostic Criteria, the Feighner criteria, and the DSM-III for diagnosing alcoholics. J Nerv Ment Dis 169:654–658, 1981

Polich JM, Armor DJ: The Course of Alcoholism: Four Years after Treatment. New York, Wiley, 1981

Robins E, Guze SB: Establishment of diagnostic validity in psychiatric illness: its application to schizophrenia. Am J Psychiatry 126:983–987, 1970

Robins LN: The diagnosis of alcoholism after DSM-III, in Evaluation of the Alcoholic: Implications for Research, Theory and Treatment, Monograph 5. Rockville, Md, National Institute on Alcohol Abuse and Alcoholism Research, 1981, pp 85–102

Rounsaville BJ, Tierney T, Crits-Christophe K, et al: Predictors of outcome in treatment of opiate addicts: evidence for the multidimensional nature of addicts' problems. Compr Psychiatry 23:462–478, 1982a

Rounsaville BJ, Weissman MM, Kleber H, et al: The heterogeneity of psychiatric diagnosis in treated opiate addicts. Arch Gen Psychiatry 39:161–166, 1982b

Segal BM: Alcohol disorders and DSM-III. J Clin Psychiatry 42:448, 1981

Siegel RK: Cocaine smoking. J Psychoact Drugs 14:321–337, 1982

Singerman B, Stoltzman RK, Robins LN, et al: Diagnostic concordance between DSM-III, Feighner, and RDC. Clin Psychiatry 42:422–426, 1981

Skinner HA: Primary syndromes of alcohol abuse: their management and correlates. Br J Addict 76:63–76, 1981

Skinner HA, Allen BA: Alcohol dependence syndrome: measurement and validation. J Abnorm Psychol 91:199–209, 1982

Smith DE, Wesson DR: Cocaine, in Cocaine. Edited by Jeri RJ. Lima, Peru, Pacific Press, 1980

Spitzer RL, Endicott J, Robins E: Research diagnostic criteria: rationale and reliability. Arch Gen Psychiatry 35:773–782, 1978

Spitzer RL, Williams JB, Skodol AE: DSM-III: the major achievements and an overview. Am J Psychiatry 137:151–164, 1980

Stockwell T, Hodgson R, Edwards G, et al: The development of a questionnaire to measure severity of alcohol dependence. Br J Addict 74:79–87, 1979

Stoltzman RK, Helzer JE, Robins LN, et al: How does DSM-III differ from the systems on which it was built? J Clin Psychiatry 42:411–421, 1981

WHO: Memorandum: nomenclature and classification of drug- and alcohol-related problems. Bull WHO 59:225–242, 1981

11 *Current review of psychosexual disorders*

DAVID P. MCWHIRTER AND MARTHA J.
KIRKPATRICK

The explosion of new data concerning human sexuality and its various forms of expression may have reached its culmination, or at least a plateau. In the past three years there has been a dearth of new findings. The pivotal contributions of Masters and Johnson (1966, 1970) followed the pioneering studies of Kinsey and associates (1948, 1953). Although much groundwork had been laid in earlier decades, the 1950s and 1960s brought the most impressive advances in our knowledge concerning human sexuality. There has been a gradual shift in perspective, with a consequent opening up of attitudes about sexuality, with less rigid guidelines, lacking the former pejorative connotations and judgmental conclusions. Old stereotypes, often reinforced by inadequately researched studies, have fallen by the wayside as more recent research has uncovered new data that defy understanding or interpretation with the old tools of psychological investigation. The physiology and neurochemistry of sexual responses are just beginning to be studied at significant levels of confidence, replicability, and accuracy. Our understanding of the roots of gender identity is only slightly less confused today than it was in the recent past.

The "Psychosexual Disorders" section of *DSM-III* has proved to be a positive step forward in the clarification of our understanding of the wide range of variations to be found in the expression of human sexuality. The diagnostic criteria have sharpened our thinking in many areas and standardized our discussions and research, and still more clarification is needed. New findings have appeared that have shed bright light in formerly dark zones. Most important, *DSM-III* has brought a new sense of neutrality to our thinking about some areas of sexual functioning. It is all too easy to allow old beliefs to continue to be used as facts, even in the face of astounding new evidence. From past experience we have learned how easy it is to manufacture new mental illnesses simply by using our authority to call them that, and in the process label a whole new group of persons as ill, without the substantive, empirical research to support our pronouncements. It seems very important, especially in the field of human sexuality, for us to tread lightly with our diagnostic acumen, leaning on the new knowledge we have while admitting our ignorance about so much.

This chapter briefly discusses some, but not all, of the issues involved in an evaluation of the "Psychosexual Disorders" section of *DSM-III*. In addition to a review of the most current literature, we present a questionnaire (Table 11.1) that was submitted to some of those on the original Psychosexual Disorders Committee for *DSM-III* and to other selected experts around the country who have been using the diagnostic manual. We also review some, but not all, of the correspondence in Dr. Spitzer's files on the more controversial portions of this section. We follow the four-division format of psychosexual disorders in *DSM-III*: gender-identity disorders, paraphilias, psychosexual dysfunctions, and other psychosexual disorders.

GENDER-IDENTITY DISORDERS

In a letter to Robert Spitzer in August 1978, Robert Stoller said:

I believe the issues are insoluble at present due to our lack of adequate information regarding syndromes to be described and because present-day thinking (theories) on sexual behavior are still so unformed. You know that I agree with you that we must nonetheless press on to develop a classification that will serve us all in our clinical work and that will form the best possible basis for further advances in research.

302.5x Transsexualism

There have been numerous articles on postoperative evaluation of individuals with the transsexual syndrome (Hunt and Hampson, 1980; Satterfield, 1982). There also have been numerous suggestions for revisions of this category. One of the major objections seems to revolve around criterion C: "The disturbance has been continuous (not limited to periods of stress) for at least two years." Some clinicians and researchers insist that this criterion has the potential to introduce persons to the category of transsexualism who are not really suitable candidates for reassignment surgery. For instance, among males, some transvestites get diagnosed as transsexual when they suddenly panic and believe that they need sex-reassignment surgery. We have been calling this condition "transsexual crisis" (Huntington, Huntington, and McWhirter, 1983). The disturbance is frequently continuous for several years and thus fits the category of transsexualism. Some propose that the two-year criterion is too brief and really should read: "The disturbance has been present in the early developmental history and continuous (not limited to periods of stress) for at least two years." This tightening of the criteria for transsexualism would force more diagnoses into the "atypical gender-identity disorder," which then would need to be expanded to include several other categories, such as the individual who lives as the opposite sex, but does not seek reassignment surgery and is not uncomfortable with his/her anatomic sex. We have been referring to this individual as a "transgenderist" (Huntington et al., 1983).

We need a diagnostic category such as "progressive gender-identity disorder," with several subtypes, such as those cross-dressing heterosexual men and those predominantly homosexual men who cross-dress, sometimes as female impersonators, who then progress on to seeking sex-reassignment surgery. There is

Table 11.1. *Questionnaire on psychosexual-disorders classification of DSM-III*

General questions
Please respond to the following questions on separate sheets of paper. Please feel free to skip those you feel unable to answer.

1. *DSM-III* provides for an axis I or principal diagnosis of psychosexual disorders, with other data contained on the other axes. Has this been helpful to you? Has this approach simplified and/or clarified diagnostic problems?
2. Is this section sufficiently comprehensive? Are there other sexual situations that you think belong here, e.g., repercussions from rape or incest?
3. Are there problems you have encountered with the diagnostic criteria for any disorder listed? Suggestions for changes?
4. What new data do you think should be incorporated in *DSM-IV?* Specifically, are there new data on any specific disorder, including clinical course, outcome, family history, or treatment response, that should be included?

Specific questions
1. Are the diagnostic criteria for transsexualism specific enough? Should there be more emphasis on the intensity of the desire, the early history, lack of precipitating factors, the insistent quality of the desire, the increase in social isolation?
2. *Paraphilias:* Is the distinction between an individual who has a wide range of fantasies during sexual relations and one who has a limiting and distressing reliance on bizarre acts or symbolic behaviors sufficiently clear? Should distinctions be made between paraphilias of behavior, such as voyeurism and exhibitionism, and those of object choice, such as pedophilia?
3. *Psychosexual dysfunctions:*
   a. This category is based on "inhibition" as the essential feature. Is this consistent with your experience? Should there be consideration of dysinhibited states, e.g., hypersexuality or compulsive masturbation?
   b. Is the division of the sexual-response cycle into appetitive, excitement, orgasm, and resolution satisfactory? Should orgasm and ejaculation be separate events for the male? Should mention be made of the difficulties that arise as a consequence of male/female sexual differences in the resolution phase?
   c. Are the categories of sexual dysfunction sufficiently comprehensive?
   d. Does your experience confirm instances of possible pathology in women who experience orgasm during noncoital clitoral stimulation but not during coitus in the absence of manual clitoral stimulation?
   e. Inhibited male orgasm is defined by a delay or absence of ejaculation. Is this satisfactory, or do you find males who have orgasm without ejaculation and those who have ejaculation without the experience of orgasm? Should these conditions be accounted for by dividing this category into inhibited male orgasm and inhibited male ejaculation?
   f. Premature ejaculation, by definition, is limited to men. Rapid "premature" orgasm also occurs in women, often in response to fear of giving up control or being dependent on the partner's actions. Should this category be changed to premature orgasm to allow inclusion of either sex?
4. *Ego-dystonic homosexuality:* How has the decision to remove homosexuality from the *DSM* and retain ego-dystonic homosexuality affected your thinking or practice? (The defining criteria of mental disorders are distress and/or dysfunction.) In your experience, are there homosexual individuals without distress or dysfunction? Are

Table 11.1. *(cont.)*

Specific questions

there subgroups of homosexual individuals, other than ego-dystonic, in whom the sexual orientation is the major expression of pathology? If so, would you briefly explain. In your experience, have homosexual individuals been more willing to consult psychiatrists for psychological problems since this change? Has this change helped broaden residency programs on sexuality by including homosexuality? Has this change supported increased research for better understanding of homosexual development and adult adjustment?

5. There are persons who are able to perform adequately and receive pleasure from sexual acts but cannot integrate the act with an affectional attachment to a specific partner. Should a category for this state be included in this section?

6. Do you have any other thoughts or suggestions regarding revision of this section?

Responses should be returned to:
David P. McWhirter, M.D.
Clinical Institute for Human Relationships
3821 Fourth Avenue
San Diego, California 92103

If you have questions and would prefer to discuss them over the telephone, contact Dr. McWhirter at (619) 542-0088

---

another subtype, as mentioned earlier: the man living as the opposite sex, but not seeking reassignment surgery.

Levine and Lothstein (1981) said that "an axis I descriptive diagnosis of either transsexualism or atypical gender identity disorder is not clinically meaningful; neither diagnosis provides the clinician with suggestions for management." And we would further add that neither diagnosis adequately describes, for further research and communication with each other, what we are seeing in the clinic.

There is considerable disagreement about the value of the fifth-digit diagnosis describing sexual behavior in conjunction with transsexualism. One thing we know quite clearly these days is that gender identity and sexual orientation or object choice are different aspects of the same person. This is one rationale for the fifth digit, but, as explained by Huntington and associates (1983) and by Levine and Lothstein (1981), we have learned much more about the disturbance and need to seriously consider revisions of the current classifications.

Paul Walker, Ph.D., past president of the International Gender Dysphoria Society, strongly recommends revision of the following sentence in the section "Course and subtypes": "Since surgical sex reassignment is a recent development, the long-term course of the disorder with this treatment is unknown." This sentence has been used in several court cases to declare sex-reassignment surgery as experimental. Surgery is hardly a recent development, because it first appeared in the medical literature in 1919. Long-term results are not unknown, although they are debated. Walker recommends omitting the foregoing sentence and substituting the following: "Fulfillment of the diagnostic criteria for transsexualism does not imply a recommended course of treatment. Psychotherapy for all transsexuals and sex-reassignment surgery for some transsexuals is the usual course of treatment. The decision to perform sex-reassignment surgery is based on criteria and standards not addressed in *DSM-III.*"

302.60 Gender-identity disorder of childhood

The diagnostic criteria for females have been challenged by some researchers (Zucker et al., 1984). Criterion B:

Persistent repudiation of female anatomic structures, as manifested by at least one of the following repeated assertions:

(1) that she will grow up to become a man (not merely in role)
(2) that she is biologically unable to become pregnant
(3) that she will not develop breasts
(4) that she has no vagina
(5) that she has, or will grow, a penis

Zucker and associates (1984) think that this criterion implies that females must be delusional to fit this diagnostic category. They do agree that some of the girls in their study showed considerable anatomic dysphoria (e.g., wanting a penis, standing to urinate), but none fit the criteria as stated in *DSM-III.*

This same criticism can be leveled at criterion B for males, except that the statements are not as factual, and there is a choice of another criterion in the section. Review by others working in this field is needed at this time for further reporting on this section.

PARAPHILIAS

This section needs review by those actively working in this field. There continues to be discussion whether or not other paraphilias should be included. The original discussions about including "rape" as a category have strong proponents and antagonists. It was not included in *DSM-III* because it is considered a crime, not a psychiatric diagnosis. On the other hand, using a category like "forced sexual activity with nonconsenting partner" is one way of looking at the possibility of including rape. Also, it has been suggested that it is a disorder of impaired impulse control and belongs in some category of that kind, because it is not really a sexual disorder, but rather a violent, impulse-ridden act.

Bullough, Bullough, and Smith (1983) have offered some new insight into the descriptions and distinctions between cross-dressers of various sorts that clarifies the differential diagnosis further. There are other questions about the differential diagnosis as presented in *DSM-III* that were discussed earlier with transsexualism.

PSYCHOSEXUAL DYSFUNCTIONS

Although the division of the sexual-response cycle into appetitive, excitement, orgasm, and resolution phases has been helpful in diagnostic classification, the individual diagnostic categories appear inadequate. For example, the section "Inhibited Sexual Desire" does not include a category for aversion or fear of all sexual behavior. It is also listed as very rare, whereas most sex therapists indicate that it is now one of the more frequent symptoms seen in the clinic.

Another example of diagnostic confusion is using ejaculation and orgasm synonymously, though ejaculation can occur without orgasm, and orgasm has occurred without ejaculation. Ejaculation is a CNS afferent process, and orgasm is a CNS efferent process, usually simultaneous and joined, but not always.

Although it is mentioned in the section "Atypical Psychosexual Dysfunction," there is mounting evidence that premature orgasm in females is a serious enough dysfunction to have a category of its own.

One of the continuing major difficulties with the psychosexual dysfunctions is the lack of a way of identifying degrees of severity and the omission of consideration of those dysfunctions that are the result of interaction of the partner's dysfunctions. For instance, inhibited desire may not be a distress for the person with the inhibition, but it does become dysfunctional for the partner. There are no categories for those dysfunctions related to disequilibrium within the dyad, such as discordant biorhythms (a night person with a morning person) or incompatibility related to unequal frequencies of desire.

Schover and associates (1982) have proposed a complete alternative to this portion of *DSM-III*, calling it a "Multiaxial Problem-Oriented System for Sexual Dysfunctions." Their classification system came out of their clinical work at SUNY, Stony Brook, and is a considerably more complex system. Its advantage is to be found in the exactitude of the description of each kind of dysfunction and the concomitant applicability to treatment.

OTHER PSYCHOSEXUAL DISORDERS

302.00 **Ego-dystonic homosexuality**

This diagnostic category is one of the most controversial and highly contested categories in all of *DSM-III*. With the elimination of homosexuality as a mental illness in 1973 and the inclusion of sexual-orientation disorder, the stage was set for the disagreements that have arisen in recent years concerning this category. The correspondence of the *DSM-III* subcommittee is contained in an article by Bayer and Spitzer (1982). There have been no subsequent reports of how useful this category has been. On the other hand, in the interim, some suggestions have been made regarding the use of the term "homophobia," which was coined by Weinberg (1972) to describe fear of homosexual persons or fear of being homosexual oneself. The use of the term "ego-dystonic homosexuality" seems to many to go against the phenomenological grain of *DSM-III*. It is the least phenomenological diagnostic category in the manual. The solution lies in adding an example under sexual disorder NOS [Section 302.89 in *DSM-IIIR*] such as persistent and marked distress about one's sexual orientation. This issue needs exploration and input from clinicians of all experiences.

SUMMARY

The opinions of the framers of the original "Psychosexual Disorders" section and a selected list of other experts in various categories within the section have been sought through the questionnaire included as Table 11.1. Many have responded, making only minor suggestions for change or correction. Others have suggested more sweeping changes.

Despite some of the conflicts and disagreements, the "Psychosexual Disorders" section in *DSM-III* has brought a new calm to the diagnosis of sexual problems in psychiatry. It has introduced a far less pejorative attitude about many behaviors formerly considered too taboo to discuss in almost any circles. *DSM-III* has helped in expanding our own understanding and the understanding of others concerning the research in this area and the research that still must be done. We submit these preliminary comments as our first exploratory step toward a useful revision of the "Psychosexual Disorders" section.

REFERENCES

Bayer R, Spitzer R: Edited correspondence on the status of homosexuality in DSM-III. J Hist Behav Sci 18:32–52, 1982

Bullough V, Bullough B, Smith R: A comparison of transvestites, transsexuals, homosexual and heterosexual men. J Sex Res 19:4, 1983

Hunt D, Hampson J: Follow-up of 17 biologic male transsexuals after sex reassignment. Am J Psychiatry 137(April):4, 1980

Huntington RP, Huntington S, McWhirter DP: Gender identity disorders – a new diagnostic proposal. Presented to Society for the Scientific Study of Sex, annual meeting, Chicago, Ill, Nov. 19, 1983

Kinsey AC, Pomeroy W, Martin C: Sexual Behavior in the Human Male. Philadelphia, WB Saunders, 1948

Kinsey AC, Pomeroy W, Martin C, et al: Sexual Behavior in the Human Female. Philadelphia, WB Saunders, 1953

Levine S, Lothstein L: Transsexualism or the gender dysphoria syndrome. J Sex Mar Ther 7:2, 1981

Masters W, Johnson V: Human Sexual Response. Boston, Little, Brown, 1966
    Human Sexual Inadequacy. Boston, Little, Brown, 1970

Satterfield S: Satisfaction with results shown best predictor of adjustment after transsexual surgery. APA News July 16, 1982

Schover LR, Friedman JM, Weiler SJ, et al: Multiaxial problem-oriented system for sexual dysfunctions. Arch Gen Psychiatry 39:32–52, 1982

Weinberg, G: Society and the Healthy Homosexual. New York, St. Martin's Press, 1972

Zucker KJ, Doering R, Brudley SJ, et al: Sex-type play in gender disturbed children: a comparison to sibling and psychiatric controls. Arch Sex Behav 11:309–321, 1984

12 Overview

GARY TUCKER

Dr. Taylor's excellent and provocative chapter on organic mental disorders raised many important questions. In the field trials of *DSM-III,* the diagnostic grouping of dementia did not fare too well, achieving only 50% reliability. It is more than likely that this poor reliability was due to poor standardization of criteria. Dr. Taylor proposed to remedy this by defining terms more clearly and through the use of various paper-and-pencil tests to evaluate organic mental diseases. The discussion centered mainly on how this proposal could be put into operation and on the types of tests that could be used.

In parallel with this desire for the clinician to begin to use neuropsychological tests in the diagnosis of organic dysfunction was the desire to use other laboratory evidence as part of the diagnostic criteria. Whether or not the field is ready for this was questioned, as it was stressed that many clinicians currently are not aware of the significance of laboratory findings in most psychiatric conditions (e.g., abnormal EEG findings in schizophrenic patients, "soft" neurological signs).

This caused considerable discussion about the theoretical implications of the name "organic mental disease," because it implies that there are psychiatric conditions that are not "organic"; such alternative names as coarse brain disease, neurologic disorder, and so on, were proposed. Most believed that the current designation is adequate and has communicative value and that it is important to keep these behavioral conditions still within the province of psychiatry, rather than sending them completely over to neurology. This led almost serendipitously to an interesting discussion of the role of etiologic factors in many "organic" diseases of the central nervous system. For example, for many "organic" disorders (e.g., seizure disorders, Alzheimer's disease) the etiologic processes are no more evident than for the affective disorders. All that is evident to the clinician are the specific symptoms. The discussion highlighted the multiple causes possible for a given phenomenologic presentation. Consequently, whereas most shared the opinion that the strict demarcation between "organic" and "functional" was arbitrary, it was recognized that, over time, enough credence and distinction have been given to the conditions dealt with in this category that little would be gained by changing the overall name, and the primary problems are standardization of terms and the potential utility of various laboratory measures in adding precision to the diagnostic process, as well as allowing us to differentiate these conditions more readily from other psychiatric categories.

There was significant agreement that there is currently enough descriptive literature to include such conditions as the postconcussion syndrome, organic anxiety syndromes, anorexia, dissociative states, and perhaps psychomotor states in the category of organic mental diseases. However, there was significant controversy about how expansive and specific we should be with the categories until identification of both anatomic and etiologic agents is possible.

Dr. Rounsaville's chapter on substance-abuse disorders noted that, particularly for alcoholism, several studies have found that in clinical use the *DSM-III* criteria reveal a high degree of validity. He also anticipated that the NIMH-sponsored Epidemiologic Catchment Area (ECA) studies now in progress at five medical centers should be very helpful in the continued refinement of the classification of substance-abuse disorders. The major problem evident in the use of the categories of substance-abuse disorders is the relationship to other diagnostic categories due to the ubiquitous use of alcohol and drugs in the general population and particularly in psychiatric disturbances. It is frequently difficult clinically to determine whether the substance abuse or the depression came first. However, epidemiologically this is a problem, because in specialized treatment centers for alcoholism and substance abuse, the non-drug-use diagnoses are often ignored. Basically, the changes suggested for *DSM-III* were not major, except for perhaps adding a primary- and secondary-category stipulation that does not lend itself to a phenomenologic orientation. Most of the suggested changes had to do with sharpening the criteria (noting the ambiguity of some terms, such as "tolerance"), making a clearer distinction between abuse and addiction, and the need for defining "dependence" on the basis of the agent, rather than overall.

Perhaps of most interest, as highlighted by the substance-abuse category, is the obvious lack of follow-up studies using the *DSM-III* criteria, especially in light of the economic implications of diagnosis with regard to reimbursement, not to mention treatment. It was believed the NIMH-sponsored ECA studies will be particularly useful in this regard. An interesting figure of 14.5% lifetime incidence of alcoholism was cited in the discussion by Dr. Helzer in their ECA study. It was also observed that some of the impairment criteria are difficult to apply to females, particularly for alcoholism, as they relate mostly to work outside the home. Another problem that relates to the nature of drug abuse is that poly-drug use is quite common, and this is difficult to stipulate in *DSM-III*. The relationships between symptoms and social impairment, dependence and tolerance, are also areas in which more study is necessary, particularly concerning which patterns and symptoms go together.

The discussion of Dr. McWhirter's chapter on psychosexual disorders again emphasized that just as alcoholism is often ignored by most psychiatrists, the area of sexual dysfunction is equally disregarded. Perhaps this is exacerbated by the lack of physiologic and pharmacologic data on sexual dysfunction. *DSM-III* has been of major utility to clinicians who treat sexual disorders. There have even been a few validating studies for the categories of transsexualism. The importance of this diagnosis for transsexual surgery was a clear stimulant to these studies. It was also noteworthy that the factors of reimbursement came up in this discussion as well, in that insurance companies will not reimburse for *DSM-III* sexual dysfunctions. Again, the absence of etiologic or even age-of-onset data in the criteria used for diagnosing psychosexual disorders was evident.

In summary, the discussions of all chapters were stimulating and useful. In general, one can say that in these three categories there was some degree of satisfaction and feeling of improvement through *DSM-III*. The conflict between those with specific research interests and the uses of the clinician was apparent throughout the discussion, with the feeling that *DSM-III* is more useful for clinicians than for researchers. The discussion also highlighted, for all of these conditions, that there have been few studies that would clarify the classifications used in *DSM-III* with regard to treatment or outcome. It is also apparent that the seeming objective nature and quantification of symptoms used by *DSM-III* obscure the process of their derivation, in that these are arbitary categories developed by a panel of "experts" and not as data-based as we would like to think. Consequently, there was some expectation that there will be significant changes and shifting between categories and criteria as more empirical studies are done using *DSM-III* as a basis and stimulus for these studies. And perhaps eventually we shall be able to remove the criteria from the realm of consensus as more etiologic data appear.

PART IV

The anxiety and somatoform disorders

The anxiety and somatoform disorders are the subjects of this section. John Nemiah traces the development of the psychoanalytic view of anxiety from its earliest origins through modern developmental concepts and theories before discussing the relation between psychoanalytic concepts and the *DSM-III* classification of anxiety disorders. David Barlow presents recent findings based on research conducted by himself and his colleagues concerning the classification of anxiety disorders. A comprehensive review of the somatoform disorders is provided by Robert Cloninger. In the "Overview," I present a commentary based on these chapters and on the discussion that followed their original presentation at the conference sponsored by the Committee to Evalute *DSM-III*.

Gerald L. Klerman

13 *The psychoanalytic view of anxiety*
Basic concepts and recent advances

JOHN C. NEMIAH

Modern psychoanalytic contributions to an understanding of anxiety derive primarily from clinical observations of adult patients and from studies by psychoanalytically oriented investigators of the psychological development of infants and children. Although these clinical and research activities have produced no revolutionary findings or concepts, they have nonetheless helped to fill in the gaps and clarify areas of obscurity in the basic theory of anxiety that was set forth during the early decades of psychoanalytic investigations. In what follows, I first trace the evolution of that theory from its beginnings to its ultimate classic formulation, then describe the modern findings that have advanced our understanding of the clinical phenomena, and conclude by briefly discussing the relation between psychoanalytic concepts and the *DSM-III* classification of anxiety disorders.

Psychoanalysis rests on two basic concepts: unconscious mental processes and psychological conflict. The notion of the unconscious long antedated Freud. It was forced on clinicians and philosophers during the latter part of the eighteenth century and the early decades of the nineteenth by the alterations in consciousness produced by "magnetic" (later termed "hypnotic") maneuvers and by the clinical observation of the "doubling of consciousness," seen in patients with multiple personalities, now included under the *DSM-III* category of the dissociative disorders.

EARLY THEORIES OF SYMPTOM FORMATION

Charcot, Janet, and dissociation

The most extensive and most systematic study of these altered states of consciousness was made by Charcot and his colleagues at the Salpêtrière as a part of their investigation of hysteria. It reached its zenith in Janet's monumental clinical observations and theoretical formulations (Janet, 1903, 1907). Charcot, Janet, and their colleagues were well aware that unconscious (or subconscious, as they would have said) memories of past emotionally traumatic events underlay and were represented by a host of consciously experienced hysterical symptoms. Similarly, they were fully cognizant of the close relation between hypnotic phenomena and hysterical symptoms, and they recognized the usefulness of hypnosis in exploring and bringing to light the unconscious determinants of the surface clinical symptoms. True to their basic biological orientation, they fashioned their explanatory theories in physiological (or, perhaps more accurately, pseudophysiological) terms. Fundamental to their thinking was the concept of nervous energy, which, it was postulated, bound together all the neurological and psychological processes of the central nervous system into a functioning, unified whole under the domination of the *ego,* which was experienced consciously as a sense of the self or personal identity. The normal person has a sufficient amount of nervous energy to maintain the integrity of the ego and its functions despite the severest assaults imposed by stressful environmental events. In some individuals, however, hereditary factors result in an abnormally low quantum of nervous energy. In the face of serious physical illness or emotionally draining events (e.g., severe frights or serious losses), the already limited energy is depleted below the critical level, leading to a series of symptoms that occur stepwise as the energy level falls lower and lower. Initially the patient experiences a loss of identity and reality, accompanied by increasing fatigue (neurasthenia); next, as the binding power of the energy is further compromised, lower-order autonomic functions escape control of the ego in the form of anxiety and related obsessional and phobic symptoms; ultimately, as the energy is yet further exhausted, complex associations of mental events and functions (memories, emotions, motor and sensory functions) fall away from the ego's domain to take up an autonomous existence beyond conscious awareness and recall. It is this eventual *dissociation,* as Janet (1907) termed it, of nervous and mental processes that sets the stage for the appearance of the rich mélange of hysterical symptoms.

Freud and psychological conflict

Freud's journey to Paris in the 1880s to study neuropathology under Charcot exposed him to the exciting new observations and ideas about hysteria that filled the air. Enchanted by what he heard and saw, Freud's interests were deflected from his original neuropathological goal, and he returned to Vienna to embark on an exploration of hysterical phenomena that laid the groundwork for the subsequent development of psychoanalysis.

In his earliest theoretical formulations (made in conjunction with his senior colleague, Breuer), Freud initially adhered to the concept of a traumatic origin of hysterical symptoms (Breuer and Freud, 1893; Freud, 1894). Similarly, he considered the pathological splitting off (dissociation) of mental complexes to be the result of spontaneous hypnoid states that followed alterations in the level of nervous energy. In one of his earliest psychological papers, however, Freud (1894) proposed an alternative explanation for the occurrence of pathological dissociation. With the introduction of the term "defense hysteria" (as opposed to hypnoid hysteria), Freud suggested that a dissociative splitting off of mental contents occurred when memories and associated feelings were so painful that the ego actively pushed (or repressed) them from conscious awareness and voluntary recall. Thus rendered unconscious, the mental events (as similarly postulated in the French conceptual scheme) then formed the source of consciously experienced hysterical symptoms. The difference between the French explanation and Freud's explanation of symptom production, it can be seen, lies not in the relation of unconscious complexes to surface symptoms (the postulated mechanisms here are the same) but in their respective views as to how dissociation occurs as the first step in the pathological process. For the French, dissociation results when mental complexes *passively* fall away from an ego weakened by an abnormal depletion of nervous energy. For Freud, dissociation results from a process of *active* exclusion of mental events from consciousness by an ego strong enough to banish those thoughts, memories, and feelings that come into open, painful conflict with it. With this explanatory model, Freud introduced a radically new idea of mental functioning (including symptom formation) – that of psychological conflict. It was this innovative concept, combined with the well-formulated ideas of unconscious mental events, that initiated the subsequent psychoanalytic elaboration of psychodynamic mental structure and process.

French theoreticians focused primarily on the *cognitive* aspect of the memories of traumatic events in the formation of hysterical symptoms. Freud similarly saw the form of the hysterical symptom as a reflection of the form of the memory's cognitive content. But he stressed the equal importance of the affective element of the memory as well. The affect not only motivated the repression of the traumatic complex but also supplied the energy for conversion of the repressed contents into the somatic hysterical symptom. By the same token, successful therapeutic removal of the hysterical symptom required the raising of both memory and affect into consciousness and the discharge of the affect in cathartic emotional expression. "Each individual symptom," he wrote (Breuer and Freud, 1893) in describing the procedure that became known as cathartic treatment, "immediately and permanently disappeared when we had succeeded in bringing clearly to light the memory of the event by which it was provoked and in arousing its accompanying affect. . . . Recollection without affect almost invariably produces no result."

INITIAL PSYCHOANALYTIC FORMULATIONS OF ANXIETY

Freud initially spoke of affect in general terms without attempting to delineate or distinguish among the individual kinds of feelings. The important feature of pathogenic affects was their painful quality, which served as the motivation for defensive dissociation. The specific coloring of the affect (whether it was one of anxiety, sadness, anger, guilt, or disgust) was of secondary importance, and no attempt was made at the start to correlate specific affects with specific kinds of symptoms. Very early in the course of his clinical observations, however, Freud's attention was drawn to the prevalence and importance of anxiety as a central affect in neurotic disorders. This presumably became evident to him as he moved from a study of hysteria, in which anxiety is less obviously connected with the symptoms, to an interest in phobic and obsessive–compulsive symptoms, in which the symptom of anxiety is of central importance. Freud (1894, 1895b) rapidly recognized that the anxiety found in these conditions was secondary – that is, that the phobic or obsessional idea was not inherently or obviously anxiety-provoking, but became so only with borrowed anxiety. The source of the anxiety lay elsewhere, having become associated with the phobic or obsessional symptom as the result of displacement. It was not until Freud specifically focused his attention on anxiety itself that he was able to formulate a theory as to its genesis.

The French school, and Janet in particular, divided neurotic disorders into two major categories, hysteria and psychasthenia. The term "hysteria" included the sensorimotor symptoms and the alterations of consciousness that resulted from the dissociation of complex mental processes. The term "psychasthenia" referred to a diffuse, kaleidoscopic collection of phobic, obsessional, neurasthenic, depressive, and anxious symptoms that were not further refined into diagnostic categories. In an early clinical paper, Freud (1895a) proposed that anxiety neurosis was a distinct clinical entity in its own right. To prove his point, he not only defined it in clinical terms but also proposed a specific cause.

Anxiety neurosis (the actual neurosis)

In the course of his clinical practice, Freud noted that his patients, both men and women, commonly developed an anxiety neurosis in association with sexual practices (continence, coitus interruptus) that precluded a discharge of libidinal energy in sexual orgasm. Although he was perhaps unwittingly putting the cart before the horse, Freud attributed the outbreak of anxiety symptoms to a mounting accumulation of undischarged libido and its eventual transformation into anxiety. Freud emphasized the fact that, in contrast to hysterical symptoms, whose production involved complex psychological mechanisms, there was no psychic elaboration in the genesis of anxiety. The transformation of libido to anxiety was a strictly somatic, physiological process. He pointed to

the extremely important fact that the anxiety which underlies the clinical symptoms of the neurosis can be traced to *no psychical origin.* Such an origin would exist, for instance, if it was found that the anxiety neurosis was based on a single or repeated justifiable fright, and that that fright had since provided the source for the subject's readiness for anxiety. But this is not so. Hysteria or a traumatic neurosis can be acquired from a single fright, but never anxiety neurosis. . . . *The mechanism of anxiety neurosis is to be looked for in a deflection of somatic sexual excitation from the psychical sphere, and in a consequent abnormal employment of that excitation.* . . . Anxiety neurosis . . . is the product of all those factors which prevent the somatic excitation from being worked over psychically. The manifestations of anxiety neurosis appear when the somatic excitation which has been deflected from the psyche is expended subcortically in totally inadequate reactions. . . . In [anxiety neurosis] *we find a psychical insufficiency, as a consequence of which abnormal somatic processes arise.* . . . Instead of a psychical working-over of the excitation, a deflection of it occurs into the somatic field. [Freud, 1895a; italics in original]

To emphasize the somatic origins of anxiety and the absence of psychical mechanisms in its genesis, Freud classified the anxiety neurosis as an "actual neurosis," in contradistinction to the psychoneuroses, like hysteria or phobic disorders, in which the symptoms were the end result of complex psychological processes.

The economic theory of anxiety

It should be noted here that in what came to be called the *transformation hypothesis* or the *economic hypothesis* of anxiety formation, the source of anxiety is traced to a basic biological drive, and the intensity and magnitude of the symptom are directly and proportionally related to the intensity and magnitude of the underlying drive of which it is a somatic transformation. It was not until some three decades later that Freud explicitly modified his conception of the nature and genesis of anxiety, but before turning our attention to the clinical observations that eventually led to this alteration in theory, we must pursue the developments in the economic hypothesis that more immediately followed these initial formulations.

We noted earlier that in his first approach to explaining the genesis of hysterical symptoms, Freud adhered to the traumatic theory of their causes that he had inherited from his Parisian teachers. After examining nearly two score young hysterical women with his newly fashioned psychoanalytic techniques, Freud (1896) generalized his findings in the form of a specific theory of the cause of hysterical neurosis. Hysteria, he said, had its origins in a traumatic sexual assault of the little girl by an older man, usually the father. With puberty, and the appearance of libido secondary to the endocrine changes associated with that phase of development, the old traumatic memories, which had become invested with libido, were intensified and became the nucleus for a major conflict over sexuality, with the repression of libido and its conversion into hysterical symptoms. Freud's theory was not spun out of thin air, but was based on the fact that each of his patients in the course of their associations had reported a childhood sexual attack. What Freud initially took as historical fact, however, could not be substantiated when he sought independent corroboration of the alleged assault.

Development of libido theory

Not without considerable inner turmoil, as the letters to Fliess (Bonaparte, Freud, and Kris, 1954) tell us, Freud abandoned his theory. After reflection, however, in concert with additional observations from patients and his self-analysis, Freud gradually came to the recognition that what his patients had told him about their childhood sexual experiences were the reports of fantasies, not factual events. From this discovery stemmed a growing awareness of an orderly development of childhood sexuality culminating in the oedipus complex (Freud, 1905). Adult neurotic disorders were then seen to be the result of conflicts over the sexual drive traceable back to disturbances in the course of childhood sexual development. Repression was invoked not against painful memories of traumatic events but against the forbidden libidinal drive itself. The traumatic theory of the neuroses gave way to the concept of their genesis in the dynamic conflict between libidinal strivings and a controlling, repressing ego. Anxiety was then seen as deriving from a transformation of libido blocked from discharge not by external circumstances but by internal psychological defenses. Anxiety, in other words, was still viewed as an economic transformation of undischarged libido. It was only the explanation of the mechanism by which libido was blocked from discharge that was altered.

At the same time, the new theoretical model provided a better explanation for the increasingly recognized fact that anxiety was a ubiquitous symptom running like a thread through all the neurotic disorders: If the controls over libidinal discharge were internal, autonomous, and automatic, rather than being under the external voluntary control over sexual behavior, there was much more likelihood that the libidinal drives would be blocked from expression, with their consequent transformation into the manifestations of clinical anxiety. In this revised model, individuals became unwilling victims of their internal psychological conflicts and less in control of their destinies.

DEVELOPMENT OF CLASSIC ANXIETY THEORY

Time does not permit us to examine all the steps by which the economic theory of anxiety was modified to become the *signal theory* of anxiety formation, and we are able to touch on only three major elements that led to this revision of the theoretical conceptualization. Mention has already been made of the growing recognition of the ubiquitousness of anxiety in neurotic disorders. The major focus of interest, as we have seen, was on the internal source of this affect, but Freud was, of course, aware that anxiety was a natural and normal response to external dangerous stimuli as well. This latter *realistic anxiety,* or *fear,* was clearly a primary and basic response of the individual to dangerous and threatening situations that could potentially cause harm. In this case, anxiety was not the manifestation of an internal transformation of psychic energy; it arose de novo as an elementary and appropriate affect in its own right. It is of interest, therefore, to note that even in his early psychoanalytic writings, Freud (1900) made occasional but isolated references to neurotic anxiety as being a response to the internal danger of the threatened emergence into consciousness of forbidden, repressed mental elements. In this context, furthermore, anxiety was seen as a motivating force for strengthening psychological defenses against the threatening unconscious drive or its derivatives.

The developmental source of anxiety

Despite Freud's empirical recognition that there was another mechanism for the production of anxiety different from that involving a transformation of libido, he did not incorporate his observations into his formal theory of anxiety formation, but persisted in his concept of anxiety as being secondary to the transformation of other, more basic psychic elements. Changes in anxiety theory occurred only after Freud had arrived at a radical revision of his concept of the nature and structure of the psychic apparatus. Before describing this conceptual alteration, however, we must first briefly note one other proposal that Freud advanced (again somewhat casually and without fully weaving it into his existing theoretical scheme) concerning the clinical manifestations of anxiety.

The transformation theory of anxiety was conceptually clear and intelligible, but it did not account for the explicit forms and nature of the clinical symptom, nor explain why it had the special and singular affective quality that characterized it. Initially, but without giving the idea much weight, Freud (1895a) suggested that anxiety resembled the physiological accompaniments of sexual orgasm. This provided an explanation of the *form* of anxiety symptoms, but gave no clues as to the reason for the intensely painful quality of anxiety, as contrasted with the ecstatic pleasures of sexual orgasm. In 1910, with hardly any warning in his previous writings and formulations, Freud proposed that anxiety was related to the infant's experience of the traumatic process of birth. "Birth," he wrote, "is both the first of all dangers to life and the prototype of all later ones that cause us to feel anxiety, and the experience of birth has probably left behind in us the expression of affect which we call anxiety." Speculative, untestable, and quite probably inaccurate as the specific elements of this hypothesis may be, it nonetheless set the stage for two important basic conceptual approaches that later became central to the consideration of anxiety. First, we note once again the view of anxiety as a reaction to external danger. But perhaps even more important is the proposition that anxiety in the adult has its roots in early life experiences that act as the template for the subsequent manifestations of the affect. Although Freud did not himself elaborate on this developmental aspect of anxiety, it has, as we see later, become an important part of modern analytic understanding of the various clinical manifestations of anxiety.

Models of the mind

The topographic model. We must now turn our attention to the alteration in the concept of psychic structure that, as we have indicated, set the stage for the revision in the theory of anxiety. In Freud's first picture of the mind (the so-called *topographic model*), the ego, endowed with self-preservative instincts, is opposed to the basic biological libidinal drive, its components, and its derivatives. The ego can be equated with consciousness, in contradistinction to the unconscious, which is composed of all those mental elements that have been subjected to repression. In this scheme, as we have seen, anxiety is the conscious experience by the ego of an affect that results from a transformation of libido that cannot be openly and directly discharged after it has been rendered unconscious by repression.

Narcissism. In his early analytic formulations, Freud paid relatively little attention to the nature of the ego or to elaborating on its structure and functions.

When, however, toward the end of the first decade of this century, he came increasingly to focus his attention on the serious disturbances in affects and cognition found in depressive disorders and the major psychoses, he was forced to expand his observations and theoretical concepts to include the phenomena of narcissism (Freud, 1914). It soon became apparent that the so-called self-preservative instincts were in fact the manifestations of libido directed not at external objects but at the self in an intense form of self-love. This recognition of the existence of narcissism leveled a severe blow at the concept of self-preservative instincts set in opposition to libidinal instincts that was central to the topographic model. If the self-preservative instincts were in fact merely libido directed toward the self, the dual theory of two separate, distinct, and qualitatively different sets of instincts in antithesis to one another was untenable, and a new model of the mind was required that would be more in keeping with the new clinical observations and the concept of narcissism that arose from them.

The structural model. The development of a new model did not come easily or quickly. Indeed, it was more than a decade before Freud proposed the *structural model* of the psyche, which has since that time remained as the basic conceptual scheme of psychic structure for analytic clinicians and theoreticians alike. The interlude between the two models was not a period of inactivity for Freud and his analytic colleagues. Indeed, it gave rise to many new observations and theories, to an explicit awareness of the fundamental importance of the aggressive drive in the production of mental disorders, and to a series of sophisticated metapsychological papers that set the stage for the ultimate development of much of modern ego psychology. We must, however, forgo a more detailed look at this period of psychoanalytic evolution and turn to a brief exposition of the structural model that was its ultimate product.

The terms "id," "ego," and "superego," used to label the various parts of the psyche, as conceived of structurally, are common parlance in modern English vocabulary, but a brief definition of each is in order as a basis for understanding their structural relations to one another, as well as the relation of anxiety to the psychic structure they comprise. The id is viewed as being the seat of the drives and their repressed derivatives. The ego is composed of a variety of functions (cognitive, sensory, executive, defensive) designed to control, modulate, and canalize the expression of the drives in conformity with the demands of the superego and external sanctions and to provide for their gratification by means of adaptive manipulations of external reality. The superego is the repository for the ego ideals and the sanctions of conscience, which guide and influence the ego in its behavior vis-à-vis the drives and external reality. In the topographic model, conscious and unconscious were seen as distinctly separate portions of the mind; in the structural model, the terms "conscious" and "unconscious" are used adjectively and refer to the quality of functioning of the three primary agencies. The id, by definition, is totally unconscious, whereas the functions of the ego and superego may be both unconscious and conscious.

Anxiety as an ego affect

In this new structural conceptual scheme, anxiety is an *ego affect*. It is generated in and experienced by the ego, as a response to realistic external danger or to the pressure for discharge of internal drives whose expression in behavior may elicit a threatening response of reprisal from the external world or the superego. When confronted with clinical anxiety, two types of questions can be asked:

1. What is the person afraid of – that is, what libidinal or aggressive behavior stemming from underlying drives is he afraid of initiating?
2. Why is he afraid of the drive and its intended action? Is he afraid of total dissolution of his ego organization if the drive escapes control into open expression (id anxiety)? Is he afraid of being abandoned by or losing the love of a person important to him (separation anxiety)? Is he afraid of retaliatory, punitive damage to his body (castration anxiety)? Is he afraid of moral condemnation and guilt arising from a punitive conscience (superego or moral anxiety)?

Anxiety theory revised: traumatic and signal anxiety

Two kinds of anxiety must be distinguished at this point. Anxiety in a particularly severe, intense, and disorganizing form ("traumatic anxiety") may occur when the individual is confronted with a highly dangerous external situation or the total loss of control of a forbidden repressed drive. In either event the person feels helplessly overwhelmed. On the other hand, the threat, rather than the actuality, of a traumatic situation leads to a lesser, milder form of anxiety ("signal anxiety") that anticipates the possibility of a state of helplessness and acts as a signal to the individual to take remedial measures – whether this be action to ward off external danger or the erection of internal psychological defenses to contain a drive threatening to get out of control. In this latter situation, anxiety motivates and results in the operation of repression and allied defenses rather than (as conceptualized in the topographic model) being the result of repression itself. Whereas *traumatic anxiety* is conceived of, in economic terms, as being a discharge of energy (both psychological and physiological) commensurate with the magnitude of the traumatic situation, *signal anxiety* is not viewed as being a discharge phenomenon (either of transformed libido or of anxiety itself), but as quantitatively small anticipatory arousal, sufficient to motivate the individual to take appropriate defensive action but not of a quality or magnitude to disorganize his executive functions or to produce a state of passive, overwhelming helplessness.

This, then, was the concept of anxiety that emerged following major revision of the psychoanalytic scheme of psychic structure (Freud, 1926), and from that time on it has proved useful for clinicians dealing with patients with psychoanalytic methods of observation and therapeutic techniques. It is congruent with the clinician's observation that anxiety is a phenomenon central to emotional disorders in general and to neurotic disorders in particular. It is consistent with the clinical distinction between overwhelming, disorganizing panic and anticipatory signal anxiety. And it fits with the repeated clinical observation that anxiety is a sensitive indicator of areas of psychological conflict and, as a corollary, that focusing in a clinical interview on areas of conflict in such a way as to bring repressed drives closer to consciousness arouses anxiety, which in turn produces an increase in defensive responses.

MODERN PSYCHOANALYTIC OBSERVATIONS AND THEORY

Subsequent clinical observations and conceptualizations have not required a major revision of these principles, nor have they diminished their usefulness for clinicians. As noted earlier, modern analytic observation and theory, particularly in the areas of developmental psychology and of the related study of psychological structural defects that characterizes current ego psychology, have broadened analysis beyond the more limited concern with psychological conflict, and in so doing have added to our understanding of symptom formation in general and of anxiety in particular. We must therefore turn briefly to these newer findings as they bear on the nature and formation of the anxiety disorders.

Developmental observation and theory

Direct observations of infants by child psychiatrists and other investigators (Zetzel, 1955; Ramzy and Wallerstein, 1958; Brody and Axelrad, 1966; Compton, 1972) have adduced a wealth of information not only about the development of behavior patterns during the early months and years of life but also about cognitive processes and affective expression that permit reasonable inferences about inner experience in the preverbal child. It is generally agreed that during the first three to four months of life the response to painful stimuli (whether their source is external or from inner needs, like hunger) is a diffuse somatomotor and autonomic discharge accompanied by an experience of unpleasure that is not as yet differentiated into specific, discrete affects, including anxiety. The disturbed arousal of the infant elicits a response from his (or her) mother or other caretakers aimed at satisfying his needs and removing painful environmental stimuli.

With the emergence of increasingly sophisticated cognitive processes, the infant develops pari passu a growing perception of his mother in specific relation to the relief of his unpleasant inner feeling; he learns, in other words, that she relieves pain and makes him comfortable, and ultimately her very presence arouses an anticipation of relief that enables him, temporarily at least, to postpone the automatic, global discharge of unpleasure. At the same time as these perceptions develop, so does the recognition that the absence of the mother puts him in danger of once again experiencing the traumatic situation that produces the painful unpleasure. His cognitive ability both to perceive and to remember provides him with the basis for experiencing a primitive form of anticipatory anxiety.

As development evolves in both physiological and psychological dimensions, this less intense form of anticipatory, or signal, anxiety becomes increasingly differentiated from the more intense, diffuse, disorganizing traumatic anxiety that results in a massive motor and physiological discharge. As a corollary of this differentiation, anxiety becomes increasingly a psychic and experiential phenomenon, and the somatic physiological concomitants become more localized, more controlled, less prominent, and less intense. At the same time, however, the developmental anlage of early traumatic anxiety remains as a potential response to situations of overwhelming internal or external danger if the anticipatory anxiety has not been successful in initiating actions that remove or modify the danger situation.

Contribution to an understanding of anxiety

The developmental view of anxiety helps to clarify a number of clinical observations about the nature and form of anxiety as it is seen in adult patients.

1. It provides a basis for understanding the twofold clinical manifestation of anxiety as overwhelming, disorganizing panic, on the one hand, and a lesser, more tolerable affect characterized by a quality of anxious expectation, on the other. And although analysts are not agreed as to whether the two forms of anxiety are qualitatively distinct (the *dual theory* of anxiety) or merely quantitatively different manifestations of a qualitatively unitary phenomenon (Rangell, 1955), they concur in viewing panic as the reemergence of the developmentally earlier state of traumatic anxiety and in viewing anticipatory, signal anxiety as being that lesser anxiety that is made possible by the development of the cognitive functions that underlie the capacity to recognize the mere threat of a danger situation carrying the potential for producing traumatic anxiety.

2. Developmental theory provides a framework for understanding the intensity of anxiety that is seen in psychotic and borderline states. It is the result of developmental defects in the cognitive functions of the ego that compromise the ego's capacity to moderate the intensity of drives and affects and to make accurate cognitive appraisals of the nature of danger situations. As a consequence, the ability to anticipate is diminished, and danger situations are more readily perceived as traumatic. The potential for experiencing traumatic anxiety is closer to consciousness, and the perception of even a slight danger will evoke a generalized, all-encompassing discharge of anxiety in an attack of overwhelming panic.

3. The heightened vulnerability of certain individuals to separation anxiety, which is a prominent feature of agoraphobia and many borderline character disorders, is viewed as a developmental arrest. The experience of anxiety retains its primitive quality and intensity because of the persistence into adulthood of an unmodified, infantile hypersensitivity to the loss of or separation from important protecting and mothering persons.

4. The emergence of traumatic neuroses in the face of suddenly occurring, overwhelmingly frightening environmental events can be understood as the tearing apart of the fabric of ego structure and the exposure of the traumatized individual to the full force of the long-submerged state of traumatic anxiety and helplessness that characterized his earliest infantile responses to traumatic situations.

5. Finally, clinical study of individuals subjected to enduring situations of terror, brutality, dehumanization, and torture (such as that suffered in the concentration camps of the Nazi holocaust and their more modern counterparts) has given rise to the concept of ego and affective regression to earlier developmental states of function. Both Schur (1955, 1958) and Krystal (1971), for example, speak of "resomatization" and "de-differentiation" of affects (including anxiety), leading to the experiencing of affect primarily in its physiological mode without an accompanying awareness of its specific psychological feeling tone. Krystal, in particular, has pointed to the high incidence of classic psychosomatic disorders (e.g., peptic ulcer, rheumatoid arthritis) in persons who have suffered such psychological regressions.

THE PSYCHOANALYTIC VIEW OF ANXIETY AND *DSM-III*

Having thus cursorily traced the development of the psychoanalytic view of anxiety from its earliest origins through modern developmental concepts and theories, let us in this final section turn to a consideration of the congruence, or lack of it, between the *DSM-III* classification of anxiety disorders and the psychoanalytic understanding of their nature and pathogenesis. Let me state at the start that in my opinion they are quite compatible.

1. In the first place, I believe that *DSM-III* correctly links together anxiety states, phobic neurosis, and obsessive–compulsive neurosis under the more general category of anxiety disorders. This is entirely consonant with the psychoanalytic view that anxiety is the central feature in each of these neuroses, both as an overt clinical symptom and as a motivation for defensive maneuvers, which are variously manifested as phobic and obsessive–compulsive symptoms.

2. The *DSM-III* division of anxiety states into panic disorder and generalized anxiety disorder coincides with the twofold nature of anxiety that is expressed in psychoanalytic language in its distinction between traumatic anxiety and signal anxiety.

3. The recognition in *DSM-III* of the anticipatory anxiety of agoraphobia and its role in arousing a secondary defensive avoidance of the phobic situation is similarly consistent with the analytic concepts not only of signal anxiety but also of the elements of learning (displacement) that result in the attachment of anxiety to the phobic object or situation.

DSM-III and psychoanalysis, then, have similar views about the clinical phenomena of the anxiety disorders. Psychoanalysis, of course, goes beyond pure phenomenology to offer explanations of the pathogenesis of symptoms, whereas such explanations are not to be found in *DSM-III*. The latter deliberately, and rightly, I think, eschews theoretical formulations and remains at a strictly phenomenological level of discourse. At the same time, there is nothing in the approach of *DSM-III* that is antithetical to psychoanalytic theories of symptom formation. It is quite possible to apply psychoanalytic concepts (unconscious mental processes, psychological conflict, anxiety as a response to internal psychological dangers, psychological defenses against drives) to an understanding of the anxiety disorders without coming into conceptual conflict with the classification that *DSM-III* proposes for these neurotic syndromes. If a conflict exists, it is with other theories of pathogenesis, not with the clinical facts. Here, too, it is a virtue of *DSM-III* that its empirical, phenomenological approach allows for a variety of theoretical views, whether these be biological or behavioral, or speak in other tongues. *DSM-III,* in other words, aptly defines and delimits the arena in which the theoretical battles are to be joined – an essential first step toward an ultimate understanding of etiology and rational treatment.

Lest I appear to end on too bellicose a note, let me say that in actuality I do not see these different theoretical schemes (psychoanalytic, behavioral, biological) as being truly at odds with one another. Each makes observations and formulations about a part, but only a part, of the entire picture. Each contributes findings at different levels of discourse. Each provides only a partial answer to the questions raised by clinical anxiety. Taken together, they complement one another in a greater conceptual whole. Using the phenomenological base of *DSM-III* as a springboard, we are enabled to explore all the dimensions of anxiety in such a way as to make valid correlations among its biological, behavioral, and psychodynamic elements in a conceptual synthesis that will make possible a more powerful explanation of the facts than each pursued in blind isolation can provide. The creation of that synthesis is an important task ahead for all of us.

REFERENCES

Bonaparte M, Freud A, Kris E. eds: The Origins of Psychoanalysis. New York, Basic Books, 1954

Breuer J, Freud S: On the Psychical Mechanism of Hysterical Phenomena: Preliminary Communication, Standard Edition . . . , vol 2, pp 3–17. London, Hogarth Press, (1893) 1955

Brody S, Axelrad S: Anxiety, socialization, and ego formation in infancy. Int J Psycho-Anal 47:218–229, 1966

Compton A: A study of the psychoanalytic theory of anxiety, II: developments in the theory of anxiety since 1926. J Am Psychoanal Assoc 20:341–394, 1972

Freud S: The Neuro-Psychoses of Defence, Standard Edition . . . , vol 3, pp 45–61. London, Hogarth Press, (1894) 1962

The Aetiology of Hysteria, Standard Edition . . . , vol 3, pp 191–221. London, Hogarth Press, (1896) 1962

On the Grounds for Detaching a Particular Syndrome from Neurasthenia under the Description "Anxiety Neurosis," Standard Edition . . . , vol 3, pp 89–115. London, Hogarth Press, (1895a) 1962

Obsessions and Phobias, Standard Edition . . . , vol 3, pp 74–82. London, Hogarth Press, (1895b) 1962

The Interpretation of Dreams; Standard Edition . . . , vol. 5, pp. 581–582. London, Hogarth Press, (1900) 1953

Three Essays on the Theory of Sex, Standard Edition . . . , vol 7, pp 130–243. London, Hogarth Press, (1905) 1953

A Special Type of Object Choice Made by Men, Standard Edition . . . , vol 11, pp 165–175. London, Hogarth Press, (1910) 1957

On Narcissism, Standard Edition . . . , vol 14, pp 73–102. London, Hogarth Press, (1914) 1957

Inhibitions, Symptoms and Anxiety, Standard Edition . . . , vol 10, pp 87–172. London, Hogarth Press, (1926) 1959

Janet P: Les Obsessions et la Psychasthénie, 2 vols. Paris, Félix Alcan, 1903

The Major Symptoms of Hysteria. New York, Macmillan, 1907

Krystal H: Trauma: considerations of its intensity and chronicity, in Psychic Traumatization. Edited by Krystal H, Niederland WG. Boston, Little, Brown, 1971

Ramzy I, Wallerstein R: Pain, fear and anxiety: a study in their interrelationships. Psychoanal Study Child 13:147–189, 1958

Rangell L: On the psychoanalytic theory of anxiety: a statement of a unitary theory. J Am Psychoanal Assoc 3:389–414, 1955

Schur M: Comments on the metapsychology of somatization. Psychoanal Study Child 10:110–164, 1955

The ego and the id in anxiety. Psychoanal Study Child 13:190–220, 1958

Zetzel E: The concept of anxiety in relation to the development of psychoanalysis. J Am Psychoanal Assoc 3:369–398, 1955

14 *The classification of anxiety disorders*

DAVID H. BARLOW

The research emphasis of the Center for Stress and Anxiety Disorders until recently has been on developing and assessing treatments for the various anxiety and stress disorders. But any treatment study requires reliable classification of patients into identifiable categories. This is particularly true for the anxiety disorders, because the phenomenology of various problems termed "anxiety" is extremely heterogeneous. Diverse phenomena, such as the somatic manifestations of panic, the percept of derealization, intrusive thoughts, and massive avoidance behavior such as that found in agoraphobia, are all subsumed under the broad heading of anxiety disorders. This heterogeneity, of course, was one of the major factors leading to difficulties with the term "neurosis," at least from the point of view of nosology. Thus, it seemed apparent to most of us in treatment-assessment research that the *DSM-III* descriptions of anxiety disorders represented major advances in diagnosis and classification, with their descriptive and in some cases empirically derived categories.

Nevertheless, it remained important to determine if patients entering our various clinical trials in the area of agoraphobia, panic disorder, generalized anxiety disorder, and social phobia could be identified with reliability and could be differentiated from one another. With the increasing specificity and complexity of diagnostic criteria, as evident in the *DSM-III*, standardized interview protocols are necessary if one is to test fairly the reliability of these categories and sample the broad range of phenomena present even in the most discrete categories, such as simple phobia. The SADS interview permitting differential diagnosis within the schizophrenic and affective disorders is probably the best example (Endicott and Spitzer, 1978, 1979). Unfortunately, neither the SADS nor other newly developed structured interviews, such as the Diagnostic Interview Schedule (DIS) (Robins et al., 1981), cover sufficient information to permit differential diagnoses among all of the anxiety disorders. For example, the DIS, designed for quite a different purpose, does not cover generalized anxiety disorder (GAD), social phobia, or posttraumatic stress disorder and, of course, is designed for administration by a lay person.

ANXIETY DISORDERS INTERVIEW SCHEDULE

In order to proceed more effectively with our own research, we began developing in 1981 a detailed structured interview specifically for the anxiety disorders that we termed the Anxiety Disorders Interview Schedule (ADIS) (DiNardo et al., 1982). The ADIS was designed not only to permit differential diagnoses among the *DSM-III* anxiety-disorder categories but also to provide data beyond the basic information required for establishing the diagnostic criteria. To this end, information such as the history of the problem, situational and cognitive factors influencing anxiety, and detailed symptom ratings provides a data base for detailed investigation of the clinical characteristics of the categories. We included questions in these areas for future studies on validity, and some preliminary data bearing on this topic are included in this chapter. Because depression is often associated with anxiety, a fairly detailed examination of depressive symptoms as well as their relationships to symptoms of anxiety disorders was included in the interview. Whereas many of the items were developed by our own staff, some items were adapted from the SADS and from the Present State Examination (Wing, Cooper, and Sartorius, 1974). Also embedded in the interview are the Hamilton Anxiety Scale and the Hamilton Depression Scale. But to ensure the continuity of the interview, the items of the Hamilton scales are grouped according to content, so that similar items can be rated simultaneously.

There are several other features of the ADIS that are relevant to data presented in this chapter. First, because one of our major goals was to gather as much detailed information as possible for purposes of later descriptive studies, there are few cutoff questions that would result in skipping sections of the interview. In this regard, we did not adhere to the hierarchical organization suggested by *DSM-III*, where, for example, any anxiety disorder such as panic disorder would be subsumed under major affective disorder if that were also found. This turned out to be an important step in describing as fully as possible the complete phenomenology of those presenting with one or another of the anxiety disorders. For example, there are many instances, it turns out, in which two anxiety disorders seem to exist independently, as in a patient who reports a long history of social fears and a recent history of panics in a wide variety of situations, many of which are not social situations. In these cases the clinician will make a distinction between a primary and a secondary disorder, based on severity and interference with functioning. The temporal relationship between or among the disorders will be noted and often will help to establish their independence, but will not in and of itself determine the primary–secondary status of the disorders. We do not assume that the more long-standing disorder necessarily is the primary problem, unless the information indicates that the more recent problem can be subsumed under the long-standing one, as described in a later section of this chapter. Furthermore, as many secondary diagnoses can be given as are ascertainable by the clinician after administration of the ADIS. Occasionally a patient will present with two distinct anxiety disorders that are both severe and are interfering with functioning. In these cases, two primary diagnoses will be given, although secondary diagnoses still can be assigned if present. On the other hand, if symptoms that meet the criteria for one anxiety disorder are clearly part of another anxiety disorder, then no separate diagnoses are given. For example, many agoraphobics report fears of heights or enclosed places because such situations represent the unavailability of an escape route in case of panic. In another example, simple phobics or obsessive–compulsives may "panic" when confronted with a specific phobic object or an intrusive thought, respectively, but these will not be diagnosed as panic disorder. Thus, the ADIS is not designed for administration by a lay person, but requires clinical judgments and some experience with the anxiety disorders.

To summarize, if one disorder can be clearly subsumed under another, the subsumed disorder is neither diagnosed nor given a secondary status. But if two anxiety disorders are judged to be independent, primary status is determined on the basis of relative severity and interference with functioning, rather than on the basis of temporal relationships or other hierarchical assumptions.

Reliability studies

With these guidelines in mind, preliminary reliability studies were undertaken on 60 patients admitted consecutively to our Phobia and Anxiety Disorders Clinic within the Center for Stress and Anxiety Disorders. A detailed description of the sample and the data is available (DiNardo et al., 1983). It is worth noting here, however, that the anxiety-disorder categories were subjected to an extremely stringent test of reliability. Each of the 60 patients was administered the ADIS at two different times by different and independent interviewers, each of whom, of course, was blind to the results of the other interview. Furthermore, diagnostic agreement was defined as an exact match of the two clinicians' primary diagnoses. For example, in our sample there were several cases in which the raters arrived at the same two anxiety diagnoses but did not agree on which of the two was the primary diagnosis. In calculating κ, these cases were scored as disagreements. When disagreements occurred, a consensus diagnosis was arrived at after detailed discussion of the case at a staff meeting. At this meeting, the apparent reasons for the disagreement were also identified, although in some cases it was necessary to examine clinicians' entries into the ADIS to clarify the source of disagreement. The preliminary reliability data are presented in Table 14.1. The kappa (κ) coefficients are good indeed, with the exception of that for generalized anxiety disorder. For example, the extremely high κ of .853 for agoraphobia with panic represents about as good an agreement as one could expect in a study of diagnostic reliability. Furthermore, we have some confidence in this particular κ, because it is based on 23 cases and because the addition of a substantial number of cases since these data were prepared has not changed the κ at all. Nevertheless, some of these categories were based on small numbers of patients. For example, there were only 6 cases of generalized anxiety disorder (GAD) and 3 cases of obsessive–compulsive dis-

Table 14.1. κ *coefficients for specific diagnostic categories*

Diagnosis	κ
Agoraphobia with panic attacks	.853
Panic disorder	.692
Generalized anxiety disorder	.467
Social phobia	.771
Obsessive–compulsive disorder	.658
Major depression	.571
Other:	.692
Bipolar disorder	
Dysthymic disorder	
Axis III	
No mental disorder	
Schizophreniform disorder	
Adjustment disorder	
with anxious mood	
with mixed emotional features	

Source: Adapted from Dinardo et al. (1983). *Arch Gen Psychiatry* 40:1070–1074. Copyright 1983, American Medical Association.

order in our first "wave" of patients. Since these data were prepared, we have added 3 more cases of obsessive–compulsive disorder for a total of 6, and the κ has increased to .825. More important, we have added 6 cases of GAD, for a total of 12, and the κ has now risen to .571. Although this is still low, it is approaching the range of respectable agreement. All other κ values have increased with the addition of more subjects, with the exception of that for panic disorder, which decreased only slightly. There were too few simple phobics to calculate a κ in the first wave, but now we have a total of 7, yielding a low κ of .558. As noted later, this somewhat surprising difficulty in agreeing on a diagnosis of simple phobia is due to the fact that almost all of our simple phobics also presented with other anxiety disorders making the clinical weighting for determining what is the primary disorder and what the secondary somewhat difficult.

Clinicians disagreed on the primary diagnosis for 17 patients in the first wave of 60 patients. A summary of clinicians' original primary diagnoses, subsequent consensus diagnoses, and sources of disagreement for all cases of diagnostic disagreement is presented in Table 14.2. In this table, the source of disagreement in the right-hand column refers to the specific reason why the clinicians disagreed. Six different reasons or categories of disagreement were identified, and the frequency of disagreement for each of these categories is presented in Table

Table 14.2. *Frequency of sources of diagnostic disagreement*

Source	Frequency
1. Subject variance	3
2. Information variance	7
3. Insufficient information provided by ADIS	0
4. Insufficient specification of criteria in *DSM-III*	2
5. Differential weighting of aspects of clinical picture	7
6. Clinician's error	1
Total	20[a]

[a]Clinicians disagreed on primary diagnosis in 17 of 60 cases. The total number of sources of disagreement is more than this, because in some cases, more than one source of disagreement was identified.

14.3. "Subject variance" refers to an actual change in the patient's condition or status between the two interviews, which occurred a median of two weeks apart, and four to five weeks or more apart in a few cases. For example, the patient may have been severely depressed during the first interview, but less depressed during the second interview several weeks later. One of the most common sources of disagreement was information variance in which patients provided different, or at least considerably more detailed, information to one clinician than to the other. The other common source of disagreement, termed "differential weighting of aspects of clinical picture," refers to situations in which both clinicians would identify the same two disorders in a patient but would have them in different orders of severity. This, of course, was scored a disagreement. During examination of the second wave of patients, currently in progress, disagreements due to differential weighting of the clinical picture have dropped considerably, but information variance is occurring at about the same rate, making this the single largest source of disagreement.

In summary, it appears that the *DSM-III* categories of anxiety disorders provide excellent descriptions of the phenomena presenting to clinicians, even without the hierarchical decision rules within the anxiety disorders suggested by *DSM-III*. The only exceptions are GAD and, somewhat surprisingly, simple phobia. But we shall be able to say more about these categories when a sufficient N is generated. Finally, it is worth noting that the first wave of 60 patients yielded no cases of agoraphobia without panic. To date we have examined a total of 41 patients with agoraphobia, and only 1 patient has met the definition of agoraphobia without panic. But it is interesting to examine the phenomenology of this case. This particular woman had had what she called her first "panic attack" at a banquet several years earlier, but the panic involved only two symptoms, severe diarrhea and perspiration. Since that time she has developed a classic agoraphobic pattern, with a very restricted range of behavior. Furthermore, her fear revolves around the possibility of diarrhea recurring

Table 14.3. *Cases involving diagnostic disagreement: diagnoses and sources of disagreement*

Subject no.	Diagnosis 1	Diagnosis 2	Consensus diagnosis	Sources of disagreement[a]
7	Axis III	Major depression	Major depression	5
10	Simple phobia	Obsessive–compulsive disorder	Obsessive–compulsive disorder	1,5
11	Schizophreniform disorder	Generalized anxiety disorder	Atypical anxiety	2
15	Major depression	Dysthymic disorder	Dysthymic disorder	1
16	Panic disorder	Social phobia	Social phobia	2,6
17	Panic disorder	Simple phobia	Simple phobia	2,5
18	Panic disorder	Generalized anxiety disorder	Panic disorder	
20	Generalized anxiety disorder	Agoraphobia with panic attacks	Generalized anxiety disorder	4
21	Agoraphobia with panic attacks	Major depression	Agoraphobia with panic attacks/major depression	1
22	Generalized anxiety disorder	Social phobia	Social phobia	5
28	Agoraphobia with panic attacks	Simple phobia	Agoraphobia with panic attacks	5
33	Panic disorder	Adjustment disorder with mixed emotional features	Adjustment disorder with mixed emotional features	2
42	No mental disorder	Generalized anxiety disorder	Generalized anxiety disorder	2
43	Panic disorder	Social phobia	Social phobia	5
56	Generalized anxiety disorder	Agoraphobia with panic attacks	Agoraphobia with panic attacks	2
58	Generalized anxiety disorder	No mental disorder	No mental disorder	5
59	Major depression	Bipolar disorder, depressed	Bipolar disorder, depressed	2

when she goes out, which in fact happens occasionally, if rarely. However, she does not present with a sufficient number of symptoms associated with panic to fit technically into the *DSM-III* category of agoraphobia with panic. Nevertheless, it is not open spaces she fears, but the somatic consequences of the fear response, which in her case are somewhat atypical. Agoraphobia without panic may well exist, as we presumed before beginning this series. But after examining 41 consecutive cases of agoraphobia, we have yet to document the existence of this category.

Distribution of additional diagnoses

Another interesting pattern of results appears when one examines the distribution of additional diagnoses among the anxiety disorders. Table 14.4 shows the numbers and percentages of anxiety-disorder cases in which additional but secondary anxiety diagnoses were assigned. As one can see, one or more additional diagnoses were assigned in a substantial number of cases, and the number of additional diagnoses appears to be related to the primary diagnosis. In approximately half of the cases of agoraphobia and social phobia, no additional diagnoses were assigned. However, there were relatively few cases of panic disorder, GAD, and obsessive–compulsive disorders in which no additional diagnoses were assigned. For example, only 12% of the panic-disorder cases and 17% of the cases of GAD did not receive an additional diagnosis. None of the cases of obsessive–compulsive disorder went without an additional diagnosis, although one must remember that only six cases are presently in this category.

Table 14.5 shows the distribution of specific additional diagnoses among the anxiety-disorder cases. The first number of each entry indicates the total number of cases in which the particular additional diagnosis was assigned by either or both raters. The parenthetical figure indicates the number of those cases in which the diagnosis was independently assigned by both raters or by consensus of the staff. GAD as an additional diagnosis may be underrepresented because of some errors in recording this particular diagnosis. At present, we are checking these reports by examining the data from each ADIS. For example, there may be cases of panic disorder in which a GAD diagnosis can also be reached, although the reverse most likely would not occur, because it is almost certain that if a panic disorder were documented, it would be rated more severe than the GAD, thus assuming the primary position among the two diagnoses. Of particular interest in this table is the frequency with which a depressive diagnosis (either major affective disorder or dysthymic disorder) appears as an additional diagnosis among the anxiety disorders. If one counts a diagnosis by either clinician of a depressive disorder, then this diagnosis occurs in 16 (39%) of the 41 cases of agoraphobia, 6 (35%) of the 17 cases of panic disorder, 4 (21%) of the 19 cases of social phobia, and 2 (17%) of the 12 cases of GAD. Finally, 4 of 6 cases of obsessive–compulsive disorder received a depressive diagnosis, and in all 4 cases both interviewers agreed that this was a major affective disorder. On the other hand, none of the simple phobics were depressed. It is shown later

Table 14.4. *Number of anxiety-disorder cases in which additional diagnoses were assigned*

Additional diagnoses	Primary diagnosis						
	Agoraphobia	Social phobia	Simple phobia	Panic disorder	GAD	Obsessive–compulsive	Major affective
0	20 (49%)	10 (53%)	3 (43%)	2 (12%)	2 (17%)	0	0
1	8 (20%)	7 (37%)	2 (29%)	11 (65%)	5 (42%)	3 (50%)	3 (50%)
2	9 (22%)	2 (11%)	2 (29%)	3 (18%)	3 (25%)	3 (50%)	2 (33%)
≥3	4 (1%)	0	0	1 (6%)	2 (16%)	0	1 (17%)

Table 14.5. *Additional diagnoses among anxiety-disorder cases*

Additional diagnoses	Primary diagnosis						
	Agoraphobia	Social phobia	Simple phobia	Panic disorder	GAD	Obsessive–compulsive	Major affective
Agoraphobia	–	0	1(1)[a]	0	2(2)	1(1)	2(0)
Social phobia	7(5)	–	2(2)	6(4)	4(2)	0	0
Simple phobia	7(4)	1(1)	–	5(4)	5(3)	1(1)	3(3)
Panic disorder	0	0	1(1)	–	0	1(0)	1(0)
GAD	1(0)	1(1)	0	0	–	1(1)	1(0)
Obsessive–compulsive	3(1)	2(2)	0	1(1)	0	–	1(1)
Major affective disorder	6(4)	1(1)	0	2(2)	0	4(4)	–
Dysthymic disorder	10(3)	3(2)	0	4(1)	2(0)	0	0
Somatization disorder	0	0	0	1(1)	0	0	0
Axis III	2(2)	1(1)	1(1)	0	4(1)	0	1(1)
Alcohol abuse	0	1(1)	0	0	0	0	1(1)
Conversion	0	0	0	0	0	1(1)	0
Cyclothymic	0	1(1)	0	0	0	0	0
Axis II	2(1)	0	1(1)	0	0	0	0

[a]Additional diagnoses assigned independently by both raters or by staff consensus appear in parentheses.

that the incidence of depression in these categories roughly parallels clinicians' ratings of the severities of the anxiety disorders.

It seems clear from these data that a number of distinct anxiety disorders varying in severity may occur at the same time in any one individual. These additional diagnoses also seem to have important treatment implications in many cases. For example, one agoraphobic in one of our groups also presented with a distinct blood and injury phobia, which would be categorized under a specific phobia. This complicated her treatment by graduated exposure, because when confronted with a specifically phobic object, such as a dead squirrel in the road during her practice sessions, she experienced the bradycardia and hypotension that paradoxically are characteristic of this particular specific phobia (Connolly, Hallam, and Marks, 1976; Yule and Fernando, 1980), and she occasionally would faint – something agoraphobics, of course, almost never do. In this case, the specific phobia had to be treated before substantial progress could be made with the agoraphobia.

Preliminary validity studies

Anxiety and depression. Reliability, good as it is, is not the same as validity. Examination of the validity of diagnostic categories requires evidence of qualitative, or at least quantitative, differences among categories and/or differential treatment responses or courses. There are few data at the present time bearing on the validity of the *DSM-III* anxiety-disorder category, which is, of course, quite new. One area of particular interest concerns the relationship between anxiety and depression. This is too large a topic to cover fully in this chapter (Barlow and Maser, 1984). Leckman and associates (1983) studied first-degree relatives of individuals with major depression, either with or without an anxiety disorder. Their findings indicated that the relatives of individuals with major depression plus an anxiety disorder were at greater risk for major depression as well as anxiety disorders than were the relatives of individuals with major depression without an anxiety disorder. Furthermore, this risk was present whether or not the anxiety disorder occurred solely in association with episodes of major depression. These findings, of course, do not support the assumption that anxiety occurring at the same time as an episode of major depression should not be diagnosed.

Coming at this problem from the anxiety-disorders side, we have had 10 consensus diagnoses of major affective disorder in the past year in patients who were either self-referred or referred by their primary-care physicians for treatment of anxiety. A typical case concerned a 35-year-old mother of two who reported feeling panicky almost continually, both at home and while outside of her house. The panic attacks included onset of rapid heartbeat, tightness in the chest, feelings of unreality, and fear of doing something uncontrolled. She also reported feeling immobilized during the attacks. A brief history revealed that the attacks were of relatively recent origin (three months) and were predated by depression associated with her divorce three months prior to the first panic attack. Facing the prospect of providing for her family alone, she became anxious about trying to handle day-to-day chores and decisions. Detailed questioning concerning the attacks revealed that they occurred anytime she was faced with a decision, even as minor as making out a grocery list or selecting an article of clothing for the day. Therefore, the fear of being outside of her house was mediated not by fear of having a panic attack but fear of being faced with a situation in which she would have to make a decision. All other aspects of her clinical picture and behavior during the interview suggested that depression was the primary diagnosis, and, in fact, depression was independently diagnosed by both clinicians. In view of the severity of the disorders in this group of depressed patients with anxiety, implied in the data of Leckman and associates (1983), we were curious to compare Hamilton anxiety and Hamilton depression scores for this group with all other subcategories of the anxiety disorders. The results are presented in Table 14.6. As one can see, following univariate analyses of variance and appropriate post hoc testing, both those with major affective disorder and obsessive–compulsive disorder scored high on the depression scale and were significantly more depressed than those with any of the remaining anxiety disorders, whose scores did not differ from one another.

Patients with major affective disorders also demonstrated the most anxiety on the Hamilton Anxiety Scale. Obsessive–compulsives and agoraphobics were equally anxious on this scale and not significantly less anxious than those with major affective disorders, whereas simple phobics, as one might expect, were the least anxious. In regard to our population with major depression, one must remember that this group was skewed in that they were referred to an anxiety-disorder clinic with obvious symptoms of severe anxiety. Thus, though they do not represent a typically depressed group, they are a good group for comparison for our purposes.

Finally, Table 14.7 takes a closer look at individual items on the Hamilton Depression Scale that best discriminate among the two highest groups, major affective disorder and obsessive–compulsive disorder, and the other diagnostic groups. On three items, retardation, helplessness, and suicidal thoughts, those with major affective disorders had a significantly higher rating than any other group. There were no significant differences on these items among the anxiety-disorder groups. On other items there was little to choose between obsessive–compulsive and depressed populations. With increased power, which we estimate should occur with $N = 15$ per group, and the ability to perform discriminant-function analyses, differential patterns among these groups should become clearer.

Detailed analysis of the relationship between anxiety and depression is difficult both conceptually and methodologically. One of the major problems is that rating scales or self-report inventories measuring depression and anxiety often use similar items (Foa and Foa, 1982). For example, the Hamilton scales, if examined closely, overlap approximately 60%, ensuring what may be a somewhat spurious correlation. This problem has been attacked on a number of fronts, with some of the more promising results coming from investigators such as Akiskal (1983) in the sleep laboratory. For example, it may not be enough to

Table 14.6. *Hamilton-scale scores and severity of the primary diagnosis[a] for the diagnostic groups*

Diagnosis						
	Agoraphobia	Social phobia	Simple phobia	Panic disorder	GAD	Obsessive–compulsive	Major affective
Anxiety	25.7_{cd}	20.7_{ab}	17.4_a	22.4_{abc}	23.3_{bc}	25.2_{bcd}	29.8_d
Depression	16.4_a	12.8_a	13.7_a	13.8_a	12.6_a	24.0_b	26.8_b
Mean severity	5.63_b	5.63_g	5.00_{ab}	5.18_{ab}	4.50_a	6.00_b	6.17_b

Note: Means with similar subscripts are not significantly different.
[a]The mean of two clinicians' judgments of severity on a 0–8 scale.

Table 14.7. *Hamilton depression items for the diagnostic groups*

Item	Diagnosis						
	Agoraphobia	Social phobia	Simple phobia	Panic disorder	GAD	Obsessive–compulsive	Major affective
Mood	2.00_a	1.84_a	1.36_a	1.71_a	1.67_a	2.58_b	3.25_b
Insomnia early	1.62_{ab}	1.24_a	1.64_{ab}	1.21_a	1.50_{ab}	1.92_{bc}	2.42_c
Work	2.33_a	2.05_a	1.79_a	1.79_a	1.92_a	2.50_{ab}	3.42_b
Retardation	1.09_a	1.13_a	1.00_a	1.00_a	1.00_a	1.25_a	1.58_b
Suicide	1.55_b	1.50_{ab}	1.36_{ab}	1.18_a	1.13_a	1.33_{ab}	2.33_c
Helplessness	1.79_a	1.55_a	1.57_a	1.58_a	1.45_a	2.00_a	2.67_b

Note: Means with similar subscripts are not significantly different.

say that anxiety either does or does not accompany depression and leave it at that. In the case described earlier, anxiety clearly accompanied depression, but a secondary diagnosis of panic disorder was not made, because the panic was predictably associated with the cue of making decisions, much as occasional panic in a simple phobic is reliably associated with specific phobic cues. On the other hand, in several depressives there was an independent diagnosis of panic disorder, as well as several other independent anxiety disorders (Tables 14.4 and 14.5). Although considerably more work will be required to ascertain patterns of additional anxiety diagnoses in this group, it may be important at least to determine the type of anxiety present (e.g., GAD versus panic) and to determine whether the panic is an independent disorder or is predictably associated with depression cues. Naturally, different treatment implications may result.

The phenomenon of panic. One of the most important developments in the study of anxiety disorders during the past several years, in addition to the appearance of the *DSM-III* itself, has been the focus on panic as a possible qualitatively different anxiety phenomenon. Credit for this is due to Klein (1981) and his colleagues, who have demonstrated in their initial work the differential responses to pharmacological treatment observed for panic versus the more general or anticipatory anxiety (Zitrin, Klein, and Woerner, 1980; Zitrin, 1981; Zitrin et al., 1983). In addition, the preliminary observation that lactate produces panic only in those with panic disorders in remission, but not in normals, lends further support to the importance of the phenomenon of panic. Recently, in a preliminary experiment evaluating the effects of psychosocial treatments on intense anxiety versus background anxiety, we also found that a combination of relaxation and cognitive restructuring procedures affected intense anxiety, but not background anxiety, lending some further support to Klein's pharmacological dissection work (Barlow and Beck, 1984; Waddell, Barlow, and O'Brien, 1984). Finally, there is preliminary evidence of different developmental antecedents for panic versus GAD (Raskin et al., 1982), and one cannot ignore the fact that patients report these types of anxieties to be qualitatively different. On the other hand, some investigators have found panic and GAD to look very much alike on the whole (Hoehn-Saric, 1981), whereas others believe that panic and GAD are at different points on a dimension of severity (Barlow and Maser, 1984).

Another important step in the validation process includes ascertaining the prevalence and phenomenology of panic across various diagnostic categories, and we have completed a preliminary analysis with our initial patients. The *DSM-III*, of course, lists 12 symptoms that may contribute to identification of panic, along with sudden occurrences of discrete periods of apprehension and impending doom, and notes that the presence of any four or more is necessary to label the event a true panic. In addition to detailed questions on specific diagnostic criteria for panic, the ADIS requires that the clinician review and rate each of the 12 symptoms on a 0-to-4 scale, where 0 indicates the absence of the symptom, and 4 indicates that the symptom is very severe and grossly disabling. Table 14.8 presents some data from this analysis.

Table 14.8. *Incidence of panic across diagnostic categories*

	Agoraphobia with panic	Social phobia	Simple phobia	Panic disorder	GAD	Obsessive–compulsive	Major affective
Percentage of symptoms	83.5[b]	57.6[a]	59.4[a]	83.3[b]	50.0[a]	75.2[ab]	61.6[ab]
Panic frequency	10.47[a]	4.68[a]	2.28[a]	6.00[a]	4.33[a]	19.67[a]	67.67[b]
Diagnosis on *DSM-III* panic criteria	74%	50%	33%	82%	29%	100%	100%
Diagnosis met except for panic frequency	98%	84%	85%	100%	75%	83%	83%
Reports of panic	98%	89%	100%	100%	83%	83%	83%

Note: a and *b* indicate significant Duncan groupings.

If one looks at the percentages of the 12 symptoms experienced in each of the anxiety-disorder categories as well as the category of major depression, it is evident that all categories have at least 50% (or 6 of these symptoms), including generalized anxiety disorder. Although some statistically significant differences emerge, panic disorder or agoraphobia with panic do not differ significantly from obsessive–compulsive disorder or even major depression on a number of these panic like symptoms. In fact, looking at the last row in the table, there are no differences among patient reports of panic attacks among the diagnostic categories. Even if one goes to the frequency of panics in the past three weeks, one can find little to choose at the present time, with the exception of major depression, in which several patients reported experiencing numerous panics, thereby inflating the results for this category. Finally, if one looks at only the data from the ADIS and averages the responses across two raters, which gives a slightly different picture than the final consensus diagnoses, one can see that a substantial percentage of most anxiety-disorder categories will meet the diagnostic criteria for panic disorder, the only exceptions being simple phobia and GAD, but even here approximately 30% will qualify. If one drops the criterion of three panic attacks in a three-week period of time, then almost everyone in each category will otherwise qualify for the diagnosis of panic.

But some intriguing differences emerge when one examines individual symptoms making up the panic diagnosis. For example, reports of dizziness are most severe and do not differ among the categories of agoraphobia with panic, panic disorder, and obsessive–compulsive disorder. Reported symptoms of dizziness among patients with GAD are somewhat lower, but still significantly higher than among patients with social phobia, simple phobia, or major depression. This more detailed analysis is currently in progress and should be available in the near future for all preliminary patients. Achieving an adequate sample size, and therefore sufficient power, will also be an important goal in obtaining the fullest picture of the phenomenon of panic.

If these data hold up, then one might speculate that the occurrence of panic is a dimension of all anxiety disorders as well as major depression, with differences occurring only in frequency across some of the disorders. But these panic attacks would not indicate the existence of a panic disorder as we now conceive it in each of these categories. Within the category of simple phobia, the cues are clear, both to the patient and to the therapist, and therefore the panics are predictable. Within the category of major depression, we have already discussed the patient for whom the cues, in this case decision making, were not clear to the patient initially, although they became clear on examination. One major difference between biological and psychological conceptions of panic lies in assumptions concerning the presence of cues in patients for whom panic is otherwise occasionally unpredictable. Although most investigators agree that cues or antecedents for panic exist in most anxiety-disorder categories, diagnoses such as panic disorder and agoraphobia with panic often seem characterized by a lack of clear antecedents to panic, accounting for patients' reports of the unpredictable nature of these events. Searches for either biological determinants of panic or the presence of psychological (or physiological) antecedents are under way in a number of centers and may well influence our notions on the classification of panic in the years to come. Our own impression is that cues for panic in our agoraphobics are most always associated with mild exercise, sexual relations, sudden temperature changes, stress, or other cues that alter physiological functioning in some discernible way, albeit out of the patient's awareness. But these are only clinical impressions at the present time.

CONCLUSIONS

In summary, the *DSM-III* classification of anxiety disorders has proved extremely useful and will, we predict, be very important in facilitating research into the nature of anxiety in the years to come. Whether or not the current categories reflect the truth about anxiety disorders awaits further research, but the fact that at least we can all agree on what we are talking about, in a descriptive sense, is an absolutely necessary first step. Our research and clinical experience to date would be consistent with almost all of the revisions in these categories recently proposed by Spitzer and Williams (1985) – specifically, the dropping of a hierarchical system of assigning diagnoses so that multiple anxiety-disorder categories may exist in individuals, with ratings of severity as the only determinant of primary versus secondary status. Particularly intriguing and consistent with our experience is the possibility of deemphasizing the term "agoraphobia" in favor of "panic disorder," with varying amounts of avoidance, which in our experience seems determined by environmental contingencies. As noted earlier, we have not seen any true agoraphobics without panics, only an agoraphobic with atypical "panics." The time period in which panics may have occurred in relation to the time of the interview should also be specified, even if in an arbitrary way. Currently, in our own system, if a patient has met the criteria for panic disorder, but panics have not occurred in the past year, that patient is assigned to the category panic disorder, past episodes. Any assumption that once a panic disorder always a panic disorder, of course, implies specific underlying etiological mechanisms.

Finally, the nature of GAD is still fuzzy. At present we are undertaking a major analysis of the relationship of GAD to other anxiety-disorder categories, but the data are not yet in. There seems little question that one month is too short a time to accurately classify these people, to the extent that they exist. We suggest one year as being more appropriate. Also, the very criteria for GAD are a bit vague. For example, we have come to rely on quantifiable rating scales of severity on the various dimensions of GAD to differentiate these cases more clearly from "no mental disorder." Despite this fact, GAD was the competing diagnosis in both of the cases in which one interviewer had opted for the "no mental disorder" designation. In most other cases, in our experience, people who end up in the category of GAD have subclinical phobias or panics. It seems that if one looks closely at patients with GAD, most of their anxiety either has situational determinants or is characterized by subclinical panics, but the anxiety is not severe enough or frequent enough to meet the criteria for another *DSM-III* anxiety-disorder category. If this turns out to be the case in most patients with GAD, it may be more useful to categorize them in one of the other categories and simply indicate by severity ratings the impairment caused by the symptoms. On the other hand, it is possible that the GAD category is more in line with a personality disorder characterized by chronic and severe worrying accompanied by some autonomic responding.

Finally, it is entirely possible that anxiety disorders are dimensional rather than categorical and may take many forms, depending on environmental contingencies, personality variables, levels of stress, and so on. In this sense, the variety of anxiety disorders may simply be variations on a theme, with the particular form (e.g., obsession panic) changing over time. Clinically this seems to happen (Barlow and Maser, 1984), but formal studies of the courses of these disorders are essential.

REFERENCES

Akiskal HS: Diagnosis and classification of affective disorders: new insights from clinical and laboratory approaches. Psychiatr Dev 1:123–160, 1983

Barlow DH, Beck JG: The psychosocial treatment of anxiety disorders: current status, future directions, in Psychotherapy Research: Where Are We and Where Should We Go? Edited by Williams JBW, Spitzer RL. New York, Guilford, 1984

Barlow DH, Maser JD: Psychopathology in anxiety disorders: a report on an NIMH workshop, 1984

Connolly J, Hallam RS, Marks IM: Selective association of fainting with blood-illness-injury fear. Behav Ther 7:8–13, 1976

DiNardo PA, O'Brien GT, Barlow DH, et al: Anxiety Disorders Interview Schedule (ADIS). Available from Phobia and Anxiety Disorders Clinic, Drawer 107, SUNY–Albany, 135 Western Avenue, Albany, NY 12222

Reliability of DSM-III anxiety disorder categories using a new structured interview. Arch Gen Psychiatry 40:1070–1074, 1983

Endicott J, Spitzer RL: A diagnostic interview: the Schedule for Affective Disorders and Schizophrenia. Arch Gen Psychiatry 35:837–844, 1978

Use of the Research Diagnostic Criteria and the Schedule for Affective Disorders and Schizophrenia to study affective disorders. Am J Psychiatry 136:52–56, 1979

Foa EB, Foa UG: Differentiating anxiety and depression: Is it possible? Is it useful? Psychopharmacol Bull 18:62–68, 1982

Hoehn-Saric R: Characteristics of chronic anxiety patients, in Anxiety: New Research and Changing Concepts. Edited by Klein DF, Rabkin J. New York, Raven Press, 1981

Klein DF: Anxiety reconceptualized, Anxiety: New Research and Changing Concepts. Edited by Klein DF, Rabkin J. New York, Raven Press, 1981

Leckman JF, Merikangas KR, Pauls DL, et al: Anxiety disorders associated with episodes of depression: family study data contradict DSM-III convention. Am J Psychiatry 140:880–882, 1983

Raskin M, Peeke HVS, Dickman W, et al: Panic and generalized anxiety disorders: developmental antecedents and precipitants. Arch Gen Psychiatry 29:687–689, 1982

Robins LN, Helzer JE, Croughan J, et al: National Institute of Mental Health Diagnostic Interview Schedule: its history, characteristics, and validity. Arch Gen Psychiatry 38:381–389, 1981

Spitzer RL, Williams JBW: Proposed revisions in the DSM-III classification of anxiety disorders based on research and clinical experience, in Anxiety and the Anxiety Disorders. Edited by Tuma AH, Maser J. Hillsdale, NJ, Lawrence Erlbaum Associates, 1985

Waddell MT, Barlow DH, O'Brien GT: Cognitive and relaxation treatment for panic disorders: effects on panic versus "background" anxiety. Behav Res Ther 22:393–402, 1984

Wing JK, Cooper JE, Sartorius N: The Measurement and Classification of Psychiatric Symptoms. Cambridge University Press, 1974

Yule W, Fernando P: Blood phobia – beware. Behav Res Ther 18:587–590, 1980

Zitrin CM: Combined pharmacologic and psychotherapeutic treatment of phobias, in Phobia: Psychological and Pharmacological Treatment. Edited by Mavissakalian MR, Barlow DH. New York, Guilford, 1981

Zitrin CM, Klein DF, Woerner MG: Treatment of agoraphobia with group exposure in vivo and imipramine. Arch Gen Psychiatry 37:63–72, 1980

Zitrin CM, Klein DF, Woerner MG, et al: Comparison of imipramine hydrochloride and placebo. Arch Gen Psychiatry 40:125–139, 1983

15 *Diagnosis of somatoform disorders*
A critique of DSM-III

C. ROBERT CLONINGER

One of the most important innovations in the third edition of the American Psychiatric Association's *Diagnostic and Statistical Manual of Mental Disorders (DSM-III)* is its classification of psychiatric disorders in which the most prominent symptoms suggest physical illness. The multiaxial system permits specification of distinct aspects of clinical symptoms, personality, physical illness, and psychosocial stress for each patient. This permits the comprehensive description that is so often needed in liaison psychiatry (Linn and Spitzer, 1982), as well as distinctions among groups of patients that in the past had often been confused (Hyler and Spitzer, 1978).

DSM-III distinguishes five groups of disorders according to the roles of known pathophysiological mechanisms, psychological conflict, and voluntary control over symptoms (Table 15.1). The term "somatoform disorders" refers to illnesses in which there is no known physical disorder or pathophysiological mechanism to explain symptoms and in which psychological conflicts lead to involuntary formation of physical signs and symptoms. In *DSM-III* these disorders include somatization disorder (formerly called chronic hysteria or Briquet's syndrome), conversion disorder (or hysterical neurosis, conversion type), psychogenic pain disorder, hypochondriasis (or hypochondriacal neurosis), and other atypical somatoform disorders. These disorders are distinguished on axis I of *DSM-III* from dissociative, anxiety, and affective states that had been grouped together as neuroses in earlier classifications. Associated personality disorders such as histrionic personality disorder are noted on axis II, if present. When psychological factors are important in the initiation, exacerbation, or maintenance of a somatoform disorder with a known physical disorder, this is noted on axis I, and the physical disorder is specified on axis III. Symptoms explained by a known pathophysiological mechanism – such as vasovagal reflex for fainting, or muscle spasm for tension headaches or backaches – are treated as physical disorders, not as somatoform disorders. Thus, *DSM-III* attempts to be conceptually consistent in the principles used to subdivide disorders with prominent physical symptoms.

Overall, *DSM-III* also seeks to avoid assumptions about causes, but a major exception is made in the criteria for conversion disorder and psychogenic pain disorder. Based on the assumptions of current psychodynamic theory, judg-

243

Table 15.1. *DSM-III inclusion and exclusion criteria used in differential diagnosis of symptoms suggesting physical illness*

Classification	Physical mechanism explains the symptoms	Symptoms are linked to psychological factors	Symptoms initiation is under voluntary control	Obvious recognizable environmental goal
Somatoform disorders	No	Yes	No	Variable
Factitious disorders	Variable	Yes	Yes	No
Malingering	Variable	Variable	Yes	Yes
Psychological factors affecting physical condition	Yes	Yes	No	Variable
Undiagnosed physical illness	Variable	Variable	No	No

Source: Hyler and Spitzer (1978). *Am J Psychiatry* 135:1500–1504, 1978. Copyright 1978, the American Psychiatric Association. Reprinted by permission.

Table 15.2. *DSM-III diagnostic criteria for conversion disorder*

A. The predominant disturbance is loss of or alteration in physical functioning suggesting a physical disorder.
B. Psychological factors are judged to be etiologically involved in the symptoms, as evidenced by one of the following:
   1. There is a temporal relationship between an environmental stimulus that is apparently related to a psychological conflict or need and the initial symptom or exacerbation of the symptom.
   2. The symptom enables the individual to avoid some activity that is considered noxious.
   3. The symptom enables the individual to get support from the environment that otherwise might not be forthcoming.
C. It has been determined that the symptom is not under voluntary control.
D. The symptom cannot, after appropriate investigation, be explained by a known physical disorder or pathophysiological mechanism.
E. The symptom is not limited to pain or to a disturbance in sexual functioning.
F. Not due to somatization disorder or schizophrenia.

ments about primary gain and secondary gain are required for diagnosis of conversion symptoms and psychogenic pain.

In this chapter I review the available data concerning the utility and validity of the criteria for each somatoform disorder. In addition, the justification for many innovations in the general system for classifying patients with prominent physical symptoms is considered. Finally, some revisions for the current criteria are proposed based on available data. Questions that will require the most urgent attention in future work are identified.

CONVERSION DISORDER

Conversion disorder is considered first because it illustrates most clearly the theoretical and practical problems inherent in the diagnosis of somatoform disorders. The issues include the types of symptoms considered as conversion symptoms, methods for exclusion of medical illness as an explanation of the symptoms, and the inclusion criteria for psychopathology or psychological conflict. The current *DSM-III* criteria for conversion disorder are shown in Table 15.2.

Types of symptoms

In conversion disorder, *DSM-III* requires loss of or alteration in physical functioning, not simply complaints of physical symptoms. Such loss or alteration most often involves the classic symptoms suggesting neurological disease, such as paralysis, blindness, aphonia, ataxia, or anesthesia. *DSM-III* also includes disturbances in the autonomic nervous system (e.g., psychogenic vomiting or fainting) or in the endocrine system (e.g., pseudocyesis) as conversions. When conversion symptoms are limited to pain or sexual dysfunction, conversion disorder is not diagnosed even if the underlying mechanism is presumed to be similar to that for conversion disorder.

The distinction between patients with classic pseudoneurological symptoms and those with psychogenic pain has a basis in historical tradition and the natural history of the symptoms. Among patients without physical disorder in follow-up studies, psychogenic pain is often chronic (Blumer and Heilbronn, 1982), whereas individual pseudoneurological symptoms are usually transient (Gatfield and Guze, 1962). However, recent work has found that psychogenic vomiting usually has a chronic, nondebilitating course (Rosenthal, Webb, and Wruble, 1980; Wruble, Rosenthal, and Webb, 1982). With the availability of radioimmunoassays for serum prolactin, most patients with symptoms suggestive of false pregnancy (pseudocyesis) can now be shown to have an objective endocrine disturbance, most often a prolactinoma (Cohen, 1982). Combining such disparate types of symptoms as transient paralysis and chronic psychogenic vomiting in one category has no apparent advantage for prediction of outcome or choice of treatment. Accordingly, consideration should be given to recognizing subtypes of conversion disorder, distinguishing classic pseudoneurological syndromes, autonomic disturbances, and endocrine disturbances, or to categorizing autonomic and endocrine disturbances with other symptoms, such as tension headaches, when the pathophysiological mechanism is known.

Medical exclusion criteria

The major problem in the diagnosis of conversion symptoms is the exclusion of physical disorder. This discrimination can be extremely difficult early in the course of a medical disorder, especially if the signs and symptoms are atypical and/or are combined with a "functional overlay" of psychiatric symptoms. Judgments concerning whether or not signs and symptoms follow what are considered to be known anatomic and physiological boundaries are notoriously unreliable because of limitations in our knowledge of pathophysiology, natural variations in the presentations of physical disorders, and limited methods for objective assessment. Patients with undiagnosed physical disorders often are in distress and may exaggerate or misrepresent their symptoms. For example, Slater (1965) found in his follow-up of 85 patients diagnosed as having conversion symptoms that 59% had developed organic disorders that explained the original complaint. Similarly, Gatfield and Guze (1962) found that 21% of 24 patients diagnosed as having conversion reactions on a neurology service had definite neurological diseases to explain the original symptoms 3 to 10 years later. Gatfield and Guze observed that all these errors were due to temporary partial improvement during medical evaluation or sedation that falsely suggested psychiatric illness. Thus, *DSM-III* is clearly justified in noting the inadequacy of such observations and emphasizing the necessity for positive inclusion criteria for diagnosing psychiatric illness.

Table 15.3. *Utility of psychiatric criteria for distinguishing conversions and physical disorders*

Putative diagnostic criteria	Predicts no physical disorder	References[a]
Prior history of conversions	Yes	1–4,6–8
Prior history of recurrent somatic complaints	Yes	1–4,6–8
Prior model for symptoms	Yes	4
Current anxiety or dysphoria	No	5
Emotional stress prior to onset		
(a) any	No	4,5
(b) previous history of conversions with conflict resolution	Yes	4
(c) with symbolism	No	4,8
Secondary gain	No	4
Improvement with suggestion or sedation	No	1
MMPI profile type	No	5
Histrionic personality		
(a) with prior history of conversions	Yes	1,4,8
(b) no prior history of conversion	No	1,4,8
La Belle indifference	No	4,8

[a]Reference numbers: 1 (Gatfield and Guze, 1962), 2 (Slater, 1965), 3 (Perley and Guze, 1962), 4 (Raskin et al., 1966), 5 (Watson and Buranen, 1979), 6 (Purtell et al., 1951), 7 (Guze et al., 1971a,b), 8 (Bishop and Torch, 1979).

Psychiatric inclusion criteria

The requirement of positive evidence of psychopathology or psychological conflict adopted in *DSM-III* requires a clinical judgment that the etiological mechanism for the symptoms is primary gain (evidenced by item B1 in Table 15.2) and/or secondary gain (evidenced by item B2 and B3 in Table 15.2). Fortunately, several studies are available that provide an empirical test of the utility of these and other criteria for distinguishing conversion symptoms from physical disorders. These include follow-up studies that test what clinical features distinguish patients who do or do not prove to have physical disorders (Gatfield and Guze, 1962; Perley and Guze, 1962; Slater, 1965; Raskin, Talbott, and Meyerson, 1966; Watson and Buranen, 1979) and cross-sectional comparisons of the clinical features that distinguish patients with conversion reactions from other psychiatric and medical disorders (Purtell, Robins, and Cohen, 1951; Lader and Sartorius, 1968; Guze, Woodruff, and Clayton, 1971b; Bishop and Torch, 1979). Several clinical criteria have been evaluated in these studies and are summarized in Table 15.3.

Isolated conversion reactions are uncommon, and a previous history of conversion symptoms is useful in distinguishing patients with conversion symptoms from those with undiagnosed physical disorders (Purtell et al., 1951; Gatfield and Guze, 1962; Perley and Guze, 1962; Slater, 1965, Raskin et al., 1966; Guze et al., 1971b; Bishop and Torch, 1979). Patients with true conversions more often have a previous history of multiple unexplained somatic symptoms than do those with undiagnosed physical disorders (Purtell et al., 1951; Gatfield and Guze, 1962; Perley and Guze, 1962; Slater, 1965; Raskin et al., 1966; Guze et al., 1971b). Such a previous history of conversion and/or somatic complaints is the most reliable predictor of the absence of physical disorders.

In contrast, evaluation of emotional stress has proved difficult and of limited utility. Events that are obviously stressful often antecede the onset or exacerbation of physical disorders as well as various psychiatric disorders and do not distinguish true conversions from initially undiagnosed physical disorders (Raskin et al., 1966; Watson and Buranen, 1979). Nevertheless, Raskin and associates (1966) reported success in distinguishing conversion symptoms from physical disorders by judgments about whether or not the symptoms were being used to solve a conflict brought about by a precipitating stress. However, their judgment was highly dependent on the patient's report of prior conversion symptoms and somatic complaints: That is, an event that would be trivial for an average individual was judged to be significant because it was reportedly associated with somatic symptoms in the past. *DSM-III* also notes that etiological inferences about psychogenic stress are secure only when the sequence of events is repeated, but this confounds etiological assumptions with observed recurrence. Raskin and associates (1966) found that prior history of such somatic symptoms was more sensitive in identifying conversion symptoms, was more readily evaluated, and was equally specific.

Stricter definitions of primary gain as the effectiveness of a conversion symptom in reducing anxiety by a mechanism of symbolic expression of the repressed wish also are of limited utility. In practice, evaluation of symbolism is difficult or impossible in brief consultations (Raskin et al., 1966). Also, patients with conversion reactions often can be shown to experience marked anxiety in objective physiological tests (Lader and Sartorius, 1968; Mears and Horvath, 1972).

Secondary gain is present as often in patients coping with known physical disorders as in patients coping with conversion symptoms. Raskin and associates found that neither primary nor secondary gain was useful in distinguishing conversion and physical disorders. Similarly, there was no difference between such patients in regard to profiles on the Minnesota Multiphasic Psychological Inventory (MMPI) and the frequency of an attitude of indifference (Raskin et al., 1966; Watson and Buranen, 1979).

The diagnosis of conversion disorder is often suspected if patients are dramatic or suggestible. Such traits are associated with conversions, but are not a sufficient basis for diagnosis in the absence of a previous history of conversions and unexplained somatic complaints. Gatfield and Guze (1962) found that diagnosis based on histrionic behavior or temporary incomplete improvement with suggestion or sedation often led to misdiagnosis or organic disorders. There is evidence that patients with conversion symptoms report a history of similar

Table 15.4. *Suggestions for revised diagnositic criteria for conversion disorder*

A.   The predominant disturbance is loss of or alteration in physical functioning suggesting a neurological disorder.
B.   Similar or different types of losses or alterations in neurological function are recurrent over a period of at least six months.
C.   It has been determined that the symptoms are not under voluntary control.
D.   The symptoms cannot, after appropriate investigation, be explained by a known physical disorder or pathophysiological mechanism.
E.   The symptoms are not limited to pain, a disturbance in sexual functioning, or autonomic or endocrine disturbances.
F.   Not due to somatization disorder.

prior physical disorders in themselves or other role models (Raskin et al., 1966; Lazare, 1981), but such a history is not sufficiently specific as a solitary criterion.

In summary, in the absence of somatization disorder, the most reliable psychiatric inclusion criterion for distinguishing patients with true conversions from those with physical disorders is a previous history of conversion disorder. Explicit revised criteria are given in Table 15.4. This has the advantage of being purely descriptive and free of etiological assumptions. In addition, the suggested revision does not refer to any isolated symptom as a disorder, but requires a pattern of symptoms over an extended period. The diagnosis is limited to disturbances suggesting neurological disorders. Even when autonomic and endocrine disturbances have a psychogenic or apparent symbolic value, the pathophysiology of the symptoms involves known mechanisms. Patients have different courses of illness, much as do those with tension headaches. Thus, psychogenic autonomic and endocrine disturbances may be considered psychophysiological disorders, with the physical disorder specified on axis III and psychological factors affecting physical illness noted on axis I. The only psychiatric exclusion is for somatization disorder. No other disorders, such as schizophrenia, are associated with recurrent conversions; so it is useful to note both diagnoses when they coexist.

PSYCHOGENIC PAIN DISORDER

The *DSM-III* criteria for psychogenic pain disorder are identical with those for conversion disorder, except that the symptoms are limited to pain. This means that nearly all the concerns noted for conversions apply at least equally to psychogenic pain. In one follow-up of patients diagnosed prior to *DSM-III* as having psychogenic pain, most proved to have physical disorders (Slater, 1965). To determine if some patients with chronic unexplained pain had been falsely diagnosed as having psychogenic pain disorder, Hendler, Uematsu, and Long (1982) used thermography to evaluate 224 consecutive patient with no radiologic, neurologic, orthopedic, or laboratory abnormalities. Abnor-

Table 15.5. *Clinical features of pain-prone disorder*

Somatic complaint
  Continuous pain of obscure origin
  Hypochondriacal preoccupation
  Desire for surgery
Solid citizen
  Denial of conflicts
  Idealization of self and of family relations
  Ergomania (prepain): "workaholism," relentless activity
Depression
  Anergia (postpain): lack of initiative, inactivity, fatigue
  Anhedonia: inability to enjoy social life, leisure, and sex
  Insomnia
  Depressive mood and despair
History
  Family (and personal) history of depression and alcoholism
  Past abuse by spouse
  Crippled relative
  Relative with chronic pain

Source: Blumer and Heilbronn (1982). © by Williams & Wilkins, 1982.

mal results from thermography in 19% led to revised diagnoses of reflex sympathetic dystrophy, never root irritation, and thoracic outlet syndrome. Thus, dysfunction of the sympathetic nervous system may be easily misdiagnosed as psychogenic pain unless specialized tests like thermography are carried out.

Williams and Spitzer (1982) also have noted that evidence suggesting primary or secondary gain is often not discernible in patients with unexplained pain. Bishop and Torch (1979) noted that evidence of secondary gain was more frequent in 80 patients with idiopathic pain than in 94 other neurotic patients (36% vs. 4%). However, secondary gain is equally common in patients with physical disorders, as noted for conversion symptoms. Thus, the differential diagnosis to distinguish psychogenic pain from physical disorders requires revision of the diagnostic criterion for evidence of psychological factors, just as does conversion disorder.

Blumer and Heilbronn (1982) evaluated a consecutive series of 129 patients with idiopathic chronic pain and compared them to 36 patients with chronic rheumatoid arthritis who were receiving gold therapy. They noted that such patients had a hypochondriacal preoccupation with the painful body parts, inability to appreciate and verbalize their feelings (alexithymia), a previous history of relentless overactivity ("workaholism" or "ergomania"), and current depression, with anergia, insomnia, and anhedonia. They proposed the name "pain-prone disorder" and suggested that it was a variant of depressive disease (Table 15.5). However, only 12% of the patients had a history of depression prior to onset of pain. The controls were often responsive to gold therapy; so

Table 15.6. *Suggestions for diagnostic criteria for idiopathic pain disorder*

A. Preoccupation and severe pain of at least six months' duration is the predominant disturbance.

B. The pain presented as a symptom is inconsistent with the anatomic distribution of the nervous system; after extensive evaluation, no organic abnormality or patho-physiological mechanism can be found to account for the pain; or, when there is some related organic abnormality, the complaint of pain is grossly in excess of what would be expected from the physical findings.

C. Not due to somatization disorder, schizophrenia, or major depression.

Source: William and Spitzer (1982). © by Williams & Wilkins, 1982.

differences in frequencies of depressive symptoms are not surprising. Other differences were not sensitive or specific enough for use as diagnostic criteria. Measures of "ergomania" were significant, but the strength of the associations were still low: Idiopathic patients had engaged in more prepain work and chronic overtime (50% vs. 28%) and more often took no annual vacation (48% vs. 22%).

Based on the findings of Blumer and Heilbronn and their own findings about the inadequacy of the psychological criterion for psychogenic pain, Williams and Spitzer suggested revisions to the *DSM-III* category. They proposed that the name be changed to "idiopathic pain disorder," because positive evidence of psychogenicity often is not discernible. They also would add a duration requirement of six months. Their proposed revised criteria are shown in Table 15.6.

The proposed revisions by Williams and Spitzer for pain disorder and by me for conversion disorder are similar in requiring chronic or recurrent symptoms. Other features do not have the sensitivity or specificity required of diagnostic criteria. They differ in regard to which psychiatric disorders should be excluded. I would suggest the following principle for exclusion rules: The only disorders that should be considered mutually exclusive should be those with such frequent overlap in symptoms that they would otherwise be strongly associated in general samples. That is, impose exclusion rules only when the use of multiple labels would be largely redundant.

SOMATIZATION DISORDER

Validity of Briquet's syndrome

Briquet's syndrome has been described by Guze and his associates as a chronic syndrome of recurrent symptoms in many different organ systems that begins before age 30 and is associated with psychiatric distress but no physical disorder (Guze, 1967; Woodruff, 1967; Guze et al., 1971b). It is associated with excessive surgery and medical attention for a wide variety of medically unexplained complaints. Characteristic symptoms include frequent bodily pains, gastrointestinal symptoms, pseudoneurological conversion symptoms, sexual and mental problems, anxiety and depressive symptoms, and the belief that they have been sickly most of their lives. Perley and Guze (1962) described 59 symptoms in 10 groups as characteristic of Briquet's syndrome and required at least 20 medically unexplained symptoms in 9 groups for diagnosis (Table 15.7). When thus defined, follow-up studies have shown that the clinical picture will remain unchanged over time in 90%, and no other medical or psychiatric disorder will develop to explain the symptoms (Perley and Guze, 1962; Martin, Cloninger, and Guze, 1979). The disorder is diagnosed predominantly in women, but occasional cases occur in men (Guze, Woodruff, and Clayton, 1972).

Clinical and family studies have shown the independence of Briquet's syndrome from anxiety disorders and affective disorders. Briquet's syndrome is associated with greater risks for juvenile delinquency (Guze, Woodruff, and Clayton, 1971a) and adult criminality (Cloninger and Guze, 1970) than are anxiety disorders and primary affective disorders, even though anxiety and depressive symptoms commonly occur in Briquet's syndrome.

Furthermore, the male relatives of women with Briquet's syndrome are at increased risk for antisocial personality and alcohol abuse, whereas their female relatives have an excess of Briquet's syndrome predominantly (Cloninger, Reich, and Guze, 1975; Woerner and Guze, 1975). In contrast, family studies of anxiety disorders have found no excess of antisocial personality (Cloninger et al., 1981). Patients with Briquet's syndrome frequently attempt suicide but rarely are successful (Guze, 1967). These observations are important evidence supporting the decision in *DSM-III* to separate somatoform disorders, anxiety disorders, and affective disorders.

The validity of Briquet's syndrome was supported by an independent principal-component analysis of hypochondriacal psychiatric patients (Bianchi, 1973) and a neurophysiological study (Flor-Henry et al., 1981) that distinguished "acute hysteria" from "chronic hysteria." However, neither study used the explicit criteria recommended by Guze.

Need for medical judgment

Guze's criteria require a judgment as to whether or not each of the possible 59 symptoms can be medically explained. This judgment requires medical training to develop the skill to make critical assessments of the description of the symptoms, diagnostic evaluations, and putative physical diagnoses. Psychiatrists and other physicians can do this reliably even in patients wtih multiple chronic medical illnesses (Woodruff, 1967). However, patients with Briquet's syndrome often attribute symptoms to a variety of physical disorders, and nonphysicians are unable to evaluate such assertions adequately. As a result, when nonphysicians accept medical explanations offered by patients (without

Table 15.7. *Symptom items for Guze's criteria for Briquet's syndrome*

Group 1	**Group 6**
Headaches	Abdominal pain
Sickly most of life	Vomiting
Group 2	**Group 7**
Blindness	Dysmenorrhea
Paralysis	Menstrual irregularity
Anesthesia	Amenorrhea
Aphonia	Excessive bleeding
Fits or convulsions	**Group 8**
Unconsciousness	Sexual indifference
Amnesia	Frigidity
Deafness	Dyspareunia
Hallucinations	Other sexual difficulties
Urinary retention	Vomiting nine months of pregnancy or hospitalized
Ataxia	for hyperemesis gravidarum
Other conversion symptoms	**Group 9**
Group 3	Back pain
Fatigue	Joint pain
Lump in throat	Extremity pain
Fainting spells	Burning pains of the sexual organs, mouth, or
Visual blurring	rectum
Weakness	Other bodily pains
Dysuria	**Group 10**
Group 4	Nervousness
Breathing difficulty	Fears
Palpitation	Depressed feelings
Anxiety attacks	Need to quit working or inability to carry on
Chest pain	regular duties because of feeling sick
Dizziness	Crying easily
Group 5	Feeling life is hopeless
Anorexia	Thinking a good deal about dying
Weight loss	Wanting to die
Marked fluctuations in weight	Thinking of suicide
Nausea	Suicide attempts
Abdominal bloating	
Food intolerances	
Diarrhea	
Constipation	

attempting to judge their plausibility), Briquet's syndrome is underdiagnosed (Robins et al., 1981). The sensitivity for nonphysicians, compared with psychiatrists, is 55% using Guze's criteria and 41% using *DSM-III* criteria. Specificity remains high (97%–99%) for nonphysicians for both the Guze and *DSM-III* criteria.

Abridged criteria in DSM-III

Use of Guze's criteria in routine clinical practice has been inhibited by their length and complexity. For each of the 59 symptoms in Table 15.7, decisions must be made whether or not the complaint is severe enough to require medical attention or to interfere with the patient's life and whether or not the complaint can be medically explained. To reduce the effort, a sensitive screening interview involving only 14 items was developed in 1973 (Woodruff et al., 1973). No shorter criteria were found that were both highly sensitive and specific, and so the full criteria were retained to establish a definite diagnosis.

Another effort was made in 1979 by Drs. Lee Robins, Sam Guze, John Helzer, and Jack Croughan (pers. commun.) to develop criteria that were simpler and shorter for *DSM-III*. Data were available on all 59 variables for 1,116 women in five clinical studies, including relatives of outpatients ($N = 475$), outpatients ($N = 324$), emergency room patients ($N = 177$), and inpatients ($N = 140$). The frequency of Briquet's syndrome varied from 2% among relatives of outpatients to 23% among inpatients. First, the 59 variables were screened to eliminate those that poorly discriminated patients with and without Briquet's syndrome. Nineteen variables were dropped: all 10 symptoms in group 10 in Table 15.7, headache, fits, hallucinations, fatigue, anorexia, weight loss, constipation, amenorrhea, and other sexual difficulties. The reduced criteria set consisted of 40 symptoms in nine groups (as well as onset before age 30). Next, three levels of groups (6+, 7+, 8+) and six levels of symptoms (14+ to 19+) were tested alone and in all possible combinations in each study separately and in all studies combined. The combination was selected that misclassified the fewest subjects as having Briquet's syndrome or not having it, as diagnosed by Guze's criteria. The best agreement was obtained by merely requiring 14 symptoms regardless of the number of groups. This criterion showed good overall agreement ($\kappa = .80$), but modestly overestimated somatization disorder among healthier populations and underestimated it among inpatients (Table 15.8). From another viewpoint, among those diagnosed as having somatization disorder by *DSM-III*, the percentages who did not fulfill Guze's original criteria were 7% of 27 inpatients, 12% of 17 emergency patients, 25% of 32 outpatients, and 38% of 13 relatives of outpatients. Among those diagnosed as Briquet's syndrome by Guze's criteria, the percentages negative by *DSM-III* is 0% of 8 relatives of outpatients, 8% of 26 outpatients, 7% of 16 emergency patients, and 22% of 32 inpatients.

Further modifications of the criteria were introduced ad hoc. "Seizures" was returned to the list of items, and "anesthesia" was omitted. Panic or "anxiety attacks" were omitted to avoid overlap with panic disorder. Distinctions were dropped between "faints" and "unconsciousness" and between "paralysis" and "weakness." "Dysphagia" was substituted for "lump in throat." "Diplopia" was substituted for "other conversions" because it was the most common other conversion. Overall, the number of distinct items was reduced from 40 to 37. The criteria for men were based on the work with women, with two fewer symptoms

Table 15.8. *Comparison of* DSM-III *and Guze's criteria for somatization disorder*

Population	No. of women	% Positive Guze	% Positive DSM-III	DSM-III sensitivity (%)	DSM-III specificity (%)
Relatives of outpatients	475	2	3	100	99
Outpatients	324	8	10	92	97
Emergency room	177	9	10	94	99
Inpatients	140	23	19	78	98
Total	1,116	7	7	88	98

required because of ineligibility for the four gynecologic items. Such changes appear rather minor, but data are needed to validate the final criteria adopted in *DSM-III* for both men and women. Though there appears to be good overall agreement between Guze's criteria and *DSM-III* criteria, research using both is needed so that discrepant cases can be evaluated. Results should be available soon from a follow-up and family study of Washington University outpatients.

HYPOCHONDRIASIS

In a recent review of hypochondriasis, Barsky and Klerman (1983) noted that there are data to support four different ways of conceptualizing hypochondriasis:

1. It is a psychiatric syndrome composed of "functional" somatic complaints, fear of disease, bodily preoccupation, and the persistent pursuit of medical care despite reassurance.
2. According to psychodynamic theory, the patient is disturbed by problems of anger and hostility, orality and dependency, low self-esteem, or guilt and masochism.
3. The cognitive set the patient uses to assess bodily sensations tends to amplify and augment normal bodily sensations, so that the patient has a low threshold and tolerance for physical sensations, often misinterpreting normal sensations as an indication of disease.
4. Hypochondriasis is socially learned sick-role behavior and indirect interpersonal communication that is reinforced by success in eliciting caretaking and other secondary gains from the sick role.

These features are all characteristic of the somatoform disorders in general, and serious doubt exists whether or not there is a discrete disease entity corresponding to hypochondriacal neurosis.

The *DSM-III* criteria for hypochondriasis or hypochondriacal neurosis require preoccupation with an unrealistic fear or belief of having a serious disease and impaired social or occupational function despite medical evaluation and reassurance (Table 15.9). The concept that such patients have an augmenting perceptual style and often misinterpret normal sensations is mentioned in the description, but is not part of the criteria. This is unfortunate, because it could encourage the use of objective tests such as measurements of pain threshold and tolerance or event-related electroencephalographic potentials.

The *DSM-III* criteria are essentially the same as those proposed in 1928 by Gillespie, who believed that hypochondriasis was an independent discrete disease entity. However, Kenyon (1976) concluded from an extensive literature review and a controlled study of 512 psychiatric patients with hypochondriacal symptoms that hypochondriasis was always a secondary part of another syndrome, usually a depressive illness. In addition, Bianchi (1973) carried out a principal-components analysis of 235 psychiatric patients and identified one component that corresponded to a distinct group of female patients who had a syndrome of multiple somatic complaints, unnecessary surgery, and psychogenic pain associated with a low pain threshold. Bianchi concluded that these women had Briquet's syndrome or somatization disorder. He also concluded that other aspects of hypochondriasis were ancillary symptoms of other primary psychiatric disorders. For example, those scoring high on his disease-conviction component usually had endogenous depressions, and those with disease phobias usually had anxiety neuroses.

Recent work in the Stockholm adoption study has led to identification of two discrete somatoform disorders that differ in the frequency and diversity of their somatic complaints (Cloninger et al., 1984). Type 1 has low diversity of complaints, but a high frequency of psychiatric, abdominal, and back complaints. This is similar to the belief that was prevalent until the late nineteenth century that hypochondriasis was associated specifically with complaints involving the hypochondriac region of the abdomen (that is, below the costal cartilages), rather than with nonspecific morbid disease preoccupation. Type 2 has high diversity of complaints, despite lower overall frequency, similar to the diversity characteristic of somatization disorder. Discriminant functions have been derived showing that each patient group falls in discrete components separated by antimodes; that is, there are natural boundaries distinguishing the syndromes. Also, different genetic and environmental factors have been shown to be important in these disorders, further justifying a multicategory system. However, more detailed clinical studies are needed to develop explicit psychiatric criteria.

It is important to note that the Swedish studies were done in a general population sample rather than in psychiatric patients. It may well be that few patients with hypochondriacal neurosis ever see psychiatrists. Studies with general or primary-care populations are needed. Until then, there is heuristic value in retaining the category of hypochondriasis to stimulate further research.

ATYPICAL SOMATOFORM DISORDERS

This is a residual category, but dysmorphophobia is said to be a common example. Caution in diagnosing patients with dysmorphophobia must be

Table 15.9. *DSM-III diagnostic criteria for hypochondriasis*

A. The predominant disturbance is an unrealistic interpretation of physical signs or sensations as abnormal, leading to preoccupation with the fear or belief of having a serious disease.
B. Thorough physical evaluation does not support the diagnosis of any physical disorder that can account for the physical signs or sensations or for the individual's unrealistic interpretation of them.
C. The unrealistic fear or belief of having a disease persists despite medical reassurance and causes impairment in social or occupational functioning.
D. Not due to any other mental disorder such as schizophrenia, affective disorder, or somatization disorder.

---

exercised. Many such patients are delusional (Bishop, 1980) and should not be categorized as having somatoform disorders.

SUMMARY AND CONCLUSIONS

In its general features, *DSM-III* represents a major advance over *DSM-II* and *ICD-9* in its system for classifying patients whose chief complaints suggest physical disorders. The separation of somatoform disorders from other groups of disorders introduces much needed conceptual clarity as well as descriptive distinctions that are justified by differences in symptom patterns, courses of illness, responses to treatment, and patterns of familial aggregation. The recent demonstration that genetic factors are important in the development of some somatoform disorders (Cloninger et al., 1984) means that the distinction concerning whether or not pathophysiological mechanisms are known will ultimately be self-defeating for psychiatry. The true issue is not whether or not there is an objective pathophysiological mechanism but whether assessment and treatment are better carried out by psychiatrists and related professional groups or by surgeons, internists, and other physician groups. This is not an urgent problem, but eventually it will need revision.

Despite advances in general features, much more work is needed to validate the criteria for each of the individual somatoform disorders. In particular, the criteria for conversion disorder and psychogenic pain disorder need immediate revision, because the evidence for psychological conflict requires etiological inferences that are neither reliable nor useful in distinguishing physical and psychiatric disorders. Further clinical studies are needed among patients with *DSM-III* somatization disorder who do not fulfill Guze's original criteria for Briquet's syndrome because of possible differences in risks of medical illness, suicide, and treatment responses. This information will become available soon from ongoing research at Washington University in St. Louis. Finally, the category of hypochondriasis has no empirical data to support its distinctness from other syndromes, but probably should be retained for its descriptive and heuristic value.

REFERENCES

Barsky AJ, Klerman GL: Overview: hypochondriasis, bodily complaints, and somatic styles. Am J Psychiatry 140:273–283, 1983

Bianchi GN: Patterns of hypochondriasis: a principal components analysis. Br J Psychiatry 122:541–548, 1973

Bishop ER Jr: Monosymptomatic hypochondriasis. Psychosomatics 21:731–747, 1980

Bishop ER Jr, Torch EM: Dividing "hysteria": a preliminary investigation of conversion disorder and psychologia. J Nerv Ment Dis 167:348–356, 1979

Blumer D, Heilbronn M: Chronic pain as a variant of depressive disease: the pain-prone disorder. J Nerv Ment Dis 170:381–406, 1982

Cloninger CR, Guze SB: Psychiatric illness and female criminality: the role of sociopathy and hysteria in the antisocial woman. Am J Psychiatry 127:303–311, 1970

Cloninger CR, Martin RL, Guze SB, et al: A blind follow-up and family study of anxiety neurosis, in Anxiety: New Research and Changing Concepts. Edited by Klein DF, Rabkin J. New York, Raven Press, 1981, pp 137–150

Cloninger CR, Reich T, Guze SB: The multifactorial model of disease transmission, III: familial relationship between sociopathy and hysteria (Briquet's syndrome). Br J Psychiatry 127:23–32, 1975

Cloninger CR, Sigvardsson S, von Knorring A-L, et al: An adoption study of somatoform disorders, II: identification of two discrete somatoform disorders. Arch Gen Psychiatry 41:863–871, 1984

Cohen LM: A current perspective of pseudocyesis. Am J Psychiatry 139:1140–1144, 1982

Flor-Henry P, Fromm-Auch D, Tapper M, et al: A neuropsychological syndrome of the stable syndrome of hysteria. Biol Psychiatry 16:601–626, 1981

Gatfield PD, Guze SB: Prognosis and differential diagnosis of conversion reactions (a follow-up study). Dis Nerv Syst 23:1–8, 1962

Gillespie RD: Hypochondria: its definition, nosology, and psychopathology. Guys Hosp Rep 78:408–460, 1928

Guze SB: The diagnosis of hysteria: what are we trying to do? Am J Psychiatry 123:491–498, 1967

Guze SB, Woodruff RA, Clayton PJ: Hysteria and antisocial personality: further evidence of an association. Am J Psychiatry 127:957–960, 1971a

A study of conversion symptoms in psychiatric outpatients. Am J Psychiatry 128:643–646, 1971b

Sex, age, and the diagnosis of hysteria (Briquet's syndrome). Am J Psychiatry 129:745–748, 1972

Hendler N, Uematesu S, Long D: Thermographic validation of physical complaints in "psychogenic pain" patients. Psychosomatics 23:283–287, 1982

Hyler SE, Spitzer RL: Hysteria split asunder. Am J Psychiatry 135:1500–1504, 1978

Kenyon FE: Hypochondriacal states. Br J Psychiatry 129:1–14, 1976

Lader M, Sartorius N: Anxiety in patients with hysterical conversion symptoms. J Neurol Neurosurg Psychiatry 31:490–495, 1968

Lazare A: Current concepts in psychiatry: conversion symptoms. N Engl J Med 305:745–748, 1981

Linn L, Spitzer RL: DSM-III: implications for liaison psychiatry and psychosomatic medicine. JAMA 247:3207–3209, 1982

Martin RL, Cloninger CR, Guze SB: The evaluation of diagnostic concordance in follow-up studies, II: a blind follow-up of female criminals. J Psychiatr Res 15:107–125, 1979

Mears R, Horvath T: Acute and chronic hysteria. Br J Psychiatry 121:653–657, 1972

Perley M, Guze SB: Hysteria – the stability and usefulness of clinical criteria. N Engl J Med 266:421–426, 1962

Purtell J, Robins E, Cohen M: Observations on clinical aspects of hysteria. JAMA 146:902–909, 1951

Raskin M, Talbott JA, Meyerson AT: Diagnosis of conversion reactions: predictive value of psychiatric criteria. JAMA 197:102–106, 1966

Robins LN, Helzer JE, Croughan J, et al: National Institute of Mental Health Diagnostic Interview Schedule: its history, characteristics, and validity. Arch Gen Psychiatry 38:381–389, 1981

Rosenthal RH, Webb WL, Wruble LD: Diagnosis and management of persistent psychogenic vomiting. Psychosomatics 21:722–730, 1980

Slater E: Diagnosis of hysteria. Br Med J 1:1395–1399, 1965

Watson CG, Buranen C: The frequency and identification of false positive conversion reactions. J Nerv Ment Dis 167:243–247, 1979

Williams JBW, Spitzer RL: Idiopathic pain disorder: a critique to pain-prone disorder and a proposal for a revision of the DSM-III category psychogenic pain disorder. J Nerv Ment Dis 170:415–419, 1982

Woerner PI, Guze SB: A family and marital study of hysteria. Br J Psychiatry 114:161–168, 1975

Woodruff RA: Hysteria, an evaluation of objective diagnostic criteria by the study of women with chronic medical illnesses. Br J Psychiatry 114:1115–1119, 1967

Woodruff RA, Robins LN, Taibleson M, et al: A computer assisted derivation of a screening interview for hysteria. Arch Gen Psychiatry 29:450–454, 1973

Wruble LD, Rosenthal RH, Webb WL: Psychogenic vomiting: a review. Am J Gastroenterol 77:318–321, 1982

16   *Overview*

GERALD L. KLERMAN

The decision to discontinue a category for neurotic disorders and disaggregate them into affective, anxiety, dissociative, and somatoform disorders was one of the most controversial decisions made by the creators of the *DSM-III*. While *DSM-III* was being formulated, during 1978–9, considerable discussion, often polemic, was exchanged about the intent and consequences of eliminating the grouping of neurotic disorders.

> First, it represented a significant discontinuity with the past, going against many of the traditions of *DSM-I* and *DSM-II*.
>
> Second, it put the American classification at variance with the World Health Organization, International Classification of Diseases (WHO–ICD), which has the distinction between psychotic and neurotic disorders as one of its basic classification principles.
>
> Third, and perhaps most important, by eliminating the grouping of neurotic disorders, the *DSM-III* rejected the widely held presumption that these disorders have a common psychogenesis, in defenses against anxiety, and possibly etiology, in psychological developments.

The *DSM-II* had stipulated that psychoneurotic conditions are based on defenses against underlying anxiety. In most of European psychiatry, psychoneuroses are considered to be based on personality and/or psychosocial factors, in contrast to the psychoses, which are believed to be based on constitutional, usually genetic, causes.

The *DSM-III* formulators concluded that the evidence in favor of this presumed etiology was inconclusive and that more scientific credibility would be gained by adopting an "atheoretical" approach, and therefore they grouped disorders together on the basis of dominant psychopathology rather than presumptive causes or pathogenesis.

Since 1980, much of this controversy has subsided. Within the United States, the proponents of the concept of neuroses, mainly psychoanalytically and psychodynamically oriented psychiatrists, have accepted the *DSM-III*. Whereas the focus of psychodynamic and psychoanalytic interest and psychotherapeutic treatments in previous decades was on "symptom neuroses," such as neurotic

260

depression, anxiety states, hysteria and obsessive–compulsive neurosis, the current focus has shifted to personality disorders, especially the narcissistic and borderline personality disorders.

OBSESSIVE-COMPULSIVE DISORDER

There is general satisfaction with the concept of obsessive–compulsive disorders and with the *DSM-III* criteria. Intensive research is now under way to evaluate new forms of behavior therapy and drug treatment with tricyclic antidepressants, particularly clomipramine and MAO inhibitors (Jenike, 1983). In addition, we are beginning to see family studies of obsessive–compulsive disorders and also studies of neurotransmitter metabolism. These studies are increasingly using the *DSM-III* criteria. In epidemiologic studies, the *DSM-III* criteria are embodied in the Diagnostic Interview Scale, and the preliminary reports from the Epidemiologic Catchment Area study indicate a six-month incidence of about 1% in the three communities reported on in New Haven, St. Louis, and Baltimore.

SOMATOFORM DISORDERS

The status of somatoform disorders remains a subject of considerable discussion. There is still uncertainty regarding the relationship of "real" physical disorder to conversion disorders. Similar problems arise with regard to hypochondriasis. Because the hypochondriacal attitudinal triad (disease-conviction, disease-fear, and help-seeking behavior) often occurs in patients with diagnosed physical illnesses (in which case the hypochondriasis may be considered secondary and is diagnosed by evaluation by clinicians), the patient's attitudinal responses may be out of proportion to the diagnosed organ abnormality and the internist's expectation of the level of distress and disability.

Within the somatoform disorders, somatization disorder has received considerable attention, particularly because of the extensive work by the St. Louis group on the concept of Briquet's syndrome, as an alternative to the classic concept of hysteria. There is a high degree of overlap between the St. Louis concept of Briquet's syndrome and *DSM-III* somatization disorder. However, about 20% of patients who meet the criteria for *DSM-III* somatization disorder do not meet the St. Louis criteria for Briquet's syndrome. Further research is needed on the prognostic significance of various symptom sets, particularly the ability to distinguish physical from psychologic disorders. Some studies indicate that a high proportion of patients diagnosed with conversion disorder will have developed medically diagnosed physical disorders on follow-up. It would be highly desirable to have criteria with better predictive validity to differentiate conversion disorder from symptoms that are the prodrome of neurologic and medical conditions. The current concept of psychogenic pain disorder was criticized because of the presumption of cause, and the suggestion was made to rename the disorder idiopathic pain disorder.

ANXIETY DISORDERS

The most far-reaching psychopathologic debates have followed Klein's proposal to separate panic states and agoraphobia from other anxiety disorders and group them together. This proposal, parts of which are embodied in the *DSM-III* classification (American Psychiatric Association, 1980) of anxiety disorders, represents a departure from the consensus concerning anxiety and anxiety disorders that characterized the field following the end of World War I. That consensus viewed anxiety, phobias, and anxiety states on a continuum, with normal anxiety and fear at one end, and anxiety symptoms, anxiety neurosis, and phobic states at the other end. In that model, the clinical states were aligned on a continuum, and the gradations between them were seen as gradations of intensity of distress and degree of social impairment.

In the mid-1970s, this continuum model was challenged by a number of researchers, particularly Klein (1980), who emphasized the crucial role of the panic attack in the pathogenesis of agoraphobia. Additional evidence derived from the differential responses of anxiety states to pharmacologic agents. A new model emphasizing discontinuity emerged, with panic disorders and agoraphobia related to each other, but separate from normal fear, anxiety, and anxiety neurosis.

This new discontinuity model was partially incorporated in the *DSM-III* classification of anxiety disorders, a decision that has led to considerable controversy within the United States and between American investigators and those in Europe, particularly those who follow *ICD-9*. The divergence between American and European traditions is described in detail by Jablensky (1985). These differences involve more than terminology. They represent a basic difference in scientific thinking about anxiety.

Jablensky (1985) and Roth (1984) have pointed out that attention to the clinical states that today are called anxiety disorders did not emerge until the second half of the nineteenth century. Psychiatry as a medical specialty began in the late eighteenth century with the appointment of the medical authority in the asylums and mental hospitals. Given that historical context, it is understandable that the initial efforts in scientific psychopathology would focus on "insanity" and "lunacy" conditions, which now are regarded as "psychotic." In the last decades of the nineteenth century, physicians in major cities in Western Europe and North America began to observe a group of noninstitutionalized patients who, though not psychotic, suffered from distressing bodily symptoms and irrational thoughts and behaviors. Prominent symptoms among these patients were fearfulness, distress, bodily complaints, sweating, and palpitations.

Various terms were applied to these patients – neurasthenia, hypochondriasis, and hysteria. Clinical descriptions by Westphal (1871) were incorporated by Kraepelin in his concept of "Schenkenneurosie." Beard (1880), in the United States, had described "neurasthenia" as the "American disease of civilization," because he speculated that the increased frequency of this disorder was due to the pace of civilized living, particularly in urbanized and industrialized countries. The term "anxiety" did not come into general intellectual and clinical use until the latter part of the nineteenth century, and its adoption was heavily influenced by the philosophical ideas of Kierkegaard.

Freud's psychoanalytic theories were widely applied to clinical psychoneurosis. In 1894, he proposed separating anxiety neurosis from neurasthenia. A number of psychoanalysts have reconstructed Freud's thinking about the clinical phenomenology of the anxiety state (Michels, Frances, and Shear, 1985). They note that Freud's early papers contain excellent clinical descriptions of phenomena that would now be considered panic attacks. He also described the role of panic in initiating phobic behavior. Freud was the Kraepelin of the psychoneuroses, having described disorders such as obsessive–compulsive states and phobia, and having related these clinical states to normal fear and anxiety. In an attempt to develop a comprehensive theory, in 1923 Freud formulated his signal theory of anxiety – whereby he postulated that anxiety arose in the ego and served as a signal to mobilize the defenses against internal drives (in the psychoneuroses) and against external threats (in normal fear). Based on these clinical writings, as well as the theoretical implications of the work of Pavlov and Cannon, the consensus emerged as a continuity model of anxiety and anxiety disorders. This continuity model was held by biologists, psychoanalysts, and behaviorists. All agreed with the essence of the model, though they emphasized different etiologies.

In 1960, a number of factors led to questions about the continuity model.

1. The terms used failed to convey precise meaning. David Sheehan has identified 37 different nosologic terms that overlap with anxiety (Sheehan and Sheehan, 1982).

2. Two classes of drugs – the MAO inhibitors and the tricyclics, which by the conventional logic of psychopharmacology are called "antidepressants" – were shown to be effective for anxiety disorders. On phenomenologic grounds, these disorders were different from depression.

3. Certain forms of anxiety disorders, particularly agoraphobia, did not respond to neuroleptics or benzodiazepines, the prototypic antianxiety drugs. This was paradoxical. Why should the most intensive anxiety states not respond to even powerful neuroleptic drugs?

In response to these observations, a new diagnostic model emerged in the early 1970s. This model proposed bringing panic disorder and agoraphobia together and separating this complex of conditions from the other anxiety states. This model emphasized the discontinuity of panic and agoraphobia from other anxiety states.

A central feature of this model was that a panic attack was a unique psychic experience, not a more intense form of normal fear and anxiety. A panic attack occurs as the sudden onset of intense fear and anxiety, with a sense of dread and foreboding and fear of being trapped. These cognitive elements were combined with awareness of physiologic change, particularly autonomic arousal manifested by sweating, palpitations, a feeling of lightheadedness, and so on.

The initial panic attack and the onset of the episode occur spontaneously without apparent environmental precipitant. The repeated episodes of spontaneous panic attacks postulated to drive phobia avoidance behavior are not based on a classic Pavlovian conditioning model. In contrast, the panic attack is regarded as the initiator of the avoidant behavior.

Clinical, therapeutic (Klein, 1980), genetic-familial (Noyes et al., 1978; Crowe et al., 1980, 1983; Leckman, et al., 1983; Surman et al., in press), and pathophysiologic (Fink, Taylor, and Volavka, 1969; Ackerman and Sachar, 1974; Lapierre, Knott, Gray, 1984) evidence supports the new diagnostic model. There is a psychopathologic cluster composed of panic attacks, agoraphobia, and extensive phobic avoidance. This cluster constitutes a separate psychopathologic entity, different from other forms of phobia, generalized anxiety, and obsessive–compulsive disorders.

All forms of anxiety disorders share some similarities, particularly the symptoms of anxiety, dread, and foreboding. The complex of panic disorder, agoraphobia, and phobic disorder is different from other disorders; the unique feature is the panic attack. The panic attack not only is the sine qua non for diagnosis but also is considered the driving force in the pathogenesis of the phobic and avoidant behavior. Phobic and avoidant behavior, anticipatory anxiety, and help-seeking behavior are important features of the syndrome, but are seen as responses of the individual to the aversive experience of the panic attack.

CONCLUSIONS

Revisions of the classic concept of psychoneuroses, as embodied in the *DSM-III,* have stimulated considerable controversy. Even more important is empirical research, which in general has supported the validity and utility of the decision to disaggregate psychoneuroses into anxiety disorders, dissociative disorders, and somatoform disorders. Psychoneurotic depression has been aggregated with other affective disorders, and the *DSM-III* is the first official nomenclature to have a separate category for affective disorders. The field is now in a period of intense empirical research, and within the next decade it is likely that many of the questions about the validity of certain diagnostic classes and the specificity of symptom sets will be resolved.

REFERENCES

Ackerman S, Sachar E: The lactate theory of anxiety: a review and re-evaluation. Psychosom Med, 36:69–81, 1974

American Psychiatric Association: Diagnostic and Statistical Manual of Mental Disorders, third edition. Washington, DC, APA, 1980

Beard G: A Practical Treatise on Nervous Exhaustion (Neurasthenia). New York, William Wood, 1880

Crowe RR, Noyes R, Pauls DL, et al: A family study of panic disorder. Arch Gen Psychiatry 40:1065–1069, 1983

Crowe RR, Pauls DL, Slymen DJ, et al: A family study of anxiety neurosis. Arch Gen Psychiatry 37:77–79, 1980

Fink M, Taylor M, Volavka J: Anxiety precipitated by lactate. N Engl J Med 281:1429, 1969

Jablensky A: Approaches to the definition and classification of anxiety and related disorders in European psychiatry, in Anxiety and the Anxiety Disorders. Edited by Tuma AH, Maser J. Hillsdale, NJ, Lawrence Erlbaum Associates, 1985

Jenike MA: Obsessive-compulsive disorder. Compr Psychiatry 24:99–115, 1983

Klein DF: Anxiety reconceptualized. Compr Psychiatry 21:411–427, 1980

Lapierre YD, Knott VJ, Gray R: Psychophysiological correlates of sodium lactate. Psychopharmacol Bull 20:50–57, 1984

Leckman JF, Weissman MM, Merikangas KR, et al: Panic disorder and major depression: increased risk of depression, alcoholism, panic, and phobic disorders in families of depressed probands with panic disorder. Arch Gen Psychiatry 40:1055–1060, 1983

Michels R, Frances A, Shear MK: Psychodynamic models of anxiety, in Anxiety and the Anxiety Disorders. Edited by Tuma AH, Maser J. Hillsdale, NJ, Lawrence Erlbaum Associates, 1985

Noyes R Jr, Clancy J, Crowe R, et al: The familial prevalence of anxiety neurosis. Arch Gen Psychiatry 35:1057–1059, 1978

Roth M: Agoraphobia, panic disorder and generalized anxiety disorder: some implications of recent advances. Psychiatr Dev 2:31–52, 1984

Sheehan DV, Sheehan KH: The classification of anxiety and hysterical states, part I: historical review and empirical delineation. J Clin Psychopharmacol 2:235–243, 1982

Surman OS, Sheehan DV, Fuller TC, et al: Panic disorder in HLA identical sibling pairs. (in press)

Westphal C: Die agoraphobie; eine neuropathische erscheinung. Arch Psychiatr Nervenkr 3:138–161, 1871

PART V

The personality disorders

Part V is devoted to the personality disorders found on axis II of the *Diagnostic and Statistical Manual of Mental Disorders,* third edition. Ten of the 11 personality disorders are reviewed. Only antisocial personality disorder is not covered in Part V.

Allen Frances and Thomas Widiger review the research evidence and clinical opinion regarding the borderline, avoidant, dependent, and passive-aggressive personality disorders. They indicate areas for future research, changes in terminology, and ideas regarding the diagnostic criteria, and they offer general suggestions that apply to all the axis II diagnoses. Arnold Cooper describes the current psychiatric literature and opinion regarding histrionic, narcissistic, and compulsive personality disorders, and Larry Siever and Kenneth Kendler discuss the paranoid, schizoid, and schizotypal personality disorders, personality disorders that share common criteria reflecting social distance and emotional contriction.

Normund Wong

17   *A critical review of four DSM-III*
personality disorders
Borderline, avoidant, dependent, and passive-aggressive

ALLEN FRANCES and THOMAS A. WIDIGER

We apply a double standard in our review of these four *DSM-III* personality disorders. We begin with a fairly extensive discussion of borderline personality disorder (BPD) and then provide only brief comments on the avoidant, dependent, and passive-aggressive personality disorders. This apportionment of attention reflects the widespread interest among clinicians and researchers in BPD and the fact that among the other *DSM-III* personality disorders only the schizotypal and antisocial have received any substantial systematic investigation. Our critique of the evidence supporting BPD is much more demanding than that applied to the other personality disorders. This takes into account the fact that ambitious claims have been made for BPD as a "validated" separate diagnostic entity, and much more evidence is available for critical review. We do not mean to imply that BPD is any less validated than other personality disorders, but only to introduce caution into the interpretation of the limited data that are available.

How may we understand the recent fascination engendered by BPD and the relative lack of interest in the other personality disorders? Several, perhaps interacting, factors may be responsible:

1. BPD probably has the highest incidence of the personality diagnoses, both among inpatients and among outpatients.
2. BPD patients suffer and cause suffering, usually in an open and flamboyant manner.
3. BPD has possibly important interactions or overlaps with "bordering" axis I conditions like affective disorder, substance abuse, attention deficit, episodic dyscontrol, brief reactive psychosis, and schizophrenia.
4. BPD is of interest because of psychoanalytic conceptions that it represents the external manifestations of an intrapsychic structure that, developmentally and functionally, is midway between proposed psychotic and neurotic structures.
5. BPD's vague boundaries and widely distributed, but relatively nonspecific, definitional features make it a wastebasket category in diagnostic situations that are otherwise fuzzy and uncertain (Widiger, 1982a).

For each of the four disorders under consideration, we describe the incidence and reliability, review critically the available research evidence and clinical opinion, and then make suggestions for future research, terminology, and additions to or alterations in the *DSM-III* diagnostic criteria. The chapter closes with a series of suggestions that apply to axis II in general.

BORDERLINE PERSONALITY DISORDER

Because so much has been written about borderline conditions, we cannot hope to provide an exhaustive review. We concentrate attention on those systematic studies that have specifically examined BPD patients as defined in *DSM-III*. We are most interested in studies that contribute to knowledge about the convergent and discriminant validity of the BPD criteria set as manifest in clinical description, family, course and test data, and treatment response. Our conclusion is that the BPD category is a useful inclusion in *DSM-III*, but that exaggerated claims have been made on the basis of preliminary findings subject to alternative interpretations.

Prevalence and reliability

Studies reporting the prevalences of individual personality disorders have used so many different methods and samples that the absolute percentages they offer do not seem very meaningful. Therefore, in most instances, we report the rank order of prevalence for each personality disorder under consideration in comparison with the other 10 listed in the *DSM-III* section on personality disorders.

BPD has been ranked as the most common of the personality disorders in most studies (Koenigsberg, 1982; Kass et al., 1983; Frances et al., 1984; Stangl et al., 1985) or close to the top (Mellsop et al., 1982). When consecutive inpatients have been tested with the Diagnostic Interview for Borderlines (DIB), between 15% and 20% (Kroll et al., 1982) have scored in the borderline range in both the United States and the United Kingdom (but note that the DIB is more inclusive than *DSM-III*). Patients meeting the criteria for BPD tend to be female, with a 2:1 to 9:1 ratio, depending on the sample. The reliability of the *DSM-III* BPD criteria has been reported as .72 (Frances et al., 1984), .81 (Stangl et al., 1985), and .29 (Mellsop et al., 1982).

Descriptive validity

Although this has not yet been tested extensively for the *DSM-III* criteria set, numerous recent studies have investigated the ability of other instruments to discriminate BPD patients on descriptive grounds from comparison groups that have included patients with schizophrenic, affective, and other personality disorders. By far the best-studied instrument is the DIB, developed by Gunderson and Kolb (1978; Kolb and Gunderson, 1980). It has performed well in discriminating BPD patients in both inpatient and outpatient samples and with various comparison groups in a half dozen different centers (e.g., Soloff,

1981a,b). The DIB selects for a population of patients that probably includes both the schizotypal and BPD categories as these are defined in *DSM-III*.

Other investigator-rated or patient- or family-rated instruments tapping similar items have been developed and studied by groups under the direction of Perry and Klerman (1980), Sheehy, Goldsmith, and Charles (1980), Pfohl (Stangl et al., 1985), Hyler (Hurt et al., 1984), and Kernberg and associates (1981). Because different efforts at instrument development have resulted in similar item sets, and because the mean scores on many of these items have been significantly higher in BPD than in comparison groups, some of the more optimistic investigators have concluded that BPD has been proved to have discriminant validity and is best considered a separate diagnostic entity.

There are several reasons to be extremely cautious about this conclusion. The methodological limitations of current efforts at descriptive validation of BPD are serious and are discussed in some detail later. Moreover, the available results remain equivocal and subject to the opposite interpretation that BPD is anything but a distinct entity. Although BPD items do load in BPD groups, they seem to follow a continuous distribution without sharp cutoff points to delineate the disorder. Moreover, every study that has looked for overlaps between BPD and other axis I and axis II disorders has found them, and in spades (e.g., Klein, 1975; Murray, 1979; Andrulonis et al., 1981; Soloff, 1981b; Snyder et al., 1982b; Resnick and Schultz, 1983). BPD patients have strikingly high simultaneous incidences of affective disorder, of other personality disorders (especially schizotypal), and of evidence of organic dysfunction (at least for male inpatients). It is difficult to accept claims based on group-mean data that BPD has been successfully discriminated from other disorders when so many BPD patients simultaneously satisfy the criteria for these same disorders. The burden of proof would seem to be on the argument that such association is no more than coincidental.

We can report some data on the *DSM-III* criteria set that were gathered with colleagues at New York Hospital (Clarkin et al., 1983; Frances et al., 1984, in press). We found that all eight BPD items were significantly more likely to be present in BPD outpatients than in comparison patients meeting the criteria for other personality disorders. With the exception of intolerance of being alone, all BPD items had substantial incidences in the BPD group (67%–89%), with κ values varying from .48 to .70. Several methods of measuring conditional probability (positive predictive power, sensitivity, and specificity) demonstrated that all eight criteria, alone or in combination, were useful and deserved retention in future BPD definitional sets (Widiger et al., 1984). Two additional contenders for possible future inclusion (depersonalization/derealization and brief psychotic episodes) were not useful discriminators in this sample. BPD patients were quite likely to meet criteria for affective disorders in spite of our efforts to recruit a primarily axis II sample, and two-thirds of BPD patients also met the criteria for another axis II diagnosis (most commonly schizotypal, dependent, histrionic, or narcissistic). *DSM-III* correlated highly with the DIB (.76) and had about equivalent overall reliability (.72 vs. .78). A DIB score of 7 provided the most efficient cutoff, but did not occur at a point of rarity, so that patients with scores of 6 and 7 were equally and arbitrarily likely to be assigned to *DSM-III* BPD and non-BPD groups.

In summary, our interpretation of the results of available studies is that groups of BPD patients differ from groups of non-BPD patients on items that substantially agree across criteria sets. However, BPD also overlaps so inextricably with so many other conditions that it is impossible to conclude that descriptive validity has been established (and probably optimistic to assume that it ever can be).

Family data

Several investigators (Stone, 1980; Andrulonis et al., 1982; Loranger, Oldham, and Talis, 1982; Siever, 1982; Pope et al., 1983; Soloff and Millward, 1983a) found high incidences of affective disorder (30%–40%) among first-degree relatives of BPD probands, but they did not find any significant increase in schizophrenia. It seems clear that the BPD criteria select for patients who are more on the affective than the schizophrenic spectrum. The consistency of this result is a bit puzzling, considering the high degree of overlap between BPD and schizotypal personality disorder, especially because the latter has a likely (if controversial) genetic relation to schizophrenia (Gunderson, Siever, and Spaulding, 1983).

The findings most consistent with BPD as a separate syndrome come from the studies of Loranger and Pope. Loranger and associates (1982) found that relatives of BPD inpatient probands were 10 times more likely to meet BPD criteria than were relatives of schizophrenic or affective probands, although the families of BPD patients also loaded for affective disorder. Similarly, Pope and associates (1983) found increased incidences of personality disorder among relatives of BPD probands and increased affective disorder among relatives of patients who met the criteria for both BPD and affective disorder. More work is necessary, particularly to determine the degree to which BPD breeds true and the genetic pattern for patients who meet the criteria for both BPD and schizotypal personality disorder.

Family data have also been used to test psychosocial hypotheses that BPD patients have been either overinvolved with or neglected by their families (or both). These studies are retrospective and have inherent methodological problems. They cannot provide conclusive support for a familial cause for the BPD syndrome, because it is just as likely that the family's behavior has been in response to having to raise a difficult child as it has been a cause of the difficulty. Moreover, a retrospective report is subject to all sorts of distortions, especially under the sampling conditions used in the available studies. Nonetheless, it is of some interest that the early empirical findings on DIB-defined borderlines (Gunderson, Kerr, and Englund, 1980; Frank and Paris, 1981; Gunderson and Englund, 1981) support the emotion-deprivation hypothesis and provide no support for the family-enmeshment hypothesis.

Test data

Two types of test data – biological and psychological – might provide support for the construct validity of the BPD diagnosis and/or evidence of its overlap with specific other syndromes. It must be remembered that psychological tests vary in the degrees to which they are sufficiently different from standard clinical assessments to have power as independent validators.

Several laboratories (Akiskal et al., 1980; Andrulonis et al., 1981; Carroll et al., 1981; Soloff, George, and Nathen, 1982) are attempting to find biological markers for BPD, and some early findings are available. Carroll's group found an unusually high level (62%) of DST nonsuppression in BPD patients and suggested that BPD may be linked biologically to affective disorder even if the overt clinical manifestations of the two disorders sometimes differ. Unfortunately, the specificity of the DST has recently been questioned by many investigators, and another interpretation of Carroll's findings might be that they add to the mounting evidence that DST results are nonspecifically abnormal in patients with a wide variety of psychiatric conditions. Moreover, two other studies (Kroll, Sines, and Martin, 1981; Soloff et al., 1982) found positive DST results in fewer than 20% of BPD patients even though many of those patients met the criteria for concurrent affective disorder.

Akiskal's group reported REM latencies in a small number of BPD patients that were equivalent to the shortened latencies in depressed patients and significantly different from the normal latencies that occurred in control patients with diagnoses of other personality disorders. Andrulonis is studying motion sickness and EEG profiles as possible markers of subtypes of the BPD syndrome.

There have been repeated suggestions in the literature that borderline patients characteristically do well on structured (WAIS-like) psychological tests, but show bizarre thinking on unstructured (Rorschach-like) tests (Carr et al., 1979; Singer and Larson, 1981). Unfortunately, the hypothesis has not clearly been tested for *DSM-III*-defined BPD patients, and it may not apply well to them. Because the *DSM-III* definition of BPD does not include milder manifestations of thought disorders (this is reserved for the schizotypal category), *DSM-III* schizotypals are more likely than borderlines to respond bizarrely on unstructured tests. Moreover, Widiger (1982b) recently criticized the methods used in the studies that supported the impression that borderlines can be discriminated by their behavior in structured and unstructured test situations.

There have been five studies contrasting the MMPI profiles for BPD patients with those for various comparison groups (Kroll et al., 1981; Snyder et al., 1982a; Gustin et al., 1983; Lloyd et al., 1983; Hurt et al., 1985). The consistent finding is that BPD patients have strikingly high F scores and high scores on a number of subscales (although the particular scales vary a bit from study to study). There are two competing interpretations of these data. Gustin and associates attempted to eliminate possible contamination from various sources of response bias and concluded that BPD patients have high scores on numerous scales because they suffer a great deal and are polysymptomatic. However, Hurt and associates found that BPD outpatients had even higher scores than BPD inpatients, suggesting that the high scores on the self-report MMPI may be more closely related to help-seeking behavior. In all MMPI studies, the mean profiles for BPD patients closely approximated the mean profiles for comparison groups, the only difference being one of severity. Thus far, the MMPI has not discriminated a characteristic BPD profile or item set. We can conclude that the data from biological and psychological tests are sparse and provide little support for or against the validity of BPD as a separate syndrome.

Course data

The *DSM-III* BPD definition is only a few years old, and obviously there has not been sufficient time to do long-term prospective course studies. Several bits of evidence are available, however. Pope and associates (1983) performed a follow-up study (four to seven years) of patients who received *DSM-III* BPD diagnoses on chart review. None of the patients develped schizophrenia, but many developed or continued to experience affective disorder. The BPD personality diagnosis remained fairly stable over time, as did the patients' other additional personality-disorder diagnoses (note that histrionic personality disorder was a particularly frequent overlap in this sample). The outcome for BPD patients was much worse overall than that for affective-disorder patients and approached that for schizophrenics, except on occupational function. This confirms earlier findings of Werble (1970) and Gunderson, Carpenter, and Strauss (1975) that BPD patients (defined by other criteria sets) experienced sustained serious morbidity. Akiskal (1981) also found that BPD patients frequently developed affective disorders during follow-up, but did not show vulnerability to schizophrenia.

Review of the developmental histories of BPD patients is another way of studying the course of the disorder. Soloff and Millward (1983b) tested three hypotheses about the early developmental histories of BPD patients (defined by DIB, not *DSM-III*, criteria). They could not confirm Andrulonis's finding of an increased incidence of neurodevelopmental deficits, but they did find support for the hypothesis of early family separation and family conflict. As Soloff and Millward pointed out, however, their conclusions are limited by the retrospective nature of the design and may pertain to all character disorders rather than applying specifically to BPD. Our data (Gilmore et al., in press), comparing the developmental histories of BPD outpatients and those for patients with other personality disorders, indicate an opposite result. Hyperactivity, learning problems, and irritability were the most discriminating features in the developmental histories of BPD patients.

Treatment response

There had been no systematic studies at the time this chapter was written of the responses of *DSM-III*-defined BPD patients to psychotropic drugs or psychotherapeutic interventions. Lykowski and Tsuang (1980) suggested that the *DSM-III* BPD criteria set selects such heterogeneous groups of patients that it is unlikely by itself to be a good guide for treatment. Patients likely to meet BPD criteria have been treated with various kinds of antidepressants, lithium, low doses of neuroleptics, stimulants, and antiepileptics, but in an uncontrolled fashion (Cole and Sunderland, 1982) and without conclusive results. Moreover, many other authors have counseled against the use of psychotropic drugs in BPD patients. It is likely that some medications will be effective for particular target symptoms, but that no single medication will be uniformly effective for all BPD patients. This whole question requires much additional study.

Comment

The available evidence confirms that operational criteria sets and semistructured instruments have facilitated, in their different ways, reliable diagnosis of BPD. This is a major and necessary advance. On the other hand, the usefulness and validity of the construct have not been demonstrated, notwithstanding the occasional claims to the contrary. Studies that have claimed to "validate" BPD as a distinct entity have shared a research strategy that is beset by serious methodological and conceptual limitations. Typically, groups of patients are diagnosed as having BPD by one or another systematic, or not so systematic, clinical method and then are found to display group-mean differences versus comparison groups on descriptive measures that are similar to and on the same descriptive level of abstraction as was the clinical diagnosis. Such a procedure allows some confidence in the reliability among instruments, but it must be remembered that in most instances the different assessments are drawing on the same clinical features in ways that are only slightly different. This problem is greatly compounded when, as is often the case, the different assessments are not made blind to one another and when BPD patients also often meet the criteria for other disorders. Similarly, self-report measures tapping clinical symptoms and behaviors (e.g., the PDQ, MMPI) are able to provide a measure of reliability across assessment methods, but do not by themselves validate the construct or demonstrate its meaningfulness.

The available research also has paid insufficient attention to the possible important influences on results exerted by sample selection, base rates, and choice of comparison groups. Findings may vary depending on whether the sample consists of inpatients or outpatients, how they are referred for study, the nature of the hospital's reputation and diagnostic habits, the base rates for different diagnoses and symptoms in the general hospital population, whether the comparison groups consist of patients meeting the criteria for an axis I or axis II condition (or both), and whether or not social class, sex, intelligence, and other variables are controlled. The question of comparison groups is particularly important. It may be no great trick to distinguish BPD from schizophrenia or affective disorder. It must be demonstrated that the distinction is based on something that has to do specifically with "borderlineness" and is not inherent in the fact that all personality-disorder patients are likely to differ in all sorts of ways from those meeting the criteria for schizophrenic and affective disorders. This requires that BPD patients also be compared with those meeting the criteria only for other personality disorders.

Another problem results from the fact that the available studies have established their "validation" by demonstrating group-mean differences between the BPD and comparison groups. This procedure is becoming increasingly unpopular among psychometricians because it loses information and can be misleading in its suggestion that entities are "distinct." By ignoring the distribution of individual scores, the method of reporting group means may fail to reveal what is a continuous distribution with much overlap at the artificial boundaries between categories. More individual approaches (i.e., those that report conditional probabilities) save information and provide a less distorted picture that demonstrates the inevitable presence of fuzzy boundaries around personality categories. Also in this regard, there has been insufficient attention to and reporting of the dimensional characteristics of BPD. It remains entirely consistent with the available data that BPD is a dimensionally and widely distributed marker of nonspecific instability and severity and is therefore anything but a validated, distinct entity (Frances et al., 1984, in press; Widiger, 1982a).

No convincing body of evidence is available to document that the BPD construct meaningfully and differentially predicts important aspects of course, family history, biological functioning, treatment response, or etiology. We can conclude on the available data that BPD describes a more or less descriptively recognizable group of patients, but we have no basis to conclude what the particular description means or implies. It must be recognized, in this regard, that descriptive homogeneity does not by any means guarantee homogeneity in etiology, course, treatment response, and so on (e.g., fever and headache symptoms may result from influenza or meningitis or brain tumor). There are good reasons to suppose that the BPD rubric is markedly heterogeneous, because it can be reached in so many different ways (i.e., 93 combinations of five or more of eight criteria) and because it overlaps with affective, schizotypal, organic, and other personality disorders (Widiger and Kelso, 1983). Claims that descriptive validation establishes BPD as a separate diagnostic entity are being made just prior to what we predict will be its gradual dismemberment into underlying component parts and/or its conversion into a dimension.

This is not to say that it was a mistake to include BPD into *DSM-III* (Spitzer and Endicott, 1979; Spitzer, Endicott, and Gibbon, 1979). The research supporting BPD, weak as it may be, is far more extensive than that for any other personality disorder. Moreover, the *DSM-III* description of the BPD patient rings true clinically and is a frequent and troubling patient presentation in all sorts of settings. The only problem with the existing literature is its tendency to jump to the conclusion that BPD is a discrete entity. Personality disorders inherently have fuzzy boundaries, and it is unwise to expect any of them (and perhaps BPD especially) to ever attain the status of discrete entity. Nonetheless, a category (or dimension) for unstable behavior is necessary, and *DSM-III* has filled this niche well with its BPD definition.

Suggestions

Future research. The methodological issues we have discussed indicate possible guidelines for future research strategies. It seems unwise to assume that the current BPD category warrants singleminded efforts at "validation." The BPD category is likely to be far too heterogeneous to survive in its current form. Research investigations should devote attention to reducing it to its several more precise component categories or to establishing its value as a dimension measuring instability and/or severity. It also seems premature to begin any vigorous exploration of the biology of BPD, both because the category remains heterogeneous and because the available biological measures and challenge tests have failed to be consistent or useful even when applied to more precisely defined conditions (e.g., affective disorders) in which there is more theoretical reason to suspect that they would be useful markers. It would also seem that we have suddenly acquired an excess of riches in the development of instruments designed to collect data for a BPD diagnosis. Different semistructured instruments have been developed by Gunderson, Baron, Perry, Pfohl, and Sheehy, all of which cover more or less the same ground, each in a somewhat different way. The instruments developed by Baron and Pfohl are specifically geared for the *DSM-III* criteria set. The DIB, developed by Gunderson and Kolb, draws a more heterogeneous sample that also includes schizotypals. A self-report instrument has also been developed by Hyler and colleagues that casts a wider net than the *DSM-III* interview (Hurt et al., 1984). It may be wise at this point to select a standard instrument for use in most studies, lest we construct an unnecessary babel of very similar tongues.

Terminology. As a member of the Personality Disorders Advisory Committe, I (A.F.) had objected to the retention in *DSM-III* of the term "borderline" because it lacked descriptive clarity and might convey the misleading connotation that the *DSM-III*-defined category was equivalent to psychoanalytic constructs. I was overruled at the time and in retrospect am pleased that an alternative term (my preference was unstable personality disorder) did not receive requisite support. We now believe that the great advantage of retaining the term BPD is that it is suitably vague and tentative and can be replaced by other terms as more data are collected. The only unfortunate aspect of the term is that, in some circles, it has become reified and is treated as an explanatory concept rather than as a vagabond and transitory boundary label.

Criteria. The evidence is clear that it was useful to provide separate BPD and schizotypal criteria sets. Although the eight items in the BPD set vary considerably in their frequency, reliability, sensitivity, specificity, and positive predictive power (Frances et al., 1984, in press), they have all performed well enough singly and in combination to warrant retention. Two additional contenders (depersonalization/derealization and brief psychotic episodes) that were expected to provide useful discrimination were not particularly helpful in our outpatient sample and deserve continued exclusion as essential criteria.

There are several small points regarding the wording of criteria that warrant attention and are easily correctable. Physically self-damaging acts are scored twice (in criterion 1 as an example of impulsivity and again on their own as criterion 6). Such overlap within a criteria set is a psychometric error that can be corrected by omitting the reference in criterion 1. The examples given for identity disturbance (e.g., "I feel like I am my sister when I'm good") are remarkably inane, and the wording is insufficiently suggestive of the enduring and unusual degree of identity disturbance (not just flightiness) that should be required. An alternative wording might read: marked and continuous identity disturbance manifested by prolonged depersonalization or derealization, feelings of personal fragmentation, frequent changes in feelings about gender identity, and inability to commit oneself to long-term goals.

AVOIDANT, DEPENDENT, AND PASSIVE-AGGRESSIVE PERSONALITY DISORDERS

These three disorders form a natural grouping for discussion. There is preliminary evidence from studies investigating the properties of the interpersonal circumplex that they correlate highly with one another and occupy adjoining territories in the lower right and lower left quandrants of the circle (Widiger and Kelso, 1983). This is not the place to present the circumplex model, especially because an excellent recent review is available (Wiggins, 1982). The point to mention here is that these disorders are all characterized by low scores on one of the two axes that generate the circumplex (i.e., dominance), but vary in their scores on the other (i.e., affiliation). All three personality disorders display submissiveness, but dependents are likely to be higher on love, whereas avoidants and passive-aggressives are likely to be higher on "hostility." Frequently a patient who meets the criteria for one of these disorders will meet the criteria for one or more of the others.

The avoidant, dependent, and passive-aggressive personality disorders also share a common problem in their *DSM-III* definitions. Each has been described by a criteria set that is too circumscribed to convey the full range of behaviors properly included within the syndrome. We suggest ways in which the *DSM-III* criteria might be broadened and enriched.

These disorders form a good part of the bread and butter of outpatient practice (especially private practice). They have received little research attention because they are unlikely to be responsible for hospitalization, they cause relatively mild impairment, and they are undramatic in presentation.

Avoidant personality disorder

Prevalence. Among the *DSM-III* personality disorders, avoidant personality disorder (APD) has been ranked second (Mellsop et al., 1982), fourth (Frances et al., 1984; Stangl et al., 1985), fifth (Kass et al., 1983), and sixth (Stangler and

Printz, 1980; Koenigsberg et al., 1983; Hurt et al., 1984). Millon (1981) suggested that, on axis II, APD overlaps most with the dependent, passive-aggressive, borderline, and schizoid personality disorders.

Comments. There have been three criticisms leveled at the *DSM-III* definition of APD. It has been claimed that the clinical picture described by the APD criteria set is only rarely encountered in clinical practice (e.g., Perry, Kernberg, Gunderson), that it is indistinguishable from schizoid personality, and that its inclusion in *DSM-III* was based on an adherence to Millon's theoretical system (e.g., Kernberg, 1984). We take up each issue in turn.

It is not at all clear to us why several distinguished colleagues find themselves making the APD diagnosis rarely or never at all, whereas APD does appear with some frequency in systematic studies, as noted earlier, and seems to be a frequent diagnosis in our own outpatient departments and in our private practice. Sampling is certainly one factor. Avoidants are rarely hospitalized and probably are more commonly encountered in private practice than in clinic settings. Moreover, avoidant behaviors are undramatic, usually are only mildly to moderately incapacitating, and often are rationalized as matters of taste. Some colleagues may be inclined to subsume such behaviors with axis I disorders (especially those related to anxiety) or within other axis II disorders (especially schizoid or dependent).

The concern that the avoidant and schizoid personalities are impossible to distinguish requires more testing than it has received. Certainly in our clinical experience, the distinction has been useful even if some patients fall at the boundary between categories (Frances, 1980). The avoidant (like the schizoid) is likely to avoid new interpersonal contacts, but (unlike the schizoid) is likely to have close and enduring relationships. Both types of patients are cautious about establishing a new relationship with the therapist, but once the therapist has become familiar, the avoidant patient is able to form a strong attachment. It should occasion no great concern that the two conditions have a degree of overlap, because this is characteristic of all personality disorders.

The notion that APD is a hothouse hybrid born of Millon's theory ignores its antecedents in an extensive psychoanalytic literature on the phobic character (Fenichel, 1945; Rado, 1969; MacKinnon and Michels, 1971) and in the descriptive literature on the hyperesthetic constitutional type (Kretchmer, 1925; Schneider, 1950). Indeed, Millon did coin the term "avoidant personality disorder" and does relate the syndrome to his theoretical notions, but it is entirely possible to find the term useful without accepting Millon's speculations about its etiology.

Our own reservation is that the *DSM-III* APD definition is too restrictive and focuses its attention on only one among many causes of avoidance (i.e., interpersonal hypersensitivity) at the expense of other equally important factors.

Suggestions

RESEARCH. APD may stand in a spectrum relationship to anxiety disorders in a fashion similar to the proposed status of the personality spectrum to the affective and schizophrenic disorders. This question deserves investigation and probably can best be approached by determining the incidence of this axis II disorder in relatives of probands who meet the criteria for anxiety disorders in comparison with its incidence among relatives of probands with another disorder, say depression. Studies might also attempt to determine the degree of overlap between the avoidant and schizoid personality disorders.

TERMINOLOGY. Two possible alternatives – phobic personality disorder and inhibited personality disorder – would be about equally good, but offer no special advantages.

CRITERIA. The *DSM-III* criteria set for APD should be broadened to include additional reasons for social withdrawal beyond sensitivity to interpersonal rejection (which is the only one now listed). Other fears that cause avoidance include fear of losing control of various impulses, fear of failure or success, fear of embarrassment, fear of being hurt, fear of overstimulation, and fear of uncomfortable body sensations. The examples might emphasize how the avoidant patient strives for familiarity and sameness – for example, the same restaurant, the same table, the same entree.

Dependent personality disorder

Prevalance and reliability. The rank order of prevalence of dependent personality disorder (DPD) among personality disorders has been reported as second (Kass et al., 1983; Frances et al., 1984, in press; Stangl et al., 1985), fourth (Stangler and Printz, 1980), and fifth (Mellsop et al., 1982). High incidences of similarly defined syndromes have been reported for military personnel both in World War II (Malinow, 1981a) and more recently (Schuckit and Gunderson, 1979). Next to histrionic personality, DPD has the highest female–male ratio. Interrater reliability has been reported as .40 (Mellsop et al., 1982) and .84 (Stangl et al., 1985).

Comments. The major problem with this category arises because the two personality features it implicity combines (i.e., dependence and submissiveness) covary much more frequently in women than in men. The implications of this have been picked up by Kaplan (1983), who uses DPD as a prime illustration in an otherwise unconvincing argument that *DSM-III* is sex-biased. Kaplan makes the interesting point that the criteria included within DPD reflect a man's view of what is pathological in dependence, that is, its associated submissiveness. *DSM-III* labels dependence as pathological only when the patient allows others to assume major responsibility for major areas of life, subordinates needs, and lacks self-confidence. Kaplan points out that "DSM-III singles out for scrutiny and therefore diagnoses the ways in which women express dependency but not the ways in which men express dependency." For example, *DSM-*

III does not have criteria for men who depend totally on their wives to maintain their homes and social lives and to care for their children. It does not note that widowed men have a greater need than do widowed women to remarry and to be cared for and that being unmarried seems to predict mental illness in men but not in women. Dependence in men, she argues, is sanctioned, unnoticed, and undiagnosed.

In their different ways, men probably are every bit as dependent as women. The difference between sexes is likely to be on another dimension (i.e., dominance–submission) included in the *DSM-III* DPD criteria set. Women more often than men have tended toward compliant expressions of dependence, men toward domineering expressions. Our society and profession are more likely to label as pathological the compliant expressions.

A second criticism comes from Kernberg (1984), who objects to the separation in *DSM-III* of the dependent and passive-aggressive personality disorders. He notes that these disorders entered *DSM-I* under more or less the same mantle and that they often coexist and express two aspects of the same underlying conflict. Although this is doubtless true, it should cause no special concern that these two personality disorders correlate with one another, as this is inevitable and common in the personality-disorders section. The two descriptions seem sufficiently different to warrant separate standing.

Suggestions

RESEARCH. The degree of correlation among the traits of dependence, submissiveness, and passivity as these are manifest in women and in men should be studied further. Because these issues touch on controversial social and political questions, it may be useful to gather additional data from the public and from psychiatrists to guide decisions about what constitutes impairment and disorder in regard to dependence, submission, and dominance.

TERMINOLOGY. The major question is deciding whether the category should emphasize dependence (in which case the current term suffices) or should emphasize aspects of the dominance–submission axis, better expressed by terms like submissive or compliant or self-effacing personality disorder. Another contender – passive personality disorder – best covers yet a third related but distinguishable component of the syndrome.

CRITERIA. A series of decisions must be made. If the focus of the *DSM-III* definition is to remain on dependence, should we broaden the criteria set to include "dominant" dependent items that occur more often in men (such as dependence on others to negotiate the household and child-rearing activities of daily life, pathological dependence on secretaries, and so forth)? Kaplan's point that prevailing attitudes determine the degree to which these behaviors are seen as pathological must be addressed in deciding whether or not such unsubmissive expressions of dependence are sufficiently distressing or disabling to warrant diagnosis as disorder and inclusion in an official nomenclature. This is a question with interesting and significant political overtones.

This problem can be avoided by altering the title and contents of the criteria set to emphasize the features of pathological submissiveness and unassertiveness. Of course, the question would immediately arise whether or not there should, in fairness, also be an autocratic personality disorder within axis II. In fact, an autocratic type has been generated in the circumplex literature (although it may be hard to distinguish from the narcissistic). Such inclusion would also meet the criticism that *DSM-III* is biased in the direction of labeling as "disordered" any exaggerations of more characteristically female behaviors, while having a much higher tolerance for exaggerations of more characteristically male behaviors. At a minimum, the *DSM-III* criteria should be broadened to include additional items that tap submissiveness, unassertiveness, lack of ambition, inability to self-start, and difficulty in separating from parents and caretakers.

Passive-aggressive personality disorder

Prevalence. Passive-aggressive personality disorder (PAD) is one of the least diagnosed of the personality disorders and is more common in males. Its rank order in prevalance studies has been reported as eighth in several studies (Stangler and Printz, 1980; Kass et al., 1983; Frances et al., 1984, in press; Stangl et al., 1985).

Comment. A number of commentators of diverse orientations have noted that the criteria set defining PAD is too narrow and restrictive. Malinow (1981b) pointed out that there was considerable reluctance to include PAD as a *DSM-III* diagnosis even though it had been a charter member in previous official nomenclatures and a popular *DSM-I* and *DSM-II* diagnosis. Spitzer and the Task Force had doubted that PAD was best regarded as a full personality syndrome and instead considered it a situationally reactive defensive maneuver or part of other symptoms. For this reason, PAD was left out of the first draft of *DSM-III* and finally was included only in response to support and pressure from its adherents. Malinow suggested that the inclusion was (perhaps appropriately enough) made in passive-aggressive fashion. The grudging quality of the acceptance of PAD is evidenced by the restrictive nature of its definition in *DSM-III* and the special stipulation in its criteria set that the diagnosis not be made in the presence of another personality disorder, an encumbrance placed only on this category among all the axis II disorders.

There were two members of the Personality Disorder Advisory Committee who argued unsuccessfully for a wider PAD definition – Millon and Frances. Millon believed that the *DSM-III* PAD definition was too narrowly focused on the single trait of resisting authority and that the broader complex of related characteristics should include irritable and erratic mood, low frustration tolerance and anger threshold, discontented self-image as evidenced by feeling misunderstood and unappreciated by others, interpersonal ambivalence around dependence/independence, and unpredictable and sulking behaviors. He proposed the terms "negativistic" or "oppositional personality disorder" to replace the name passive-aggressive.

Frances was interested in establishing a masochistic personality disorder as an official category within axis II and suggested, along with Arnold Cooper, M.D. (Frances and Cooper, 1981), that this might best be done by adding masochistic traits (e.g., self-defeating, self-punishing, second-guessing, subverting own goals, seeing the worst in oneself and others and seeing life as a constant struggle, feeling imposed upon unfairly, being rigid and intolerant of praise or success) to the description of oppositional behaviors that were already included with the PAD definition in *DSM-III*.

The argument offered against the (essentially similar) suggestions made by Millon and Frances was that the descriptions we proposed contained features that the Task Force preferred to place within the axis I criteria sets for the milder (and presumably spectrum) affective disorders. It seems to us (and seemed to A.F. then) that this argument reflects a rather naive and reductionistic conception of the possible interplay between affective and personality disorders and prejudges the question (with a biological bias) without first allowing for systematic investigation. If there is an affective contribution to personality characteristics, as one of many contributions in a multivariate system, this should not disqualify that syndrome from consideration as a personality disorder, especially when the behaviors are enduring and pervasive and have additional characteristics that are not clearly affective.

A number of authors have independently commented on the close relationship between masochistic and passive-aggressive traits and have suggested that the *DSM-III* PAD description might be expanded to include masochistic items (Vaillant and Perry, 1980; Perry and Flannery, 1982; Wiggins, 1982). Wiggins (1982) has pointed out the proximate placement of passive-aggressive and masochistic traits on the interpersonal circumplex. Perry and Flannery (1982) have suggested that there are four subgroups included within the *DSM-III* PAD category, one of which is masochistic. The only systematic studies on PAD (Whitman, Torsman, and Koenig, 1954; Small, Small, and Alig, 1970) both found many traits that may be considered masochistic (ambivalence, guilt, depression, tearful rage) to be associated with the PAD syndrome. Millon traces the history of PAD in part to Kraepelin's and Blueler's descriptions of the irritable personality and in part to psychoanalytic conceptions of the masochistic personality.

Suggestions

RESEARCH. It will be interesting to investigate more systematically the proposed relationship between oppositional ("passive-aggressive") traits and self-defeating ("masochistic") traits, as well as the relationship between these behaviors and affective disorders. Passive-aggressive and masochistic traits are particular obstacles to success and compliance in all psychiatric and medical treatments and should be major subjects of study as predictors in treatment process and outcome studies. The development of therapeutic methods of changing or working within these traits is of the utmost importance in improving treatment results.

TERMINOLOGY

1. "Passive-aggressive personality disorder" emphasizes the ambivalent coexistence of dependence and oppositionalism, but it has the problems of etiological connotation and previous misuse in military settings.
2. "Oppositional personality disorder" provides continuity with the section on childhood disorders and is interpersonally descriptive, but has an excessively narrow connotation that captures only the interpersonal aspect of the syndrome.
3. "Negativistic personality disorder" is appealingly broad and clearly descriptive, and it captures both interpersonal and intrapsychic aspects of behavior, but it is a new term without tradition.
4. "Masochistic personality disorder" captures the self-defeating aspect without adequately conveying the oppositional aspect and has an etiological connotation.

Our preference is "negativistic personality disorder" (Millon's term) despite and perhaps because of its lack of tradition. This term suggests less about etiology than the terms "passive-aggressive" and "masochistic," and it better combines aspects of both oppositionalism and self-defeatingness.

CRITERIA. The requirement that no other personality disorder coexist with PAD is nonsensical and should be dropped. Criteria should be broadened beyond oppositionalism to include some combination of the negativistic and masochistic features that have already been listed.

GENERAL AXIS II SUGGESTIONS

Although the specific assignment for this conference included only the four personality disorders we have already discussed, we would like to close our remarks with several suggestions that apply to the entire axis II personality-disorders section.

1. In its current form, the *DSM-III* definitions of some disorders (e.g., compulsive, avoidant) are monothetic – that is, patients are expected to meet all of the criteria listed for the disorder – whereas other diagnoses (e.g., borderline, schizotypal) are polythetic, in that patients are required to meet only a specific number of criteria drawn from a longer list of possibilities. It would increase consistency to use one or the other method in defining all of the personality disorders, and there is a strong theoretical argument that favors the polythetic method. A number of authors have pointed out that the definitions of the various *DSM-III* personality disorders describe diagnostic prototypes that are only imprecisely approximated by actual patients in the clinical situation (Cantor et al., 1980; Horowitz et al., 1981; Clarkin et al., 1983; Widiger and Kelso, 1983). The polythetic method better conveys the probabilistic and prototypal nature of

personality diagnosis and the inherent heterogeneity of patients defined by the criteria set for any given category. It probably would also be wise from a methodological standpoint to include approximately the same number of items in the criteria set for each of the different personality disorders.

2. Dimensional methods of personality diagnosis show great promise and have achieved wide acceptance among psychologists and psychometricians. The interpersonal-circumplex method has particularly strong appeal as a possible eventual replacement for the current axis II format (Frances, 1982; Wiggins, 1982; Widiger and Kelso, 1983). Researchers studying personality disorders probably should report their results dimensionally as well as categorically. Field trials specifically designed to test dimensional methods are warranted. Moreover, psychiatrists would do well to recognize that research and theory development on personality diagnosis and assessment have been the mainstays of clinical psychology for many decades and that the sophistication of the psychological literature on personality diagnosis far exceeds that available in psychiatric journals. Any committee organized to develop alternatives in personality-disorder classification should include much greater psychologist representation (at least as consultants) than has heretofore been the case.

3. Even if *DSM-III* and *DSM-IV* continue to retain basically their current axis II format, there is no reason to assume that the diagnostic categories that were originally selected will ultimately prove to be the most enduringly valuable. Further research must investigate the degrees of correlation among items and overlap among categories to determine if existing categories might be collapsed and/or if new ones might emerge.

4. The current placement of the possible affective spectrum disorders (the cyclothymic and dysthymic) within axis I and other possible spectrum disorders (the schizotypal, paranoid, schizoid, and avoidant) within axis II is inconsistent, betrays an etiological bias, and is reductionistic in its conception of the relationship between clinical syndromes and personality disorder. All of the conditions are best included within axis II, unless the method used in axis II is radically altered in a dimensional, interpersonal direction.

5. There has been insufficient attention to several methodological issues in axis II personality-disorder research: (a) the influences of sample selection, choice of comparison group, and base rates, (b) the fact that descriptive similarity does not by itself guarantee similarity in etiology, course, or treatment response, and (c) the probability that personality disorders are likely to be heterogeneous within their definitional boundaries and difficult to demarcate from one another. Group-mean statistics may lose information and artificially emphasize discriminations that lose meaning when one studies the distributions of individual patients.

REFERENCES

Akiskal HS: Subaffective disorders: dysthymic, cyclothymic, and bipolar II disorders in the borderline realm. Psychiatr Clin North Am 4:25–46, 1981

Akiskal HS, Rosenthal TH, Haykel RF, et al: Characterological depressions, clinical and sleep EEG findings separating subaffective dysthymics from character spectrum disorders. Arch Gen Psychiatry 37:777–783, 1980

Andrulonis PA, Glueck BC, Stroebel EF, et al: Organic brain dysfunction and the borderline syndrome. Psychiatr Clin North Am 4:47–66, 1981

Borderline personality subcategories. J Nerv Ment Dis 170:670–679, 1982

Cantor N, Smith EE, French R, et al: Psychiatric diagnosis as prototype categorization. J Abnorm Psychol 89:181–193, 1980

Carr AC, Goldstein EG, Hunt HF, et al: Psychological tests and borderline patients. J Pers Assess 43:582–589, 1979

Carroll BJ, Greden JF, Feinberg J, et al: Neuroendocrine evaluation of depression in borderline patients: Psychiatr Clin North Am 4:89–98, 1981

Clarkin JF, Widiger TA, Frances A, et al: Prototype typology and the borderline personality disorder. J Abnorm Psychol 92:263–275, 1983

Cole JO, Sunderland PL: The drug treatment of borderline patients, in Psychiatry 1982: Annual Review. Edited by Grinspoon L. Washington, DC, APA Press, 1982

Fenichel O: The Psychoanalytic Theory of Neurosis. New York, Norton, 1945

Frances A: The DSM-III personality disorder section: a commentary. Am J Psychiatry 137:1050–1054, 1980

Categorical and dimensional systems of personality diagnosis: a comparison. Compr Psychiatry 23:516–527, 1982

Frances A, Clarkin J, Gilmore M, et al: Reliability of criteria for borderline personality disorder: a comparison of DSM-III and DIB. Am J Psychiatry 141:1080–1084, 1984

Frances A, Clarkin J, Hurt S, et al: Borderline personality disorder: category or dimension. (in press)

Frances A, Cooper A: Descriptive and dynamic psychiatry: a perspective on DSM-III. Am J Psychiatry 138:1198–1202, 1981

Frank H, Paris J: Recollections of family experience in borderline patients. Arch Gen Psychiatry 38:1031–1034, 1981

Gilmore J, Frances A, Clarkin J, et al: Developmental histories of DSM-III borderline personality disorder patients. (in press)

Gunderson JG, Carpenter WJ, Strauss JS: Borderline and schizophrenic patients: a comparative study. Am J Psychiatry 132:1257–1264, 1975

Gunderson JG, Englund PW: Characterizing the families of borderlines. Psychiatr Clin North Am 4:159–168, 1981

Gunderson JG, Kerr J, Englund BW: The families of borderlines. Arch Gen Psychiatry 37:27–33, 1980

Gunderson JG, Kolb JE: Discriminating features of borderline patients. Am J Psychiatry 138:792–796, 1978

Gunderson JG, Siever LG, Spaulding E: The search for a schizotype. Arch Gen Psychiatry 40:15–22, 1983

Gustin Q, Goodpaster W, Sajadic, et al: MMPI characteristics of the DSM-III borderline personality disorder. J Pers Assessment 47:50–59, 1983

Horowitz LM, Post D, French R, et al: The prototype as a construct in abnormal psychology. J Abnorm Psychol 90:575–585, 1981

Hurt SE, Clarkin J, Frances A, et al: The discriminant validity of the MMPI for borderline personality disorder. J Pers Assessment 49:56–61, 1985

Hurt SE, Hyler SE, Frances A, et al: Assessing borderline personality with self-report, clinical interview, or semi-structured interview. Am J Psychiatry 141:1228–1231, 1984

Kaplan J: A woman's view of DSM-III. Am Psychol 38:786–792, 1983

Kass F, Spitzer RL, Williams JBW: An empirical study of the issue of sex bias in the diagnostic criteria of DSM-III axis II personality disorders. Am Psychol 38:799–801, 1983

Kernberg OF: Severe Personality Disorders. New Haven, Yale University Press, 1984

Kernberg OF, Goldstein EG, Carr AC, et al: Diagnosing borderline personality. J Nerv Ment Dis 169:225–231, 1981

Klein DF: Psychopharmacology and the borderline patient, in Borderline States in Psychiatry. Edited by Mack JE. New York, Grune & Stratton, 1975

Koenigsberg HW: A comparison of hospitalized and nonhospitalized borderline patients. Am J Psychiatry 139:1292–1297, 1982

The relationship between syndrome and personality disorder in DSM-III: experience with 2009 patients. (in press)

Koenigsberg HW, Kernberg OF, Schomer J: Diagnosing borderline conditions in an outpatient setting. Arch Gen Psychiatry 40:49–58, 1983

Kolb JE, Gunderson JG: Diagnosing borderline patients with a semistructured interview. Arch Gen Psychiatry 37:37–41, 1980

Kretchmer E: Physique and Character. London, Kegan Paul, 1925

Kroll J, Carey K, Sines L, et al: Are there borderlines in Britain? Arch Gen Psychiatry 39:60–63, 1982

Kroll J, Sines L, Martin K: Borderline personality disorder: construct validity of the concept. Arch Gen Psychiatry 38:1021–1026, 1981

Lloyd C, Overall J, Kinsey L, et al: A comparison of the MMPI profiles of borderline and nonborderline outpatients. J Nerv Ment Dis 171:207–215, 1983

Loranger AW, Oldham JM, Talis EH: Familial transmission of DSM-III borderline personality disorder. Arch Gen Psychiatry 39:795–799, 1982

Lykowski JC, Tsuang MT: Precautions in treating DSM-III borderline personality disorder. Am J Psychiatry 137:110–111, 1980

MacKinnon RA, Michels R: The Psychiatric Interview in Clinical Practice. Philadelphia, WB Saunders, 1971

Malinow KL: Dependent personality, in Personality Disorders: Diagnosis and Management. Edited by Lion J. Baltimore, Williams & Wilkins, 1981a

Passive-aggressive personality, in Personality Disorders: Diagnosis and Management. Edited by Lion J. Baltimore, Williams & Wilkins, 1981b

Mellsop G, Varghese F, Joshua J, et al: Reliability of Axis II of DSM-III. Am J Psychiatry 139:1360–1361, 1982

Millon T: Disorders of Personality: DSM-III: Axis II. New York, Wiley, 1981

Murray JE: Minimal brain dysfunction and borderline personality adjustment. Am J Psychiatry 33:391–403, 1979

Perry JC, Flannery RB: Passive aggressive personality disorder. J Nerv Ment Disease 170:164–173, 1982

Perry JC, Klerman GL: Clinical features of the borderline personality disorder: Am J Psychiatry 137:165–173, 1980

Pope HG, Jonas JM, Hudson JE, et al: The validity of DSM-III borderline personality disorder. Arch Gen Psychiatry 40:23–30, 1983

Rado S: Adaptational Psychodynamics. New York, Science House, 1969

Resnick RJ, Schulz P: Borderline personality disorder: symptomatology and MMPI characteristics. J Clin Psychiatry 44:289–292, 1983

Schneider K: Psychopathic Personalities. London, Cassell, 1950

Schuckit M, Gunderson EK: The clinical characteristics of personality disorder subtypes in naval service. J Clin Psychiatry 40:29–35, 1979

Sheehy M, Goldsmith L, Charles E: A comparative study of borderline patients in a psychiatric outpatient clinic. Am J Psychiatry 137:1374–1379, 1980

Siever LJ: Genetic factors in borderline personalities, in Psychiatry 1982: Annual Review. Edited by Grinspoon L. Washington, APA Press, 1982

Singer MT, Larson DG: Borderline personality and the Rorschach test. Arch Gen Psychiatry 38:693–698, 1981

Small I, Small J, Alig V: Passive aggressive personality disorder. Am J Psychiatry 126:973–981, 1970

Snyder S, Pitts WM, Goodpaster WA, et al: MMPI profile of DSM-III borderline personality disorder. Am J Psychiatry 139:1046–1048, 1982a

Snyder S, Sajidi C, Pitts WM, et al: Identifying the depression border of borderline personality disorder. Am J Psychiatry 139:814–817, 1982b

Soloff PH: Concurrent validation of a diagnostic interview for borderlines: a replication study. Arch Gen Psychiatry 38:686–692, 1981a

Affect, impulse, and psychosis in borderline disorders: a validation study. Compr Psychiatry 22:337–349, 1981b

Soloff PH, George AW, Nathen RS: The dexamethasone suppression tests in borderline personality disorder. Am J. Psychiatry 139:1621–1623, 1982

Soloff PH, Millward JW: Psychiatric disorders in the families of borderline patients. Arch Gen Psychiatry 40:37–44, 1983a

Developmental histories of borderline patients. Compr Psychiatry 24:574–588, 1983b

Spitzer RL, Endicott JL: The justification for separating schizotypal and borderline personality disorders. Schizophr Bull 5:95–104, 1979

Spitzer RL, Endicott H, Gibbon M: Crossing the border into borderline personality and borderline schizophrenia. Arch Gen Psychiatry 36:17–24, 1979

Stangl D, Pfohl B, Zimmerman M, et al: A structured interview for the DSM-III personality disorders. Arch Gen Psychiatry 42:591–596, 1985

Stangler RS, Printz AM: DSM-III: psychiatric diagnosis in a university population. Am J Psychiatry 137:937–940, 1980

Stone M: The Borderline Syndromes. New York, McGraw-Hill, 1980

Vaillant G, Perry JC: Personality disorders, in Comprehensive Textbook of Psychiatry III. Edited by Freedman A, Kaplan R, Saddock B. Baltimore, Williams & Wilkins, 1980

Werble B: Second follow-up study of borderline patients. Arch Gen Psychiatry 23:3–7, 1970

Whitman R, Torsman H, Koenig R: Clinical assessment of passive-aggressive personality. Arch Neurol Psychiatry 72:540–549, 1954

Widiger TA: Prototype typology and borderline diagnosis. Clinical Psychology Review 2:115–135, 1982a

Psychological tests and the borderline diagnosis. J Pers Assessment 46:227–238, 1982b

Widiger TA, Hurt S, Frances A, et al: Diagnostic efficiency and DSM-III. Arch Gen Psychiatry 41:1005–1012, 1984

Widiger TA, Kelso K: Psychodiagnosis of axis II. Clinical Psychology Review 3:491–510, 1983

Wiggins J: Circumplex models of interpersonal behavior in clinical psychology, in Handbook of Research Methods in Clinical Psychology. Edited by Kendall P, Butcher J. New York, Wiley, 1982

18 *Histrionic, narcissistic, and compulsive personality disorders*

ARNOLD M. COOPER

The *DSM-III,* providing a new nosologic organization for considering the personality disorders, and attempting to provide clear criteria for diagnosis, has stimulated all psychiatrists to reexamine their premises and to scrutinize their clinical experience, and it has given some the opportunity to attempt new research in personality disorders. In reviewing the histrionic, narcissistic, and compulsive personality disorders, several themes emege repeatedly, as do suggested areas for revision.

I note, in beginning, that the names given to the three disorders I am discussing refer to different levels of observation and inference. "Histrionic" refers to an overt behavioral style, presumably readily observable. I believe that "narcissistic" refers to a complex theoretical conception with a range of behaviors that derive from a central intrapsychic difficulty. "Compulsive" has aspects of both an overt behavior and a theoretical formulation. This difference in the level of label assignment illustrates one of the problems in classifying the personality disorders: We cannot easily separate direct observations and low-level inference.

HISTRIONIC PERSONALITY DISORDER

Incidence ranges from 7% to 19% have been described: The latter figure derives from the *DSM-III* field trials (Kass, Spitzer, and Williams, 1983), and the former from a study by Koenigsberg and associates (1985). This disorder has the most clearly predominant female-to-male ratio, as high as 8:1. This has led some to question whether the traits under consideration reflect abnormality in any absolute sense or only cultural bias. I return to this issue later.

Reliability

Field trials and the study by Mellsop and associates (1982) indicate poor reliability.

290

Discussion

The histrionic personality is a new category replacing the previous "hysterical," presumably because of the unavoidable historical baggage attached to the term "hysterical" – implying everything from wandering uterus to wandering eye. The term "histrionic" emphasizes one of the character traits associated with this constellation, although the trait is not, in itself, sufficient to define the disorder. Millon (1981), for example, prefers the label "gregarious" to "histrionic" for the type under consideration.

Chodoff and Lyons, as far back as 1958, described the hysterical personality as characterized by dependence, egocentricity, emotionality, exhibitionism, and fear of sexuality, sexual provocativeness, and suggestibility. Various descriptions since that time have not differed much. Other trait studies have suggested such additional descriptors as dependence, and rejection of others (Lazare et al., 1966; Lazare, 1971; MacKinnon and Michels, 1971; Vandenberg and Helston, 1975; Blacker and Tupin, 1977).

It is interesting that, contrary to the traditional view of the hysterical personality, the histrionic criteria sets never mention sex – not seductiveness nor provocative behaviors nor sexual fears nor sexual hyperactivity. We might recall that the treatment of Anna O. by Breuer was broken off when she developed pseudocyesis and the conviction that she was going to bear Breuer's child. I believe that many clinicians, in consonance with the trait studies mentioned, continue to find sexuality an important and specific form of the histrionic display of many of the patients under discussion, and it is a significant transference issue in treatment.

The omission of sex from the criteria points to several difficulties in the defining criteria:

1. There really are only two criteria. Set A contains five different descriptions of the term "histrionic." Set B contains five descriptors of infantile or immature interpersonal relationships. There is a paucity of descriptors indicating any richness to the syndrome. What is being described is an individual who is dramatically infantile. That does not capture the full flavor of the hysteric.

2. The psychiatric literature has long discussed the severity spectrum of the histrionic personality. Easser and Lesser (1965) and Kernberg (pers. commun.), for example, have suggested a discontinuity between the healthier hysteric and the more "infantile" hysteric or "hysteroid." Tupin (1981), drawing on a number of studies of trait clusters, diagrammed "good" and "bad" versions of histrionic personality traits. The "good" histrionic is, among other things, ambitious, competitive, vain, insensitive, coquettish, emotionally expressive and labile, impulsive, adherent to strict standards of behavior, competitive-destructive with men, and uneasy with women. The "bad" histrionic person has low self-esteem, and diminished guilt, frequently complains of physical problems, and is passive, dependent, pouty, unpredictable, sensitive, communicatively unclear, compliant, demanding, and helpless.

Kernberg (pers. commun.) has suggested that the histrionic personality disorder in *DSM-III* confuses what he would prefer to call an "infantile" personality disorder with what is properly and traditionally referred to as the hysterical personality disorder. The work of Easser and Lesser on the hysteroid tends in the same direction.

Marmor (1953), in a similar vein, suggested that one distinguish the "genital" hysteric from the "oral" hysteric.

I support the view that these are significantly different personalities, not easily handled by judging them in terms of severity. Many of the traits that are judged infantile or oral also will be found in the more severely narcissistic, dependent, and passive-aggressive individuals.

I would emphasize that the "higher-level" histrionic, in my experience, is capable of sustained, although crisis-prone, relationships; can, in a genuine crisis, put aside histrionic defenses to carry out adaptive tasks; is capable of genuine mourning; and will, in treatment, form multilevel transferences that carry continuity and depth as well as clinging seductiveness.

One might question whether the higher-level histrionics have a disorder or are merely exhibiting traits. Clinical experience demonstrates that many of these patients suffer from their compulsive need for approval and their inability to sustain their self-esteem without constant outside support and are aware of the inappropriateness of their behaviors as they begin to lose their looks and their youth. They present to clinicians with feelings of depression and emptiness, fears of intensification of their sexual histrionics, and guilty feelings of depression concerning the hollowness of their own drama, and, of course, they experience crises after disappointments in love.

The issue of higher- or lower-level histrionic personality disorder hinges around the stability of self and the capacity for object relations – in similarity to the issues that influence narcissistic behavior. I would suggest that revised criteria consider two disorders, or, at least, present clear indicators of "better" and "worse," which would be coded.

3. The diagnosis currently is made on a choice of three items from column A and two from column B. This Chinese-menu selection seems arbitrary, at least. I can think of no reason why not four and two, or any other combination. A revised set of criteria would include references to sexuality, and, specifically, to sexuality as a mode of relating to others.

Sex bias

Chodoff (1982), Tupin (1981), and others have considered the problem of why there is such an excess of females over males in all studies. Only antisocial personality disorder shows a similar, although reversed, sex ratio. It has been suggested that hysterical behaviors are labeled "pathological" more readily in women than are the culture-determined counterpart behaviors in men. "Macho" defenses or male caricatures do not achieve nosologic status as readily as do female caricatures. Chodoff suggests that caricatures of sex roles are culturally determined, are present in both male and female, and lead to "sociopathic" behavior in males and hysteria in females. The question of how much is biological is left open. In Chapter 17, Dr. Frances alluded to the dispute between Kaplan and Spitzer and associates concerning sex bias in *DSM-III;* I do not repeat his discussion here.

NARCISSISTIC PERSONALITY DISORDERS

The classification of narcissistic personality disorder is entirely new in *DSM-III,* reflecting the intense interest of the profession in issues of narcissism. This interest has been fanned by the work of psychoanalysts, primarily Kohut (1971) and Kernberg (1975), and the views of prominent sociologists such as Christopher Lasch (1978) and Spiro Agnew. An enormous psychoanalytic literature has shed a great deal of light on theories of narcissism, its normal and pathological forms of presentation, and methods of treating narcissistic disorders. No studies validating the *DSM-III* criteria are available, and opinions on the *DSM-III* category range from the view of Kernberg that the description of the narcissistic personality disorder is "essentially satisfactory" and "includes recent contributions from psychoanalytic studies and acknowledges the descriptive criteria derived from psychoanalytically oriented clinical investigation" (O. F. Kernberg, pers. commun.) to the view of Vaillant and Perry (1980) that "in the authors' opinion, unless more empirical criteria are involved and a more rational basis for the diagnosis is reached, it will be well to drop narcissistic personality disorder from the nomenclature." The difference could not be sharper.

The incidence studies tend to reveal rather low diagnostic rates. In the *DSM-III* field trials, narcissistic personality was the least diagnosed personality disorder, and in the Vanderbilt Clinic study reported by Kass and associates (1983) it ranked eighth in frequency. Mellsop and associates (1982), in their study of 77 patients diagnosed as having personality disorders, never diagnosed a narcissistic personality. Koenigsberg and associates (1985) found 2% in their sample. Stangl and associates found 3%, and Stangler and Printz (1980) found 8%. Part of the variability is due to large sample variability and differences in methods of study. The rather low diagnostic rate is particularly interesting because psychiatrists seem to believe that narcissistic personality disturbances are common.

Reliability

Raskin and Hall (1981), in an effort to establish reliability for the narcissistic personality disorders, constructed an inventory designed to measure differences in the quantity of narcissism according to *DSM-III* criteria. Comparing their results with those from the Eysencks' personality questionnaire, they found that narcissism was positively and significantly correlated with the extroversion and psychoticism scales. It is difficult to know how to interpret this result, but it may confirm the rather narrow definition given the narcissistic personality disorder in *DSM-III*.

Discussion

The difficulty in assessing the category of narcissistic personality disorder will provide an opportunity to focus on an inherent difficulty of all the *DSM-III* personality disorders. As I have already indicated in discussing histrionic personality, the effort to define a disorder in terms of a set of behaviors without reference to an underlying unifying idea poses great problems. Whether one adheres to psychodynamic theory, social-learning theory, cognitive theory, or even behavioral theory, there remains a problem of specifying which of two or more alternative behaviors will emerge from underlying processes or the earlier history. The narcissistic personality disorder, if it exists, surely derives its coherence from a set of theoretical propositions.

If, for example, we conceive of the narcissistic personality disorder as broadly relating to some difficulties with the sense of self and the regulation of self-esteem, we cannot predict which self-presentation will be used to defend against painful exposure of these areas of weakness. *DSM-III* emphasizes the overt grandiosity, ambition, exhibitionism, and cool entitlement and exploitiveness of the narcissistic personality disorders. There is a group of patients for whom this is clearly the case. There is, however, another group of patients whose overt characteristics are shyness, an often charming dependence on grander others, an inability to express rage overtly, and ready shame and humiliation when confronted with criticism, often followed by significant feelings of depression. These patients, after some period of psychotherapy or extended exploration – often requiring 5 to 10 meetings – will reveal that beneath their surface shyness and modesty lie fantasies of exhibitionistic grandiosity, denigration of their heroes, and burning envy and rage. Even after these traits are quite apparent to the interviewer, the patient may continue to deny their existence or their import. The problem is not which patient is more narcissistic. The difference lies in whether more aggressive or more passive masochistic defenses are used to protect against fears of recognition of their sense of shrunken and meager self-representation and object relations. It is worth noting that Kernberg and Kohut, who have contributed the most to our modern ideas of the narcissistic personality disorder, share the view that diagnosis cannot be made by overt presentation; rather, diagnosis requires the experience of the therapeutic situation and organization of those data through a psychodynamic frame of reference.

Similar points are made in several recent reviews. For example, Bursten (1982) suggests that two dimensions – the firmness of the sense of self and the intensity of the focus on the self – define the "narcissistic personality." He suggests that these central defining dimensions are given clinical expression in a variety of clusters not always readily recognizable: "One has to listen a bit to the patient in order to distinguish the features. The narcissistic aspects of the personality may not be immediately apparent." Bursten describes five different personality types that represent different ways of playing out narcissistic tendencies – exhibitionistic, paranoid, antisocial, dependent, and avoidant. In his view, these personality types represent the intersections of intense narcissism with other personality dimensions.

The views of Millon (1981) deserve special consideration, because he takes credit for formulating the basic document from which the current criteria set was derived, with "minor revisions" (p. 166). We note that Millon's relevant chapter is entitled "Narcissistic Personality: The Egotistic Pattern." Millon, after a review of the shifting use of the concept of narcissism in psychoanalytic thinking, from the early 1930s, when narcissistic personalities were described as successful models of leadership, to the more recent literature, in which narcissistic characteristics are seen as complex derivatives representing failures of regulation of self-esteem, opts for the earlier view in describing the clinical picture he chooses to label the narcissistic personality. He states that "narcissists convey a calm and self-assured quality in their social behavior" (p. 166). In my experience, some do, but most do not.

Recent emphasis on narcissism as a normal personality characteristic – usually referring to egotistic or active modes of self-assertion and self-confidence – has confused the effort to delineate the pathological syndrome, as if abnormality consisted only of too much of what was normal. That seems to be Millon's view. This view does not allow for description of the transformations of original tendencies to opposites and the compromise formations that occur during psychic development. Pathological narcissism – whether one believes in Kernberg's, Kohut's, or someone else's views – is surely not too much self-confidence, even on the phenomenologic level, and may in fact show as depression and low self-esteem. Even the lack of empathy, usually agreed on as a trait, can be extremely subtle, with a presenting surface of a kindly listener and an empathic charmer. Only deeper understanding of the person's character may reveal his lack of interest in the other person, whom he may, in fact, have understood.

A recent review by Akhtar and Thompson (1982) deserves special mention. They emphasize key areas of deficit: (a) in self-concept, (b) in interpersonal relations, and (c) around superego functions. They derive several dimensions to be examined, and for each of these they describe overt and covert behaviors. For example, under self-concept, they describe:

Overt: inflated self-regard; haughty grandiosity; fantasies of wealth, power, beauty, brilliance; sense of entitlement; illusory invulnerability.
Covert: inordinate hypersensitivity; feelings of inferiority, worthlessness, fragility; continuous search for strength and glory. (p. 20)

It is this polarity that *DSM-III* fails to convey. I would go a step further than Akhtar and Thompson and suggest that either of these descriptions can be overt, with the other covert, or in fact they can be multilayered.

A syndrome believed to be of such importance by major groups of clinicians cannot easily be abandoned at this point. This first attempt at definition in *DSM-*

III is expectably overly one-dimensional. The next round of classification may be better served by abandoning an effort at simple description of overt characteristics. It may be better to attempt a double description of "overt" and "covert," not entirely the same as conscious and unconscious.

It would also be useful to grade the criteria in terms of severity rather than offering a random selection adding up to a required number. The criteria ought to indicate both quantity (how much of the personality is engulfed in narcissistic abnormality) and quality (how immature and fragile are the defensive modes).

Pathological narcissism is involved in all pathological behaviors, and singling out the disorders of the self for primary scrutiny is an enterprise rooted in theories and derived from the experience of transference.

Addition of an axis VI for defense or dynamic mechanisms should permit much better description of the range of pathological behaviors that may stem from a central difficulty in self-esteem regulation and differentiation of self and other.

COMPULSIVE PERSONALITY

This new title replaces the obsessive–compulsive personality of *DSM-II*. This disorder is particularly interesting because it is one of the few personality disorders for which there has been a quite consistent description over many decades. As Millon (1981) describes, the predictions and descriptions derived from psychoanalytic study have been well confirmed.

Incidence

Incidence figures vary widely for reasons not entirely apparent. Mellsop and Koenigsberg, in their separate studies, found about a 2% incidence. The *DSM-III* field trials diagnosed 22%.

Reliability

The reliability of diagnosis is probably poor.

Discussion

I question the wisdom of changing the name from obsessive–compulsive to compulsive. Shapiro (1965, 1981) and Millon, like others before them, emphasize the constant sense of "should" that underlies all the activities of these individuals. This "should," besides removing the pleasure from the activity, can result in either compulsive (i.e., fearful and conforming) behaviors or obsessional (i.e., ambivalent, or formes frustes of defiant) behaviors. Compulsive characters are often consciously filled with obsessional doubts, ambivalence, and worry.

One of the five criteria for compulsive personality disorders in *DSM-III* is "indecisiveness: decision-making is either avoided, postponed, or protracted, perhaps because of an inordinate fear of making a mistake, e.g., the individual cannot get assignments done on time because of ruminating about priorities."

This is such an excellent description of what is usually meant by obsessional personality characteristics that it seems unnecessarily confining, and perhaps confusing, to have removed obsessive from the title of the disorder. Clinical experience indicates that individuals are rarely simply compulsive. The surface compulsive may be secretly personally untidy or even dirty, and some seemingly well-ordered compulsives are barely hiding the fact that they are unable to sort out the disorder in their minds and therefore dare not leave anything out.

Furthermore, retaining the name obsessive–compulsive disorder would encourage further research into the question of the connection between the personality abnormalities and the symptom disorders. Most clinicians believe that they are connected, although Sandler and Hazari, in a study in 1960, claimed that obsessional traits and symptoms did not covary and formed separate clusters.

Finally, I again emphasize the desirability of using the full extent of our psychiatric knowledge in trying to understand complex syndromes. The obsessive–compulsive personality, regardless of theoretical bias, is seen by almost all clinicians (perhaps, in fact, all) to represent the expression of underlying conflicts over obedience or defiance toward nursery rules, and the unresolvable oscillations between rage against authority and fear of authority. This understanding provides a rich range of behavior clustering. Any given instance of the disorder may present a facade of pathological orderliness or of untidiness, seemingly stupid stubbornness or pathological conformism, severe constriction of any overt emotion or periods of clinging attachment and dependence.

Despite the usual facade of emotional barrenness, the obsessive–compulsive personality is object-dependent, while desperately trying to control affective expression. Well-integrated compulsive characters suffer from their emotional constriction. They experience depression, anxiety, hypochondriasis, and sadness, are prone to paranoia, and may even have temper outbursts or explosions of "fun" under the influence of a drink or two. They are capable of or require intensely dependent relationships. The term "compulsive" fails to capture the struggle of ambivalence that may be observable in the surface obsessional traits and is always an underlying issue. The criteria, as given, are unexceptionable and follow tradition, but divorced from a developmental perspective, they are narrow. The low incidences reported in most of the studies suggest that it is grossly underdiagnosed by current criteria, when compared with our experience with colleagues and friends.

SUMMARY REMARKS

DSM-III has presented us with a superb study opportunity. The personality-disorders section suffers from low reliability and, in my opinion, from poor description in several categories. Suggested improvements are as follows:

1. The full range of psychiatric clinical experience should be used in describing

syndromes in terms both of developmental characteristics and of low-level theories that the profession shares.

2. An axis of defenses would help in the effort to understand the interaction of sources of anxiety or damaged self-esteem with available defensive modes.
3. A scaling of criteria according to severity.
4. A dimensional approach, as suggested by Frances and others.
5. Opportunities should be provided for indicating covert, or even unconscious, inferred or discovered wishes and fantasies that may, over time, oscillate in any given individual and certainly will find different expressions in a population.

At the heart of trying to understand personality disorders on the basis of a small list of overt behaviors is the unsolved problem of symptom choice. Given a conflict, or a deficit of structure, or a problem of cognitive dissonance, or a faulty learning, one is unable to predict the combination of defenses that are likely to be adopted. Because defensive modes are limited, people may or may not resemble each other on the surface in ways that will be useful in understanding the disorder for purposes of ultimately understanding etiology, or for preparing treatments, or for making predictions. I am not suggesting that descriptive clusters be abandoned. I am suggesting that the descriptions include more of what most psychiatrists, rightly or wrongly, do include – their inferences that derive from their low-level theories and their lengthier contacts with patients.

REFERENCES

Akhtar S, Thompson JA: Overview: narcissistic personality disorder. Am J Psychiatry 139:12–20, 1982
Blacker KH, Tupin JP: Hysteria and hysterical structures: developmental and social theories, in Hysterical Personality. Edited by Horowitz MD. New York, Aaronson, 1977, pp 95–142
Bursten B: Narcissistic personalities in DSM-III. Compr Psychiatry 26:409–420, 1982
Chodoff P: Hysteria and women. Am J Psychiatry 139:545–551, 1982
Chodoff P, Lyons H: Hysteria, the hysterical personality, and "hysterical" conversion. Am J Psychiatry 144:734–740, 1958
Easser BR, Lesser SR: Hysterical personality: a re-evaluation. Psychoanal Q 34:389–405, 1965
Kass F, Spitzer RL, Williams JBW: An empirical study of the issue of sex bias in the diagnostic criteria of DSM-III, axis 2, personality disorders. Am Psychol 38:799–801, 1983
Kernberg OF: Borderline Conditions of Pathological Narcissism. New York, Aaronson, 1975
Koenigsberg HW, Kaplan RB, Gilmore MM, et al: The relationship between syndrome and personality disorder in DSM-III: experience with 1995 patients. Am J Psychiatry 142:207–212, 1985
Kohut H: The Analysis of the Self. New York, International Universities Press, 1971
Lasch C: The Culture of Narcissism: American Life in an Age of Diminishing Expectation. New York, Norton, 1978
Lazare A: The hysterical character in psychoanalytic theory – an evolution and confusion. Arch Gen Psychiatry 25:131–137, 1971

Lazare A, Klerman G, Armor B, et al: Obsessive and hysterical personality patterns: an investigation of psychoanalytic concepts by means of factor analysis. Arch Gen Psychiatry 14:624, 1966

MacKinnon R, Michels R: The Psychiatric Interview in Clinical Practice. 1971, pp 110–146

Marmor J: Orality in the hysterical personality. J Am Psychoanal Assoc 1:656–671, 1953

Mellsop G, Varghese F, Joshua S, et al: The reliability of axis 2 of DSM-III. Am J Psychiatry 139:1360–1361, 1982

Millon T: Disorders of Personality, DSM-III: Axis 2. New York, Wiley, 1981

Raskin R, Hall CS: The narcissistic personality inventory: alternate form reliability and further evidence of construct validity. J Pers Assess 45:159–162, 1981

Sandler J, Hazari A: The obsessional: on the psychological classification of obsessional character traits and symptoms. Br J Med Psychol 33:113–122, 1960

Shapiro D: Neurotic Styles. New York, Basic Books, 1965
    Autonomy and Rigid Character. New York, Basic Books, 1981

Stangler BS, Printz AM: DSM-III: psychiatric diagnosis, university population. Am J Psychiatry 137:937–940, 1980

Tupin JP: Histrionic personality, in Personality Disorders: Diagnosis and Management, second edition, revised for *DSM-III.* Edited by Lion JR. Baltimore, Williams & Wilkins, 1981, pp 85–96

Vaillant GE, Perry JC: Personality disorders, in Comprehensive Textbook of Psychiatry, III. Edited by Kaplan HI, Freedman AM, Sadock BJ. Baltimore, Williams & Wilkins, 1980, pp 1562–1590

Vandenberg PJ, Helstone FS: Oral, obsessive, and hysterical personality patterns: a Dutch replication. J Psychiatr Res 12:319, 1975

19 An evaluation of the DSM-III categories of paranoid, schizoid, and schizotypal personality disorders

LARRY J. SIEVER AND
KENNETH S. KENDLER

The *DSM-III* criteria for paranoid, schizoid, and schizotypal personality disorders represent an attempt to formalize criteria for a group of characterologic patterns that have been linked historically or phenomenologically, although not necessarily empirically, with schizophrenia. Because of their eccentricities and social aloofness, individuals with these disorders often are set apart from others and thus are considered "peculiar" or "odd." They are thus grouped together in *DSM-III* as the "odd" cluster. All of these disorders share criteria reflecting social distance and emotional constriction. Both paranoid and schizotypal personality disorders are also characterized by suspiciousness, hypersensitivity, and exaggerated expectation of external threat. Thus, one might expect overlap in the diagnoses of these personality disorders.

We briefly review the historical underpinnings of each of these disorders in order to define the reasons for considering them as separate and clinically useful diagnostic categories. It is important, however, to recognize that with the exception of several studies on schizotypal personality disorder, little empirical research has been reported on the reliability or validity of the *DSM-III* criteria for these disorders. We cannot know at this time whether or not the selection of these particular diagnostic categories for inclusion in *DSM-III* and the use of the specific *DSM-III* criteria for these disorders represent the most valid and clinically useful means of characterizing individuals with this subgroup of personality disorders. We review the currently available empirical evidence and draw on our clinical experience in order to help frame the relevant future investigations that will be required to develop more meaningful criteria for these disorders.

PARANOID PERSONALITY DISORDER

Historical considerations

The hallmark of paranoid personality disorder is extreme suspiciousness or exaggerated expectation of threat from others. Although the term has been in use since the time of the ancient Greeks as a term for general psycho-

300

pathology, it acquired more specific meaning in the writings of descriptive psychiatrists in the nineteenth century such as Kraepelin (1913). He used the term "paranoia" to describe highly systematized delusions in the absence of a general psychiatric deterioration, which would be currently categorized by *DSM-III* as paranoid disorder. He considered individuals with paranoid personality disorder to be predisposed to the development of paranoid conditions and characterized by perversive mistrust of others. Thus, the term "paranoid" has been linked phenomenologically and historically to psychotic disorders, especially schizophrenia, because paranoid ideation occurs in paranoid schizophrenia, in delusional or paranoid disorder, and even in the psychotic affective disorders such as mania. In all these disorders, however, the symptoms are acute and of psychotic proportions. The question remains whether the paranoid symptoms observed in all these disorders reflect common etiologic antecedents or are etiologically distinct. We address this question in reviewing studies of paranoid personality disorder.

Diagnostic criteria and differential diagnosis

The *DSM-III* criteria for personality disorder include three categories of long-term characteristics: (1) pervasive, unwarranted suspiciousness and mistrust of people, (2) hypersensitivity, and (3) restricted affectivity. Individual inclusion criteria for each of these characteristics range from four to eight items. Many of these are inferential, as well as difficult to define operationally and verify, such as "searching for confirmation of bias," "absence of passive, soft, tender, and sentimental feelings," "exaggerating of difficulties," or "readiness to counterattack." They are also less specific to paranoid personality disorder and could reflect a broad spectrum of psychopathology rather than a specific diagnostic picture of paranoid personality. Because no specific empirical studies have been done to examine the validity of these criteria, they must be considered to represent the clinical consensus of the architects of *DSM-III* at the time of its formulation.

There is a fair amount of overlap between the criteria for paranoid personality disorder and those for other personality disorders. Suspiciousness and paranoid ideation are also characteristic of schizotypal personality disorder. Cool, constricted affect is shared with schizoid, schizotypal, and compulsive personality disorders. Rigidity is a common characteristic of both paranoid and compulsive personality disorders.

Thus, it is not surprising that these related disorders frequently overlap. For example, in a preliminary study of 57 character-disordered patients hospitalized in a Veterans Administration (VA) hospital acute inpatient unit and diagnosed by the Structured Interview for *DSM-III* Personality Disorders (SIDP) (Stangl et al., 1985), 20 of 57 satisfied the criteria for paranoid personality disorder (L. J. Siever, H. Klar, et al., unpublished data). Sixteen of those 20 satisfied the *DSM-III* criteria for schizotypal personality disorder as well, and 6 satisfied the criteria for compulsive personality disorder, 5 for borderline personality disorder, 4 for avoidant personality disorder, and 1 for antisocial personality disorder. All patients in the sample satisfied at least four inclusion criteria for paranoid personality disorder, and a number of those who did not meet the criteria satisfied a comparable number of inclusion criteria as those who did meet the *DSM-III* criteria, largely because of the distribution of items. Although the exact character of the overlap depends, of course, on the characteristics of the sample population, which in this case was an inpatient sample in whom severe psychopathology might be expected, the data suggest that frequent overlap exists between paranoid personality disorder and other *DSM-III* axis II diagnoses.

In another study (J. G. Gunderson, M. Zanarini, et al., unpublished data), 42 patients were diagnosed using the Personality Disorder Questionnaire (PDQ) and Diagnostic Interview for Personality Disorders (DIPD), which includes the Diagnostic Interview for Borderlines (DIB) as well as a structured interview for the personality disorders. There was low reliability between the two instruments. As in the previous study, most individuals satisfied the criteria for more than one personality disorder (average 3.3). By the PDQ, 6 (25%) of 24 patients in their borderline sample as diagnosed by the DIB satisfied the *DSM-III* criteria for paranoid personality disorder, and by the DIPD, 12 (33%) of 36 met the criteria for this disorder. In general, it was diagnosed less frequently than schizotypal or borderline personality disorder, but more frequently than schizoid personality disorder. Individuals with paranoid personality disorder in their sample (14 of 36) were also frequently diagnosed as having borderline personality disorder (78% by PDQ), compulsive personality disorder (56% by PDQ), dependent personality disorder (56% by PDQ), histrionic personality disorder (71% by DIPD, 56% by PDQ), and schizotypal personality disorder (57% by DIPD, 56% by PDQ). This study as well suggests considerable overlap between paranoid personality disorder and other personality disorders in an inpatient sample, including several from the "dramatic" cluster.

Reliability studies, although not providing information as to the specificity of individual criteria, suggest that reliability for paranoid personality disorder is low. Reliability for the axis II diagnoses as a whole is only modest (κ coefficient .61 for joint interview reliability, .54 for test–retest reliability) (Spitzer, Forman, and Nee, 1979b). Another study by Mellsop and Varghesi (1982) using three raters found a low reliability for paranoid personality disorder (κ coefficient .35), although somewhat higher than those observed for most other personality disorders, including the others in the "odd" cluster. As was observed in the VA study, a large proportion of their patients (63%) with axis II diagnoses satisfied the criteria for more than one personality disorder. Paranoid personality was diagnosed relatively less frequently (13% of all personality-disorder subjects) than schizotypal personality disorder (47%), but more frequently than schizoid personality disorder (5%), consonant also with previously presented results. The degree of overlap between these diagnoses could not be ascertained from this report.

Epidemiology

The exact incidence of this disorder in the population remains to be determined, particularly using *DSM-III* criteria. Results of the midtown Manhattan study (Srole et al., 1962) suggest that paranoid perceptions are found frequently in an urban population: 23.2% of respondents acknowledged feeling that people are against them without any good reason. Estimates of the incidence of paranoid personality disorder in the general population may be derived from studies of control populations in family studies of schizophrenia. One study of psychiatric diagnoses in the relatives of schizophrenics and nonschizophrenics found that paranoid personality, characterized by a consistent display of hostility to the interviewer, acquaintances, neighbors, and so on, was observed in 3 (4.3%) of 69 relatives of controls (Stephens et al., 1975). In the only study to systematically apply *DSM-III* criteria, Kendler and Gruenberg (1982) reviewed the case records of 138 personally interviewed relatives of control adoptees and found one case of paranoid personality disorder (0.7%). A study based on one outpatient clinic showed a greater incidence in males than in females (Kass, Spitzer, and Williams, 1983). More accurate estimates of the population incidence and sex ratio for paranoid personality disorder await prospective studies using operationalized interviews to evaluate the *DSM-III* criteria for paranoid personality disorder in a representative sample of the population.

Genetic studies

Two studies have raised the possibility that paranoid personality is genetically related to schizophrenia. In one study, Stephens and associates (1975) found that paranoid personality disorder was observed with an incidence of 9.0% in the interviewed first-degree relatives of schizophrenics, versus 4.3% among interviewed first-degree relatives of controls. They did not use *DSM-III* criteria, and the difference observed did not reach statistical significance. Another study by Kendler and Gruenberg (1982), using the *DSM-III* criteria for paranoid personality disorder, did find a significantly increased incidence in the interviewed biological relatives of schizophrenic adoptees (3.8%) than in the interviewed biological relatives of control adoptees (0.7%) or the interviewed adoptive relatives of the schizophrenic adoptees. Baron (1983) found paranoid personality disorder, by *DSM-III* criteria, to be modestly but significantly more common in the parents and siblings of schizophrenics than in those of controls.

A second study by Kendler, Masterson, and Davis (1985) used a definition for paranoid personality disorder that was broadly equivalent to the *DSM-III* criteria, although not including the specific inclusion criteria. They defined paranoid personality disorder as a "consistent pattern of suspiciousness or distrustfulness inappropriate to social circumstances, evidence of paranoid ideation, with undue social anxiety and hypersensitivity to imagined criticism." They applied this definition blindly in a family-history study of the first-degree relatives of schizophrenics and controls from the Bronx VA Hospital and found an incidence of zero among 119 first-degree relatives of controls and 0.8% among 330 first-degree relatives of schizophrenics, a nonsignificant difference. However, their system was hierarchical, such that individuals with suspiciousness, but in addition having schizotypal characteristics, were considered to have schizotypal personality disorder only, not paranoid personality disorder.

Kendler and associates (1985) did find an incidence of 4.8% for paranoid personality disorder among first-degree relatives of patients with nonschizophrenic paranoid psychosis (delusional disorder), significantly greater than the incidence among either the first-degree relatives of the schizophrenics or of the controls. This study differed from the first in that *DSM-III* criteria were not applied, probands were not adopted, only first-degree relatives were diagnosed, relatives were not interviewed directly, and diagnoses were hierarchical such that paranoid diagnoses were excluded if schizotypal personality disorder was present. These studies considered together, however, suggest that a weak familial link may exist between paranoid personality disorder and schizophrenia, but it does not appear to be as strong as the familial link between paranoid personality disorder and delusional disorder. The latter, according to the Kendler VA study, although including only a small sample of paranoid relatives, may be particularly specific for nonschizotypal paranoid individuals.

Biological markers

Biological markers have not been systematically studied in paranoid personality disorder.

Psychological testing

Although few studies have been done using psychological testing in individuals with paranoid personality disorder, a number of studies have examined the paranoid–nonparanoid distinction in schizophrenia (Silverman, 1964). For example, paranoid schizophrenics may respond more sensitively to nonverbal cues (LaRusso, 1978), perhaps accounting for their exaggerated attribution of malicious intent to others. The applicability of such studies to paranoid personality disorder, however, remains to be determined.

Course of illness and treatment response

We are aware of no empirical studies regarding treatment response in paranoid personality disorder. Because this personality disorder, by definition, reflects long-term characteristics, remissions and exacerbations presumably are rare. However, whether or not individuals with paranoid personality disorder go on to develop delusional disorder or schizophrenia or even schizotypal personality disorder has not been systematically examined. Although there are no good empirical studies, to our knowledge, of treatment response in this group, psychotherapy and, under some circumstances, low-dosage neuroleptics may have limited benefit in these disorders.

Considerations for future research

The inclusion criteria for paranoid personality disorder are numerous and appear to be relatively nonspecific as presently formulated. It is not clear that the multiplicity of criteria and the minimum requirements for each of the three major categories of characteristics add to the diagnostic usefulness of the *DSM-III* criteria for this disorder. More careful study of the paranoid-personality-disordered relatives of individuals with delusional disorder may be helpful in defining more valid criteria, and, of course, studies are needed regarding the discriminating features of this disorder in the psychiatric population and its treatment responsiveness.

SCHIZOID PERSONALITY DISORDER

Historical considerations

The term "schizoid personality" originally gained currency with Bleuler (1978) and later was elaborated by other descriptive psychiatrists in the early part of this century. It was considered to represent a clinical picture often observed in schizophrenics remitted from psychosis, in schizophrenics prior to the onset of psychosis, and in relatives of schizophrenics. The most prominent features of this syndrome were thus social isolation and constricted affect. Over time, the term "schizoid" came to apply more broadly to psychopathology characterized by relative detachment and limited intimacy and thus lost its specificity as a diagnosis related to schizophrenia.

Diagnostic criteria and differential diagnosis

Three inclusion criteria are required for schizoid personality disorder: (1) emotional coldness and aloofness, and absence of warm, tender feelings for others, (2) indifference to praise or criticism or to the feelings of others, and (3) close friendships with no more than one or two persons, including family members. The rest of the criteria are exclusionary, ruling out individuals with eccentricities characteristic of schizotypal personality disorder, individuals with schizophrenia or paranoid disorder, and individuals under 18 years meeting the criteria for schizotypal disorder of childhood or adolescence. These criteria emphasize the central characteristic of the schizoid personality: the limited capacity for social relationships. This characteristic is also central for schizotypal personality disorder, but that diagnosis requires, in addition, some evidence of unusual perceptions, speech, or behaviors that are milder than, but akin to, psychotic symptoms.

There have been no systematic studies of the *DSM-III* criteria for schizoid personality disorder. Gunderson, Siever, and Spaulding (1983), however, found that the biological relatives of schizophrenic adoptees who were diagnosed originally as having "borderline schizophrenia" were marked more by social isolation and constricted affect than by perceptual or cognitive distortions such as those included in the *DSM-III* for schizotypal personality disorder (Spitzer, Endicott, and Gibbon, 1979a). This issue will be discussed in greater depth in relation to schizotypal personality disorder, but it raises the issue of where the dividing line should be drawn between schizoid and schizotypal personality disorders. If psychoticlike distortions of perceptions, thought, and behavior are less characteristic of the schizotypal individual than are isolation, suspiciousness, and aloofness, the characteristics of schizotypal individuals will be difficult to discriminate clinically from those of schizoid personality disorder as currently defined.

Criteria for schizoid personality disorder are difficult to establish – for example, "absence of warm, tender feelings" or "indifference to the feelings of others." These characteristics are, in our experience, not often noted by patients or those relatives or friends who know them well, even in those who are socially isolated. When these characteristics are absent, social isolation is often attributable to fear of rejection, as in avoidant personality disorder. When characteristics such as indifference to feelings or absence of warm feelings are present, decreased rapport, suspiciousness, and other criteria for schizotypal personality disorder are often observed. Thus, the two new diagnostic categories largely preempt the category of schizoid personality disorder. Perhaps for these reasons, Mellsop and Varghesi (1982) diagnosed schizoid personality disorder in only 3 of 64 personality-disordered patients. Preliminary results of L. J. Siever, H. Klar, and associates (unpublished data) and J. G. Gunderson, M. Zanarini, and associates (unpublished data) suggest that schizoid personality disorder is not observed among inpatients, but its applicability to outpatients or nonpsychiatric patients is unknown.

Epidemiology

Little is known of the epidemiology of schizoid personality disorder in the general population. In Mellsop's study it was diagnosed less frequently in an inpatient population than most other conditions, including the other diagnoses in the "odd" cluster. A similar infrequency was observed among outpatients in the Vanderbilt Clinic in New York City, but not in the larger field trials (Kass et al., 1983).

Genetic studies

We are not aware of any studies examining the family histories or genetics of probands diagnosed as having schizoid personality disorder by *DSM-III*. Most studies that have examined this issue have done so from the vantage point of studying the genetics of schizophrenia. Kety and associates (1968) did not find any significantly increased incidence of *DSM-III* schizoid personality disorder among biological relatives of schizophrenics, as compared with the biological relatives of controls or adoptive relatives of schizophrenics. However, their definition was broad and included individuals with inadequate personality and mild psychopathology. Stephens and associates (1975) did find increases in the incidences of schizoid and paranoid personalities among relatives of schizophrenic patients, as compared with controls, but they used a definition that included two distinct groups: the first having social isolation and lack of tender feelings, and the second having eccentricity and digressive communication. Particularly the latter group might currently be considered to have schizotypal personality disorder.

Schizoid personality has been hypothesized to be the premorbid personality of future schizophrenic individuals. Although studies of this question have not been undertaken using the *DSM-III* criteria for schizoid personality disorder, several studies have suggested that this may not be the characteristic premorbid personality of schizophrenics, although its presence may predict a less favorable outcome (Gittelman-Klein and Klein, 1969; Longabaugh and Eldred, 1973; Roff, Knight, and Wertheim, 1976; Siever, 1981).

Biological markers

There have been no studies, to our knowledge, examining biological markers in individuals specifically diagnosed as having schizoid personality disorder by *DSM-III*.

Psychological testing

The psychological characteristics of individuals with schizoid personality disorder have been a focus of investigation in part because of its presumed relationship to schizophrenia prior to the advent of the *DSM-III* criteria for schizoid personality disorder. However, we are not aware of any studies specifically examining individuals meeting the *DSM-III* criteria for schizoid personality disorder. Because most of the earlier studies were attempting to identify characteristics related to schizophrenia, they may more appropriately be considered under schizotypal personality disorder. However, several studies have suggested impairment of empathy in schizoid children and adults (Chick, Waterhouse, and Wolff, 1979; Wolff and Chick, 1980).

Course of illness and treatment response

Clinical experience suggests that schizoid patients usually are not motivated to seek treatment, and even if they do they are unlikely to change dramatically. However, empirical studies are needed in this area.

Considerations for future research

Schizoid personality disorder, as presently defined in *DSM-III*, may have been largely subsumed by the two new personality disorders: schizotypal personality disorder and avoidant personality disorder. Others with paranoid and compulsive personality disorders also may meet the criteria for schizoid personality disorder. Individuals in these four diagnostic groups may be characterized by social isolation and apparent aloofness. In the avoidant personality, the social distance and isolation are functions of a deep-seated fear of disappointment in relationships, rather than a true inclination to be a "loner." In the severe compulsive personality, constricted affect and difficulty with tender feelings frequently limit the scope of interpersonal relatedness. In this disorder, however, these characteristics seem to be associated with excessive rigidity, perfectionism, and desire for control over the ambiguities that affective experiences elicit. Such individuals often display a sensitivity to criticism from others, in contrast to the apparent indifference of the schizoid individual. Paranoid personalities may be isolated and constricted, in addition to their mistrust and suspiciousness of others. Finally, individuals with schizotypal personality disorder are isolated and constricted, but usually appear eccentric and suspicious as well. Would a case group of schizoid-personality-disordered individuals remain if these diagnoses are systematically excluded? Especially when one considers that perceptual and cognitive distortions only infrequently accompany other criteria in the schizotypal relatives of schizophrenics, would one find "loners" without tender feelings and indifference to others without, in essence, being schizotypal as well – for example, suspicious with inadequate rapport? This question remains to be researched, but it is our experience in both clinical and nonclinical (e.g., volunteer) populations that it is rare to find such individuals who do not exhibit some of the schizotypal characteristics observed in the relatives of schizophrenics. Thus, the schizoid personality disorder needs to be more clearly demarcated from these other disorders, particularly schizotypal personality disorder, and consideration should be given to collapsing these two disorders.

It is rare to find individuals whom one can confidently assess as having an "absence of tender feelings" and "indifference to praise and criticism." In the preliminary study at the VA, even schizotypal individuals have acknowledged these characteristics, whereas schizoid individuals have rarely been observed. Thus, these criteria must be reevaluated in empirical studies. There is another group of individuals similar to "as-if" personalities (Deutsch, 1942) who might have been considered schizoid under previous clinical psychodynamic formulations (Guntrip, 1968; Siever and Gunderson, 1983). Such individuals may not appear isolated, in that they may have spouses and superficial friends, but they appear to be affectively impoverished, particularly in their capacity for intimacy, and to have no internal sense of identity, with their behavior being tied specifically to the immediate external milieu. All of these patients may not be sufficiently isolated to satisfy the criteria for schizoid, nor are they self-destructive or impulsive enough to satisfy the criteria for borderline, and yet they may suffer from a profound sense of emptiness, difficulty in intimacy, and diffuse identity disturbance. Should these patients be characterized as having personality disorder?

More specific investigations of character-disordered probands, with attention to overlap between criteria and specificity of criteria, are required to ascertain the applicability of the diagnosis of schizoid personality disorder. Family history, biological markers, and other external validating criteria should be employed to determine the definition and usefulness of this category.

SCHIZOTYPAL PERSONALITY DISORDER

Historical considerations

Rado (1953, 1962) introduced the terms "schizotype" and "schizotypal" as condensations of the term "schizophrenic genotype." He applied them to individuals who might be related genetically to schizophrenics. Meehl (1962) elaborated on possible psychological deficits in schizotypes that include anhedonia and social aversiveness, as well as cognitive slippage. Spitzer and Endicott (1979) revived this term in their attempt to delineate diagnostic categories in the area of personality disorders. They wished to define a personality disorder, which they termed schizotypal personality disorder, that might be more specifically related to schizophrenia in the absence of overt psychosis and to demarcate these patients from individuals who were primarily unstable, whom they designated as having borderline personality disorder, and from those who were merely socially isolated, whom they designated as having schizoid personality disorder. Of the three diagnoses, this is the most recent to emerge, and the only one with empirical supporting evidence.

Diagnostic criteria and differential diagnosis

Spitzer and associates (1979a) attempted to characterize the "borderline schizophrenics" in the adoptive studies of Kety and associates (1968) as a basis for this new disorder. These individuals had schizophrenialike characteristics and were found more frequently among the biological relatives of schizophrenic adoptees than among their adoptive relatives or among the biological relatives of control adoptees. They examined the records of "schizophrenic spectrum disorders," including certain and uncertain borderline schizophrenia, uncertain schizophrenia, as well as schizoid and inadequate personalities. From these records they derived eight items pertaining to social isolation, constricted affect and social distance, referential ideation and suspiciousness, and deviant perception that they found to discriminate between "borderline schizophrenics" and their relatives. They found a sensitivity of 86% and specificity of 95% in characterizing the relatives of schizophrenics, although they used a cutoff of three out of eight items, rather than four, as is required under the current *DSM-III* criteria. They cross-validated their items in the sample of Danish adopted-away offspring of schizophrenics (Rosenthal et al., 1968) and found a lower sensitivity (63%) and higher specificity (100%). They then tested these criteria in the clinical population at large by sending a multiple-choice questionnaire, including criteria for schizotypal personality disorder and borderline personality disorder (then unstable personality disorder), to 4,000 randomly selected members of the American Psychiatric Association. They asked them to rate a borderline patient and a control patient. They performed a factor analysis and found that most of the unstable items loaded on one factor and the schizotypal items on another. However, the two factors accounted for only a small proportion of the variance (33%) of the combined sample. On the basis of the sensitivity and specificity of the items for the 222 patients given the clinical diagnosis of borderline schizophrenia, they developed a cutoff of four of the eight items that provided maximum specificity and sensitivity in distinguishing these patients from the other patients.

Although this study represented an important start in characterizing this new disorder, the question remains whether or not these criteria constitute a valid entity that represents a clinically meaningful category. A major impetus for defining this diagnosis was an attempt to characterize a group of patients with phenomenological and perhaps genetic and psychobiological relatedness to schizophrenia. In fact, though, the way the criteria were derived leaves open the possibility that they may not have best characterized the psychological attributes of individuals related to schizophrenics. Criteria were defined ad hoc from an examination of the adoptive-study records, which included not only borderline schizophrenics but also schizoid or inadequate personality disorders, as well as uncertain schizophrenics. They were applied again to the same sample and to a second sample from the same set of studies. However, Spitzer and associates used a cutoff of three of eight items to determine their specificity and sensitivity, raising the possibility that only a minority of the criteria may characterize any particular borderline schizophrenic relative of a schizophrenic proband.

Reider and associates (1975) applied the *DSM-III* criteria for schizotypal personality disorder to 9 borderline schizophrenics from the study of Kety and associates (1968), 10 borderline schizophrenics from the study of Rosenthal and associates (1968), and 11 borderline schizophrenics from their own study of the offspring of schizophrenics. They found that 73% of them satisfied the *DSM-III* criteria for schizotypal personality disorder, but again used three rather than four criteria. Most of the patients satisfied the criteria for other personality disorders as well. Again, it would appear that many of these relatives satisfy only a few of the criteria for schizotypal personality disorder.

Similarly, Khouri and associates (1980) derived another similar set of criteria and applied it to borderline schizophrenics from the Rosenthal adopted-away studies (Rosenthal et al., 1968). Using a cutoff of 2 out of a possible 16 symptoms, 11 of the 14 original borderline schizophrenic patients were considered borderline schizophrenic by their criteria, whereas none of the controls were. Although the separation is impressive, the low cutoff score suggests that these criteria might include items that do not well characterize the majority of relatives of schizophrenics.

In an attempt to address this question, Gunderson and associates (1983) examined the case records of the Danish adoptive study in an attempt to determine which criteria best separated borderline schizophrenics from relatives with non-schizophrenia-related personality disorders. This study suggested that emotional detachment, social isolation, eccentric appearance, social dysfunction, and somatic problems better distinguished the borderline schizophrenics, particularly those related to a chronic schizophrenic proband, from the controls than did psychoticlike symptoms such as recurrent illusions or magical thinking.

Kendler, Gruenberg, and Tsuang (1983) reported similar results from an examinaton of the relatives of the Iowa 500 schizophrenic probands. They suggested that the "negative" symptoms such as decreased rapport and social isolation better distinguished these relatives from those of controls than did the "positive" symptoms such as recurrent illusions, magical thinking, and cognitive distortions. Such "positive" symptoms are observed relatively infrequently in the relatives of schizophrenics, and they often accompany the "unstable" symptoms that are part of the *DSM-III* criteria for borderline personality disorder. In fact, the majority of the patients in Spitzer's survey met the criteria for both disorders. These may be related to affective instability as well as schizotypy and thus seem to be less specific for relatedness to schizophrenia.

In a preliminary study at the Bronx VA Hospital (L. J. Siever, H. Klar, et al., unpublished data) we found that 29 of 57 patients satisfied the *DSM-III* criteria for schizotypal personality disorder according to the SIDP. Of these 29, 13 were diagnosed as having borderline personality disorder. These patients also satisfied the criteria for personality disorders such as histrionic ($N = 7$) and/or antisocial personality disorders ($N = 5$). Conversely, half of the patients diagnosed as having borderline personality disorder (13 of 27) had a concomitant diagnosis of schizotypal personality disorder. Antisocial, histrionic, and paranoid personalities were each observed in a substantial proportion of the schizotypal patients. Thus, in this inpatient population, schizotypal personality disorder frequently coexisted with other disorders, particularly borderline personality disorder. Eighteen of 29 satisfied the RDC criteria for major depressive disorder, although most remitted within the first week of hospitalization. These overlaps may be partially due to the fact that schizotypal individuals may be unlikely to present to a psychiatric inpatient facility unless they have coexisting affective and/or impulse-related psychotherapy.

In another study, J. G. Gunderson, M. Zanarini, and associates (unpublished data) found schizotypal personality disorder to be present in 25% of their borderline sample diagnosed by the DIB, a considerable overlap. Of 15 schizotypal patients, all had borderline personality disorder as well by the DIPD, 67% were histrionic by the DIPD (80% by the PDQ), and 70% were dependent (also by PDQ).

The reliability of this diagnosis, according to Mellsop and Varghesi (1982), is also quite low (κ coefficient of .19). It is diagnosed more frequently in their inpatient population than most other axis II disorders, with the exception of borderline, histrionic, and avoidant personality disorders, and is observed 10 times more frequently than schizoid personality disorder. In the *DSM-III* field trials it was observed slightly more frequently in males than in females, although this difference was not significant (Kass et al., 1983). In contrast to the other studies, it was diagnosed to a lesser degree than schizoid personality. A smaller study of adult outpatients in the Vanderbilt Clinic suggests that it is diagnosed relatively infrequently, as are other disorders of the "odd" cluster. Because of the differing natures of the clinic populations, the low reliability for the diagnosis, and the lack of an operationalized interview in the last study, they are difficult to compare or interpret.

Epidemiology

The epidemiology of schizotypal personality disorder as diagnosed by *DSM-III* is also unknown. Kendler, Gruenberg, and Strauss (1981) found a low incidence among the biological relatives of controls (1.5% for unscreened controls) in the Danish adoptee studies, but this, of course, represented an atypical sample.

Genetic studies

Studies demonstrating a genetic relationship between "borderline" or "latent" schizophrenia and chronic schizophrenia have for the most part been discussed earlier. Kendler and associates (1981) were the first to demonstrate that schizotypal personality disorder, as diagnosed by *DSM-III*, had a higher incidence among the interviewed biological relatives of schizophrenics than among the interviewed biological relatives of controls or the interviewed adoptive relatives of schizophrenics. However, they found that the *DSM-III* criteria for schizotypal personality diagnosed only about half of those designated by Kety and associates (1968), suggesting again that these criteria are not very sensitive for the characteristics observed in the relatives of schizophrenics. Baron (1983) found an increased incidence of schizotypal personality disorder among parents and siblings of schizophrenics, as compared with controls, with two schizotypal parents having a substantially increased risk for schizophrenia in their offspring. Torgerson (1984) observed a higher incidence of schizotypal personality disorder among monozygotic co-twins than among dizygotic co-twins of schizotypal probands, but no cases of schizophrenia in the co-twins. These results suggest that genetic factors are important in the causation of schizotypal personality disorder and that these factors are more likely to result in schizotypal than in schizophrenic psychopathology. Thus, although it appears that the current criteria for schizotypal personality disorder may identify a disorder related, at least in some individuals, to schizophrenia, it may not most sensitively capture the characteristics of these individuals.

Biological markers

Because of the relatedness of schizotypal personality disorder to schizophrenia, which has been studied extensively from a psychobiological vantage point, biological markers have been evaluated in schizotypal individuals to a greater degree than for the other diagnoses in this cluster. Several studies suggest a link between smooth-pursuit eye movement (SPEM) dysfunction and schizotypal characteristics. SPEM dysfunction has been observed rather consistently with a high incidence among schizophrenics (Lipton and Levy, 1983), whereas its presence in the affective disorders has not been clearly evaluated. It may be observed in schizophrenics in remission (Iacono, Tuason, and Johnson, 1981) and appears to be under genetic control (Holzman et al., 1980), suggesting that it may represent a genetic marker for schizophrenia.

Poor eye tracking in a population of normal twins has also been correlated with psychoticism on the Differential Personality Inventory (Iacono and Lykken, 1979) and social introversion and related psychopathology in two separate samples of college volunteers (Siever et al., 1982b). A recent study by Siever and associates (1982a) using the "high-risk strategy" (i.e., identifying individuals on the marker and evaluating their clinical characteristics) demonstrated that the incidence of schizotypal personality disorder was significantly greater in a group of low-accuracy trackers than in a group of high-accuracy trackers in the same college volunteer population. Thus, at least a subgroup of schizotypal individuals share a biological marker with schizophrenics. In this study, low-accuracy trackers were more likely to show characteristics of social introversion, suspiciousness, and decreased rapport than perceptual aberrations or unusual thought patterns, just as was observed in the studies of relatives of schizophrenics.

Baron and associates (1980, 1983) have demonstrated an association between low platelet and plasma monoamine oxidase (MAO) activities and schizotypal personality disorder in the relatives of schizophrenics and in volunteers. Low platelet MAO activity has also been observed in schizophrenics, although this finding may be in part a function of medication.

Braff (1981) examined a cohort of nonmedicated schizotypal patients, as diagnosed by *DSM-III,* with a tachistoscopic backward-masking task and found an information-processing deficit, but not a visual-input defect, in these individuals, similar to that observed in paranoid schizophrenics. Similar results were reported by Sterenko (1978) in schizotypal subjects identified by a schizophreniform 2-7-8 profile on the MMPI.

These studies, although not all using *DSM-III* criteria, converge in suggesting that many schizotypal individuals share psychobiological abnormalities with schizophrenic individuals.

Psychological testing

Investigators have searched for several decades for a psychological test that might identify individuals related to schizophrenics, the "schizoids" or "schizotypes." These have generally not employed the *DSM-III* criteria for schizotypal personality disorder. Golden and Meehl (1979) attempted to identify a "schizoid factor" from the MMPI that would distinguish nonschizophrenic individuals with schizophrenialike characteristics from other nonschizophrenic psychiatric inpatient populations. That profile, however, did not prove useful in distinguishing schizophrenics themselves from controls in another study (Miller and Streinger, 1982).

Chapman, Edwell, and Chapman (1980) have also attempted to develop psychological scales measuring psychosis-proneness. Their physical-anhedonia scale evaluates the degree to which an individual has a deficit in experiencing pleasure, and their perceptual-aberration scale measures the degree of perceptual distortions. Students who score high on the perceptual-aberration scale either may be schizotypal or may show signs of affective lability, whereas those who score high on the physical-anhedonia scale tend to be socially isolated and schizotypal, but may not show perceptual distortions. Thus, it would appear that perceptual aberrations may not be specific for schizotypal individuals, but may also identify individuals with disorders in the affective realm. Furthermore, they do not correlate with physical anhedonia. Simons, MacMillan, and Ireland (1982) have shown that individuals with elevated scores on either of these scales, but particularly on the perceptual-aberration scale, show increased reaction-time crossover, which is characteristic of schizophrenics as well. Decreased electrodermal responsiveness (Simons, 1981) and evoked potentials (Simons, 1982) have also been demonstrated in individuals with physical anhedonia.

Eckblad (1983) identified a group of students on the basis of a magical-ideation scale and found that a significantly greater number of those scoring high on this scale showed schizotypal features, which include magical thinking, by RDC, as compared with controls. His scale correlated highly with perceptual aberration, but not with physical anhedonia. However, his criteria included many items such as "strangers are reading my mind" that might be considered referential, not just magical. Thus one might wonder if it is referential thinking that is truly being assessed on this scale.

Other studies have shown mild memory deficit (Koh and Peterson, 1974) and loosening of personal constructs over time (Higgins and Schwartz, 1976) in schizotypic individuals identified by their aberrant MMPI profiles.

These studies suggest that individuals with schizotypal characteristics can be identified in a volunteer population, although there does not seem to be one scale that will identify these individuals. These individuals show neuropsychological and psychophysiological test responses similar to those of schizophrenics. Perceptual distortions or thought disorder will apparently identify a perhaps more disordered subgroup of schizotypal individuals, but will also identify individuals with affective symptoms, whereas other individuals characterized by constricted affect and social withdrawal may not show perceptual aberrations.

Course of illness and response to treatment

Clinical experience suggests that these patients have a chronic course but may gain limited benefit from psychotherapy. Stone (1983) suggested helping such patients come to terms with their solitary mode of existence and using a reliable, cautious, and systematic approach to therapy without unduly great expectations. Using such an approach with schizotypal patients diagnosed by *DSM-III*, he found that the greater their schizophrenialike symptoms, such as social avoidance or suspiciousness, the less their tendency to improve. However, they were not likely to worsen unless they had marked impairment in reality testing. Prior to the advent of *DSM-III*, numerous dynamically oriented clinicians discussed the problems of psychotherapy with psychotic characters, pseudoneurotic schizophrenia, or borderline states (Frosch, 1964; Knight, 1983), all similar clinically to the current *DSM-III* diagnosis of schizotypal personality disorder, and emphasized the need to protect these patients from psychotic disorganization, rather than attacking defensive systems. However, empirical study of *DSM-III* schizotypal-personality-disordered patients is needed to more objectively evaluate these patients' responses to psychotherapeutic interventions.

There have been few published reports on psychopharmacologic treatment of schizotypal patients. Pseudoneurotic schizophrenics and schizoid patients have been noted to respond to antidepressants, particularly when depressed (Klein, 1967; Hedberg, Houck, and Glueck, 1971), and to neuroleptics when decompensation is pending, although they may show little improvement in more long-standing cognitive disorganization. A recent study of patients with borderline schizotypal personality disorders selected by DIB scores greater than 7 suggested that patients on either haloperidol or imipramine showed greater symptomatic improvement than did those on placebo at 14, 21, and 28 days, but not at 35 days (Soloff et al., 1983). The beginning of a trend for affective instability in the borderlines to respond better to haloperidol than to imipramine has been noted (P. H. Soloff et al., unpublished data).

Considerations for future research

Although more research has been done on schizotypal personality disorder than on the other two personality disorders reviewed here, a number of important questions remain unanswered. It does not appear that items such as magical thinking or recurrent illusions are useful criteria for this disorder, and modifications for these criteria have been suggested (Gunderson et al., 1983). With such a modification of schizotypal personality disorder, is there any further need for schizoid personality disorder, or should the two be collapsed?

Furthermore, psychoticlike symptoms are demonstrable in both borderline and schizotypal personality disorders, but are now included only in the criteria for schizotypal personality disorder. Perhaps the character of the psychoticlike symptoms might distinguish schizotypal patients from borderline patients, just as, for example, the mood congruence of the delusions of grandeur in manic patients can be distinguished from the persecutory delusions observed in paranoid schizophrenics. Persistent referential ideas are more common in schizotypal patients, whereas transient regressions to magical thinking or ideas of reference in the context of frustration in a close interpersonal relationship characterize borderline patients. Individuals with borderline personality disorder having primarily affective psychopathology may show the latter phenomena and thus may satisfy the criteria (e.g., referential, magical thinking) for schizo-typal personality disorder. However, these borderlines often are not socially iso-lated and show no genetic relationship to schizophrenia (Siever and Gunderson, 1979; Siever, 1982), so that, at least in these individuals, a concurrent diagnosis of schizotypal personality disorder may represent a diagnostic misclassification. More research into the discrimination of psychoticlike symptoms in individuals with schizophrenia-related traits from those in individuals with affective or impulse-related psychopathology may prevent such misclassification and improve the separation between borderline and schizotypal personality disorders.

As yet, there have been few systematic studies of family history, biological markers, and responses to treatment among patients with *DSM-III* schizotypal personality disorder. Such studies will be invaluable for better understanding the diagnostic boundaries of this disorder and how it may be treated.

CONCLUSION

Systematic empirical studies of the personality disorders have only recently been initiated, and this is in part because of the attempt to standardize the criteria for these disorders in *DSM-III*. However, most of the criteria for the disorders reviewed here have only limited, if any, empirical basis. We must thus be prepared to modify our diagnostic classifications and criteria signifi-cantly in the face of emerging evidence from empirical studies.

For the three disorders discussed here, it is unclear that the multiplicity of items adds diagnostic sensitivity or specificity for any of these disorders. For example, it is not clear that paranoid personality, defined more simply in terms of a consistent pattern of suspiciousness or mistrust inappropriate to the realistic circumstances and an unwillingness to revise perceptions in light of new infor-mation, would be any less clinically applicable or valid. The manner in which criteria such as these might be operationalized in an interview format will undoubtedly ultimately determine their usefulness. Currently, reliability for the *DSM-III* criteria without such an operationalized interview is low. Although there exist no external validators for paranoid personality disorder, paranoid personality disorder is found in the relatives of patients with delusional disorder. Perhaps an examination of such relatives might permit development of criteria for a more genetically homogeneous population.

Exclusionary criteria might be employed more frequently. For example, in clinical practice, paranoid and schizotypal personality disorders frequently coexist. However, when Kendler and associates (1985) used a hierarchical diag-nostic system in which paranoid personality disorder was diagnosed only in the absence of schizotypal features, paranoid personality disorder was observed more frequently among the relatives of patients with delusional disorder than among the relatives of schizophrenics, in whom the incidence did not differ from that for control relatives. Thus, it may be useful to have the presence of schizotypal personality disorder be an exclusionary criterion for paranoid per-sonality disorder.

It is also not clear that, as currently defined, schizoid personality disorder will prove to be a useful or valid diagnostic category independent of schizotypal or avoidant personality disorder. Schizoid and schizotypal personality disorders might be merged, with social isolation, diminished rapport, constricted affect, and suspiciousness providing the key criteria. Other individuals with relative social isolation might be subsumed under other personality disorders or, if there is no evidence of interpersonal or occupational dysfunction, not considered personality-disordered. Psychoticlike symptoms appear not to be good discriminators for schizotypal personality disorder and are relatively less frequently observed than other criteria for this disorder.

The boundaries between schizotypal and borderline personality disorders also require further clarification, as they overlap in 25%–60% of borderline patients according to current studies. This overlap may in part be attributable to the fact that the psychoticlike symptoms, as they are defined in the *DSM-III* criteria for schizotypal personality disorder, may not be specific for individuals with a personality disorder genetically or even phenomenologically related to schizophrenia. These symptoms apparently may be observed in borderlines with predominantly affective or impulse-related psychopathology, causing unnecessary blurring of boundaries between these disorders. We need careful empirical studies to delineate the character of these symptoms, their mood congruence, and their responsiveness to shifts in relationships. For example, transient referential ideation in relation to the loss of an important other person in borderline personality disorder with cyclothymic features may reflect a different cause than pervasive consistent suspiciousness of others, as observed in some relatives of schizophrenics. Loading psychotic items in the criteria for schizotypal personality disorder may result in the same kind of error that was observed when psychotic symptoms were presumed to be pathognomonic of schizophrenia, and patients with other disorders such as delusional disorder or affective disorder were thus mistakenly diagnosed as having schizophrenia.

It must be emphasized that sample characteristics may have profound influences on the categories of personality disorders and their degrees of overlap observed in a clinical population. Thus, inpatients may differ from outpatients, and some personality disorders may be more common in nonpsychiatric populations.

These suggestions are only tentative, but raise issues for further study in the attempt to better characterize the personality disorders. An attempt to define these disorders by validators such as family history, biological markers, course, and treatment responsiveness will ultimately prove most useful in redefining the criteria for these disorders.

REFERENCES

Baron M: Schizotypal personality disorder: family studies, in Abstracts of the 136th annual meeting of the American Psychiatric Association, 1983, p 141
Baron M, Asnis L, Gruen R, et al: Plasma amine oxidase and genetic vulnerability to schizophrenia. Arch Gen Psychiatry 40:275–282, 1983

Baron M, Leavitt M, Perlman R: Low platelet monamine oxidase activity: a possible biochemical correlate of borderline schizophrenia. Psychiatr Res 3:329–335, 1980

Bleuler M: The Schizophrenic Disorders. Translated by Clemens SM. New Haven, Yale University Press, 1978

Braff DL: Impaired speed of information processing in nonmedicated schizotypal patients. Schizo Bull 7:499–508, 1981

Chapman LJ, Edell WS, Chapman JB: Physical anhedonia, perceptual aberration and psychosis proneness. Schizo Bull 6:639–653, 1980

Chick J, Waterhouse L, Wolff S: Psychological construing in schizoid children grown up. Br J Psychiatry 135:425–430, 1979

Deutsch H: Some forms of emotional disturbance and their relationship to schizophrenia. Psychoanal Q 11:301–321, 1942

Eckblad M: Magical ideation as an indicator of schizotype. J Consult Clin Psychol 51:215–225, 1983

Frosch J: The psychotic character: clinical psychiatric considerations. Psychiatr Q 38:81–96, 1964

Gittelman-Klein R, Klein D: Premorbid asocial adjustment and prognosis in schizophrenia. J Psychiatr Res 7:35–53, 1969

Golden R, Meehl P: Detection of schizoid taxon with MMPI indications. J Abnorm Psychol 88:217–233, 1979

Gunderson JG, Siever LJ, Spaulding E: The search for a schizotype: crossing the border again. Arch Gen Psychiatry 40:15–22, 1983

Guntrip H: Schizoid phenomena, in Object-Relations and the Self. Edited by Sutherland JD. London, Hogarth Press, 1968

Hedberg DL, Houck JH, Glueck BC: Tranylcypromine-trifluoperazine combination in the treatment of schizophrenia. Am J Psychiatry 127:114–146, 1971

Higgins K, Schwartz JC: Use of reinforcement to produce loose construing: differential effects for schizotypic and nonschizotypic normals. Psychol Rep 38:799–806, 1976

Hoch P, Polatin P: Pseudoneurotic forms of schizophrenia. Psychiatr Q 23:248–276, 1949

Holzman PS, Kringler E, Levy DL, et al: Deviant eye tracking in twins discordant for psychosis. Arch Gen Psychiatry 37:637–641, 1980

Iacono WG, Lykken DT: Eye tracking and psychopathology. Arch Gen Psychiatry 36:1361–1369, 1979

Iacono WG, Tuason VB, Johnson RA: Dissociation of smooth-pursuit and saccadic eye tracking in remitted schizophrenics. Arch Gen Psychiatry 38:991–996, 1981.

Kass F, Spitzer RL, Williams JBW: An empirical study of the issue of sex bias in the diagnostic criteria of DSM-III axis II personality disorders. Am Psychol 38:799–801, 1983

Kendler KS, Gruenberg AM: Genetic relationship between paranoid personality disorder and "schizophrenic spectrum" disorders. Am J Psychiatry 39:1185–1186, 1982

Kendler KS, Gruenberg AM, Strauss JS: An independent analysis of the Copenhagen sample of the Danish adoption study of schizophrenia, II: the relationship between schizotypal personality disorder and schizophrenia. Arch Gen Psychiatry 38:982–987, 1981

Kendler KS, Gruenberg AM, Tsuang MT: The specificity of DSM-III schizotypal symptoms, in Abstracts of the 136th annual meeting of the American Psychiatric Association, 1983, p 140

Kendler KS, Masterson CC, Davis KL: Psychiatric illness in first-degree relatives of patients with paranoid psychosis, schizophrenia and medical illness. Br J Psychiatry 147:524–531, 1985

Kety SS, Rosenthal D, Wender PH, et al: The types and prevalence of mental illness in the biological and adoptive families of adopted schizophrenics, in The Transmission of Schizophrenia. Edited by Rosenthal D, Kety SS. Oxford, Pergamon Press, 1968

Khouri PJ, Haier RJ, Reider RO, et al: A symptom schedule for the diagnosis of borderline schizophrenia: a first report. Br J Psychiatry 137:140–147, 1980

Klein DF: Importance of psychiatric diagnosis in the prediction of clinical drug effects. Arch Gen Psychiatry 16:118–126, 1967

Knight R: Borderline states. Bull Menninger Clin 17:1–12, 1983

Koh SD, Peterson RA: Perceptual memory for numerousness in "non psychotic schizophrenics." J Abnorm Psychol 83:215–226, 1974

Kraepelin E: Psychiatrie. Leipzig, 1913

LaRusso L: Sensitivity of paranoid psychosis to nonverbal cues. J Abnorm Psychol 87:463–471, 1978

Lipton R, Levy D: Eye movement dysfunction in psychiatric patients: a review. Schizo Bull 9:13–32, 1983

Longabaugh R, Eldred SH: Premorbid adjustments, schizoid personality and onset of illness as predictors of post-hospitalization functioning. J Psychiatr Res 10:19–29, 1973

Meehl PE: Schizotaxia, schizotypy, schizophrenia. Am Psychol 17:827–838, 1962

Mellsop G, Varghesi F: The reliability of axis II of DSM-III. Am J Psychiatry 139:1360–1361, 1982

Miller H, Streinger D: Use of the Golden-Meehl indicators in the detection of schizoid-taxon membership. J Abnorm Psychol 91:55–60, 1982

Rado S: Dynamics and classification of disordered behavior. Am J Psychiatry 110:406–416, 1953

Theory and therapy: the theory of schizotypal organization and its application to the treatment of decompensated schizotypal behavior, in Psychoanalysis of Behavior, Vol 2. Edited by Rado S. New York, Grune & Stratton, 1962, pp 127–140

Reider RO, Rosenthal D, Wender PH, et al: The offspring of schizophrenics: fetal and neonatal deaths. Arch Gen Psychiatry 32:200–211, 1975

Roff JD, Knight R, Wertheim E: A factor analytic study of childhood symptoms antecedent to schizophrenia. J Abnorm Psychol 85:543–549, 1976

Rosenthal D, Wender PH, Kety SS, et al: Schizophrenics' offspring reared in adoptive homes, in The Transmission of Schizophrenia. Edited by Rosenthal D, Kety SS. Oxford, Pergamon Press, 1968

Siever LJ: Schizoid and Schizotypal Personality Disorders. Baltimore, Williams & Wilkins, 1981, pp 32–64

Genetic factors in borderline personalities, in American Psychiatric Review. Edited by Grinspoon L. Washington, DC, American Psychiatric Press, 1982, pp 437–456

Siever LJ, Coursey RD, Lees R, et al: Physiologic and psychologic correlates of deviant-eye tracking, in Biological Markers in Psychiatry and Neurology. Edited by Hanin I, Usdin E. New York, Pergamon, 1982a, pp 359–370

Siever LJ, Gunderson JG: Genetic determinants of borderline conditions. Schizo Bull 5:59–86, 1979

The search for a schizotypal personality: historical origins and current status. Compr Psychiatry 24:199–212, 1983

Siever LJ, Haier RJ, Coursey RD, et al: Smooth pursuit eye movements in nonpsychotic populations: relationship to other "markers" for schizophrenia and psychological correlates. Arch Gen Psychiatry 39:1001–1005, 1982b

Silverman J: The problem of attention in research and theory in schizophrenia. Psychol Rev 71:352–379, 1964

Simons RF: Electrodermal and cardiac orienting in psychometrically high-risk subjects. Psychiatr Res 4:347–356, 1981

Physical anhedonia and future psychopathology: a possible electrocortical continuity. Psychophysiologia 19:433–441, 1982

Simons RF, MacMillan FW 3rd, Ireland FB: Reaction-time crossover in preselected schizotype subjects. J Abnorm Psychol 91:414–419, 1982

Soloff PH, George AWA, Nathan RS, et al: Pharmacotherapy of borderlines: an empirical trial, in Abstracts of the 136th annual meeting of the American Psychiatric Association, 1983, p 230

Spitzer RL, Endicott J, Gibbon M: Crossing the border into borderline personality and borderline schizophrenia: the development of criteria. Arch Gen Psychiatry 36:17–24, 1979a

Spitzer RL, Forman JBS, Nee J: DSM-III field trials, I: initial interrater diagnostic reliability. Am J Psychiatry 136:815–817, 1979b

Srole L, Langer TS, Michael ST, et al: Mental Health in the Metropolis: The Midtown Manhattan Study. Series in Social Psychiatry, Vol 1. Edited by Rennie TAC. New York, McGraw-Hill, 1962

Stangl D, Pfohl B, Zimmerman M, et al: A structured interview for the DSM-III personality disorders. Arch Gen Psychiatry 42:591–596, 1985

Stephens DA, Atkinson MW, Kay DWK, et al: Psychiatric morbidity in parents and sibs of schizophrenics and non-schizophrenics. Br J Psychiatry 127:97–108, 1975

Torgersen S: Genetic and nosological aspects of schizotypal and borderline personality disorders: a twin study. Arch Gen Psychiatry 41:546–554, 1984

20 *Overview*

NORMUND WONG

In the preceding chapters, four prominent authorities have undertaken the difficult task of reviewing 10 of the 11 *DSM-III* personality disorders. There was extensive discussion from the audience following their presentations. Because of the breadth and comprehensiveness of the authors' approach to so complex a subject, I believe it is useful to provide a descriptive précis of each presentation before summarizing the discussion that was generated.

BORDERLINE, AVOIDANT, DEPENDENT, AND PASSIVE-AGGRESSIVE PERSONALITY DISORDERS

Frances and Widiger regard the inconsistency in how the personality disorders are defined as a major problem. Some of the disorders require that individuals must possess all of the *DSM-III* criteria and therefore use a monothetic approach, whereas other disorders use a polythetic perspective; that is, persons need fulfill only a specific number of all the possible criteria. The definitions of avoidant, dependent, and passive-aggressive personality disorders follow the monothetic principle, whereas the definition of the borderline personality disorder uses the polythetic approach. For greater accuracy, Frances urges the adoption of the polythetic approach for all axis II diagnoses because it conveys the inherent heterogeneity of patients in any given category.

Frances and Widiger devote considerable attention to the borderline personality disorder (BPD), claiming that it has attracted much interest from both clinicians and researchers, in contrast to the other *DSM-III* personality disorders, which have received little systematic investigation. In fact, since the introduction of BPD in *DSM-III,* no other personality disorder has provided as much research data.

Frances and Widiger believe that the classification of BPD is a useful inclusion in *DSM-III* but that its claims as a valid and useful category are overly exaggerated. Not surprisingly, in the current studies, BPD now ranks as the most common of the personality disorders. They attempt to explain this phenomenon by pointing out that the criteria for BPD overlap inextricably with a variety of other personality disorders; even more interesting, it is possible to arrive at the diagnosis of BPD by 93 different ways and still satisfy five of the eight criteria. Therefore, BPD is markedly heterogeneous in its makeup. In light of such overlap and heterogeneity, Frances and Widiger argue that it is not possible at this time to say that descriptive validity has been established for BPD.

In their examination of the existing biological and psychological test data, Frances and Widiger state that at present there is "little support for or against the validity of BPD as a separate syndrome." Long-term prospective studies are not yet available for BPD patients as defined by *DSM-III*. Existing studies support earlier conclusions that BPD patients continue to experience serious impairment and that they may develop an affective disorder but do not develop schizophrenia.

The results of research regarding the developmental history of BPD patients have been contradictory. Some studies have found an increased history of neurodevelopmental deficits, but this conclusion has not been supported by other studies. Instead, a few investigators have found evidence of early family separation and family conflict.

Frances and Widiger also review the treatment modalities and point out that despite the wide range of approaches, there had been "no systematic studies at the time this chapter was written of the responses of *DSM-III*-defined BPD patients to psychotropic drugs or psychotherapeutic interventions." In their concluding comments, they state that a reliable diagnosis can be easily established with the ready availability of operational criteria sets and semistructured instruments; however, although the instruments are reliable, they do not necessarily validate the construct of BPD. Important variables not yet fully accounted for by research include "insufficient attention to the possible important influences on results exerted by sample selection, base rates, and choice of comparison groups." Frances and Widiger believe that the BPD construct does not predict "important aspects of course, family history, biological functioning, treatment response, or etiology." However, no such claims can be said for any of the other personality disorders.

A point made by many of the authors in the chapters on personality disorders is that a patient who meets *DSM-III* criteria for one of the personality disorders may also satisfy the criteria for one or more of the others. Thus, a patient meeting the criteria for an avoidant, dependent, or passive-aggressive personality disorder may also satisfy the criteria for other personality disorders. Frances and Widiger caution that the criteria for each personality disorder are "too circumscribed to convey the full range of behaviors properly included within the syndrome."

The avoidant personality disorder (APD), like other personality disorders, overlaps with other disorders in that category. Frances and Widiger contend that the frequency of this disorder is far greater than reported by their colleagues. They believe that the difference may be due to overlapping of axis I and axis II categories and also that there may be difficulty in clearly distinguishing between the avoidant and schizoid personalities.

A major critique of the *DSM-III* APD definition is that it may be too restrictive, focusing unduly on interpersonal hypersensitivity as the stated cause of the disorder while ignoring equally important factors. Several other interesting questions are raised by Frances and Widiger in discussing the APD. Might APD be but one station in a spectrum of anxiety disorders? Is there significant and real overlap between APD and schizoid personality disorder? In fact, Frances and Widiger suggest broadening the *DSM-III* criteria for APD to include additional causative factors for social-withdrawal behavior besides extreme sensitivity to personal rejection. For example, consideration should be given to one's fear of losing control of certain impulses, of being hurt, and so forth.

In their discussion of dependent personality disorder (DPD), Frances and Widiger point out that some critics believe that the *DSM-III* definition is too sex-biased. Men may be as dependent as women, but their expressions of dependence may differ. They refer back to *DSM-I* and raise the question whether the separation of dependent and passive-aggressive personality disorders is justified. In their opinion, the two categories are sufficiently different to be treated separately. In future definitions of DPD, additional clinical and research data would be of help in developing meaningful criteria regarding what constitutes impairment or a disorder when discussing dependence, submission, and dominance. Conceivably, the description of DPD might be changed so that a different label such as "passive personality disorder" could be used. The present criteria need to be altered to highlight the characteristics of pathological submissiveness and unassertiveness. Finally, Frances and Widiger suggest including additional items for this disorder, such as lack of ambition, unassertiveness, and submissiveness.

In their discussion of the passive-aggressive personality disorder (PAD), Frances and Widiger believe that the criteria for this disorder are too confining and narrow. They call attention to the restrictiveness of the PAD definition. It is only in this disorder that the diagnosis cannot be made in the presence of another personality disorder. They argue for removal of such a strict and seemingly nonsensical requirement. In order to expand the present set of criteria, some masochistic items should be included because of the frequently observed connection between masochism and passive-aggressive traits.

HISTRIONIC, NARCISSISTIC, AND COMPULSIVE PERSONALITY DISORDERS

Arnold Cooper, in reviewing these three personality disorders, establishes early in his discussion that these disorders refer to different levels of observation and inference. The histrionic label refers to "an overt behavioral style, presumably readily observable," the narcissistic refers to "a complex theoretical conception," and the compulsive describes "aspects of both an overt behavior and a theoretical formulation." In systematic fashion, Cooper describes the current incidence and diagnostic reliability for these disorders and shares the current psychiatric literature and opinion concerning each disorder.

Although the *DSM-III* histrionic personality disorder has replaced the *DSM-*

II hysterical personality disorder, Cooper points out that nowhere in the criteria for the histrionic personality disorder is there any mention of sex, seductiveness, provocative behaviors, sexual affairs, or sexual hyperactivity, which runs contrary to the traditional view of this condition. The absence of sexual criteria disturbs many clinicians who regard sexuality as an important conflict with the histrionic patient. He takes further issue with the *DSM-III* definition of histrionic personality disorder, claiming that the current description fails to describe the clinical richness of the syndrome. As it now stands, the term "histrionic personality disorder" describes what Cooper calls a "dramatically infantile" personality and does not convey the full sense and flavor of the hysteric personality.

And because the current histrionic personality disorder basically describes an infantile personality, the full spectrum of the severity of this disorder is not accurately conveyed. The psychiatric literature distinguishes between a "good" and "bad" histrionic personality, the "genital" hysteric and the "oral" hysteric, and the "higher-level" histrionic and the "lower-level" histrionic disorder. To better define the *DSM-III* histrionic personality, Cooper suggests that the disorder be subdivided into two categories with separate criteria to indicate the "better" and "worse" histrionic personalities.

Cooper points out the arbitrary nature by which the diagnosis is made. The polythetic principle used in this disorder requires a choice of three items from column A and two items from column B. He wonders why the combination cannot be changed to four items from column A and two items from column B or "any other combination." But, above all, references to sexuality need to be made, "specifically, to sexuality as a mode of relating to others."

Like BPD, the narcissistic personality disorder (NPD) has captured the interest of the profession. Like BPD, NPD lacks studies to validate the *DSM-III* criteria, but unlike BPD this disorder has fewer studies assessing its reliability. Cooper notes that some outstanding authorities such as Kernberg consider the current *DSM-III* description of the narcissistic personality disorder to be "essentially satisfactory," whereas others (e.g., Vaillant and Perry) think "it will be well to drop narcissistic personality disorder from the nomenclature."

Cooper argues that there are great problems in attempting to define a disorder in terms of set behaviors alone without referring to an underlying or unifying idea or theory. He believes that the current definition of NPD is too one-dimensional and that the attempt to describe this disorder through overt characteristics is inadequate. The addition of an axis VI, to include defense or dynamic mechanisms, may be required to afford a more adequate description of the range of pathological behaviors that stem from difficulties in self-esteem regulation and in differentiation of self and other.

The current literature on NPD emphasizes that these patients show difficulties with the sense of self and regulation of self-esteem. Cooper adds that it is not possible to predict "which self-presentation will be used to defend against painful exposure of these areas of weakness." *DSM-III* describes one group of patients who show overt grandiosity, ambition, exhibitionism, and cool entitlement and exploitiveness, but ignores another group whose overt characteristics may be the reverse. According to Cooper, these individuals demonstrate overt characteristics such as "shyness, an often charming dependence on grander others, an inability to express rage overtly, and ready shame and humiliation when confronted with criticism, often followed by significant feelings of depression." Other authorities (e.g., Bursten, Akhtar, and Thompson) suggest that there are several dimensions to be considered when defining NPD and that both overt and covert behaviors must be taken into account when making the diagnosis.

In his review of the *DSM-II* definition of compulsive personality, Cooper questions the need for or wisdom of changing the label of obsessive–compulsive to compulsive. Compulsive characters also suffer from obsessive doubts, ambivalence, and worry. Among the current *DSM-III* criteria, the item "indecisiveness" is "an excellent description of what is usually meant by obsessional personality characteristics," and removing the term "obsessive" from the disorder creates confusion. Cooper claims that the label "obsessive–compulsive disorder" is more clinically accurate and meaningful than just compulsive personality. The term "compulsive" does not adequately emphasize the extreme ambivalence that is readily observable in obsessional traits and "is always an underlying issue." In summary, he finds the *DSM-III* criteria for compulsive personality too narrow and confining.

PARANOID, SCHIZOID, AND SCHIZOTYPAL PERSONALITY DISORDERS

Siever and Kendler discuss the paranoid, schizoid, and schizotypal personality disorders that have been grouped in *DSM-III* as the "peculiar" or "odd" cluster. Because they all share common criteria that reflect social distance and emotional constriction, these personality disorders exhibit much overlap. The authors examine the historical considerations, diagnostic criteria, differential diagnoses, epidemiology, biological markers, psychological test results, course of illness, treatment progress, and considerations for future research for all three disorders.

There has been little empirical research on the reliability or validity of the *DSM-III* criteria for these conditions, except for the schizotypal personality disorder. The polythetic approach is followed for paranoid personality disorder, and the inclusion criteria fall into three categories, each of which contains four to eight items. Because some of the items are inferential, they are difficult to define operationally and to verify. Clinical studies demonstrate frequent overlap between paranoid personality disorder and other *DSM-III* axis II diagnoses.

The epidemiological studies for paranoid personality disorder show low reliability. Siever and Kendler state that prospective studies using operationalized interviews are required before accurate estimates of the incidence and sex ratio for paranoid personality disorder can be made. Although some studies have suggested that paranoid personality might possibly be genetically related to schizophrenia, Siever and Kendler contend that "a weak familial link may exist between paranoid personality disorder and schizophrenia, but it does not appear to be as strong as the familial link between paranoid personality disorder and delusional disorder." As yet, biological markers have not been systematically studied in paranoid personality disorder. On examining the studies of the paranoid–nonparanoid distinction in schizophrenia, the authors conclude that "the applicability of such studies to paranoid personality disorder, however, remains to be determined." Apparently, no empirical studies exist regarding treatment responses in paranoid personality disorder.

Siever and Kendler claim that the diagnostic usefulness of the *DSM-III* criteria is not enhanced by the multiplicity of criteria and the minimum requirements for each of the three major groupings of characteristics for paranoid personality disorder. They believe that more careful studies of patients with paranoid personality disorder who have relatives with delusional disorder may be helpful in developing valid criteria. They also suggest further studies to refine the features of this disorder and to determine the effectiveness of various treatment modalities.

In their discussion of schizoid personality disorder, Siever and Kendler stress the lack of systematic studies of the *DSM-III* criteria for schizoid personality disorder and point out that the criteria for the disorder are difficult to confirm clinically. They find that the *DSM-III* criteria such as "absence of warm, tender feelings" or "indifference to the feelings of others" are infrequently noted, but when present warrant the diagnosis of avoidant personality disorder or schizotypal personality disorder. No genetic studies of the *DSM-III* schizoid personality disorder have been reported. It is noteworthy, however, that some studies (e.g. Siever, Gittelman-Klein and Klein, and Roff et al.) have suggested that the schizoid personality is not the characteristic premorbid personality of schizophrenics, although it may forecast a less favorable outcome.

No studies to date have examined biological markers in schizoid personality disorders as defined by *DSM-III*, nor have there been studies of psychological tests of individuals who meet the *DSM-III* criteria for schizoid personality disorder. Empirical studies are needed to determine course of illness and treatment response for schizoid patients, but schizoid patients usually are not motivated for treatment and are unlikely to show dramatic change even when treated.

Siever and Kendler think that schizotypal personality and avoidant personality disorders have largely subsumed the schizoid personality disorder. They believe "the schizoid personality disorder needs to be more clearly demarcated from these other disorders, particularly schizotypal personality disorder, and consideration should be given to collapsing these two disorders." There is also the need to develop a category for individuals who are not sufficiently isolated to satisfy the criteria for schizoid personality disorder, but who suffer from a sense of emptiness, difficulty with intimacy, and diffuse identity disturbance; however, they also do not exhibit sufficient self-destructive or impulsive behavior to satisfy the criteria for BPD.

Spitzer and his colleagues have revived the term "schizotypal personality disorder" for *DSM-III*, but Siever and Kendler question whether or not the current criteria describe a valid and clinically distinct category because of the great overlap with other personality-disorder diagnoses when attempting to diagnose schizotypal patients. Siever and his colleagues found a high frequency of anti-social, histrionic, and paranoid personality disorders coexisting in their schizo-typal patients. Gunderson and his colleagues also found that schizotypal per-sonality and borderline personality disorders diagnosed by the DIB showed considerable overlap. The low reliability for diagnosis of schizotypal personality may be explained by the different patient populations studied and the lack of an operationalized interview.

Epidemiological studies of schizotypal personality disorder are lacking; how-ever, there appears to be a genetic relationship between borderline schizophre-nia or schizotypal personality disorder and chronic schizophrenia. Siever and Kendler are careful to state that although the *DSM-III* criteria for schizotypal personality disorder may identify a disorder related to schizophrenia, it still may not capture the essential characteristics of these individuals.

Schizotypal personality disorder has been reviewed more extensively from a psychobiological perspective than have the other personality disorders. Siever and Kendler cite numerous studies that suggest a link between dysfunction in smooth eye-pursuit movement and schizotypal characteristics, studies that describe an association between low platelet and plasma monoamine oxidase activities and schizotypal personality disorder, and studies of the presence of an information-processing deficit similar to that observed in paranoid schizophre-nics. As for psychological tests, the authors conclude that "individuals with schizotypal characteristics can be identified in a volunteer population, although there does not seem to be one scale that will identify these individuals." Schizo-typal personalities appear to have a chronic clinical course and may gain some limited help from psychotherapy. Few published reports have examined psy-chopharmacological therapy for patients with schizotypal personality disorder. Although not diagnosed according to *DSM-III* criteria, some patients labeled with earlier classifications analogous to schizotypal personality disorder have responded to antidepressants and to neuroleptics, but have shown little long-term cognitive improvement.

Siever and Kendler end their review of the schizotypal personality by urging that some items be changed in the current *DSM-III* diagnostic criteria. They state that the items "magical thinking" or "recurrent delusions" are not useful. They question that there is a genuine need to maintain the category of schizoid personality disorder and instead suggest that the schizotypal and schizoid per-sonality disorders be collapsed into one diagnosis. Finally, they stress the need for research to discriminate patients with psychoticlike symptoms with schizo-phrenia-related traits from those persons showing affective- or impulse-related psychopathology and to clarify the boundaries between schizotypal and border-line personality disorders.

SUMMARY OF DISCUSSION FOLLOWING PRESENTATIONS

There was extensive comment on the overlap among many of the per-sonality disorders, such as borderline, histrionic, narcissistic, schizoid, and schizotypal. One suggested solution to resolve this problem was to enlarge or increase the number of dimensions to be considered in making the diagnosis of a personality disorder. The advantages of using an expanded dimensional approach would be as follows: Graduated scales could be used to show the merger between normal personality functioning and the personality disorders; correlations could be made between characteristic items found in the personality disorders and external validators to help explain the overlap between the presence of several personality disorders in one individual; the interaction between the several kinds of vulnerability existing in axis II diagnoses that might be related to the formation or presence of axis I diagnoses could be explained; a more faithful approach could be made to correspond to clinical reality; by offering several dimensions to describe the clinical findings, personality style, and the severity of the disorder, additional data for research purposes could be obtained, particularly if scales could be assigned to each dimension; and lastly, unifying conceptions that would lend a sense of coherence to the items making up the personality disorder could be provided.

Discussants emphasized that a dimensional approach need not be mutually exclusive or contrary to the use of a categorical system. A dimensional system provides a great deal of data that can be readily converted to a categorical system. The dimensional system would describe the personality, and the categorical system would be used to identify the specific pathological syndromes.

An objection was raised that applying the use of a dimensional model to more accurately describe and explain the personality disorders might be useful for the researcher but would prove too cumbersome for the practicing clinician. However, several studies asking clinicians to quantify the severity of a personality syndrome or disorder via the use of rating scales have been carried out without difficulty. Other examples describing successful employment of a dimensional approach were mentioned. Still, many clinicians apparently prefer not to be burdened by additional demands on their time.

As a side issue, one discussant mentioned that defining "personality" is itself intrinsically difficult and that *DSM-III* relies on items such as "significant" impairment in the individual before the diagnosis of a personality disorder can be made. It is also hard to define what is meant by "significant." Its definition implies an understanding of what is enduring and the acceptance that a graded spectrum of disability exists. At present, these concepts remain unclear and are ill-defined in *DSM-III*.

The group acknowledged that many of the personality disorders have not been sufficiently researched and are not being diagnosed as frequently as the anecdotal literature would suggest. A discrepancy exists between what the clinicians intuitively feel they are treating and what they eventually record as the *DSM-III* diagnosis. Perhaps the heated issue of insurance coverage for these disorders has added to the confusion between an actual understanding of the individual and standard diagnostic labeling practice.

In order to arrive at better and more accurate definitions of personality disorders, more sources of information besides questionnaires are necessary. There must be observations of any given patient in a variety of situations over a period of time. A correct diagnosis requires obtaining a sufficient psychiatric history, carrying out longitudinal follow-up, and using external observers or informants.

Further work must be done to arrive at more valid and reliable criteria for the personality disorders. Instead of the current Chinese-menu approach to some personality disorders, perhaps the existing dimensions for all personality disorders should be reexamined consistently and systematically. For example, when making a diagnosis of narcissistic personality disorder, we look at the individual's self-esteem, impulsivity, avoidance and dependence behaviors, and degree of suspiciousness. These and other items should be considered when studying all personality disorders. In addition, in order to provide a coherent approach, we need to focus on clearly defined exclusionary features as well.

Above all, a dimensional approach should provide the clinician and researcher with unifying concepts, not just more data or additional categories that stand alone. We need to differentiate between two types of personality instruments: One type of instrument might measure defense mechanisms and impulse regulation, whereas another type might measure behavior and be operational in nature.

The question was raised whether or not axis II was being overloaded because demands are made on it not only to describe the definition of "personality" but also to indicate the kinds of personality disorders. These issues may be different. Certain personality features that are more clinically salient than other personality characteristics may become part of the personality disorder, whereas the other items may not. Can we describe the relevant and clinical characteristics of personality without implying the existence of psychopathology? Can we then accurately identify specific symptom or item clusters that qualify as syndromes or categories of disorders? To unburden axis II, an additional axis, axis VI, would look specifically at coping mechanisms, characterological patterns, and adaptive and maladaptive behaviors that might cluster into specific personality disorders. Accomplishing these objectives would require the use of graded scales.

The point was made that axis I disorders often can confuse or mask axis II diagnoses. The lack of clarity regarding the overlap between axis I and axis II may interfere with an accurate description of the severity of axis II diagnoses. We might view the personality disorders in a different light and consider placing them into two instead of three clusters as is currently done. At present, the personality clusters consist of the odd or eccentric cluster (paranoid, schizoid, and schizotypal personality disorders), the dramatic or erratic cluster (histrionic, narcissistic, antisocial, and borderline personality disorders), and the anxious or fearful cluster (avoidant, dependent, compulsive, and passive-aggressive personality disorders). Under the new arrangement, the personality disorders would cluster around the psychoses and variations of normal personality. Some personality disorders appear to be related to the psychoses and variations of normal personality. Some personality disorders appear to be related to the psychoses, whereas others bear a resemblance to disorders of normal adaptation. A few personality disorders are quite discontinuous and distinct from patterns of normal adaptation and may require different research methods for their study. In any event, in place of the four or five personality instruments now in use, we should adopt one standard instrument in order to better coordinate our future research.

Another important issue raised during the discussion was the relationship between adult and childhood disorders. If we consider personality features as blending into personality disorders, how do such concepts apply to children? It is difficult to apply some *DSM-III* criteria to children when trying to arrive at an axis II diagnosis. Current research has shown that some personality disorders may be the residue of axis I affective disorders. Thus, these disorders may not be separate categories. Up to now, the philosophy of the planners of *DSM-III* has been that childhood conditions show less stability than adult disorders. The predictive power in childhood has been less than the predictive power in adulthood. Therefore, the *DSM-III* committee purposely made it difficult to diagnose personality disorders in children. It follows that if a personality disorder appears to be present following an episode of affective illness, it should not be diagnosed separately, but its features should be included under the affective disorder.

There are also cases in which a personality disorder may precede, or result from, or be an expression of, another disorder. In some instances, the existence of an affective disorder in personality disorder may be coincidental. *DSM-III* has attempted to adopt an atheoretical approach and asks that clinicians focus on clinical observation and avoid making assumptions about a disorder's cause in light of our current knowledge. However, it must be conceded that personality disorders do not arise de novo overnight, and they should be traceable back to childhood.

An array of questions and comments focused on specific personality diagnoses. One person pointed out that the *DSM-III* BPD is in many ways similar to the picture of the histrionic personality. The borderline, histrionic, and infantile personality disorders tend to overlap in their descriptions. Using the *DSM-III* criteria, it is possible to make a diagnosis of three or four personality disorders in an individual. One wonders if the overlap of numerous personality disorders is valid and logical. The comment was made that perhaps the high frequency of BPD found in clinical surveys may be related more to sample selection and base rates than to the actual incidence of the disorder. The incidence of BPD is much higher among those patients in intensive psychotherapy, in contrast to the low incidence of BPD found among patients not in intensive treatment. Although there appears to be a positive and strong correlation between BPD and affective disorder, we should be careful not to equate unhappiness and sadness with an affective disorder.

The diagnosis of narcissistic personality disorder should be reserved for individuals whose primary adaptive mode centers around the issue of self-esteem. We should remember that problems of self-esteem are present in every severe form of psychopathology. Ascertaining the underlying conflict of the narcissistic disorder frequently is quite difficult.

The diagnosis of avoidant personality, unlike the situation for the other personality disorders, relies on the presence of a single mechanism – a conditioned avoidance behavior. However, there may be different drives or affects underlying the avoidant behavior. It is important to distinguish between phobic avoidance and other kinds of avoidance. In phobic avoidance, the adversant effect of anxiety is being avoided. But people may avoid because of other affects, such as shame, shyness, or embarrassment. In addition, the response in the avoidant personality is almost entirely related to interpersonal relationships in which people attempt to govern their behavior by avoiding certain affective states. We should also keep in mind that a great deal of avoidant behavior in depressives overlaps with social phobia on axis I.

A plea was made for formal recognition of the existence of many low-level inferences and basic dynamic theory that help us understand our clinical observations about personality disorders. They should not be ignored, and perhaps even additional inferences should be included in the *DSM*. There is clinical agreement about many underlying issues that exist within the personality disorders. For example, most clinicians assume the presence of underlying fear and rage in patients with obsessive–compulsive disorders. In histrionic personalities functioning at a high level, we see sexual issues; in low-level-functioning histrionic patients, we encounter many infantile issues. Similar problems exist for narcissistic personality disorders.

Finally, the suggestion was made that the revised *DSM* include a masochistic personality disorder and depressive personality disorder. There are significant clinical distinctions between the masochistic and depressive personality disorders, although both disorders may be mixed in a given patient. One of the differentiating features between patients with depressive personality disorder and those with masochistic personality disorder is that the former tend to be in agony, suffering from self-torture, whereas the latter tend to provoke punishment from others and engage ultimately in self-defeating behavior.

REFERENCES

Frances A: The DSM-III personality disorder section: a commentary. Am J Psychiatry 137:1050–1054, 1980

Categorical and dimensional systems of personality diagnosis: a comparison. Compr Psychiatry 23:516–527, 1982

Frances A, Cooper AM: Descriptive and dynamic psychiatry: a perspective on DSM-III. Am J Psychiatry 138:1198–1202, 1981

Kendler KS, Gruenberg AM, Strauss JS: An independent analysis of the Copenhagen sample of the Danish adoption study of schizophrenia, II: the relationship between schizotypal personality disorder and schizophrenia. Arch Gen Psychiatry 38:982–987, 1981

Kendler, KS, Gruenberg AM, Tsuang MT: The specificity of DSM-III schizotypal symptoms, in Abstracts of the 136th annual meeting of the American Psychiatric Association, 1983, p 140

Mellsop G, Varghese F, Joshua S, et al: The reliability of axis 2 of DSM-III. Am J Psychiatry 139:1360–1361, 1982

Millon T: Disorders of Personality DSM-III: Axis 2. New York, Wiley, 1981

Siever LJ: Genetic factors in borderline personalities, in American Psychiatric Review. Edited by Grinspoon L. Washington, DC, American Psychiatric Press, 1982, pp 437–456

Siever LJ, Gunderson JG: Genetic determinants of borderline conditions. Schizophr Bull 5:59–86, 1979

The search for a schizotypal personality: historical origins and current status. Compr Psychiatry 24:199–212, 1983

Siever LJ, Haier RJ, Coursey RD, et al: Smooth pursuit eye movements in non-psychotic populations: relationship to other "markers" for schizophrenia and psychological correlates. Arch Gen Psychiatry 39:1001–1005, 1982

PART VI

Disorders of infancy, childhood, and adolescence

It is safe to say that all the problems inherent in assessing, classifying, and diagnosing psychopathology in adults also exist in children. Problems of reliability and validity of diagnostic criteria, boundary problems between diagnoses, the influence of age of onset on the phenomenology of a particular disorder, and the complex interaction among psychopathology, personality, and environmental stressors are among the more important issues that have been highlighted in this volume. In child psychiatry, these issues are complicated still further by the fact that children (for this discussion, "childhood" encompasses infancy through adolescence unless otherwise specified) are rarely self-referred. Whereas it is always useful to obtain information about an adult patient from significant others, it is imperative that one do this for children. Moreover, the younger children are, the more difficult it is to obtain diagnostically meaningful information from them. Therefore, assessment techniques, with all the reliability and validity issues related to them, must be used for parents, teachers, and children. In addition, the way one elicits information from a 3-year-old is very different than for a 15-year-old. On the other hand, it has become clear that children are important sources of information regarding their own thoughts and feelings and must be questioned precisely, rather than simply having impressions drawn from their play. Finally, there is the question whether or not the phenomenology elicited from a child at one age has the same diagnostic significance at another age. Setting a place at the table for the imaginary friend of a 4-year-old has a very different implication than it does for a 16-year-old.

In spite of these complexities, there is no doubt that childhood is in the same continuum of growth as adulthood. There is no single, arbitrary time (except those that are imposed legally) when childhood ends and adulthood begins. Thus, the *DSM-III* implication in delineating the childhood-disorders section as "disorders usually first evident in infancy, childhood, or adolescence" is that these may and in fact often do continue in adulthood. On the other hand, there is also the implication (and in some cases the frank statement) that other disorders (e.g., organic mental disorders, substance-use disorders, schizophrenic, "neurotic," and personality disorders) are not first evident in childhood or adolescence. This is, of course, untrue. Personality disorders do not sprout de novo at age 18, nor does it make sense to change the name of a problem depending on the person's age. In addition, developmental disorders often do not disappear. Although the *DSM-III* clearly states that specific developmental disorders in children "should be noted when an adult still has clinically significant signs of the disorder," I doubt that this occurs. A 25-year-old woman who has been in the mental health system since age 18, when her self-mutilating behavior came to light, had been diagnosed simply as "borderline." In *DSM-III* terms, she could be seen to fit in two categories: schizotypal personality disorder (occasional spells of magical thinking; illusions of her dead mother, who committed suicide; odd speech; hypersensitivity to criticism) and borderline personality disorder (episodes of intense anger, affective instability, self-mutilation, intolerance of being alone). In reality, this woman has had episodes of major depression and hypomania (and, on lithium, her episodic psychotic symptoms were considerably abated), but, in addition, she has such severe developmental language problems that the neuropsychologist who tested her was amazed that she was functioning at all. Although she is not retarded, her receptive and expressive language abilities were at a level for someone five to eight years old. Oddities of speech, frustration, intolerance, and sensitivity to criticism are not surprising under the circumstances. Nowhere in her three-volume record was any mention made of this (except to say that her spelling, grammar, and handwriting were bad). Nor had anyone asked her about her school history, which had included "special classes for dyslexia from grade school through high school." The question where and how to match symptoms with criteria (e.g., Is it appropriate to take symptoms that were used to meet criteria for major depression and language disorder and reinterpret them for a personality disorder?) has not been addressed in regard to adult or child psychopathology. When signs and symptoms have to be viewed with a developmental perspective, lack of knowledge about that perspective muddies the water still further.

Given the complexities associated with the diagnosis and classification of psychological disorders in children and adolescents, it would be extremely difficult to cover all the disorders found in *DSM-III*. Rather, we have elected to focus on three areas in this Part VI: childhood psychosis, depression in children, and conduct disorder. We think the issues raised by the authors in all three chapters can be generalized to the other childhood (and adult) disorders as well.

Gabrielle A. Carlson

21 Pervasive developmental disorders and schizophrenia occurring in childhood

A review of critical commentary

LYNN WATERHOUSE, DEBORAH FEIN,
JUDY NATH, AND DENISE SNYDER

Even as the *DSM-III* diagnostic criteria for subclassifying pervasive developmental disorders (PDD) and schizophrenia occurring in childhood (SOC) are beginning to be more widely used in both research (Table 21.1) and clinical practice, and even though these criteria have been lauded for their clarity and specificity by both researchers (Rutter and Shaffer, 1980) and clinicians, various problems with these diagnostic criteria are beginning to be identified. Current critical thinking includes proposals for additions to and formal reorganizations of diagnostic categories and criteria, as well as specific criticisms of categories and criteria. The proposals and criticisms can be grouped into five general areas of concern, as follows:

1. There exist children whose types of psychiatric-developmental impairment either have not been represented or have been inadequately represented in *DSM-III*, and therefore additional diagnostic subcategories or additional diagnostic criteria may be needed (Cantor, Trevenen, and Postuma, 1979; Cantor et al., 1980, 1981, 1982; Rutter and Shaffer, 1980; Noll and Benedict, 1982; Petty et al., 1984).
2. There are important issues concerning developmental processes and cognitive developmental delay that have not been adequately addressed in the *DSM-III* criteria (Rutter and Shaffer, 1980; Tanguay, 1984).
3. There are criteria that define subcategories and criteria that provide diagnostic boundaries between subcategories of PDD, and between PDD and SOC, that may be difficult to interpret and apply (Brown, 1983; Waterhouse and Snyder, 1983).
4. There are low interrater reliabilities for the subcategories of PDD and SOC and for the general PDD category as a whole (Cantwell et al., 1979a,b; Mattison et al., 1979; Williams and Spitzer, 1980; Hyler, Williams, and Spitzer, 1982).
5. Other empirically derived sets of subcategories could be constructed that might distinguish groups of children with severe psychopathology with greater validity than those presently proposed in *DSM-III* (Achenbach, 1980; Rutter and Shaffer, 1980; Waterhouse and Snyder, 1983; Tanguay, 1984; Fein et al., 1985; Ornitz, 1985; Waterhouse, Wing, and Fein, in press).

These criticisms are not unique to the *DSM-III* diagnostic criteria for subcategories of PDD and SOC. In fact, similar criticisms were voiced for nearly

335

Table 21.1. *Survey of diagnostic systems employed in research on severe childhood psychopathology published during five years (1978–82) in 10 journals*[a]

	1978	1979	1980	1981	1982	1978–82
Total number of relevant articles	22	23	29	27	28	129
Total number of diagnostic systems	38	27	48	35	43	191
Type of diagnosis						
Autism	31	19	39	27	35	151
Researcher-selected features	2	4	3	5	3	17
Clinical interview	2	4	3	3	1	13
DSM-III (1980)	1	0	7	7	9	24
Creak (1961, 1963, 1964)	5	0	2	1	1	9
Kanner (1943)	4	1	4	2	4	15
Ornitz and Ritvo (1968, 1976)	2	0	4	1	0	7
Ritvo and Freeman (NSAC) (1978)	1	0	3	1	3	8
Rutter (1966, 1968, 1972, 1974, 1977, 1978)	11	8	4	7	11	41
All others	3	2	8	1	3	17
Other childhood psychoses	7	8	9	8	8	40
Researcher-selected features	2	1	3	3	2	11
Clinical interview	3	3	1	3	2	12
DSM-II (1968)	0	1	1	0	0	2
DSM-III (1980)	0	0	0	2	1	3
Creak (1961, 1963, 1964)	2	1	2	0	3	8
All others	0	2	2	0	0	12

[a]*American Journal of Orthopsychiatry, Archives of General Psychiatry, Brain and Language, Developmental Medicine and Child Neurology, Journal of Abnormal Child Psychology, Journal of the American Academy of Child Psychiatry, Journal of Autism and Developmental Disorders, Journal of Child Psychology and Psychiatry and Allied Disciplines, Journal of Nervous and Mental Disease,* and *Schizophrenia Bulletin.*

all prior sets of criteria delineating syndromes of severe childhood psychopathology (DeMyer et al., 1971; Rimland, 1971; Bomberg, Szurek, and Etemad, 1973; Prior et al., 1975; Goldfarb, 1977; Cohen et al., 1978; Evans-Jones and Rosenbloom, 1978; Freeman et al., 1978). However, because the *DSM-III* criteria for subgrouping serious childhood psychopathology (Table 21.2) to some degree reflect the problematic state of diagnostic classification that currently

Table 21.2. *DSM-III classifications for severe childhood psychopathology*

Term	Onset	Diagnostic criteria
Pervasive developmental disorders		

Infantile autism
  Full syndrome
  Residual state
	Before 30 months	Serious lack of social response; gross language deficit; bizarre features of speech; absence of thought disorder

Childhood-onset pervasive developmental disorder
  Full syndrome
  Residual state
	30 months to 12 years	Severely disturbed emotional relationships; three or more of the following: excessive anxiety, inappropriate affect, resistance to change, oddities of motor movement, prosodic abnormalities, abnormal sensitivity to sensory stimuli, self-mutilation; absence of thought disorder

Atypical pervasive developmental disorder	Not specified	Distortions in the development of multiple basic psychological functions; does not meet the diagnostic criteria for IA or COPDD
Schizophrenia occurring in childhood[a]		

Schizophrenic disorders in childhood (types)
  Disorganized
  Catatonic
  Paranoid
  Undifferentiated
  Residual
	Deterioration from a previous level of functioning	Presence of at least 1 of 10 patterns of hallucinations, delusions, or loosening of associations or poverty of content of speech if associated with aberrant affect, delusions or hallucinations, or catatonic or other grossly disorganized behavior; impairment of 2 or more routine functions; duration of state of at least six months

[a]As per schizophrenic disorders outlined for adults.

exists within the field, the *DSM-III* PDD and SOC syndromes and their attendant criteria have thus naturally inherited the critical concerns of those working in the field. Whether or not changes in the structure or criteria of these classifications can address these concerns at the present time without further research is the central focus of this chapter.

In examining the five major critical concerns outlined earlier, we consider four types of information relevant to evaluating these concerns. First, the particulars of the criticisms of the *DSM-III* classifications are outlined. Second, where a concrete proposal concerning possible new diagnostic criteria or subcategories has been made, the relationship of this proposal to any *DSM-III* PDD syndrome is considered. Third, the viewpoint inherent in the criticism is explored from a historical perspective. Finally, the potential functional changes in PDD and SOC subcategories that might be effected by implementation of new criteria or procedures are evaluated.

PROPOSALS FOR ADDITIONS

Recent articles have called for explicit addition of two distinct sets of criteria: one for a "new" syndrome of PDD and another for an elaboration of the SOC classification proposed within *DSM-III*. Noll and Benedict (1982) argued that the category "developmental psychosis" should be added to the sub-categories of PDD, and Cantor and associates (1979, 1980b, 1981, 1982) argued that the *DSM-III* criteria for SOC are inadequate because there exist children who manifest symptoms typical of schizophrenia but in whom such disorders were manifested quite early in life, without being preceded by a period of ade-quate functioning. Both Noll and Benedict and Cantor and associates argued that for the groups of children they studied (Noll and Benedict, 1982, $N = 6$; Cantor et al., 1982, $N = 7$), there are no *DSM-III* syndromes that accurately capture critical features of onset and developmental and behavioral disorders common within these groups.

In addition to these two claims, Rutter and Shaffer (1980) asserted that the category of disintegrative psychosis is poorly served in *DSM-III* by being shifted to classification by coding under dementia. They claimed that the clinical fea-tures of disintegrative psychosis are different from the clinical features of adult dementia. They also claimed that the requirement of diagnostic certainty about organic brain disease for determining dementia will exclude children who would be diagnosable as having disintegrative psychosis on the basis of behav-iors, but who show no evidence of organic brain damage (Evans-Jones and Rosenbloom, 1978).

Developmental psychosis

Noll and Benedict argued that there exists a subgroup of children who "show a developmental pattern of autistic symptoms followed by schizophrenic symptoms" (1982, p. 187). They further claimed that whereas any child with severe psychopathology seen after the age of three years but before the age of seven years may appear to be either more "autistic" or more "schizophrenic," in order for that child to be classified as having developmental psychosis, the child should show a course of developmental symptomatological change during this period (age three to seven years) such that predominantly autistic behaviors give way to predominantly schizophrenic behaviors. Furthermore, they pro-posed that to receive a diagnosis of developmental psychosis, a child should not suffer from "significant cognitive retardation" (Noll and Benedict, 1982, p. 189). In addition, these authors claimed that because a majority of children they have identified as having developmental psychosis come from homes where severe psychopathology has been found in other family members (65% of siblings, 22% of fathers, 46% of mothers), the presence of attendant family psychopathology – though not to be a diagnostic requisite – should serve as a possible index for differential diagnosis.

A child with developmental psychosis would not meet the diagnostic criteria for childhood-onset pervasive developmental disorder (COPDD), because COPDD symptoms have a later onset (between 30 months and 12 years) than would be seen in developmental psychosis; nor would such a child meet the diagnostic criteria for SOC, because the *DSM-III* criteria for SOC include the specification of "deterioration from previous level of functioning" – something that could not be said to be true of a child identified as having developmental psychosis unless all previous pathological symptoms were to be ignored. At present, apparently, such a child would have to be assigned the diagnosis of atypical pervasive developmental disorder (APDD).

There are two limitations that affect the strength of Noll and Benedict's claim for the existence of developmental psychosis: sample size and diagnostic criteria. Noll and Benedict identified only six children and presented only a single case study in their report, and the behaviors they interpreted as evidence of schizophrenic symptoms included fragmented speech, irrelevancies, verbalized fantasies, distorted grammar, and obsessive play. Whether or not such behaviors can be interpreted as meeting the (implied) *DSM-III* criteria for evidence of schizophrenia in these children is not clear.

Despite these limitations, the category of developmental psychosis as defined by Noll and Benedict does include three criterial features that support a distinction made earlier in work done by Goldfarb (1961, 1964). In a study of 30 severely psychotic children, Goldfarb divided the children into two groups on the basis of presumptive cause: organic and nonorganic. Whereas both groups had an early onset of symptoms, the nonorganic group had higher (though still delayed when compared with normal children) cognitive functioning than did the organic group, and the nonorganic group had a greater incidence of impaired family functioning. Thus, children thought by Noll and Benedict to have developmental psychosis share with Goldfarb's nonorganic severe psychotics the triad of early onset, higher cognitive functioning (including early expression of some language skills), and more family disorders.

Although Goldfarb's finding of an organic–nonorganic distinction was not replicated (Gittelman and Birch, 1967), it may nonetheless be true that Noll and Benedict have identified a nonorganic population similar to that identified earlier by Goldfarb.

Recently, we found a subgroup of children, previously identified as autistic or schizophrenic (though not by *DSM-III* criteria) who had better language skills than other children in the sample studied and also showed evidence of family disorders (Waterhouse and Snyder, 1983). We also found a significant contingency coefficient for association between past clinical diagnoses of autism and present clinical diagnoses of schizophrenia in the same sample (where we did not find the reverse – schizophrenia diagnosed earlier and then autism later – to be significant). However, though we did follow these children longitudinally, our research focus was on cognitive development; so we have no behavioral-observation data that might address the question of change in symptoms over time.

It is important to consider that before Goldfarb's research, Bender (1953, 1956) argued that infantile autism is an early state of schizophrenia, and she applied the term "early autistic schizophrenia" to her study populations. Ten years ago, Bender and Faretra (1973) designated autism as a subsyndrome of childhood schizophrenia and claimed that childhood schizophrenia does lead to adult schizophrenia.

It is also important to note that there has been a wide range of theoretical constructs proposed to explain the possible relationship between infantile autism and childhood schizophrenia. Whereas Kanner, in his seminal article (1943), argued that autism can be distinguished from schizophrenia in both children and adults by being innate, he later hypothesized that autism represents the "earliest possible manifestation of childhood schizophrenia" (Kanner, 1949, p. 421) and concluded that autism is not separable from the schizophrenias. Rimland (1964) argued that autism and schizophrenia are polar variants of an inability to relate new stimuli to new or remembered experiences, and Ornitz and Ritvo (1968, 1976) postulated that early infantile autism, childhood schizophrenia, and other psychoses of childhood are all variants of a unitary disease impairing homeostatic regulation of sensory input and disrupting perceptual integration.

At present there is no clear pattern of empirical evidence outlining either the relationship between infantile autism and childhood schizophrenia or the relationship between these two childhood psychoses and adult schizophrenia. Whereas there are researchers who have argued that adult schizophrenics and child "psychotics" share similar deficits (Fish, 1977), there are other researchers who believe that they have found significant differences in symptoms between the two groups (DeMeyer et al., 1973; Piggot and Gottlieb, 1973). According to DeMyer, Hingtgen, and Jackson (1981), "whether [or not] infantile autism is the earliest expression of schizophrenia" must be addressed by "systematic longitudinal study and comparison of adult autistics and adult schizophrenics, a study that has never been done" (DeMyer et al., 1981, p. 397).

It must be noted, however, that Noll and Benedict did not define a category that changes with the transition from childhood into adulthood, but rather defined symptoms in a group of children who, they believe, cross from autism to schizophrenia in early middle childhood.

Petty and associates (1984) reported that they found three children who had been diagnosed as autistic before the age of 5 years, but who "lost" their autistic symptoms between ages 5 and 12 and developed symptoms of schizophrenia during that period. Petty and associates claimed that the three children had early symptoms that would support a diagnosis of infantile autism, but that subsequently all three children developed symptoms criterial to a diagnosis of schizophrenia, including hallucinations, delusions, and various forms of thought disorders. According to Tanguay, who discussed their findings, "In such instances the children could be diagnosed initially as autistic, later as autistic residual, and even later as schizophrenic, but one wonders what such a metamorphosis may imply about the specificity of each of these labels" (Tanguay, 1984).

Noll and Benedict did not offer any vision of ultimate prognoses for children diagnosed as having developmental psychosis, but they did suggest that family and individual therapy might help these children more than such intervention would help autistic children.

If added to the *DSM-III* PDD section, Noll and Benedict's proposed subcategory might stand alone as a wholly separate syndrome or could represent a special subdivision of infantile autism, or it might even define an elaboration of SOC. In whatever form the syndrome might be included, its attendant diagnostic criteria would have to consist of (1) an outline of the explicit developmental symptom changes expected, (2) some boundary specification of the "higher language and general cognitive functioning" that would be expected, and (3) some note of the possible presence of family disorders.

Childhood schizophrenia

In a recent series of articles, Cantor and associates (1979, 1980b, 1981, 1982) identified a group of children who show both symptoms criterial to schizophrenia and evidence of neuromuscular dysfunction. These researchers believed that both the psychiatric disorder and the motor disorder stem from a common pathogenic origin – cholinergic dysfunction (Cantor et al., 1980b). They labeled these children as hypotonic schizophrenics.

In a sample of 30 adolescents, Cantor and associates (1982) found that 7 of the 30 had clearly documented onset of psychotic symptoms before the age of 30 months, and only 6 of the 30 had histories of normal language development. Cantor and associates claimed that childhood schizophrenia does exist and should be explicitly defined in *DSM-III* within the PDD section. Implicit in their argument is the idea that the criteria for onset for SOC (when defined within the PDD section) should indicate that the onset could be at any time from very early childhood to puberty.

Cantor and associates asserted that "DSM-III has placed thought disorder . . . in children within the group of schizophrenias. However, since one of the inclusion criteria for a diagnosis of schizophrenia is 'deterioration from a previous level of functioning,' the small number of children with schizophrenia-like illness whose development has been disordered since infancy . . . are not accounted for" (1982, p. 758).

These researchers further argued that though they found some differences in clinical pictures for younger and older childhood schizophrenics, these symptoms were functions of developmental effects, not expressions of different disorders.

In their description of the sample of 30 children, however, Cantor and associates (1982) did not offer any analysis that compared the symptoms and behaviors of the 7 children found to have onset before 30 months with those of the 23 children and young adults who showed evidence of onset between 30 months and 12 years of age. Furthermore, when Cantor and associates (1982, Table 2, p. 759) did report frequencies of previously determined schizophrenic symptoms for their population of 30 children (4 individuals had shown incoherence, 4 had shown "thought disorder," and 5 had shown hallucinations or delusions), their report did not make clear whether the three symptom subgroups (of 4, 4, and 5 individuals) included the same individuals who had expressed a wide range of symptoms or if each instance indexed a separate individual. Also, it is not clear if any of the 7 early-onset children are included among the three symptom subgroups. An additional problem is that they did not specify exactly what behaviors of the children were coded as evidence for the presence of incoherence, "thought disorder," hallucinations, or delusions.

Most important, however, is that for neither previously determined symptoms (their Table 2) nor presently determined symptoms (their Table 4) did these researchers outline the symptoms for the 7 early-onset individuals separate from the symptoms for those 23 for whom later onset was reported. Although they clearly showed that all 30 children in their sample had good eye contact and thus would be unlikely to be accurately diagnosed as autistic, it would be of great interest to see what differences might have been found in autistic versus schizophrenic symptoms for early- and later-onset groups within their sample.

It is important to note that Cantor and associates stated that they did not find any children who showed evidence of schizophrenia who did not also show evidence of neuromuscular dysfunction. However, they saw "the converse – children who manifest the physical signs but who are not psychotic. Such children have an assortment of learning, language and behavioral disturbances" (1982, p. 762). What they have thus suggested is that there is a continuum of cholinergic dysfunction, the primary symptoms of which are manifested neuromuscularly, with a continuum of attendant psychopathology.

Just how this group of children may relate to previously identified groups of schizophrenic children is not clear. Both Bender (1953) and Fish (1961) identified hypotonia in schizophrenic children and infants at risk for schizophrenia. Historically, however, because the label childhood schizophrenia has been attached to a rather wide variety of diagnostic criteria (Werry, 1979; DeMyer et al., 1981), it is not possible to determine if Cantor and associates' hypotonic schizophrenics would form a subgroup of the previously defined childhood schizophrenics. Furthermore, given that the *DSM-II* label childhood schizophrenia was a more global label than the presently outlined SOC in *DSM-III*, and given the fact that researchers working in the past five to seven years have concentrated nearly all their investigative efforts on studying groups of children classified as having infantile autism (Table 21.1), information concerning the possible character of childhood schizophrenia is both scant and confusing.

Cantor and associates themselves argued that the earlier, more global deficit of childhood schizophrenia proposed by Creak (1964), which "subsumed three diagnoses [of *DSM-III*], i.e., Infantile Autism, Childhood Onset Pervasive Developmental Disorder, and Schizophrenic Disorder" (Cantor et al., 1981, p. 8), was the most adequate diagnostic scheme for describing their sample of 8 children. Creak and the British working party, however, intended their nine-point diagnostic scheme for determining childhood schizophrenia to serve as a means of identifying all children who had childhood psychosis. Still more confusing, the Creak nine-point checklist has been used as a means to differentially diagnose autism, schizophrenia, and childhood psychosis (Table 21.1) (Schopler et al., 1980; Freeman and Ritvo, 1981).

If the category of hypotonic schizophrenia were to be added to *DSM-III*, the diagnostic criteria for the category should include (1) a stipulation that functioning might have deteriorated or might have been consistently poor throughout development and (2) a careful description of the neuromuscular problems outlined by Cantor and associates. However, if a specific SOC set of diagnostic criteria were to be outlined (whether within or outside the PDD), it is not clear, given the sample size of Cantor and associates' studied group, whether hypotonic schizophrenia might supplant all of SOC or whether such a syndrome might be seen as a subclassification of SOC. Beyond these possible considerations, the fact that Cantor and associates saw Creak's criteria as a reasonable means of diagnosis for their sample's syndrome suggests that the diagnosis of hypotonic schizophrenia would have to cross PDD diagnostic boundaries rather than simply occupy a position within SOC.

Disintegrative psychosis

Rutter and Shaffer (1980) argued that the category of disintegrative psychosis should be treated as it is in *ICD-9* (World Health Organization, 1978), rather than being shifted to coding under dementia as it is in *DSM-III*. They based their claim largely on research done by Evans-Jones and Rosenbloom (1978). Evans-Jones and Rosenbloom studied 10 children diagnosed as having disintegrative psychosis. They defined the syndrome as one in which "normal or near normal development for the first 2½ years is followed by a severe disintegration involving severe disorder of emotions, behaviour and relationships and often a loss of speech" (1978, p. 462). These authors traced the history of identification of this syndrome from Heller (1930) to Anthony (1958) to Kolvin (1971).

Despite their stated definition of disintegrative psychosis, however, Evans-Jones and Rosenbloom included in their sample of 10 children three for whom onset of symptoms had occurred before the age of 2½. Furthermore, though the syndrome was originally outlined to identify children who were thought to have serious organic brain disease with associated developing psychopathology, of the sample of 10 children studied by Evans-Jones and Rosenbloom, only half showed any signs of organic brain abnormalities. All of the 10 were severely mentally retarded, with some "islets of cognitive skill" remaining. These authors further associated the onset of symptoms for 8 of the 10 children with a point of life stress, variously determined as "sister's marriage," "hospital admission," and "birth of a sibling" (1978, Table II, p. 463).

Of the three children who showed onset earlier than usually described for the syndrome, one had normal EEG results, another had grossly abnormal EEG results, and the third apparently was not tested. Neither of the two children who were given EEGs were reported to have experienced any serious life stress near the time of onset of symptoms, but the child not given an EEG had suffered a head-injuring fall immediately prior to onset of symptoms.

The problems with this study – as with that of Noll and Benedict and those of Cantor and associates – were small sample size and problematic presentation of symptoms. The combination of few subjects and symptoms that were either loosely described or described in a fashion that did not permit unequivocal interpretation did not allow for clear confirmation of the syndrome defined.

The syndrome of "disintegrative psychosis" as outlined by Evans-Jones and Rosenbloom, if added to the *DSM-III* PDD section, would bridge across infantile autism (IA), COPDD, and possibly APDD, as well as (adult) dementia and SOC. If inserted in the PDD section it most likely would necessitate the creation of another PDD syndrome, and that syndrome would have to have two subdivisions. The new category, "disintegrative psychosis–dementia type," would include those children with clear evidence of brain damage, and "disintegrative psychosis–presumptively non-dementia type" would include those children with no clear evidence of brain damage. Both types of disintegrative psychosis would have to include for diagnosis children with a wide range of symptoms, and would have to specify some range of onset for those symptoms.

Conclusions

The work of Cantor and associates, Noll and Benedict's case study, and Rutter and Shaffer's proposal for disposition of the syndrome outlined by Evans-Jones and Rosenbloom, taken together, point to a core problem in the study of severe child psychopathology – a problem left unresolved by *DSM-III's* PDD and SOC syndromes and criteria: What is the nature of the relationship among syndromes proposed? What is the relationship between IA and SOC, or IA and COPDD? Of the four major syndromes of severe childhood psychopathology outlined in *DSM-III* – IA, COPDD, APDD, and SOC – only the criteria for diagnosing IA have a reasonable prior history of use in the field. The classificatory syndromes COPDD and APDD appear to be artifacts of an effort to create determinable boundaries between syndromes. Until 1980, no researcher or clinician would have diagnosed a child as having "childhood-onset pervasive developmental disorder" or "atypical pervasive developmental disorder." Furthermore, the syndrome proposals for "developmental psychosis" and "hypotonic schizophrenia" we have examined here suggest that the adult diagnostic features for SOC that were intended to provide boundary conditions between IA and SOC are overridden by the apparent presence of diagnostic features of both IA and SOC within individuals, either at one point in time or over a period of development.

In a recent careful and exhaustive review of research on IA between 1970 and 1980, DeMyer and associates (1981) interpreted the *DSM-III* PDD and SOC syndromes and criteria in terms of the previous use of syndrome labels and diagnoses as follows:

"Childhood psychoses" does not appear at all. Instead of the old generic term "childhood schizophrenia," DSM-III gives us "pervasive developmental disorders" ... childhood schizophrenia is nowhere mentioned, but we are advised to speak of "schizophrenia in childhood." DSM-III also resurrected an old term that has appeared seldom in the literature of the 1970s – namely, "atypical" – and applied it to pervasive developmental disorder whose relationship to "schizophrenia in children," the authors say, is disputed. But what is its relation to infantile autism, with which it shares a generic heading? ... The answer awaits future research. [DeMyer et al., 1981, p. 392]

In addition to the review by DeMyer and associates, a number of other excellent reviews (Prior, 1979; Werry, 1979; Freeman and Ritvo, 1981) concerned with the complex and confusing relationships betwen diagnostic criteria and diagnostic labels attest the fact that the problem is not one of semantics. There simply is no set of subsumptive, clinically observed and empirically justified syndromes with differentiating criteria that would adequately serve to either classify or diagnose children with severe (or pervasive) developmental disorders (or psychopathology) (Waterhouse et al., in press).

Even if we ignore this critical underlying issue and accept the manner in which *DSM-III* PDD syndrome delineations include reifications of problematic diagnostic boundaries, as well as portmanteau categories that are artifacts of the need for distinct boundaries between syndromes, the work of Cantor and associates, Petty and associates, Noll and Benedict, and Evans-Jones and Rosenbloom still raises questions about two specific boundary criteria in the PDD section: time of onset of symptoms, and presence of symptoms criterial to schizophrenia.

Noll and Benedict claimed to have found six children whose developmental symptom shifts moved them from a diagnosis of autism to a diagnosis of schizophrenia. Cantor and associates claimed to have found seven children who were diagnosable as having SOC, but who had not deteriorated from some prior level of functioning, and who instead had shown evidence of disordered development from very early ages. Evans-Jones and Rosenbloom's study showed a range of symptoms appearing between 14 and 41 months of age in 10 children, 5 of whom showed evidence for organic disease, and 5 of whom did not.

There are several possible positions to take concerning these proposals for *DSM-III*. One is to dismiss all of them on the grounds that these proposed syndromes were all defined on the basis of research involving insufficient sample sizes and problematic diagnostic criteria. Another is to see support for these syndromes in the range of previous research findings to which they are related, and then justify adding them to *DSM-III* as additional possible "true" diagnostic categories that had not been adequately outlined before the creation of *DSM-III*. Still another position is to view these proposals as illustrative of the problems in the basic conceptualization of syndromes and criteria within the *DSM-III* PDD section and SOC, and then to review these problems in a wider fashion.

If – as the findings discussed earlier appear to suggest – autism may become schizophrenia, and schizophrenia may be identified at any age, and distintegrative psychosis may be diagnosed in children whose symptom onset was either before or after 30 months (and in whom evidence for organic brain disorder may be found or not found), given the problematic validity of reports of time of onset (Chess and Thomas, 1977; DeMyer et al., 1981), and the even more problematic process of interpreting the presence of symptoms criterial to schizophrenia across a developmental continuum from toddlerhood to puberty, it may be that the present *DSM-III* criteria and syndromes for classifying severe childhood psychopathology could compromise both clinical diagnoses and research classifications. Even if study populations for research can be selected with reliability using such boundary criteria as are presently included in *DSM-III* PDD, given the findings reviewed here, it seems likely that such samples may be too heterogeneous to permit the discovery of potentially crucial information concerning behavior patterns, clinical course, prognosis, and etiology. In clinical practice, where differential diagnosis may lead to differences in treatment plans, syndrome validity is also crucial. Furthermore, when diagnosis may hinge on symptoms or behaviors that are difficult to interpret or unreliable, clinicians may create idiosyncratic diagnostic formulas in an effort to cope with such problematic diagnostic boundaries.

DEVELOPMENTAL CONSIDERATIONS

Two articles have directed attention to cognitive/developmental considerations for PDD and SOC syndromes that the authors of those articles believed to have been inadequately addressed in *DSM-III*. Rutter and Shaffer argued that mental retardation should not have been included on the first or "psychiatric" axis, as "logically the decision on a child's intellectual level is of an entirely different kind from those involved in assessing whether he is suffering from a depressive condition . . . " (1980, p. 380). Tanguay (1984) claimed that another important consideration has been ignored in *DSM-III* categories: He argued that children's basic developmental changes must constitute crucial considerations in diagnosis, as developmental profile differences in physical, cognitive, and social developmental patterns may be criterial for diagnosis.

Both of these concerns have been central to critical thinking about psychiatric diagnosis in severe childhood psychopathology for some time (Capute et al., 1975; Bartak and Rutter, 1976; Eisenberg, 1977; Freeman et al., 1978; Prior, 1979; Waterhouse and Fein, 1984). Unfortunately, both issues have remained rather thorny, for different reasons.

Mental retardation and PDD syndromes

Rutter and Shaffer (1980) compared *DSM-III* to *ICD-9* (World Health Organization, 1978). They concluded that there is an inadequate introduction to and rationale for the axial system in *DSM-III*, and they further critically analyzed the axial system in relation to the PDD section of *DSM-III*. Most important in terms of the history of diagnosis of severe childhood psychopathology is their criticism that mental retardation should not have been established as a category within the first axis, but rather should have been put on an independent axis. These authors stated that "the central problem with two diagnoses on the same axis is that one tends to be chosen at the expense of the other" (1980, p. 381), and they refuted an argument made for inclusion of mental retardation on axis I (Russell et al., 1979), saying that "it is not true that mental illness and mental retardation concern similar disorders . . . the essential distinction between illness and retardation is that the former is primarily defined in terms of abnormal type of mental functioning, whereas the latter is primarily defined in terms of abnormal level of mental functioning" (pp. 380–1). They further asserted that "the inclusion of mental retardation on axis I was both based on false logic and also likely to be damaging in practice" (p. 381).

Despite these strong assertions, prior research suggests a more complex interpretation of the relationship between "mental illness" and mental retardation for children with pervasive developmental disorders, and within PDD, for IA in particular. Bartak and Rutter (1976) reported that the autistic children they studied who had IQ scores above 70 showed a slightly different set of behaviors than did autistic children with IQs below 70, and Capute and associates (1975) found that the severity of autistic symptoms was positively associated with the severity of mental retardation. Freeman and Ritvo (1981) found that when 23 normal, 30 autistic, and 30 mentally retarded children's rated behaviors were considered together for analysis, autistic behavioral symptoms so overlapped behaviors seen in retarded children that a discriminant-function analysis of items from the research team's Behavior Observation Scale failed to discriminate children diagnosed as autistic from children diagnosed as mentally retarded.

Because of these findings, it has been argued (Prior, 1979) that there are two distinct groups of children with infantile autism: those with IQs over 70 and those with IQs below 70. There are two parts to this thesis: (1) Those children whose IQs are above 70 will have a better prognosis for development; (2) Those children whose nonverbal IQs are near normal will express the syndrome of autism "in a 'pure' form, not associated with mental retardation" (Rutter, 1983, p. 521).

Although it is probably often true that the higher the IQ of any child diagnosed as having any syndrome of PDD or SOC, the better are that child's chances of developmental improvement, nonetheless this possibility does not serve to clarify the relationship between mental retardation and PDD. Furthermore, although the second part of the thesis – that normal-IQ autistics are expressing a "pure" form of the disorder – has a certain amount of intuitive appeal, unfortunately, given what is presently known about possible links among prenatal, perinatal, and neonatal factors and PDD, and given the essential complexity of the human brain, it is unlikely that such a simple additive formula (autism + mental retardation vs. autism − mental retardation) obtains.

We know that the vast majority of children diagnosed as autistic or schizophrenic by any previous scheme of diagnosis have IQs below 70 (DeMyer et al., 1981; Wing, 1981), and we also know that many of the behaviors shown by children diagnosed as having some form of severe pervasive developmental disorder, particularly IA, are often shown by children whose primary diagnosis is mental retardation (Schain and Yannet, 1960; Freeman and Ritvo, 1981).

To decide whether clinicians and researchers must list two diagnostic categories for one child on the same axis or provide the same information on two axes may help to resolve what is a structural expression of the problem of the relationship of mental retardation to PDD, but it will not help our understanding of the problem in any way. Furthermore, if it can be shown that there are clear differences in prognoses and symptoms for higher- and lower-IQ autistic children, then to assert that IQ should be coded on another axis reflects a tacit logical problem. If children diagnosed as autistic do constitute two distinct groups on the basis of IQ (Bartak and Rutter, 1976; Prior, 1979), then it may be that the syndrome devolves on something centrally affecting both the level of cognitive skill and behavioral symptoms. And if therefore – as has been argued for time of onset – a specific IQ cutoff point will be of help to differential diagnosis, then logically the level of IQ should neither be coded on a separate axis nor be used as a second diagnosis on the same axis, but should be included in the diagnositic criteria of the syndrome directly, thus creating two distinct forms of IA. If, however, IQ is a continuum expressed against a static set of symptoms, and IQ is theorized to be an index of cognitive functioning fairly independent of such psychiatric symptoms, then it would be best to have it coded on a separate axis.

An example of the empirical complexity that provides a counterargument to any step toward such a diagnostic bifurcation, however, is found in the data reported by Wing (1981), who demonstrated that although children with autisticlike symptoms exhibited a wide range of IQ, nonetheless the greatest number of affected children and those who showed the most "autistic" symptoms were concentrated in the IQ range of 20–50 in the sample.

A further complication lies in the present twofold use of the term "mental retardation." Its first use is as a syndrome label for "diagnosing" individuals who show a range of developmental delays – including motor, social, and cognitive delays – but in whom severe impairment of social relatedness is not observed. The second use of the term "mental retardation" is specifically as an index of cognitive retardation or delay. It is the first use that appears on axis I of *DSM-III*, but it is the second use that is thought to be critical for diagnosis of PDD.

Our own research (Waterhouse and Fein, 1982a,b, 1984; Fein et al., 1984) does not support the notion of an IQ-determined bifurcation in either an IA- or COPDD-diagnosed sample. We have found wide ranges of verbal IQ in children with similar symptoms, and we have found extreme ranges of nonverbal IQ in children sharing a significant number of symptoms. Furthermore, we have found that among a sample of children we are currently studying, there is a set of differentiable cognitive-skill profiles, and these profiles are largely independent of association with other "psychiatric" symptoms (Fein et al., 1985).

Although it is certainly possible that there is some unitary "cognitive deficit in autism ... closely linked with the social and behavioral features of the condition" (Rutter, 1983, p. 524), we nonetheless concur with Tanguay (1984) and DeMyer et al. (1981), who have argued that understanding the profiles or patterns of cognitive skills both across development and at a single point in time – in relation to social and affective behaviors, as well as independent of such behaviors – is going to be the more productive way of generating a better understanding of the complex nature of "mental retardation" in PDD.

Developmental change

Tanguay (1984) outlined a tentative framework for a new classification system for severe childhood psychopathology based on cognitive developmental considerations. He posited that there may be two basic underlying forms of cognition – sequential and holistic – each of which may unfold separately in the development of an individual. He argued that sequential processing involves linear, logical, and linguistic skills that appear later in a child's development (as per the Piagetian stage-model hypothesis), whereas he suggested that the concept of holistic thinking is a reflection of Piaget's notion of syncretic thought that develops early in life (between the second and seventh years).

Tanguay claimed that "autistic children show a dissociation in the normal pattern of development: mild to moderate impairments of posturo-motor development, moderate to severe impairments in development of holistic processing skills, and very severe impairments in development of language and sequential processing skills" (Tanguay, 1984). He also claimed that schizophrenic children experience "a moderate degree of sequential processing deficiency, and ... a lesser impairment in holistic processing" (Tanguay, 1984).

Although Tanguay did not suggest possible onset boundaries for either autism or childhood schizophrenia, he asserted that in his system schizophrenic children can be differentially distinguished from adult schizophrenics, in that individuals who develop schizophrenia in childhood will have failed to acquire various cognitive skills, whereas adult- or adolescent-onset schizophrenics will have developed normal cognitive skills that then become impaired as a function of their disorder.

Beyond these two definitions, Tanguay proposed that a third type of disorder may exist "in which the child may have relatively good sequential and holistic processing ability, but in whom the expected degree of Piagetian 'formal operations' fail to develop" (1984). He suggested that a child diagnosed as having this third form of disorder would appear odd and mannered and somewhat dissociated, but would show signs of reasonable cognitive development and some motivation for social relatedness. The proposed syndrome apparently would describe children similar to those diagnosable as having schizoid disorder.

Although the use of a theoretical framework to differentiate syndromes is both elegant and appealing, unless developmental outcomes have rigid and clearly sequenced behavioral antecedents, developmental patterns – despite their possible clinical face validity – cannot function pragmatically as diagnostic criteria in a clinical setting in which a diagnosis may have to be made on the basis of one or two clinical interviews and a review of whatever developmental history may be available. Nonetheless, developmental patterns are critical concerns in understanding PDD.

It is important to note that proposals considered in this section reflect a tension between typological and dimensional modeling of PDD. Whereas mutually exclusive syndromes are by definition typological (Kendell, 1975), a single criterion listed for a diagnostic category may capture what is expressed symptomatologically as a continuum of behaviors – requiring dimensional judgments by diagnosticians. Furthermore, individuals may be seen as fitting a given set of criteria by scalar "degrees." If five criteria are listed, some individuals may show all five, and some may show four, three, two, or one. Furthermore, developmental changes themselves may be seen as typological shifts, or as points on a continuum. This is not a methods or procedures problem, but a reflection of how little we know about the nature of development and the disorders attendant on that development.

Prior to Tanguay's proposal, Ritvo and Freeman (1978) and James and Barry (1981) had suggested ways to consider developmental issues internal to and external to diagnostic criteria. Ritvo and Freeman (1978), in drawing up the diagnostic criteria for autism for the National Society for Autistic Citizens (NSAC), included four essential features, the first of which was "disturbances of developmental rates and sequences." Ritvo and Freeman proposed that there are three developmental "pathways" – motor, social-adaptive, and cognitive – and three general types of disturbances of these developmental pathways: (1) dissociation of development within the motor pathways; (2) delay and dissociations across the three pathways; and (3) arrests, delays, or regression within a pathway.

None of the sets of criteria for syndromes within PDD or SOC address the dissociations of motor, cognitive, and social impairments of development that may occur in PDD – but it is precisely these dissociations that are so salient in children diagnosable as having PDD. We have all seen children with good fine motor skills and poor gross motor skills; children with phenomenal rote memory and primitive motor abilities; and children who are acutely socially withdrawn but who have normal pattern-recognition skills.

Although such descriptive information may not provide boundary conditions between syndrome groups because it reflects such a wide range of individual variability, there should be some way to index the existence of such dissociations in development. Ritvo and Freeman (1978) noted their existence in the NSAC definition of autism; Tanguay proposed that such dissociations in development be used as a means to define syndromes. Although it is clear from recent reviews of the current understanding of stage models of various aspects of normal development (Kagan, 1979; Thomas, 1981) that knowledge of motor, cognitive, social, and affective patterns of normal development is incomplete, there must, nonetheless, be some way to incorporate diagnostic information on development within the criteria for PDD and SOC within the *DSM-III*.

James and Barry (1981) reviewed the difficulties that variability in deficits, delays, and regressions in development pose for research in "early onset psychosis." They concluded that because such a broad band of behaviors is affected developmentally, it is not a reasonable strategy to try to eliminate these problematic developmental effects from consideration by studying only those children who do not show such a wide range of developmental delays and deficits. They argued that careful use of both mental-age-matched (MA) and chronological-age-matched (CA) control groups is preferable to an IQ-based (and thus severely limiting) selection of samples of chldren with PDD.

Although it is exactly the sort of research comparisons they proposed that should enable us to better elucidate the nature of developmental effects, and ultimately lead to knowledge that can be coded criterially for diagnosis, there are some difficulties with their proposals. First, they recommended selection of mentally retarded MA-matched control subjects, but because children diagnosed as mentally retarded cannot be viewed as having a set of even or homogeneous developmental delays, such matches may lead to distorted findings. Second, children diagnosed as having PDD or SOC have been found to have very uneven cognitive-skill profiles (DeMyer et al., 1981; Fein et al., 1985). Thus, matching on any given measure of MA will match the high point in one child's battery and the low in another's, leading to confounded and confusing conclusions. Third, as noted in the NSAC definition of autism, there may be many clinically complex dissociations not only of cognitive development but also of social and motor development in a given individual. There clearly is no way to select a control sample of normal children whose development will show these dissociations and yet will except the particular deficit that is being studied.

Conclusions

It is obvious that deficits, delays, and dissociations in various aspects of development are inherent in the symptoms of most children diagnosable as having some syndrome of PDD. There is, however, no currently existing typology that would both isolate differential patterns and offer sufficient predictive validity to provide stage-specific criteria as a means to dignose children at a single point in time. A model such as Tanguay recently proposed may, when elaborated, offer such information. At present, however, it would seem that taking notice of the existence of such variant patterns, as per Ritvo and Freeman's (1978) NSAC definition of autism, and attempting, in however limited a way, to control for such variations in the conduct of research, as James and Barry have suggested, is all that can be done to address the issue.

EFFECTIVENESS OF DIAGNOSTIC CRITERIA

There are two key boundary variables in the creation of distinctions among PDD syndromes and between PDD syndromes and SOC: the time of onset of symptoms, and the presence of symptoms criterial to schizophrenia. Early onset – before 30 months of age – is critical in distinguishing IA and COPDD, and the presence of symptoms that will support a diagnosis of schizophrenia is critical in distinguishing SOC from IA, COPDD, and APDD. In addition to the problems raised concerning the validity of these boundary criteria in determining syndrome borders, as discussed earlier, several problems arise in regard to reliable interpretation and application of these criteria to individual children and to populations of children with PDD.

Onset

A valid interpretation of early onset (i.e., before 30 months of age) can be made only if a child has had a clinical evaluation prior to 30 months. However, this requirement is not strictly observed either in research or in clinical practice. It is a tacitly accepted procedure to admit parental, family, or guardian report of early symptoms as evidence of early onset. Although it may be true that family members can be sensitive to abnormal variations in developmental stages, inherent in this accepted practice is the obvious problem of backward masking after a diagnosis has been made or serious symptoms have been noticed, as well as the normal, human (expected) uncertainty of recall.

Most critical are borderline cases. Given the fact that the recall of nonprofessionals is the basis for much of the diagnostic determination of onset, what can be said of situations of borderline onset, wherein, typically, a parent reports taking the child to a pediatrician when the child was "about three" because the child was appearing more withdrawn, or was not developing normal speech?

The problematic nature of parental or guardian reports of onset and the frequent absence of consistent early clinical evaluations press the researcher or diagnostician from two sides. Because few of these children will have solid clinical workups until "onset" is noticed (or, more likely, until some time after onset is noticed), in order to have a reasonable sample to study, or in order to establish a diagnosis, recall of family members must be considered, but the uncertainty of recall may make the character of the sample selected, or the diagnosis as established, somewhat suspect.

It is the very absoluteness of the age cutoff for onset that not only ensures the continued presence of critical borderline problems but also ensures that onset cannot be a valid syndrome boundary. When children with parallel symptoms are to be diagnosed, because it is patently untrue that one month's difference in reported onset can determine whether a child "has" IA or COPDD, or IA or APDD, diagnosticians cannot maintain any belief in the validity of the onset cutoff.

In addition to the question of the reliability of determinations of onset, there are the issues raised when samples might be able to be differentiated well, except for the fact that onset limitations provide a procrustean bed for a sample. In a recent article that concluded that *DSM-III* PDD subcategories may be valid and distinct, Rescorla and Dahl (1983) looked at behaviors of 92 children previously diagnosed at the Yale Child Study Center. Because the children had had a variety of diagnoses from different clinicians who had seen different subsets of these children, the authors grouped the children's varying diagnoses into two categories that they created: "severe atypical" and "mild atypical." Rescorla and Dahl found that the behaviors of the two groups of children were distinguishable by differential loadings of behavior scores on derived factors. Despite the clear differentiation found between the "severe atypical group" (which met the diagnostic criteria for PDD IA approximately) and the "mild atypical group" (which showed COPDD symptoms), early onset (before 30 months) was apparently typical of the severe atypical group, but had also been reported for many of the children in the mild atypical group.

The fact that behaviors could be reliably distinguished between their two groups, but that onset of symptoms before 30 months characterized many of the children in their COPDD-parallel group, suggests that strict adherence to the criterion of post-30-month onset of symptoms for the COPDD diagnostic group of *DSM-III* PDD could present a serious stumbling block for future empirical research.

In real terms, of course, given the wide range of variation seen in even normal stages of development, it is quite clear that specification of a boundary criterion for onset, either before or after 30 months of age, is arbitrary. It may also be diagnostically dysfunctional. The history of this cutoff for onset of symptoms stems largely from an early-onset/late-onset distinction of symptoms within the population of a single study (Kolvin, 1971), and it was then espoused by Rutter (1974, 1978) as a critical component in his widely used (Table 21.1) criteria for determination of autism. Our own research suggests that early onset may be a clue to severity in a certain subset of symptoms – not all of which are diagnostic criteria for IA. However, as can be seen in the findings of Rescorla and Dahl (1983), early onset may also be associated with mild COPDD-like symptoms, or, as is suggested in the research of Cantor and associates (1982), early onset may be associated with the presence of symptoms criterial to schizophrenia.

Because onset before 30 months may be both unreliable and invalid as a boundary condition, it may be better either to provide an "axis" for onset within the PDD section of *DSM-III* or to allow for some specified range of onset for the various syndromes outlined in PDD.

Symptoms criterial to schizophrenia

Cantor and associates (1982) argued that they found evidence of hallucinations, delusions, incoherence, and loosening of associations in young children, but Tanguay (1984) argued that the presence of such symptoms can be diagnosed only in a child whose mental age is at least six or seven years.

Of all the criteria posited for severe childhood syndromes, the criteria for SOC are the most problematic. Taken in concert with the position that SOC should be diagnosed – as per adult diagnoses of schizophrenia – only when a state of adequate functioning precedes the onset of some deterioration of functioning, such criteria not only limit SOC diagnosis to late-onset cases but also appear to provide an unintended "loophole" that may vastly broaden the range of symptoms acceptable for those diagnoses of SOC that may be made.

The loophole is the fact that although the boundary criteria distinguishing IA and COPDD from SOC are outlined as "hallucinations, delusions, incoherence and loosening of associations," if a diagnostician turns to the adult section on diagnosis of schizophrenia, it is clear that schizophrenia may be indexed by such open-ended symptoms as "poverty of content of speech" in association with "blunted affect." Most children with almost any form of PDD will show both poverty of content of speech and blunted affect. This means that, technically, all children who achieve some level of initial adequate functioning, even where this functioning may be seen to "deteriorate" when the child is very young, may be diagnosed as having SOC.

If, however, the crucial criteria for diagnosis of SOC are interpreted to be exactly those symptoms that are boundary limits for IA and COPDD (i.e., hallucinations, delusions, incoherence, and loosening of associations), then problems of interpretation of these mental states and behaviors in children must be addressed.

During a series of recent conference presentations (Cantor, 1983; COSAC, 1983; Brown, 1983), one of the authors of this chapter (Waterhouse) watched videotape presentations of young children described as having PDD or SOC syndromes. The children were taped in test/play sessions. In each case, a child was shown blinking several times and turning his head, moving around a bit and shifting focus away from the task. This same piece of behavior in three different children was interpreted variously in the three talks as possible evidence for (1) repetitive-compulsive ritualistic behaviors, (2) hallucinations, and (3) seizuring.

If the behaviors of children with PDD or SOC are open to such a wide range of interpretation, how are critical aberrant mental states to be clearly indexed in this population? If blinking and inattention can index hallucinations, can verbal perseveration of names of people or things index delusions?

Can schizophrenia be assumed to exist in children who cannot talk about their hallucinations or delusions, or should all children with severe developmental disorders be considered to be schizophrenic because they all show poverty of content and blunted affect? The implicit possible extreme variation in coverage permissible in using either the *DSM-III* PDD boundary criteria or those key descriptive criteria for schizophrenia could easily lead to different diagnoses for the same child at the same point in time and certainly would negate the possibility of researchers being able to believe that they are studying comparably diagnosed groups of chldren. These criteria must either be "tightened up" and made more explicit or eliminated as a boundary condition within PDD.

Furthermore, the range of coverage suggested by SOC criteria in *DSM-III* causes problems for differential diagnosis of SOC, schizoid disorder, and schizotypal personality disorder. Differential diagnosis of schizoid disorder in children depends on the absence of psychotic symptoms. If inferences concerning the possible presence of psychotic symptoms cannot be made reliably, then there can be no adequate boundary between SOC and schizoid disorder. Furthermore, there are also serious problems for isolation of SOC from schizotypal personal disorder in children, as well as schizoid from schizotypal personality. Examination of the diagnostic criteria for the three syndromes suggests that a 14-year-old who is suspicious, withdrawn, and without friends, and who exhibits blunted affect, with vague speech with poverty of content, could be given all three diagnoses.

Although judgments of psychiatric symptoms are problematic, there are other diagnostic criterial judgments that must be "operationalized" and that also can cause difficulty in interpretation. Both the "pervasive lack of responsiveness to other people" outlined as criterial for IA in PDD and the "hyper- or hyposensitivity to sensory stimuli" outlined as criterial for COPDD pose difficult problems for interpretation of the presence of these symptoms. All five sources of diagnostic unreliability (subject, occasion, information, observation and criterion variance) outlined by Spitzer, Endicott, and Robins (1975) contribute to difficulty in interpreting whether or not these two symptoms may be present in individuals.

In some children, responsiveness to others is situation-specific; in other children, responsiveness may even be person-specific. By means of intensive behavior-modification training programs, some children may be trained to meet the gaze of another person in response to a set phrase: "Look at me" or "Look at her." Does this mean they have developed a responsiveness to people? Even when two clinicians observe the same piece of behavior in the same child at the same time, they may differ in reporting its significance as an indication of abnormality in responsiveness. As professionals are now being trained in the use of *DSM-III*, the lack of sufficient operationalized specificity for the two diagnostic criteria concerning responsivity may lead to training-center differences, because prototypical cases used in teaching will reflect the addition of (needed) idiosyncratic information for interpretation and application of these criteria.

Conclusions

Because of the great difficulties inherent in using the two major and critical boundary criteria and two crucial descriptive criteria, we cannot support Williams and Spitzer's (1982) notion of the "good news" and "bad news" about *DSM-III* where PDD and SOC are concerned. They say that the good news is that for the first time "research investigators . . . can have some assurance that different researchers using these criteria mean the same thing" and that the bad news is that "these new DSM-III criteria are, for the most part, based on limited knowledge" (p. 1289). Unfortunately, it would seem that for PDD and SOC within *DSM-III,* this must be translated into the "bad news" and the "still more bad news."

We do agree with the goals for research diagnostic criteria that were outlined by Feighner and associates (1972) – that criteria should be narrowly defined, so that groups may be "pure," and explicitly operationalized to ensure that groups can be formed reliably. It can only be hoped that changes in present PDD criteria may help to meet these goals.

RELIABILITY

To date, there have been two studies concerned with the reliability of a *DSM-III* PDD diagnosis in relation to other possible (*DSM-III*) diagnoses of children: (1) phases 1 and 2 of the field trials for *DSM-III* diagnostic categories, as reported in *DSM-III* itself (Williams and Spitzer, 1980), and (2) a field trial comparison of case- and interview-based reliabilities (Hyler et al., 1982). Both of these studies investigated the reliability of the PDD section of *DSM-III* versus other possible diagnoses. Also, there has been a multipart study that explored the reliability of individual *DSM-III* PDD and SOC syndrome diagnoses (Cantwell et al., 1979a,b; Mattison et al., 1979; Russell et al., 1979).

In reporting on their study of the frequency of agreement among raters examining the same cases, Cantwell and associates (1979a) stated that "a major issue with DSM-III, as with all classification systems, will be its reliability. It is striking that neither DSM-II nor several other proposed childhood classification outlines [as summarized by the Group for the Advancement of Psychiatry (GAP)] have ever been tested for reliability on cases of child psychiatric disorders" (p. 1209). Unfortunately, the reliability studies done so far have reported what can best be described as mixed results.

In phase 1 of the field trials (American Psychiatric Association, 1980, Table 2, p. 471), the κ coefficient of agreement on diagnosis of a PDD disorder was .85; in phase 2, the κ coefficient was $-.01$. Hyler and associates (1982) reported that for disorders first evidenced in infancy, childhood, or adolescence, whereas κ for case-study-based reliability was only .44, the κ indexing interview reliability was 1.00. Mattison and associates (1979) reported good interrater reliability for PDD as a category (.76), but a wide range of reliabilities across different cases examined – from a low for schizophrenia, paranoid type (.45), to a high for infantile autism (1.00).

For Cantwell and associates (1979a), who asked 20 clinicians to evaluate 4 cases (among a group of 24 cases) for which the investigators had previously established various PDD or SOC diagnoses, the derived frequency of agreement ranged from a low of 25% (only 5 clinicians agreeing on the expected diagnosis) to a high of 100%.

Cantwell and associates (1979a) expected clinicians to rate their case 1 as both early childhood psychosis (apparently COPDD) and mental retardation, but only 5 of the 20 clinicians double-diagnosed this case. The expected diagnosis for case 2 was IA, and all 20 clinicians diagnosed that case as presenting IA. The researchers had set case 7 as SOC, but only 5 clinicians diagnosed this case as such, and most of the remaining clinicians labeled the case with the classification "early childhood psychosis." The last case, number 21, had been established by the investigators as schizophrenic, paranoid type. Only 9 of the 20 clinical raters agreed, but there was no clear consensus among the remaining clinicians on an alternative diagnosis.

Although Cantwell and associates stated that no other systems for classifying children with "psychoses" have been tested for reliability, Beitchman and associates (1978) explored interrater reliability for the GAP (1966) classification system for children's disorders. These investigators had 73 clinicians assign diagnoses to 41 cases. They reported that the intraclass coefficient for diagnosis of the category of psychiatric disorder was .71. After a review of all their findings, however, the authors concluded that "unless revisions and improvements are made in the GAP diagnostic schema, its usefulness as a system of classification in child psychiatry may be supplanted by the DSM-III" (Beitchman et al., 1978, p. 1465).

Because no subgroup breakdowns were reported by Hyler and associates (1982), we are left to conclude that perhaps as few as nine cases expressing PDD or SOC symptoms (*DSM-III* phase 1 field trials, 4 cases; *DSM-III* phase 2 field trials, 1 case; Cantwell et al., 4 cases) have been examined for either section or syndrome interrater reliability. Both the small number of cases considered and the fact that subgroup breakdowns were not investigated for reliability in the field trials mean that no firm conclusions can be drawn regarding the reliability of PDD and SOC diagnostic categories.

Conclusions

It may be that it is reasonably easy for clinicians to agree that a child has some form of PDD, especially if that child shows some of the features that have been outlined for IA. It is apparently difficult for clinicians to agree on subcategories of PDD or SOC. Rutter and Shaffer (1980) stated that similar findings have been reported for reliabilities for child psychiatric disorders in *ICD-9*. A recent review (Parks, 1983) of five checklist systems for diagnosing autism concluded that reliabilities for the systems (.55 to .95) were generally adequate. However, previous comparisons of other diagnostic systems for severe childhood psychopathologies (DeMyer et al., 1971; Rimland, 1971; Cohen et al., 1978) suggested that whereas a general disordered – nondisordered distinction can be made reliably, subgroup membership within the general disordered category (where this general category is either "childhood psychoses" or "pervasive developmental disorders") cannot be reliably determined.

Clearly, problems with reliability are not unique to *DSM-III*, but are to be expected as a function of the nature of present knowledge in the field as it overlaps with individual clinicians' internalized personal histories of diagnostic constructs.

CLINICAL, EMPIRICAL, AND THEORETICAL VALIDITY

Achenbach (1980) argued that creation of empirically derived psychiatric diagnostic syndromes is a different facet of the same endeavor represented by *DSM-III*, but Spitzer and Cantwell (1980) argued that psychiatric syndromes are not identified first by purely empirical means and then later shown to have clinical validity. Spitzer and Cantwell asserted that face validity – or clinical awareness of similar clusters of symptoms occurring in different individuals – is the starting point for identification of clinical syndromes.

Achenbach claimed, however, that the *DSM-III* childhood classifications largely reflect extrapolation of nosologic constructs from adult disorders, and he also claimed that this is a function of the fact that "the study of childhood psychopathology lags a century behind the study of adult psychopathology" (1980, p. 396). He further offered reasons why parallels to adult taxonomies are inadequate for classification of childhood disorders: Adult disorders do not have clear counterparts in children, and children's disorders impair developmental progress, whereas adults' disorders interfere with an already achieved set of cognitive and social skills.

In the case of the PDD syndromes and SOC, in absolute terms there is only one diagnostic category – IA – that reflects a syndrome that was derived from the face validity of previous clinical experience. Of the other three syndromes (COPDD, APDD, and SOC), COPDD and APDD appear to be artifacts of the process of creating a "tight" system as per the Feighner and associates (1972) goals for diagnostic criteria, whereas SOC represents an attempt to impose adult diagnostic criteria on children. COPDD, as defined in *DSM-III*, has no history of diagnosis as a syndrome under the name COPDD and in fact is currently interpreted in a variety of ways by researchers to reflect a range of previously defined clinical syndromes: (1) childhood schizophrenia (DeMyer et al., 1981), (2) mild atypical disorder (Rescorla and Dahl, 1983), (3) high-functioning autism, (4) Creak's schizophrenia, and (5) early-onset psychosis. It may also be used where the history of onset is unclear to define a group as having "late-onset" autism.

APDD is a diagnostic remainder category, the existence of which has been lauded by Rutter and Shaffer (1980), who argued that having some sort of open-ended "other" category is valuable for any set of related diagnostic criteria. The term "atypical," however, does give rise to comparisons of APDD with previously identified syndromes of the same name and may cause those in the field to speculate not only on the choice of descriptive criteria for APDD but also on the choice of that term in particular (DeMyer et al., 1981).

The *DSM-III* syndrome of SOC is not developmentally extrapolated from adult classification – to be diagnosed as having SOC, a child must be considered as an adult and must show symptoms that meet the criteria for schizophrenia in adults. As discussed earlier, the use of adult criteria is both inappropriate and problematic, generating serious concerns for syndrome validity and reliability.

We conducted two surveys of diagnostic practice. Table 21.1 reports findings from a survey of five years (1978–82) of empirical research on PDD and SOC reported in 10 journals. It reveals an increase in the research use of *DSM-III*. However, as can be seen from the ratio of the number of diagnoses to the number of studies shown in Table 21.1, most studies reviewed for this survey reported multiple diagnoses for the same population, suggesting that there may be some degree of uncertainty concerning diagnostic systems. Standard use of a single system would mark an improvement in PDD research.

We also conducted an informal survey of 20 clinicians around the country (including child psychologists, child psychiatrists, and neurologists), all of whom had extensive clinical experience with children with PDD and SOC. Although these clinicians found the *DSM-III* diagnostic criteria to be clearly laid out and easy to teach, and although they generally voiced appreciations of the atheoretical basis of these criteria, and although they considered *DSM-III* to be a great improvement over *DSM-II*, nonetheless, this group of clinicians did express a number of serious concerns.

First, though in general the clinicians' concerns both echoed and extended the concerns already discussed in this chapter, none of the clinicians suggested that there were any new PDD/SOC categories that should be added to *DSM-III*. Several clinicians, however, did suggest that the level of intellectual retardation should be coded, and others recommended that the existence of developmental dissociations be indexed in some fashion. Third, PDD and SOC diagnostic criteria received a great deal of criticism. Time of onset, presence of symptoms criterial to schizophrenia, degree of social responsiveness, and character of responsiveness to stimuli all were judged very difficult to interpret.

Fourth, the syndromes themselves were the targets of the greatest number of criticisms. Many clinicians wondered why such "ineffective" and "nonpredictive" and "unreliable" categories with "no implications for treatment" were adopted in *DSM-III*. Most clinicians had difficulty fitting children into *DSM-III* categories, and they specified the following types of cases as not being diagnosable:

1. children who met all the IA criteria except that they showed "reasonably" good language skills,

2. children who met all but the onset criteria for IA,
3. children who met all the criteria for any PDD category or SOC except that they had a mild expression of one or more symptoms,
4. early-onset schizophrenics,
5. children with mixed IA, COPDD, and SOC symptoms.

The survey also revealed that clinicians are interpreting the various categories in a variety of ways. IA in *DSM-III* is variously interpreted as both broader and narrower than Kanner's original notion. COPDD is being clinically interpreted in at least four ways: (1) as childhood schizophrenia (Creak), (2) as mild autism, (3) as late-onset autism, and (4) as partial autism. Furthermore, SOC is being variously interpreted as "impossible to diagnose in a pre-adolescent because of the requirement for thought disorder" or useful as a means to categorize late-onset, high-functioning children.

Many clinicians commented on the heterogeneity of samples formed by syndrome diagnostic criteria, and a number of clinicians suggested that all of PDD and SOC should be collapsed into a single category. A number of those surveyed said that only a small fraction of the children they see can be adequately diagnosed using *DSM-III* criteria. One clinician also found a problem with the decision tree (American Psychiatric Association, 1980, pp. 340–1) that begins with the behaviors that are ultimately excluded from the resultant diagnosis.

In summary, it is our impression that clinicians believe that there is little clinical face validity for any syndrome considered here, with the exception of IA. It is also our impression that among the 20 clinicians interviewed there exists a wide range of clinical prototypes for the classificatory label "infantile autism."

A review of the recent history of the field suggests that it is essentially Rutter's criteria (1968a,b, 1974, 1978) for autism (Tables 21.1 and 21.2) that provide the basis for the *DSM-III* diagnostic criteria for IA, despite the continuing problems with the criterion of time of onset, and despite the absence of any clear evidence for validity for the syndrome (Freeman et al., 1979; Wing, 1981; Waterhouse and Snyder, 1983; Tanguay, 1984; Waterhouse et al., in press). A social-psychological interpretation of the belief in autism as a syndrome and in Rutter's criteria as the means to identify it might be that IA is accepted not because it has clinical-syndrome validity but rather because applying the criteria results in a level of coverage that justifies diagnosticians' belief in the existence of the syndrome. In the case of IA, it is possible that a scheme earlier proposed by Rimland was not adopted partly because it appeared to provide too little coverage, and for childhood psychoses, Creak's classification system was criticized in part because it appeared to include too many individuals.

As presently used, the *DSM-III* IA criteria are satisfactory precisely because of this element: Samples selected may be very heterogeneous in basic symptoms, but reasonable samples can be selected. But being able to make a diagnosis or classify a child on the basis of some set of criteria is a measure of reliability: It is not the basis for syndrome validity.

Rutter's influence also appears to be reflected in the absence of any specific criteria designated solely for children for the diagnosis of SOC. It was essentially Rutter's persuasive arguments (1972, 1974) against the existence of schizophrenia in children as unique to children that apparently paved the way for elimination of childhood schizophrenia as a general category and led to the diagnosis of SOC being based entirely on adult diagnostic criteria. Although it is certainly clear that to some extent the diagnosis of childhood schizophrenia has been replaced by the diagnosis of IA plus remainder diagnoses (American Psychiatric Association, 1968; Freeman and Ritva, 1981), thus creating the impression that diagnostic labeling problems are largely semantic, it is possible to theorize that there may be a variety of syndromes composing childhood psychoses, including both IA and childhood schizophrenia.

Rutter and Shaffer (1980) argued that to "deserve" diagnostic delineation, a syndrome should be serious, identifiable, handicapping, and valid (p. 383) and that identification of the syndrome through diagnostic criteria should be reliable. They further claimed that though "few diagnostic categories have been validated satisfactorily . . . of course autism is a well-established condition which differs from other psychiatric disorders in numerous respects" (1980, p. 384).

Despite this assertion, and despite the general sense of the clinical face validity of autism as a diagnostic category, patients diagnosed as autistic have never been shown to have even reasonably homogeneous symptoms (Waterhouse and Snyder, 1983; Tanguay, 1984; Waterhouse et al., in press). Tanguay, in fact, recently concluded that autism is a "man-made" syndrome. Many researchers have found it difficult to distinguish autism from other diagnosable conditions and syndromes (Capute et al., 1975; Freeman et al., 1978; Wing, 1981), and the vast majority of research that has been done to examine aspects of the behavior and development of children diagnosed as autistic has not yielded results supportive of etiological, descriptive, or predictive validity (L. Waterhouse et al., unpublished data).

Wing (1981) identified a clear triad of behaviors including "abnormalities of social interaction, verbal and nonverbal communication, and imaginative activities" (1981, p. 37), but she found that when a large sample of children showing the triad of behaviors was studied, it appeared that subgroups formed on the basis of syndromes of early childhood psychosis – including autism – made arbitrary divisions of the sample.

Our own work supports Wing's finding. Although we did not study imaginative play or activities, nonetheless, using a technique pioneered by Jenkins and Glickman in 1946 as a first step to examining relationships among behaviors and symptoms, we did find three distinct groups of behaviors in a large sample of children with severe childhood psychopathology, and the first of the three groups showed parallels to the triad outlined by Wing. This first group of behaviors included abnormalities of social relatedness and severe verbal and nonverbal language deficits. The second group of behaviors included a variety of what could be interpreted as ritualistic and compulsive behaviors. The third group included a set of symptoms indexing sensorimotor irritability. These groups of behaviors did not subserve any group of diagnostic criteria, but instead cut across groups formed by Rimland, Rutter, Creak, and past and present clinical diagnoses of both autism and childhood schizophrenia.

We are now in the process of determining how these distinct groups of behaviors sort out in the repertoire of individual children.

Achenbach (1980) claimed that the need for empirically derived diagnostic categories comes from the essential complexity of the behaviors seen in childhood psychopathology. He asserted that "the diversity of potentially relevant behaviors, complicated further by the variability of each child's behavior, poses a much more massive information processing task than (simply) the detection of clinical anomalies" (1980, p. 398), and we concur with this judgment.

However, although Achenbach's rationale for moving from organized clinical impressions to empirically derived groupings is correct and well justified by the current problematic state of diagnosis for syndromes of severe childhood psychopathology, nonetheless it is also true, as Lessing, William, and Gil (1982) argued, that "statistically defined taxonomies are as vulnerable to problems of reliability and validity as systems of psychiatric diagnosis" (p. 472).

Conclusions

Unfortunately, the picture we must draw for the state of clinical and empirical validity for the PDD and SOC classifications is as bleak as that drawn for reliabilities associated with their use. Furthermore, despite the strong possibility that these syndromes may not be valid, there are presently no viable replacements for these syndromes and criteria in sight. Still more unfortunately, because of the complexities inherent in the deficits and developmental dissociations shown by children diagnosable as having forms of PDD and SOC, it will have to be both through the process of statistical (empirical) derivation and by means of some better organization of epidemiologically based clinical impressions that new categories are formed. As Achenbach has argued, clinical impressions alone, however valid, have not been a match for the presence of so much variability.

OVERALL CONCLUSION

It is our conclusion that *DSM-III* PDD and SOC classifications as presently outlined have little chance of being either valid in construct or reliable in use. In particular, the boundary criterion of time of onset and the presence of symptoms criterial to schizophrenia, as well as the boundary problem inherent in the frequent need for double diagnosis on the first axis, will all, we believe, present severe and persistent problems for diagnosis. Furthermore, it must also be pointed out that these problems do not represent problems to which clinicians can ultimately adjust through some period of greater exposure to *DSM-III* syndromes and diagnostic criteria (Spitzer and Cantwell, 1980), nor do they represent the kinds of problems that can be ameliorated by some greater awareness of the nature of shared diagnostic prototypes (Cantor et al., 1980a). It might be argued that the problems that are discussed here do reflect the presence of too many individuals on the "fuzzy boundaries" of the diagnostic prototypes, which in turn may reflect the sorting of individuals rather than the distinguishing of disorders. However, within PDD, and between PDD and SOC, because the diagnoses are mutually exclusive, children must be sorted. Furthermore, the presence of too many individuals at the fuzzy boundaries of categories suggests that there are problems with the categories themselves.

Despite the severity of these problems, however, there are no full-fledged alternatives at the present. If Cantor and associates' hypotonic schizophrenia, Noll and Benedict's autism becoming schizophrenia, and Evans-Jones and Rosenbloom's disintegrative psychosis were all to be added into the PDD section, it is not clear that the diagnostic process of using the PDD section would then become either more valid or more reliable. And it is not really possible to state in a diagnostic manual "syndromes to be announced at some future date."

If present PDD and SOC classifications for children with severe psychopathology are arbitrary, it is clear that this is not a function of diagnostic fiat. It is rather a mixture of clinical habits, the need for pure and distinct categories, and lack of knowledge about what the real syndromes may be. Given that no major valid alternatives exist now, we are able only to suggest some specific changes. First, intellectual retardation should be demarcated as distinct from mental retardation as a syndrome, and two miniaxes should be created within the PDD section itself, one for designation of the verbal and nonverbal IQ or MA of the child, and one for designation of time of onset in some approximate ranges. Second, APDD should be clearly labeled for what it is – a diagnostic remainder category that should be used when all else fails (but only in those cases in which the clinician still believes the child has symptoms that fit the general PDD category). Third, SOC should be defined within the bounds of the PDD section, even if adult criteria are to be used, and the criteria outlined for differential diagnosis of SOC must be expressed in a fashion that firmly controls for possible variability in coverage of the criteria by idiosyncratic interpretation. Fourth, the diagnostic criteria for onset of SOC should be spelled out in a clear fashion within the set of those diagnostic criteria established for SOC. Fifth, the relationship between IA and COPDD should be determined either by an onset boundary alone or by specific symptoms alone, but not by both: Because there is no research evidence that shows radical shifts in symptoms at the 30-month-onset boundary, IA should be separated from COPDD in a more clearly arbitrary fashion only by absolute time of onset, or else IA should be arbitrarily separated from COPDD (as a structurally created syndrome) by presence or absence of some single specifically designated symptom.

We agree with Tanguay that IA is a man-made syndrome, and we agree with Rutter (1978) that childhood schizophrenia has no credibility as a diagnostic entity. We further are aware that COPDD has no clinical validity and largely represents an artifact of the process of creating the PDD section. If APDD exists only as a remainder category, then the circle is complete. The next critical need in the field of severe childhood psychopathology is not to discover the "causes" of "autism" or the development patterns shown by children with "childhood-onset pervasive developmental disorders," but rather to attempt to discover what syndromes of severe childhood psychopathology really may exist (Waterhouse et al., in press).

REFERENCES

Achenbach TM: DSM-III in light of empirical research on the classification of child psychopathology. J Am Acad Child Psychiatry 19:395–412, 1980

American Psychiatric Association: Diagnostic and Statistical Manual of Mental Disorders, second edition. Washington, DC, APA, 1968

Diagnostic and Statistical Manual of Mental Disorders, third edition. Washington, DC, APA, 1980

Anthony J: An experimental approach to the psychopathology of childhood. Br J Med Psychol 31:211–223, 1958

Bartak L, Rutter M: Differences between mentally retarded and normally intelligent autistic children. J Autism Child Schizo 6:109–120, 1976

Beitchman JH, Dielman TE, Landis JR, et al: Reliability of the Group for Advancement of Psychiatry diagnostic categories in child psychiatry. Arch Gen Psychiatry 35:1461–1468, 1978

Bender L: Childhood schizophrenia. Psychiatr Q 27:663–681, 1953

Schizoprenia in childhood: its recognition, description, and treatment. Am J Orthopsychiatry 26:499–506, 1956

Bender L, Faretra G: The relationship between childhood schizophrenia and adult schizophrenia, in Genetic Factors in Schizophrenia. Edited by Kaplan AR. Springfield, Ill, Charles C Thomas, 1973, pp 28–64

Bomberg D, Szurek S, Etemad J: A statistical study of a group of psychotic children, in Clinical Studies in Childhood Psychoses. Edited by Szurek S, Berlin I. New York, Brunner/Mazel, 1973

Brown L: Neurophysiology of autism. Read before the Greater Philadelphia Chapter of the National Society for Children and Adults with Autism, Bryn Mawr, Pa, May 22, 1983

Cantor N, Smith EE, French R, et al: Psychiatric diagnosis as prototype categorization. J Abnorm Psychol 89:181–193, 1980a

Cantor S: Major psychoses of childhood. Course 53 at the American Psychiatric Association meetings, New York, May 4, 1983

Cantor S, Evans J, Pearce J, et al: Childhood schizophrenia: present but not accounted for. Am J Psychiatry 139:758–762, 1982

Cantor S, Pearce J, Pezzot-Pearce T, et al: The group of hypotonic schizophrenics: a pilot study. Schizophr Bull 7:1–11, 1981

Cantor S, Trevenen C, Postuma R: Muscle biopsy in hypotonic schizophrenic children: a preliminary report. Schizophr Bull 5:616–622, 1979

Cantor S, Trevenen C, Postuma R, et al: Is childhood schizophrenia a cholinergic disease? I: muscle morphology. Arch Gen Psychiatry 37:658–667, 1980b

Cantwell DP, Russell AT, Mattison R, et al: A comparison of DSM-II and DSM-III in the diagnosis of childhood psychiatric disorders, I: agreement with expected diagnosis. Arch Gen Psychiatry 36:1208–1213, 1979a

A comparison of DSM-II and DSM-III in the diagnosis of childhood psychiatric disorders, IV: difficulties in use, global comparison and conclusions. Arch Gen Psychiatry 36:1227–1228, 1979b

Capute AJ, Derivan AT, Chauvel PJ, et al: Infantile autism: a prospective study of diagnosis. Dev Med Child Neurol 17:58–62, 1975

Chess S, Thomas A: Temperamental individuality from childhood to adolescence. J Am Acad Child Psychiatry 16:218–226, 1977

Cohen DJ, Caparulo BK, Gold JR, et al: Clinical assessment and behavior rating scales for pervasively disturbed children. J Am Acad Child Psychiatry 17:589–603, 1978

COSAC: Council of Organizations and Schools for Autistic Children, diagnostic workshop, Rutgers University, New Brunswick, NJ, February 19, 1983

Creak M: Childhood psychosis: a review of 100 cases. Br J Psychiatry 109:84–89, 1963
Schizophrenic syndrome in childhood: further progress report of a working party. Dev Med Child Neurol 6:530–535, 1964

Creak M, Cameron K, Cowie F, et al: Schizophrenic syndrome in childhood. Br Med J 2:889–890, 1961

DeMyer MK, Barton S, DeMyer WE, et al: Prognosis in autism: a follow-up study. J Autism Child Schizo 3:199–246, 1973

DeMyer MK, Churchill D, Pontius N, et al: A comparison of five diagnostic systems for childhood schizophrenia and infantile autism. J Autism Child Schizo 1:175–189, 1971

DeMyer MK, Hingtgen JN, Jackson RK: Infantile autism reviewed: a decade of research. Schizophr Bull 7:388–451, 1981

Eisenberg L: Development as a unifying concept in psychiatry. Br J Psychiatry 131:225–237, 1977

Evans-Jones LG, Rosenbloom L: Disintegrative psychosis in childhood. Dev Med Child Neurol 20:462–470, 1978

Feighner JP, Robins E, Guze SB, et al: Diagnostic criteria for use in psychiatric research. Arch Gen Psychiatry 26:59–63, 1972

Fein D, Humes M, Kaplan E, et al: The question of left hemisphere dysfunction in infantile autism. Psychol Bull 95:258–281, 1984

Fein D, Waterhouse L, Lucci D, et al: Cognitive subtypes in developmentally disabled children. J Autism Dev Disord 15:77–96, 1985

Fish B: The study of motor development in infancy and its relationship to psychological functioning. Am J Psychiatry 117:1113–1118, 1961
Neurobiologic antecedents of schizophrenia in children. Arch Gen Psychiatry 34:1297–1313, 1977

Freeman BJ, Guthrie D, Ritvo E, et al: Behavior Observation Scale: preliminary analyses of the similarities and differences between autistic and mentally retarded children. Psychol Rep 7:357–380, 1979

Freeman BJ, Ritvo E: The syndrome of autism: a critical review, in Autism: Diagnosis, Instruction, Management, and Research. Edited by Gilliam J. Springfield, Ill, Charles C Thomas, 1981, pp 17–63

Freeman BJ, Ritvo E, Guthrie D, et al: The Behavior Observation Scale for Autism: initial methodology, data analysis, and preliminary findings on 89 children. J Am Acad Child Psychiatry 17:576–588, 1978

GAP: Psychopathological Disorders in Childhood: Theoretical Considerations and a Proposed Classification. New York, Group for the Advancement of Psychiatry, 1966

Gittelman R, Birch H: Childhood schizophrenia: intellect, neurologic status, perinatal risk, prognosis and family pathology. Arch Gen Psychiatry 17:16–25, 1967

Goldfarb W: Childhood Schizophrenia. Cambridge, Mass, Harvard University Press, 1961

An investigation of childhood schizophrenia. Arch Gen Psychiatry 11:621–634, 1964

An experience with early childhood psychoses – the variety of forms, the vicissitudes of change, the complexity of its causes. Issues Child Mental Health 5:5–51, 1977

Heller T: About Dementia Infantilis. 1930. Reprinted in Modern Perspectives in International Child Psychiatry. Edited by Howells JG. Edinburgh, Oliver & Boyd, 1969

Hyler SE, Williams JBW, Spitzer RL: Reliability in the DSM-III field trials: interview v case summary. Arch Gen Psychiatry 39:1275–1278, 1982

James A, Barry R: General maturational lag as an essential correlate of early-onset psychosis. J Autism Dev Disord 11:271–283, 1981

Jenkins RL, Glickman S: Common syndromes in child psychiatry, I: deviant behavior traits, II: the schizoid child. Am J Orthopsychiatry 16:244–261, 1946

Kagan J: The form of early development, continuity and discontinuity in emergent competences. Arch Gen Psychiatry 36:1047–1054, 1979

Kanner L: Autistic disturbances of affective contact. Nerv Child 2:181–197, 1943

Problems of nosology and psychodynamics of early infantile autism. Am J Orthopsychiatry 19:416–426, 1949

Kendell RE: The Role of Diagnosis in Psychiatry. Oxford, Blackwell Scientific, 1975

Kolvin I: Psychoses in childhood – a comparative study, in Infantile Autism: Concepts, Characteristics and Treatment. Edited by Rutter M. London, Churchill Livingstone, 1971, pp 7–26

Lessing EE, William V, Gil E: A cluster-analytically derived typology: feasible alternative to clinical diagnostic classification of children? J Abnorm Child Psychol 10:451–482, 1982

Mattison R, Cantwell DP, Russell AT, et al: A comparison of DSM-II and DSM-III in the diagnosis of childhood psychiatric disorders, II: interrater agreement. Arch Gen Psychiatry 36:1217–1222, 1979

Newsom C, Rincover A: Autism, in Behavioral Assessment of Childhood Disorders. Edited by Mash EJ, Terdal LG. New York, Guilford Press, 1979, chap. 9

Noll RB, Benedict H: Differentiations within the classification of childhood psychoses: a continuing dilemma. Merrill Palmer Quarterly 27:176–199, 1982

Ornitz EM: Neurophysiology of infantile autism. J Am Acad Child Psychiatry 24:251–262, 1985

Ornitz EM, Ritvo ER: Perceptual inconstancy in early infantile autism. Arch Gen Psychiatry 18:76–98, 1968

The syndrome of autism: a critical review. Am J Psychiatry 133:609–621, 1976

Parks SL: The assessment of autistic children: a selective review of available instruments. J Autism Dev Disord 13:255–267, 1983

Petty L, Ornitz EM, Michelman JD, et al: Autistic children who become schizophrenic. Arch Gen Psychiatry 41:129–135, 1984

Piggott LR, Gottlieb JS: Childhood schizophrenia – what is it? J Autism Child Schizo 3:96–105, 1973

Prior M, Boulton D, Gajzago C, et al: The classification of childhood psychoses by numerical taxonomy. J Child Psychol Psychiatry 16:3211–3300, 1975

Prior MR: Cognitive abilities and disabilities in infantile autism: a review. J Abnorm Child Psychol 7:357–380, 1979

Rescorla L, Dahl K: Taxonomic issues in preschool psychiatric disorders. Read before the biennial meeting of the Society for Research in Child Development, Detroit, April 1983

Rimland B: Infantile Autism. New York, Appleton-Century-Crofts, 1964

The differentiation of childhood psychoses: an analysis of checklists for 2,218 psychotic children. J Autism Child Schizo 1:161–174, 1971

Ritvo ER, Freeman BJ: National Society for Autistic Children definition of the syndrome of autism. J Autism Child Schizo 8:162–169, 1978

Russell AT, Cantwell DP, Mattison R, et al: A comparison of DSM-II and DSM-III in the diagnosis of childhood psychiatric disorders, III: multiaxial features. Arch Gen Psychiatry 36:1223–1226, 1979

Rutter M: Behavior and cognitive characteristics, in Early Childhood Autism. Edited by Wing L. Oxford, Pergamon Press, 1966, pp 51–82

Concepts of autism: a review of research. J Child Psychol Psychiatry 9:1–25, 1968a

The description and classification of infantile autism, in Proceedings of the Indiana University Colloquium on Infantile Autism. Edited by Churchill D, Alpern G, DeMyer M. Springfield, Ill, Charles C. Thomas, 1968b, pp 8–29

Childhood schizophrenia reconsidered. J Autism Child Schizo 2:315–337, 1972

The development of infantile autism. Psychol Med 4:147–163, 1974

Diagnosis and definition of childhood autism J Autism Child Schizo 8:139–161, 1978

Cognitive deficits in the pathogenesis of autism. J Child Psychol Psychiatry 24:513–531, 1983

Rutter M, Bartak L, Newman S: Autism – a central disorder of cognition and language? in Infantile Autism: Concepts, Characteristics and Treatment. Edited by Rutter M. London, Churchill Livingstone, 1971, pp 148–171

Rutter M, Hersov L (eds): Child Psychiatry: A Modern Approach. Oxford, Blackwell, 1977

Rutter M, Shaffer D: DSM-III, a step forward or back in terms of the classification of child psychiatric disorders? J Am Acad Child Psychiatry 19:371–394, 1980

Schain R, Yannet H: Infantile autism. J Pediatr 57:560–567, 1960

Schopler E, Reichler RJ, Devillis RF, et al: Toward objective classification of childhood autism: Childhood Autism Rating Scale (CARS). J Autism Dev Disord 10:91–103, 1980

Spitzer RL, Cantwell DP: The DSM-III classification of the psychiatric disorders of infancy, childhood and adolescence. J Am Acad Child Psychiatry 19:356–370, 1980

Spitzer RL, Endicott J, Robins E: Clinical criteria for psychiatric diagnosis and DSM-II. Am J Psychiatry 132:1187–1192, 1975

Tanguay PE: Toward a new classification of serious psychopathology in children. J Am Acad Child Psychiatry 23:373–384, 1984

Thomas A: Current trends in developmental theory. Am J Orthopsychiatry 51:580–609, 1981

Waterhouse L, Fein D: Language skills in developmentally delayed children. Brain and Language 15:303–315, 1982a

The left hemisphere hypothesis in autism: a critical review. Read before the International Neuropsychological Society, Deauville, France, June 1982b

Developmental trends in cognitive skills for children diagnosed as autistic and schizophrenic. Child Dev 55:236–248, 1984

Waterhouse L, Snyder D: Diagnostic criteria for infantile autism. Read before the Eden Institute annual workshop on autism, Princeton, NJ, August 31, 1983

Waterhouse L, Wing L, Fein D: Evaluating the empirical evidence for the syndrome of autism, in Autism: New Research. Edited by Dawson G, Segalowitz S. New York, Guilford Press (in press)

Werry JS: The childhood psychoses, in Psychopathological Disorders of Childhood, second edition. Edited by Quay HC, Werry JS. New York, Wiley, 1979

Williams JBW, Spitzer RL: NIMH sponsored field trial: interrater reliability, in Diagnostic and Statistical Manual of Mental Disorders (third edition). Washington, DC, American Psychiatric Association, 1980, pp 467–481

Research diagnostic criteria and DSM-III. Arch Gen Psychiatry 39:1283–1289, 1982

Wing L: Language, social and cognitive impairments of autism and severe mental retardation. J Autism Dev Disord 11:31–44, 1981

World Health Organization: International Statistical Classification of Diseases, Mental Disorders: Glossary and Guide to Their Classification. Geneva, WHO, 1978

22 *Diagnosis of depressive disorders in children*

An interim appraisal of the pertinent DSM-III categories

MARIA KOVACS

There is now increasing evidence that children suffer from depressive disorders. The presence of these disorders has been documented through the *DSM-III* (American Psychiatric Association, 1980) and the RDC (Spitzer, Endicott, and Robins, 1978) and across samples of juveniles that have varied in terms of age, sex distribution, and clinical status (Puig-Antich, 1980; Kashani et al., 1981, 1983; Kovacs et al., 1984a). The available data are therefore pertinent to an appraisal of *DSM-III* for diagnosis of depression in the preadult years.

The purpose of this chapter is to address four areas of concern: diagnostic utility and validity, the sensitivity and specificity of criterion symptoms, issues of differential diagnosis that make it especially difficult to study affective illness in children, and the interface between a developmental stage and the characteristics of the depressive disorders. The topical coverage is restricted to clinical parameters of the relevant diagnostic entities and to school-age children who have been referred to a university-affiliated pediatric medical or child psychiatric setting. The latter qualification is particularly important, because it is not yet known if the available findings can be generalized to preschoolers, to depressed children who have been treated by private practitioners, or to youngsters who have remained unreferred and untreated.

This chapter is not intended as a comprehensive review of the literature on childhood depression. Only selected research findings are summarized. Moreover, the specific data that are cited derive from only one investigation: an ongoing, naturalistic, longitudinal study of the depressive disorders in school-age children that is being conducted by the author and her collaborators. The design of the study and the characteristics of the samples have been described elsewhere (Kovacs et al., 1984a).

Preparation of this chapter was supported by grant MH-33990 from the National Institutes of Mental Health; partial support was provided by Clinical Center grant MH-30195.

BACKGROUND

Until a few years ago there was considerable controversy about the existence, symptomatic boundaries, and significance of depressive syndromes in children. It was posited, on the one hand, that "classic" depressive illness does not exist in the preadolescent years. On the other hand, proponents of the concept of childhood depression disagreed as to the manifest expression of the disorder. The theoretical issues that were debated and the various clinical characterizations that were put forth have been reviewed in detail (Conners, 1976; Gittelman-Klein, 1977; Kovacs and Beck, 1977; Lefkowitz and Burton, 1978; Welner, 1978; Kashani et al., 1981; Cantwell, 1983). Suffice it to say that there was no satisfactory way to resolve the controversy because of the diversity and ambiguity in the investigators' perspectives, diagnostic approaches, and assessment methods.

In contrast, recent studies of depressed children have been distinguished by their use of standardized clinical assessment, operational diagnostic criteria, and well-defined sampling strategies. The resultant findings have converged on at least one point: Major depression does exist and can be diagnosed in school-age children (Puig-Antich, 1980; Kashani et al., 1981). It is particularly noteworthy that the foregoing outcome was based on the use of unmodified "adult" diagnostic criteria for depression whose application to children has invited criticism.

The most poignant reservation about the adoption of "adult" DSM-III criteria has concerned the possibility that they may be too restrictive. It has been alleged that, because the definitional parameters for depression are not tailored to children, they fail to identify alternative forms of the disorder that occur in the younger years (Malmquist, 1983). The implication of this stance is that the guidelines in DSM-III are relatively insensitive to demonstrated or putative developmental features in the expressions of certain conditions. It is not surprising, therefore, that new definitions of childhood depression continue to be put forth, with an emphasis on "age-specific" symptomatic manifestations (Herzog and Rathbun, 1982).

Whereas the foregoing concerns derive from developmental psychopathology, application of the pertinent DSM-III diagnoses to children has also been questioned on the basis of standard nosologic principles. For example, when the manual was published, there was no evidence that the diagnostic categories of depression had discriminant or predictive validity in pediatric samples. Likewise, for children, the specific symptomatic criteria did not have an empirical foundation (Rutter and Shaffer, 1980).

The most parsimonious way to approach the reservations about the propriety of "adult" criteria for the diagnosis of depression in children is to examine the pertinent data. Although the issues will not be resolved fully until large-scale, multicenter psychobiological studies are undertaken and completed, the evidence so far suggests that the DSM-III categories of interest convey useful clinical information about the depressed child and that they do appear to have predictive validity.

DSM-III CATEGORIES FOR DEPRESSION: THEIR UTILITY AND VALIDITY IN JUVENILE COHORTS

The *DSM-III* contains four categories that are relevant to the diagnosis of depression: major depressive disorder (as part of a unipolar or bipolar illness), dysthymic disorder, atypical depressive disorder, and adjustment disorder with depressed mood. Most of the recent research studies of children have focused only on major depressive disorder. However, our research indicates that the various depressions can be distinguished from each other on several dimensions.

Major depressive disorder

The evidence is fairly clear that the *DSM-III,* as well as the RDC, can be used to identify major depression in school-age children. Such results have been reported in samples of prepubertal and pubertal youngsters, in inpatient and outpatient cohorts, and in normative population surveys (Puig-Antich et al., 1978; Carlson and Cantwell, 1979; Kashani and Simonds, 1979; Preskorn, Weller, and Weller, 1982; Puig-Antich, 1982; Kashani et al., 1983). Additionally, Carlson and Cantwell (1982) found that the *DSM-III* is more stringent than an earlier, developmentally oriented diagnostic schema for childhood depression with respect to the number of youngsters it identifies as depressed.

Findings from our own study indicate that among clinic-referred, school-age children, the *DSM-III* diagnosis of major depression is associated with a good recovery rate. But major depressive disorder (MDD) also has a complicated initial presentation and a high likelihood of recurrence. The most noteworthy features of major depression are the following:

1. a cumulative recovery rate of 92% within 1.5 years of onset of the index episode, and an average episode length of about 32 weeks,
2. high incidences of concurrently diagnosed affective and nonaffective disorders (dysthymia, anxiety, and conduct disorders being the most common),
3. an inverse association between the age at onset and the time to recovery from the episode – that is, the younger children are when they develop major depression, the more protracted their recovery (Kovacs et al., 1984a).

A further examination of the longitudinal courses for children with major depression reveals that this particular diagnosis has also clinically important predictive value. Over the course of five years after the onset of the first major depressive episode, there is a .72 cumulative probability of a second episode. Those youth who have recovered from "episode 1" are not likely to remain in remission for long. Within a little less than two years of initial recovery, 40% of them will have a second episode. Therefore, in our cohort, the "well time" between episodes of major depression has not yet exceeded two years. From among a number of variables that were examined, only the presence of an underlying dysthymic disorder was found to pose a significant risk for recurrent major depression (Kovacs et al., 1984b).

Our findings on the relative chronicity and comparably poor short-term prognosis for youngsters with major depression are not unprecedented. In fact, our results echo the conclusions of earlier clinical studies that relied on very different assessment strategies and diagnostic approaches (Nissen, 1971; Poznanski, Krahenbuhl, and Zrull, 1976; Chess, Thomas, and Hassibi, 1983).

Dysthymic disorder

The *DSM-III* category of dysthymic disorder (DD) is comparatively new. As it is currently defined, the criteria incorporate symptomatic features of neurotic depression, characterologic depression, or minor depression (Spitzer et al., 1978; Akiskal et al., 1980; American Psychiatric Association, 1980; Klerman, 1980). The existence of DD in the preadult years is just beginning to draw attention. There has been at least one clinical report of children who met the pertinent *DSM-III* criteria (Chess et al., 1983). Additionally, a recent epidemiological survey found that its RDC variant, namely, minor depression, could be identified in a normal population of nine-year-olds (Kashani et al., 1983).

Findings from our study indicate that among school-age outpatients, the diagnosis of dysthymia is associated with a comparatively early onset, a prolonged course and slow recovery pattern, and a high risk for superimposed episodes of major depression. More specifically, DD has the following salient features:

1. a cumulative recovery rate of 89% by a little over six years from disorder onset, with an average duration of about three years,
2. a high frequency of concurrently diagnosed *DSM-III* conditions (major depression, anxiety, attention deficit, and conduct disorders being the most common),
3. an inverse association between the child's age at onset of dysthymia and the time to recovery from the disorder (Kovacs et al., 1984a).

The predictive value of DD in school-age children is particularly interesting. During the first five years of dysthymic illness, and typically prior to its remission, these youth were found to be at high risk for the first superimposed episode of major depression (69% cumulative probability). And dysthymia was also found to pose a significant risk for a second episode of major depression. That is, children with a history of "double depression" (a previous major depressive episode that was superimposed on dysthymia) were far more likely to have a recurrent major depression than were children whose previous affective illness had entailed only major depression (Kovacs et al., 1984b).

Atypical depressive disorder

The *DSM-III* category of atypical depressive disorder apparently serves to classify clinical presentations that do not fit the definitional boundaries of the specific depressive disorders. Therefore, it is a "residual" diagnostic category. In our study of children, we have found only two general presentations so far that warrant the label of atypical depression.

One type of presentation could more accurately be designated as "atypical dysthymia." Whereas the observed phenomena were essentially dysthymic in nature, the criteria for DD were not met because of a few oddities. For example, although the duration criterion was satisfied and the required features were present, in a few cases the primary mood disturbance was irritability rather than depressed or anhedonic mood. Alternatively, a couple of children had long, unremitting histories of dysthymic symptoms, but the syndrome was always short of one criterion symptom.

The other phenomenological variant for which we used the label atypical depression was essentially an "atypical major depression." For example, at the time of the research assessment, the child met the symptomatic criteria for MDD, but the duration of the syndrome was a few days short of the required two weeks.

Therefore, the *DSM-III* category of atypical depressive disorder was found to be useful for the labeling of slightly deviant presentations among our school-age (8–13-year-old) cohort. However, the extent of the deviance from the DD or MDD prototype was not of major significance. And in our research sample, we did not find any distinctive and clearly different depressive syndromes for which "atypical depression" would have been a more appropriate designation than the other pertinent *DSM-III* labels.

Adjustment disorder with depressed mood

Because in *DSM-III* the symptomatic boundaries of adjustment disorder with depressed mood (ADDM) are not specified, in our study we required the presence of at least three clinically significant symptoms (Kovacs et al., 1984a). We presumed that this *DSM-III* category may capture two entities: bona fide adjustment disorders and "childhood equivalents" of clinically significant depressions that do not meet the stringent criteria for MDD or DD.

However, the findings to date suggest that as a diagnostic entity, ADDM bears few similarities to the more severe depressions. From among the various *DSM-III* categories of depression that we examined, ADDM emerged as the most benign, with the most favorable outcome. More specifically, the diagnosis of ADDM was associated with a rapid and early pattern of recovery: a 90% remission rate within nine months of disorder onset and an average duration of 25 weeks. ADDM patients also had the lowest incidence of other concurrent psychiatric disorders. Moreover, over the course of about five years, none of the children who previously had had ADDM subsequently developed either a major depression or a dysthymic disorder (Kovacs et al., 1984a,b).

Conclusion

Our data and the findings of others that were cited confirm the utility of *DSM-III* for diagnosis of depression in school-age clinic-referred children. Additionally, the *DSM-III* categories of depression can generally be distinguished from one another on the basis of initial presentation, clinical correlates, and subsequent course. These facts suggest that although the criteria for the various depressions were derived from adult patients, they have validity within the lower age groups.

With respect to school-age children who suffer from depression, the *DSM-III* diagnoses also convey clinically useful information about recovery and about the risk for a subsequent episode of major depression. Likewise, longitudinal study of these disorders has yielded potentially significant data on the relationship between age at onset and prognosis.

However, the foregoing conclusions must be qualified in a number of respects. First, because the utility and validity of *DSM-III* have not been studied systematically across the entire age range, it is not known if the diagnoses of depression have any heuristic value or nosologic standing among children of preschool age. Second, the findings that were cited have yet to be replicated by others. Finally, further nosologic study is clearly warranted in order to clarify several salient issues.

For example, the relationship between dysthymia and major depression in children is not yet clear (Kovacs et al., 1984a,b). If the two entities are found to be alternative expressions of the same underlying psychopathological process, then the criteria may have to be modified accordingly. Likewise, in depressed children, the presence and potential significance of coexisting psychiatric disorders need to be examined in more detail. It is unclear if this phenomenon is intrinsic to the depressive disorders in the younger years or if it reflects imprecision in the definitional criteria of *DSM-III*.

SENSITIVITY AND SPECIFICITY OF CRITERION SYMPTOMS

As noted earlier, the syndrome definitions for the depressive disorders in the *DSM-III* are applicable to and appear to be valid in school-age cohorts. However, the specific symptomatic criteria warrant closer scrutiny. For example, for DD, no rationale is provided in the *DSM-III* as to why irritability is not included as a symptom of mood disturbance (American Psychiatric Association, 1980). On the other hand, it can be questioned that certain criterion symptoms (e.g., distinct quality of depressed mood) can be assessed at all in school-age children.

A symptomatic examination of MDD versus other **DSM-III** *diagnoses*

In our study, clinical assessments of children were conducted by means of a semistructured, symptom-oriented psychiatric interview (Kovacs et al., 1984a). The interview schedule has been shown to be sufficiently reliable for use in research (Kovacs, 1985). For the purpose of the present chapter, the clinical-interview-based data were used to examine the sensitivity and specificity of selected symptoms.

Table 22.1 lists the incidences of various clinically significant symptoms in four diagnostic groups.

1. children in a "full-blown" episode of major depression (with no underlying dysthymic disorder),
2. children with pure DD to date (that is, no concurrent or previous episodes of major depression),
3. children whose diagnosis was ADDM,
4. a subsample of our psychiatric controls (children with attention deficit or conduct, oppositional, or anxiety disorders) who have been described elsewhere (Kovacs et al., 1984b).

As the data in Table 22.1 suggest, some of the symptomatic criteria for depression do not appear to have a strong empirical basis. Both within diagnostic categories and across the four groups, depressive as well as nondepressive symptoms have variable incidences. For example, excessive anger, which is a criterion symptom for DD, occurs at similar rates among children with DD, among children with the diagnosis of major depression, and among the psychiatric controls. Likewise, the presence of suicidal ideation does not distinguish the four diagnostic categories from one another.

It is instructive to examine the sensitivity and specificity of some symptoms that are supposed to be cardinal features of major depressive illness and the pertinence of other symptoms that are not required by *DSM-III*. "Sensitivity" refers to the "true positive rate" for a particular symptom – the portion of prediagnosed patients who have the variable in question. "Specificity" refers to the "true negative rate" for a symptom – the portion of prediagnosed patients who are correctly identified as not having the disorder of interest (Carroll, 1980). For the present analysis, the index diagnosis is major depression. The other two depressive disorders combined together serve as the comparison or diagnostic contrast.

According to the data, the symptom of depressed mood is a highly sensitive indicator of the diagnosis of major depression. That is, 91% of patients with this particular disorder have depressed mood. However, the symptom in question is not specific to MDD. In the diagnostic contrast group (that is, depressed children who do not have MDD), the symptom of depressed mood has only a 20% true negative rate.

On the other hand, anhedonia is a considerably more sensitive and more specific indicator of the diagnosis of major depression in children. A positive, clinically significant rating for anhedonia correctly identifies 86% of juveniles with major depression; its absence correctly identifies 90% of juveniles with the other two depressive conditions as not having a major depression.

Irritable mood, which is also a criterion symptom for major depression, has lower sensitivity and specificity than anhedonia. With respect to the index diagnosis of MDD, irritability has a sensitivity of 64%. Its specificity is 63%. That is, a negative rating on irritability correctly identifies 63% of children whose depressions do not meet the criteria for MDD.

Table 22.1. *Incidences of selected symptoms in four diagnostic groups of children* (%)

Symptom assessed in psychiatric interview	Diagnostic group			
	MDD ($N = 22$)	DD ($N = 14$)	ADDM ($N = 16$)	Psychiatric controls ($N = 30$)
Depressed mood	91	93	69	20
Feels unloved/forlorn	41	43	31	13
Anhedonia	86	0	19	0
Irritability	64	57	19	20
Anger	50	57	38	50
Temper tantrums	0	0	7	0
Disobedience	33	57	53	67
Social withdrawal	73	0	13	3
Self-deprecation	68	43	25	13
Pessimism	46	29	13	0
Reduced appetite	59	0	19	0
Increased appetite	9	21	6	3
Hypersomnia	27	7	19	3
Hyposomnia	68	21	25	10
Fatigue	68	21	12	0
Suicidal ideation	41	57	56	47
Psychomotor retardation	14	0	6	0
Psychomotor agitation	4	0	0	3
Underproductive speech	14	0	19	7
Generally uncooperative interview behavior (displays little effort/ interest; doesn't talk; is hostile)	18	0	6	7

It is of interest that whereas, according to *DSM-III,* the symptom of social withdrawal is not pathognomonic of major depression, it has considerable sensitivity and specificity for that diagnostic entity. Social withdrawal is present in 73% of patients who have florid major depression (true positive rate). Absence of social withdrawal correctly identifies 93% of the depressed diagnostic contrast group as subjects who do not have MDD.

Thus, it appears that social withdrawal should be one of the criteria for major depression in children and that irritability can readily be included in the DD category. Each of the symptoms listed in Table 22.1 (as well as others that have not been presented) can be analyzed in the manner illustrated here in order to assess its salience for the pertinent diagnostic entities.

Problems in assessment of criterion symptoms

Because of developmental factors, the presence or absence of certain depressive symptoms cannot be verified among school-age children. For example, younger patients do not seem to comprehend the gist of inquiries about whether or not their sad mood has a "distinct quality." Likewise, the symptom of "slowed thinking" cannot be elicited readily and validly from younger children.

Such difficulties in clinical assessment probably derive from the fact that many children do not have the cognitive sophistication that is required to self-monitor certain symptoms. For example, the ability to recognize "slowed thinking" in oneself presupposes an intellectual operation that has been called metacognition. Metacognition refers to the capacity to think about one's own thinking. However, the developmental literature (Kovacs, 1986) suggests that this particular ability does not emerge until the adolescent years.

Additionally, the very nature of the symptoms themselves can preclude a reasonable and face-valid clinical inquiry. Constructs such as "distinct quality" of sadness or "slowed thinking" cannot be readily objectified by examples or reformulated in simpler terms. In contrast, for instance, the related symptom of "impaired concentration" can be assessed by the use of alternative language and by a focus on the symptom's external correlates. Children can be asked about their ability "to pay attention," about teachers' and parents' comments concerning inattentiveness, or about not being able to keep one's mind on even favorite tasks or events.

It may well be that school-age children who are depressed can and do experience a distinct quality to their sadness or a change in the speed of their thinking. However, because of assessment problems, the sensitivity and specificity of such symptoms for the diagnosis of major depression cannot be determined readily. And because these phenomena are purely internal, they may elude even the parent of the depressed child.

Therefore, clinical assessment and diagnosis of children are far more complicated and problematic than among adults. This may account for the fact that in the traditional child psychiatric evaluation, symptomatic and historical data are typically gathered from adults who know the child (parents, other caretakers, teachers), whereas clinical interviews with young patients themselves generally are used to elicit process- and problem-oriented information (Puig-Antich, Chambers, and Tambrizi, 1983). Unfortunately, such an approach has considerable limitations with respect to delineation of affective disorders in children. Because depressions entail subjective experiences, symptomatic information obtained only from the parent may be incomplete or misleading.

For example, our data suggest that in separate semistructured clinical interviews concerning a child's symptoms, the parent and the child are least in agreement about the latter's affective and cognitive experiences. It has also been documented that psychiatric diagnoses based on data provided by parents are not concordant with diagnoses derived when the only informants are the children themselves (Orvaschel et al., 1981). Therefore, in order to delineate the parameters of the depressive disorders in childhood, accounts from the parents and children must be obtained and synthesized.

Conclusion

The *DSM-III* categories that apply to children have been criticized because many of the criteria therein do not have an empirical basis (Rutter and Shaffer, 1980). The analysis of selected symptoms presented here suggests that, with respect to school-age children, the criteria for the depressive disorders warrant further study.

The *syndromatic prototype* of major depression, for instance, may be relatively immune to developmental features. However, some of its manifestations that currently are not included in the diagnostic criteria could have an age-related distribution. The symptom of social withdrawal, which has high sensitivity and specificity for the diagnosis of MDD in our juvenile cohort, is one example.

Symptoms that do not appear in any of the pertinent *DSM-III* categories also warrant clinical and diagnostic attention. For example, our experiences suggest that the phenomena of severe major depression in school-age children often include loss of interest and manifest deterioration in personal hygiene. Therefore, symptomatic assessment of depressed juveniles should be broader than the criteria specified by *DSM-III*.

Moreover, in order to delimit the phenomenological boundaries of the depressive disorders in childhood, there must be a degree of uniformity in the assessment strategies of various investigators. The available evidence suggests that clinical evaluations should take into account and synthesize the data that children provide about themselves and the information that parents provide about their children.

ISSUES IN DIFFERENTIAL DIAGNOSIS

The issues encountered in differential diagnosis highlight that neither the validity of the pertinent *DSM-III* categories nor the specificity and sensitivity of the criterion symptoms can be determined easily. The major problems derive from the complex nature of psychopathology and from the fact that *DSM-III* permits multiple axis I and axis II diagnoses.

Several investigators have reported, for example, that children with major depression are likely to have other concurrent psychiatric conditions (Puig-Antich et al., 1978; Carlson and Cantwell, 1980; Puig-Antich, 1982). We have demonstrated the same phenomenon among juveniles with DD and have also shown that dysthymia and major depression often present in combination (Kovacs et al., 1984a). Whereas the various reports agree that among youngsters with MDD, separation anxiety, conduct, and attention-deficit disorders are some of the most frequent concomitant diagnoses, the incidence figures differ. Moreover, others have not yet described the combination of MDD and DD in school-age children.

Disagreements concerning the presence of multiple disorders or differentiation of one disorder from another arise partly because salient aspects of diagnostic decision making are not standardized. With respect to the depressions in childhood, there are two issues: (1) the differential between disorders that are in the same psychopathological domain (e.g., major depression versus dysthymia) and (2) the symptomatic overlap between categorically different psychiatric entities (e.g., overanxious disorder of childhood and DD).

In order to diagnose a major depression that is superimposed on DD, it is inevitable that some symptoms will be "counted" twice. For example, the presence of depressed mood qualifies the child to meet one criterion for each of the foregoing disorders. Although "double depression" has been described among adults (Keller and Shapiro, 1982), neither *DSM-III* nor the extant publications provide rules about how to weigh particular symptoms. Therefore, in our study, we had to devise an operational definition for the conditions under which such a dual diagnosis could be assigned (Kovacs et al., 1984a).

A further diagnostic problem is that in depressed children, some of the coexisting disorders entail symptoms that are similar to the manifestations of the depressive syndrome. Therefore, it is often difficult to decide if a particular complaint mirrors one or the other psychiatric entity. For example, if a major depressive episode is superimposed on attention-deficit disorder with hyperactivity, it is difficult to distinguish between hyperactive behavior and psychomotor agitation. Likewise, if separation-anxiety disorder and DD present together, the symptom of sleep disturbance could be associated with either or with both.

Similar problems arise in diagnosing a related group of disorders that have not been discussed in this chapter: the manic or hypomanic conditions. For example, restlessness, talkativeness, and distractibility are manifestations of both the hyperactive and hypomanic–manic syndromes. Likewise, if a child has had a depression and a preexisting conduct disorder, an affective shift to hypomania or mania may remain undetected because irresponsible, acting-out, "daredevil," or "nasty" behavior can be viewed as part of the conduct disorder. Differential diagnosis of bipolar illness in the preadult years is further confounded because a child's environment and daily activities often are sufficiently regimented or restricted to attenuate certain symptomatic behaviors (e.g., excessive involvement in risky or pleasurable activities).

The fact that among school-age depressed children the clinical presentation may warrant and the *DSM-III* may allow multiple diagnoses has important nosologic implications. However, the validity of particular diagnostic labels and the pertinence of criterion symptoms can be assessed only if salient aspects of the diagnostic process are formalized. Otherwise, attempts to replicate extant or ongoing work are likely to yield discordant findings.

THE INTERFACE BETWEEN DEVELOPMENT AND THE
CHARACTERISTICS OF THE DEPRESSIVE DISORDERS

According to Herzog and Rathbun (1982), as well as Malmquist (1983), the *DSM-III* criteria for the depressive disorders have limited utility in child psychiatry. The point of contention is that the guidelines do not take fully into account that the young patient's stage of development influences the expression of the depressive syndrome.

"Developmental" concerns have long dominated the field of childhood depression. Psychoanalytic, ego-analytic, cognitive, and social-cognitive theories, alone or in combination, have served as the basis of speculation about the existence and characteristics of depression in the preadult years (Conners, 1976; Kovacs and Beck, 1977; Kashani et al., 1981). For example, it has been proposed that because a child does not experience genuine guilt, the child cannot develop "classic" depression (Rochlin, 1959). According to others, depression in the juvenile years ought to be less persistent and severe than it is in adults, because children's perceptions and reactions are temporary and fleeting (Makita, 1973; Bemporad, 1978). It has also been proposed that depressed children are unlikely to experience hopelessness or self-denigration and that they will defend against the unpleasant affect by "acting out." The foregoing perspectives are delineated in greater detail elsewhere (Kovacs and Paulauskas, 1984).

Nonetheless, in spite of continued speculations along developmental lines concerning the expression of childhood depression, few of the propositions have been tested empirically. Therefore, as part of our ongoing research study, we have also examined several issues concerning developmental-stage mediation of these disorders. The hypotheses, the design, and the specific findings are described elsewhere (Kovacs and Paulauskas, 1984). In brief, two parameters of development were studied: cognitive development (assessed by means of Piagetian tasks) and somatosexual development (determined by pediatric examination). The goal of the investigation was to examine whether or not the characteristics of the depressive disorders and the type of manifest symptoms conformed to "developmental" expectations.

The findings did not support even the most common notions about developmental-stage mediation of depressive disorders in children. Instead, the results were countertheoretical and counterintuitive. For example, in our sample, the developmentally less mature children had the more chronic depressions; when in a major depressive episode, they also took far longer to recover than the more mature youngsters. Early age and prepubertal status at the onset of the depression were the two developmental markers that signaled chronicity or prolonged recovery. In this regard, the stage of cognitive development failed to emerge as a predictor.

The results were also inconsistent and contrary to expectations in regard to the relationship between developmental stage and depressive symptoms. In one set of analyses, we found no meaningful symptomatic trends. However, when the data were manipulated differently, the results revealed that the developmentally less mature children had the most pronounced anhedonia and self-deprecation. Disobedience as well as somatic complaints that presumably characterize the "masked depressions" of younger children were most evident among the cognitively and pubertally advanced youth.

Alternative explanations for these findings have been discussed (Kovacs and Paulauskas, 1984). With respect to this chapter, however, the results have several implications. First, it seems questionable that a developmental approach to the depressive disorders would facilitate a better diagnostic understanding of these entities in the school-age years. Second, the available evidence does not support the notion that depression in the juvenile years necessitates a unique nosologic category. However, the foregoing comments must be qualified in one regard: The interface between development and manifest disorder may be much more clear-cut among preschoolers. Therefore, the viability of a developmental approach to these psychiatric conditions should be examined in young children. Finally, notwithstanding our findings, a developmental perspective is pertinent and relevant to assessment of the depressive disorders. Because children's inability to report on certain symptoms may be due to maturational factors, a better understanding of cognitive and emotional development would facilitate the process of clinical evaluation and diagnosis.

FINAL COMMENT

The *DSM-III* is clearly different from previous official and unofficial systems of classification that have been used in child psychiatry. The manual's approach is primarily "nonetiologic" and descriptive. It also provides specific diagnostic criteria for the bulk of disorders contained therein. Notwithstanding the many questions about the categories that are applicable to children, the *DSM-III's* phenomenological and operational features should aid in the advancement of diagnosis and classification. At the very least, the criteria are testable and open to revision.

REFERENCES

Akiskal HS, Rosenthal TL, Haykal RF, et al: Characterological depressions: clinical and sleep EEG findings separating "subaffective dysthymias" from "character spectrum disorders." Arch Gen Psychiatry 37:777–783, 1980

American Psychiatric Association: Diagnostic and Statistical Manual of Mental Disorders, third edition. Washington, DC, APA, 1980

Bemporad JR: Manifest symptomatology of depression in children and adolescents, in Severe and Mild Depression. Edited by Arieti S, Bemporad J. New York, Basic Books, 1978

Cantwell DP: Depression in childhood: clinical picture and diagnostic criteria, in Affective Disorders in Childhood and Adolescence: An Update. Edited by Cantwell DP, Carlson GA. New York, Spectrum, 1983

Carlson GA, Cantwell DP: A survey of depressive symptoms in a child and adolescent psychiatric population: interview data. J Am Acad Child Psychiatry 18:587–599, 1979

Unmasking masked depression in children and adolescents. Am J Psychiatry 137:445–449, 1980

Diagnosis of childhood depression: a comparison of the Weinberg and DSM-III criteria. J Am Acad Child Psychiatry 21:247–250, 1982

Carroll B: Biostatistical principles of laboratory diagnostic test development. Psychopharmacol Bull 16:38–40, 1980

Chess S, Thomas A, Hassibi M: Depression in childhood and adolescence: a prospective study of six cases. J Nerv Men Dis 171:411–420, 1983

Conners CK: Classification and treatment of childhood depression and depressive equivalents, in Depression: Behavioral, Biochemical, Diagnostic and Treatment Concepts. Edited by Gallant DM, Simpson GM. New York, Spectrum, 1976

Gittelman-Klein R: Definitional and methodological issues concerning depressive illnesses in children, Depression in Childhood: Diagnosis, Treatment, and Conceptual Models. Edited by Schulterbrandt JG, Raskin A. New York, Raven Press, 1977

Herzog DB, Rathbun JM: Childhood depression: developmental considerations. Am J Dis Child 136:115–120, 1982

Kashani JH, Husain A, Shekim WO, et al: Current perspectives on childhood depression: an overview. Am J Psychiatry 138:143–153, 1981

Kashani JH, McGee RO, Clarkson SE, et al: Depression in a sample of 9-year-old children: prevalence and associated characteristics. Arch Gen Psychiatry 40:1217–1223, 1983

Kashani JH, Simonds JF: The incidence of depression in children. Am J Psychiatry 136:1203–1205, 1979

Keller MB, Shapiro RB: "Double depression": superimposition of acute depressive episodes on chronic depressive disorders. Am J Psychiatry 139:438–442, 1982

Klerman GL: Other specific affective disorders, in Comprehensive Textbook of Psychiatry III, Vol 2. Edited by Kaplan HI, Freedman AM, Sadock BJ. Baltimore, Williams & Wilkins, 1980

Kovacs M: The Interview Schedule for Children (ISC). Psychopharmacol Bull 21:991–994, 1985

A developmental perspective on methods and measures in the assessment of depressive disorders: the clinical interview, in Depression in Young People: Developmental and Clinical Perspectives. Edited by Rutter M, Izard C, Read P. New York, Guilford, 1986

Kovacs M, Beck AT: An empirical-clinical approach toward a definition of childhood depression, in Depression in Childhood: Diagnosis, Treatment, and Conceptual Models. Edited by Schulterbrandt JG, Raskin A. New York, Raven Press, 1977

Kovacs M, Feinberg TL, Crouse-Novak MA, et al: Depressive disorders in childhood, I: a longitudinal prospective study of characteristics and recovery. Arch Gen Psychiatry 41:229–237, 1984a

Depressive disorders in childhood, II: risk of a subsequent major depression. Arch Gen Psychiatry 41:643–649, 1984b

Kovacs M, Paulauskas S: Developmental stage and the expression of depressive disorders in children: an empirical analysis, in Childhood Depression (New Directions for Child Development, no. 26). Edited by Cicchetti D, Schneider-Rosen K. San Francisco, Jossey-Bass, 1984

Lefkowitz MM, Burton N: Childhood depression: a critique of the concept. Psychol Bull 85:716–726, 1978

Makita K: The rarity of "depression" in childhood. Acta Paedopsychiatrica 40:37–44, 1973

Malmquist, CP: Major depression in childhood: why don't we know more? Am J Orthopsychiatry 53:262–268, 1983

Nissen G: Depressive Syndrome in Kindes- und Jugendalter. Berlin, Springer-Verlag, 1971

Orvaschel H, Weissman MM, Padian N, et al: Assessing psychopathology in children of psychiatrically disturbed parents: a pilot study. J Am Acad Child Psychiatry 20:112–122, 1981

Poznanski EO, Krahenbuhl V, Zrull JP: Childhood depression: a longitudinal perspective. J Am Acad Child Psychiatry 15:491–501, 1976

Preskorn SH, Weller EB, Weller RA: Depression in children: relationship between plasma imipramine levels and response. J Clin Psychiatry 43:450–453, 1982

Puig-Antich J: Affective disorders in childhood: a review and perspective. Psychiatr Clin North Am 3:403–424, 1980

Major depression and conduct disorder in prepuberty. J Am Acad Child Psychiatry 21:118–128, 1982

Puig-Antich J, Blau S, Marx N, et al: Prepubertal major depressive disorder: a pilot study. J Am Acad Child Psychiatry 17:695–707, 1978

Puig-Antich J, Chambers WJ, Tabrizi MA: The clinical assessment of current depressive episodes in children and adolescents: interviews with parents and children, in Affective Disorders in Childhood and Adolescence: An Update. Edited by Cantwell DP, Carlson GA. New York, Spectrum, 1983

Rochlin G: The loss complex: a contribution to the etiology of depression. J Am Psychoanal Assoc 7:299–316, 1959

Rutter M, Shaffer D: DSM-III: a step forward or back in terms of the classification of child psychiatric disorders? J Am Acad Child Psychiatry 19:371–394, 1980

Spitzer RL, Endicott J, Robins E: Research diagnostic criteria: rationale and reliability. Arch Gen Psychiatry 35:773–782, 1978

Welner Z: Childhood depression: an overview. J Nerv Ment Dis 166:588–593, 1978

23 *An evaluation of the DSM-III diagnosis of conduct disorder*

LEE N. ROBINS

Conduct disorder is an important diagnosis in *DSM-III* because it is so commonly used. In a variety of studies of treated populations, it has been found to be the most commonly given childhood diagnosis. To learn how well pleased users are with its definition in *DSM-III*, I wrote to a number of persons who have published on conduct disorder. With one exception, there was agreement that such a diagnosis is necessary. And with unanimity the respondents did not like the current description of the disorder in *DSM-III*. However, their criticisms of it were varied. In this chapter I review the criticisms and their grounds and propose a direction for revision that I believe would satisfy most of the complaints. However, I have not circulated these suggestions to my very helpful consultants, and so am not positive that they would all agree that the proposed solution is the best possible one.

The complaints covered the following areas:

1. lack of justification for the socialized–undersocialized subtypes,
2. questions about the justification for a distinction between aggressive and non-aggressive types, and the assignment of specific behaviors to these categories,
3. adequacy of criteria for girls,
4. adequacy of criteria for preschool children,
5. absence of many common symptoms,
6. lack of precision in definition of symptoms,

This research was supported by the Epidemiological Catchment Area (ECA) program. The ECA is a series of five epidemiologic research studies performed by independent research teams in collaboration with staff of the Division of Biometry and Epidemiology (DBE) of the National Institute of Mental Health (NIMH). The NIMH Principal Collaborators are Darrel A. Regier, Ben Z. Locke, and William W. Eaton; the NIMH Project Officer is Carl A. Taube. The Principal Investigators and Co-Investigators from the five sites are as follows: Yale University, Uo1 MH 34224, Jerome K. Myers, Myrna M. Weissman, and Gary Tischler; Johns Hopkins University, Uo1 MH 33870, Morton Kramer, Ernest Gruenberg, and Sam Shapiro; Washington University, St. Louis, Uo1 MH 33883, Lee N. Robins and John Helzer; Duke University, Uo1 MH35386, Dan Blazer and Linda George; University of California, Los Angeles, Uo1 MH 35865, Richard Hough, Marvin Karno, Javier Escobar, and Audrey Burnam. This work acknowledges support of this program as well as Research Scientist Award MH 00334.

7. problems in differential diagnosis,
8. redundancy between conduct disorder and the precursor symptoms of antisocial personality and the propriety of conduct disorder as a diagnosis with adult onset.

Each of these problems is discussed in turn.

Socialized versus undersocialized

The socialized–undersocialized distinction grew out of factor analyses carried out in the 1940s by Hewitt and Jenkins with 500 case records of child-guidance patients. They identified three clusters of symptoms, two of which were the socialized and undersocialized behavior problems, and a third, internalizing disorder. However, these three scales accounted for only two-fifths of the patients. A recent study by Henn, Bardwell, and Jenkins (1980) of a delinquent sample found milder arrest records and better outcomes for the socialized delinquents. However, they did not control for the severity of the delinquency history at time of referral. If the gang membership common among socialized delinquents led to referral to court on the basis of less serious delinquency than that required for the referral of a "loner," this could explain the difference in outcome between the socialized and undersocialized delinquents.

Few studies have substantiated the distinction. Quay (1979) reviewed the literature with respect to the unpopularity of children with conduct disorder and found such unpopularity ubiquitous, suggesting that socialized conduct disorder is rare. It appeared in a study by Peterson, who found the socialized type only in juvenile delinquents and in metropolitan child-guidance clinics. Quay thinks that socialized conduct disorder may be an urban phenomenon and that the distinction does not apply elsewhere.

What support there is for the distinction seems to depend mainly on the fact that it was made in *DSM-II*. For instance, in 1975, Rutter, Shaffer, and Shepherd wrote on multiaxial classification for WHO. In that publication, they recommended classifying children as unsocialized, socialized, mixed, other, and unspecified. They said that "the category of socialized delinquency is open to dispute because the items said to characterize this disorder have not always been found to group together. Nevertheless, in view of its wide usage, as in the APA's Manual, it is probably worth retaining." Thus, the chief argument in its favor seems to be that it exists. It is questionable that a disorder seen so rarely in clinical settings is worth maintaining.

Aggressive versus nonaggressive

The next issue in the *DSM-III* classification of conduct disorder is the division into aggressive and nonaggressive types. Most analyses thus far have found that children's behaviors can be classified along a dimension that seems related to the aggressive–nonaggressive distinction, although the precise selection of symptoms found in these two categories in *DSM-III* seems not to be replicable.

Loeber and Schmaling (in press, a) carried out a factor analysis with 10,000 children. They found conduct problems to lie along a single dimension, with behaviors that they called overt or confrontive at one end, and behaviors that they called covert at the other. The overt behaviors resemble aggressive behaviors in *DSM-III*, because they include fighting and attacking others; the covert behaviors resemble the nonaggressive behavior problems in *DSM-III*, because they include running away, substance abuse, and truanting. However, fire setting and vandalism, which are part of the criteria for aggressive conduct disorder in *DSM-III*, were found among the covert behaviors. (Interestingly, the *DSM-III* text also puts them among the nonaggressive behaviors – a curious inconsistency between text and criteria.) Lying, which *DSM-III* includes among the nonaggressive behaviors, was found by Loeber and Schmaling to lie halfway between these poles. Among overt behaviors, they also found behaviors that are not part of the criteria of *DSM-III*, but are listed as associated features that apply to both aggressive and nonaggressive types – particularly, temper tantrums, irritability, and attentional difficulties.

One of the problems with the *DSM-III* division into aggressive and nonaggressive is that it leaves the nonaggressive behaviors as a residual category. The text clearly states that the nonaggressive diagnosis requires absence of aggressive symptoms. Interestingly, the diagnostic criteria for the nonaggressive subtype do not state that aggressive symptoms are a basis for excluding a diagnosis of the nonaggressive subtype.

Assuming the text is correct, and that the exclusion criterion holds, a child would be classified as aggressive if he fights, regardless of whether or not he also runs away or steals. That would be unfortunate, because Loeber and Schmaling found that the covert behaviors (which *DSM-III* classifies as nonaggressive) are more predictive of later difficulties than are the overt behaviors. For instance, delinquency is better predicted by stealing and truancy than by fighting and "sassing" the teacher. This exclusion rule thus reduces the effectiveness of the diagnosis as a prognostic tool.

Like Loeber and Schmaling, we have found the nonaggressive behaviors to be excellent predictors of later outcome. An example in point is drug abuse, the only behavior before the age of 15 that we found to be predictive of the degree of adult antisocial behavior of young black men and Vietnam veterans on its own, independent of its contribution to having a larger number of early antisocial behaviors.

Criteria for girls

The diagnosis of conduct disorder as described in *DSM-III* appeared to some researchers to be more adequate for boys than for girls. One reason appears to be the omission from the list of criterion symptoms of sexual misbehavior (other than rape), which is thought to be the behavior problem most

Table 23.1. *Correlations among conduct problems before age 15[a]*

Conduct problems	Mean correlations[b] with other 11 problems	Frequency (%)
Vandalism	.15	4
Underachievement	.15	5
Stealing	.18	19
Lying	.18	12
Runaway	.18	2
Fighting	.18	11
Arrest	.18	3
Drunk, drugs	.19	5
Sex	.20	13
Expelled/suspended	.21	7
Truant	.22	7
School discipline	.25	11

[a]ECA household sample – St. Louis.
[b]Range: .16 (vandalism vs. underachievement), .38 (discipline vs. expulsion); all are positive.

characteristic of girls. Our own research has found that very early sexual intercourse (before age 15) is one of the most common symptoms for both sexes (Table 23.1). The results in Table 23.1 come from our recent interviews with a general population sample of 3,000 adults (Robins, 1986) who were asked about 12 types of behavior problems occurring before the age of 15 as part of a diagnostic interview that included the diagnosis of antisocial personality. Note that in Table 23.1, the right-hand column shows the frequencies of these behaviors as recalled by adults. Sexual activity before age 15 was second only to stealing in the frequency with which it was reported. The first column shows the degree of intercorrelation among these behaviors. Early sexual behavior is as highly intercorrelated with other problem behaviors as are most of the behaviors that appear in *DSM-III,* suggesting that it belongs in the set of antisocial behaviors for both boys and girls.

There has been disagreement in the literature as to how greatly girls differ from boys in their pattern of behavior problems. Several studies have found that onset tends to be later in girls than in boys. This was confirmed in our study of recalled behavior problems in the general population, where the mean age of onset was slightly higher among females for 10 of the 12 behaviors inquired about (Table 23.2). Stewart and associates (1980) did not find impressive differences in symptoms by sex among inpatients diagnosed as having conduct disorder, but among outpatients, they found that there was more running away by

Table 23.2. *Courses of conduct problems before age 15*[a]

Problems in order of occurrence	Mean age of initiation before 15	
	Men	Women
School discipline	9.0	9.8
Underachievement	9.3	10.2
Fighting	9.4	10.0
Lying	9.9	9.6
Stealing	10.0	9.7
Truant	11.0	12.0
Vandalism	11.2	10.7
Drunk	11.2	11.8
Runaway	11.6	12.3
Sex	11.7	13.0
Expelled	11.8	12.1
Arrest	12.4	12.6
Drugs	12.7	13.1

[a]ECA data; $r = .87$, $z = 3.01$.

girls than by boys. We, too, found that women in the general population recalled more running away than did men, although it was rare for both sexes.

Criteria for preschool children

Another criticism of the criteria is that they are not appropriate for young children. Many of the items included simply cannot be accomplished by children below school age. Truancy is the most obvious example, but mugging, extortion, gas-station robbery, and rape all require being larger than one's victim or having the ability to use weapons. Among the studies that seem to imply that the criteria for young children are insufficient is Rachel Gittelman's finding that children who meet the criteria for hyperactivity early in life, but do not meet the criteria for conduct disorder, often develop conduct disorder later. Diagnoses that turn into something else are signs of a defect in the nosologic system (Robins and Guze, 1970). Presumably these children indeed already suffered from conduct disorder early in life, but the criteria did not allow its detection in its early form.

There is other evidence as well that conduct disorder should be detectable in very young children. Although diagnosis rarely occurs before the early school years, mothers almost always report a history of problems with compliance and aggressiveness long predating school. Presumably these children already had the disorder well before it was diagnosable by current criteria. Indeed, Mark Stewart (pers. commun.) feels that the first onset of antisocial behavior in an 11-year-old who has previously been compliant should alert the clinician to search for a diagnosis other than conduct disorder, because early onset is so much the rule. He would advocate adding an age-of-onset criterion to require emergence in early childhood.

Common symptoms

The insensitivity of the criteria for conduct disorder to conduct problems in girls and young children suggests that necessary criterion symptoms have been omitted. In addition, the criteria omit many symptoms that are commonly found in the clinical records of children with conduct disorder. Some of these appear in the *DSM-III* text, but not in the diagnostic criteria. Others may be implied, but not stated, in the criteria.

As noted earlier, sexual misbehavior seems worth including in its own right, not merely because girls' problems are underrepresented in *DSM-III*. Another common behavior problem that was noted as missing is verbal aggression. Cursing, using "bad" language, and making derogatory comments about others are some of the things that make children with conduct disorder unpopular with their peers, and this verbal aggression often appears in preschool children. Some critics believe that the *DSM-III* diagnosis is weak in assessing noncompliance, which Stewart feels is the hallmark of conduct disorder. Although *DSM-III* gives "chronic violations of a variety of important rules" as a criterion symptom for nonaggressive children, noncompliance is not absolutely required and is not even used in diagnosis of the aggressive subtype. Another omission is poor academic success despite an adequate IQ. This is almost universally found among children with conduct disorder. Cruelty is another frequently noted behavior that seems not to be fully covered by assault.

Whereas these common behavior problems are omitted, some rare ones are included. Rape and homicide are prime examples. *DSM-III* mentions that homicide is rare, but strangely makes no similar remark about rape. Both are, in fact, so rare that they are likely to be of little help in making a diagnosis.

Precise definition of symptoms

Another complaint was that the criteria for conduct disorder lack the quantifiers found in much of *DSM-III*. For instance, truancy is very specifically quantified when it serves as a precursor in the diagnosis of antisocial personality. It must occur on at least five days per year in at least two school years, not counting the last year in school. As a criterion for conduct disorder, it is simply "persistent" truancy, leaving "persistent" undefined, so that the presence of the symptom will vary with the threshold of the diagnostician. This is equally true of all the other criteria for conduct disorder.

Many children's behavior problems are considered as problems only because they are age-inappropriate – the children are either too young or too old to be behaving as they are. However, *DSM-III* provides no quantitative information about the ages at which lying, assault, and other behaviors common in very small children become pathological, nor about the age at which drinking modest amounts of alcohol is no longer "substance abuse." Again, this absence of more specific criteria will result in clinicians using varying standards.

Another lack of precision lies in failure to specify whether or not symptoms must occur in a variety of settings. One researcher-clinician noted that he would hesitate to make the diagnosis of conduct disorder if it were situation-specific. Yet pervasiveness is not required by *DSM-III*.

Differential diagnosis

Another problem cited was the difficulty in making differential diagnoses between conduct disorder and the disorders from which *DSM-III* states that it must be distinguished, particularly oppositional disorder and antisocial personality. The criteria for oppositional disorder suggest that it is in fact a mild form of conduct disorder, because it includes infractions of minor (but not important) rules and verbal (but not physical) aggression. Because children with conduct disorder have all the symptoms of oppositional disorder as well, conduct disorder preempts oppositional disorder. However, oppositional disorder seems to have no unique qualities of its own. It seems out of keeping with the general philosophy of *DSM-III* to have two diagnoses that are simply mild and severe forms of the same pattern of symptoms. (Even dysthymia requires a two-year duration, longer than major depressive disorder.)

There is the opposite kind of confusion between antisocial personality and conduct disorder. Is conduct disorder a separate diagnosis from antisocial personality, or is it an earlier and milder form? Antisocial personality is not permitted as a diagnosis for anyone under age 18, but there is no upper limit on the age at which a diagnosis of conduct disorder can be made. Because there are overlapping symptoms, some rather bizarre diagnostic results are possible: A person younger than 18 who meets the criteria for both diagnoses (other than age) will get a diagnosis of conduct disorder, but in a person 18 or older, with the identical set of symptoms, the diagnosis would be antisocial personality. If behavior problems start late in adolescence, so that the antisocial-personality criterion that says three behavior problems must occur before 15 is not met, a man or woman qualifies for a diagnosis of conduct disorder even though he or she is older than 18 and meets the adult criteria for antisocial personality.

About half the children with severe conduct disorder will later meet the criteria for a diagnosis of antisocial personality. Should children with conduct disorder change diagnoses merely because they continue their aggression, stealing, and rule breaking past age 18? At age 18, they are moved not only from one diagnosis to another but also from axis I to axis II.

Redundancy

The other awkward situation is that there are essentially two distinct diagnoses of conduct disorder: one in the section on disorders of childhood, and one in the adult section as a precursor for antisocial personality. To add to the confusion, the limitation to onset during childhood appears for conduct problems in the adult section; that is, the conduct problems that are precursors of antisocial personality must all appear before the age of 15, whereas the symptoms of conduct disorder in the section on childhood disorders presumably can begin at any age, even in adulthood.

SOME SUGGESTIONS FOR IMPROVING DIAGNOSIS OF CONDUCT DISORDER

1. There seems little reason, on the basis of existing research, to continue the distinction between socialized and undersocialized. In addition to the lack of evidence in favor of the distinction, there is a lack of agreement about what socialized conduct disorder is. If a boy has a single ally, and with this ally is engaged in hostile interactions with family, school, and peers, it is difficult to bestow on him the benevolent diagnosis of "socialized," even though he has a friend. Then what happens if the friendship ends? Does he change categories, or does he keep the designation indefinitely because the fact that he once had a friend shows that he has a capacity for friendship? The reverse can also happen, and often does in adolescence. A boy who has gotten along poorly with his male peers may develop a heterosexual relationship with some permanence once he reaches puberty. Does this shift him from undersocialized to socialized even if he continues to have no alliances with males? Between the conceptual difficulties and the scarcity of empirical support for its importance, this is a distinction that can well be dropped.

2. It seems possible to make a distinction between confrontive and covert behaviors. Whether or not this is a useful distinction we simply do not know yet. There have been no family studies to show that these behavior patterns assort within families and no attempts to determine if they have distinct psychophysiological correlates, if they are differentially associated with other disorders of childhood such as attention-deficit disorder or the anxiety disorders or childhood affective disorders, or if they have different predictive value for adult diagnoses. All we know now about their predictive value is that covert behaviors seem better predictors of juvenile delinquency. However, this is not a surprising observation, because covert behaviors include theft, which is the chief offense for which children are arrested.

So far, support for the distinction comes from factor analyses of symptoms in cross-sectional studies of general populations of schoolchildren or children diagnosed as having conduct disorder. Although the distinction is found quite consistently, all analyses also show that the two sets of behaviors are themselves highly intercorrelated; that is, confrontive children also steal and are truant. Nor are these factors uniformly found. When we factor-analyzed the childhood behavior problems reported retrospectively by adults in our general population (Table 23.3), we found a clear school-behaviors factor, which included truancy, discipline problems, expulsion, and underachievement, behaviors that come

Table 23.3. *Factor analyses of 12 conduct problems before age 15 as recalled by ECA household respondents*[a]

Girls' factors	Boys' factors		
	1	2	3
1	Sex (.54/.38)	Discipline (.70/.51[b])	
	Drunk, drugs (.43[c]/.72)	Expelled (.60/.66)	
	Fight (.36[d]/.64)	Truant (.59/.58)	
		Underachievement (.47/.63)	
2	Vandalism (.74/.60)	Lying (.66/.52)	Stealing (.51/.44)
3			Arrest (.84/.72)
			Runaway (.65[b]/.75)

[a]Girl/boy loadings.
[b]Also loads on factor 1.
[c]Also loads on factor 3.
[d]Also loads on factor 2.

from both the confrontive and covert categories if the discipline problems include open clashes with teachers. We also found fighting and substance abuse to fall on the same factor for both boys and girls, a contradiction of the distinction between confrontive and covert.

In short, the distinction between confrontive (aggressive) and covert (nonaggressive) behaviors is worthy of further study, but probably is not yet clearly enough supported to merit its use to distinguish subtypes of conduct disorder. I would recommend dropping it for the present. If it is continued, fire setting and other types of vandalism should be moved from aggressive to covert behaviors. The same should occur for breaking and entering, which usually is carried out with the intent to steal and avoid confrontation. On the other hand, chronic violation of important rules, now assigned to the nonaggressive category, often includes aggressively stated refusal to comply. It should be subdivided on the basis of confrontive versus passive disobedience.

Because the aggressive and nonaggressive behaviors are highly intercorrelated, and both are highly predictive of later distubance, neither the confrontive (aggressive) nor covert (nonaggressive) set of behaviors should be treated as a residual category, to be counted only if the other is absent. If the distinction is maintained, the most useful subtypes would seem to be the following categories:

> Conduct disorder, confrontive type
> Conduct disorder, covert type
> Conduct disorder, confrontive and covert

If the distinction is abolished, criteria could be structured as they are for anti-social personality. That is, there could be a list of symptoms, a certain number of which would be required for a positive diagnosis.

3. The missing items that appear so regularly in studies of childhood behavior problems and that appear in the text, but not in the diagnostic criteria for conduct disorder, should be added. These would include verbal aggression and direct refusal to do what an authority figure directs (confrontive), early sexual intercourse (covert), poor school achievement despite adequate IQ (covert), untrustworthiness or some synonym to capture the fact that these children often do not let their parents know where they are and do not come home on time (covert), impulsiveness and a high propensity to take risks (overt), and cruelty to animals and small children, whether physical or verbal (confrontive). Adding these items should make the criteria better applicable to girls and young children.

4. The complaint that conduct-disorder criteria are not appropriate for all ages could be handled by requiring different numbers of problems for children of different ages, with lower numbers of behaviors required for younger children. Another solution would be to obtain epidemiological data to learn what the norms are for these behaviors in children of all ages, and use these to make age-specific diagnoses. However, going this route could lead to a highly elaborate system, with separate criteria for sex and ethnic or socioeconomic statuses as well. I believe the simpler solution is preferable.

5. Each symptom should be quantified with respect to how severe it has to be, at what ages it should be considered positive, in how many situations it must occur, and what its minimum duration must be.

6. Conduct disorder should have a specified maximum age of onset. Certainly an onset age of 15, as in the criteria for antisocial personality, would not be too low. Many find it too high. Also, it probably would be advantageous to have a maximum age at which the diagnosis can be made, because at present, conduct disorder in an adult is likely to overlap with passive-aggressive personality, with disorders of impulse control, and with adjustment disorder with disturbance of conduct. Further, many of the symptoms are irrelevant for adults, particularly those associated with school performance and running away and all of those that are referred to in the delinquency literature as "status offenses," that is, behaviors that are disapproved for their precocity rather than because they are intrinsically violations of social norms. Early sex and drinking are prime examples. Because of the age-restricted content of the symptoms, it would seem reasonable to use a cutoff age not later than 21. Eighteen would also seem a reasonable limit.

7. A diagnosis of antisocial personality should be allowed in persons younger than 18. This probably would not change the pattern of diagnosis much, because few children have had the opportunity to carry out most of the criterion behaviors used to diagnose antisocial personality, such as having repeated problems on the job and incidences of wife or child beating.

8. The diagnosis of oppositional disorder should be dropped. If a child does not meet the criteria for conduct disorder, but has a few similar symptoms, the child should not receive any diagnosis. Otherwise, we are likely to be making unpleasantness equivalent to illness.

9. The childhood criteria for antisocial personality should be changed from the present form, in which 12 conduct problems are listed, 3 of which must have occurred before age 15, to the simple statement that the individual must meet the criteria for conduct disorder in childhood. This will obviate the double diagnosis of conduct disorder that now exists.

REFERENCES

Achenbach TM: DSM-III in light of empirical research on the classification of child psychopathology. J Am Acad Child Psychiatry 19:395–412, 1980

August GJ, Stewart MA: Familial subtypes of childhood hyperactivity. J Nerv Ment Dis 171:362–368, 1983

Behar D, Stewart MA: Aggressive conduct disorder of children: the clinical history and direct observations. Acta Psychiatr Scand 65:210–220, 1982

Aggressive conduct disorder: the influence of social class, sex and age on the clinical picture. J Child Psychol Psychiatry 25:119–124, 1984

Henn FA, Bardwell R, Jenkins RL: Juvenile delinquents revisited. Adult criminal activity. Arch Gen Psychiatry 37:1160–1163, 1980

Loeber R, Schmaling KB: Empirical evidence for overt and covert patterns of antisocial conduct problems. Abnormal Child Psychology (in press, a)

The utility of differentiating between mixed and pure forms of antisocial child behavior. J Abnormal Child Psychology (in press, b)

Loney J, Milich R: Hyperactivity, inattention and aggression in clinical practice. Adv Dev Behav Pediatr 3:113–147, 1982

Quay HC: Classification, in Psychopathological Disorders of Childhood, vol 2. Edited by Quay HC, Werry JS. New York, Wiley, 1979

Reitsma-Street M, Offord DR, Finch T, et al: Comparison of antisocial boys and their nonantisocial brothers. Final Report to Canadian Ministry of Community and Social Affairs. 1982

Robins E, Guze S: Establishment of diagnostic validity in psychiatric illness: its application to schizophrenia. Am J Psychiatry 126:107–111, 1970

Robins L: The consequences of conduct disorder in girls, in Development of Antisocial and Prosocial Behavior: Research, Theory, and Issues. Edited by Olweus D, Block J, Radke-Yarrow M. Orlando, Fla, Academic, 1986, pp 385–414

Rutter M, Shaffer D, Shepherd M: A Multi-axial Classification of Child Psychiatric Disorders. Geneva, World Health Organization, 1975

Stewart MA, de Blois S, Meardo J, et al: Aggressive conduct disorder of children: the clinical picture. J Nerv Ment Dis 168:604–610, 1980

Taylor E, Schachar R, Thorley G, et al: Hyperactivity, conduct disorder and attention deficit in child psychiatric patients. (in press)

Trites RL, LaPrade K: Evidence for an independent syndrome of hyperactivity. J Child Psychol Psychiatry 24:573–586, 1983

24　*Overview*

GABRIELLE A. CARLSON

DEVELOPMENTAL DISORDERS

Drs. Waterhouse, Fein, Nath, and Snyder have comprehensively reviewed both the issues to be considered in the area of childhood psychoses and the data relating to how *DSM-III* has fared. It is obvious that we need much more information about children who present with severe developmental disorders. The critical issue facing us now is whether or not we can create a diagnostic system that will provide both sufficient coverage to categorize the majority of these children and sufficiently meaningful subgroups so that homogeneous subsamples can be separated and studied. As Waterhouse and associates point out, we have yet to understand the relationship between infantile autism (IA), childhood-onset pervasive developmental disorder (COPCC), schizophrenia occurring in childhood (SOC), and schizoid and schizotypal but related personality disorders (SPD). Are these, in fact, different disorders? Do they describe only a severity dimension? Do they describe the same process with onsets at different ages? Or are they an assortment of symptoms that do not even have syndromal cohesiveness? Altogether they apparently do not provide sufficient coverage, because many children do not fit into any of these categories. This is partly because of specific criteria problems such as age of onset and presence of thought disorder. These criteria are frequently unreliable: Age of onset may be difficult to establish, and determining formal thought disorder in children, which is difficult enough, is next to impossible in children with language disorders. Similarly, hallucinations and delusions may be difficult to elicit or, when elicited, may have different implications in young children. Moreover, homogeneous samples apparently are not created even when children meet the criteria as established.

In addition to the question how these syndromes relate to each other is the question how they relate to mental retardation and other developmental delays. As Waterhouse and associates indicate, mental retardation is used both as a disorder and as a level of cognitive function. Studies suggest that mental retardation as an axis I diagnosis is ignored when autism is diagnosed. There is accumulating evidence that cognitive function belongs on a separate axis. Beyond that is the question how many of the manifestations of the autism spectrum are caused by different levels of mental retardation. Finally, among the more fascinating aspects of the pervasive developmental disorders are the inconsistencies in development across developmental lines.

Even if we could expunge the *DSM-III* criteria, it is clear that we have nothing better with which to replace them. In order not to be in that same situation by the time *DSM-IV* comes along, we need to make sure that critical pieces of information are systematically recorded. I would make three suggestions:

1. Because no major changes can be made in *DSM-III*, publish requirements for both clinical and research purposes not unlike those which Kupfer and Rush (1983) have suggested for depressive disorders. This would ensure that relevant data are not lost by coding. The records required would include:
   a. age of onset with some notation as to the reliability of that impression ("the disorder clearly began at 14 months when babbling and beginning speech totally stopped," or "at around age 3½, when nursery school started, the subject was noted to be relating abnormally," etc.),
   b. level of verbal and performance IQ,
   c. whether or not there have been fluctuations in development, including deterioration from previous levels of functioning,
   d. the level of severity of social-interactional deficits, with some attempt to create a reliable system for describing this,
   e. level of language function (absent, echolalic, sparse but communicative, communicative but peculiar prosody, etc.),
   f. presence or absence of hallucinations or delusions.
2. Use *DSM-III* more systematically. One of the points consistently made in all the discussions is that it is premature to determine that one disorder is "due to" another and thereby not code for it. Perhaps we could apply this to pervasive developmental disorders as follows: If a child meets the criteria for IA or COPDD and is pervasively retarded, the child could be noted as having both IA and mental retardation. If the child is not retarded according to performance IQ testing, then language deficits can be coded on axis II, or if the child's language problems are worse than can be explained on the basis of retardation, they can be coded on axis II even though language delay is one of the criteria for IA.
3. *DSM-III-R* should make two changes:
   a. Allow a fifth digit for notation of psychotic features, as is done for affective disorders. Then, if a child meets all the criteria for IA or COPPD but has hallucinations or delusions, the child can be given a diagnosis of atypical PDD, with psychotic features noted as axis I, presence or absence of language problems on axis II, and so forth. At least this might in part narrow the focus for some atypical PDD diagnoses.
   b. Add deviant or delayed social skills to axis II developmental disorders so that this very real line of development can be acknowledged and coded for; criteria for how to define this would need to be established by the *DSM-III-R* committee.

In summary, it is not acceptable to bemoan inadequate criteria, nor should the criteria hamper future research.

DEPRESSIVE DISORDERS

Like schizophrenia, depressive disorders in *DSM-III* are defined by criteria culled from many years of clinical experience with adults. Although the use of these criteria unmodified for children has not been conclusively validated, the bulk of research generated in the last decade, as summarized by Dr. Kovacs, suggests that such criteria can be used reliably to select a sample of depressed children (school-age and adolescent). Two conspicuous problems continue to be (1) the relationship, if any, that exists between childhood depression and adult depression and (2) whether or not, by using adult criteria, we are missing a significant population of depressed children who have different symptoms more developmentally appropriate to their age. It is hoped that by the time *DSM-IV* is written, we shall have data to answer these questions.

Dr. Kovacs also emphasizes the problem posed earlier in this section concerning how to "count" a symptom and whether or not it is appropriate to let one sign or symptom fulfill criteria for a variety of diagnoses. Although a good longitudinal history is not always available or obtainable from parents (or child), and although such histories will not clarify all circumstances, there are times when such data help. A child with attention-deficit disorder with hyperactivity may already be impulsive and irritable. If such a child then becomes dysphoric, anhedonic, and suicidal, unless it is clear on the basis of history that irritability has increased, the symptoms of the original disorder should not be "counted" to meet the criteria for depression. In other words, attention should be given to the timing of symptoms and their relationship to each other, rather than to their simple presence or absence.

Finally, as has been said before, it is important that our assumptions do not cause us to lose information. Although exclusionary criteria will ultimately be necessary to separate disorders, until we are sure what those are, multiple diagnoses may be the best way of describing patient populations. We shall never know if separation anxiety is merely another symptom of depression or an exacerbation of a child's premorbid concern that earlier was not pathological unless we can separate children with separation-anxiety disorder and major depression from those without major depression, or separate children with separation anxiety and major depression from those with major depression and conduct disorder.

CONDUCT DISORDER

Conduct disorder presents some of the same dilemmas as PDD. As Dr. Robins indicates, the relationships among disorders, in this case oppositional disorder, conduct disorder, and antisocial personality disorder, are ambiguous. This seeming spectrum tries to make allowances for the fact that not all "misbehavior" evolves into serious adult antisocial disorder. Dr. Robins has aptly pointed out, however, that there is no compelling reason to consider misbehavior or unpleasantness per se a psychiatric disorder. Without more precise quantifiers, oppositional-disorder criteria, such as temper tantrums, argumentativeness, and stubborness, would appear to have such high incidences as to make oppositional disorder an epidemic among 13–18-year-olds. On the other hand, if oppositional disorder serves to label early-onset conduct disorder, this goal might be better served, as Dr. Robins suggests, by including conduct symptoms of which younger children are capable. If the core symptom for conduct disorder and ultimately antisocial personality is, in fact, "violation of the basic rights of others or of major age-appropriate societal norms or rules," then the major question is, Should each child be assessed as to whether or not he ever understands that others have basic rights? Although conscience, morality, and empathy should be developing in preschool children, not until children are well into elementary school does society believe that children understand those issues. If conduct disorder is to be a precise cataloging of transgressions without the problem of motivation, then certainly the intensity and duration of each item would need more precise definition for each developmental stage (preschool, elementary-school, junior-high, and high-school mental ages).

Perhaps the best predictors of difficulty from preschool age to school age have been restlessness or hyperactivity and short attention span (Richman, Stevenson, and Graham, 1982; F. Earls, pers. commun.), at least in boys. Although attention-deficit disorder was not discussed during our symposium, I believe that it is important at least to mention the fact that this disorder often coexists with conduct disorder, and they may be, at early ages, indistinguishable. In fact, this important caveat was reiterated in the subsequent discussion. There is no law against giving children two axis I diagnoses, and in the case of conduct disorder it is important that diagnostic consideration not stop once the criteria for conduct disorder are fulfilled. Besides having attention disorder, children meeting the criteria for conduct disorder have been found to have coexisting mental retardation, schizophrenia, organic brain syndrome (Lewis et al., 1984), depressive disorder (Carlson and Cantwell, 1980; Puig-Antich, 1982; Kovacs et al., 1984), and attention-deficit disorder without hyperactivity (G. A. Carlson and J. Asarnow, unpublished data).

REFERENCES

Carlson GA, Cantwell DP: Unmasking masked depression in children and adolescents. Am J Psychiatry 137:445–449, 1980

Kovacs M, Feinberg TL, Crouse-Novak MA, et al: Depressive disorders in childhood, I: a longitudinal prospective study of characteristics and recovery. Arch Gen Psychiatry 41:229–237, 1984

Kupfer DJ, Rush AJ: Recommendations for depression publications (letters to the editor). Arch Gen Psychiatry 40:1031, 1983

Lewis DO, Lewis M, Unger L, et al: Conduct disorder and its synonyms: diagnoses of dubious validity and usefulness. Am J Psychiatry 141:514–519, 1984

Puig-Antich J: Major depression and conduct disorder in prepuberty. J Am Acad Child Psychiatry 21:118–128, 1982

Richman N, Stevenson J, Graham PJ: Pre-school to school: A behavioural study. New York, Academic Press, 1982

PART VII

Nosologic principles and diagnostic criteria

This section on nosologic principles and diagnostic criteria is intended to address some of the structural and theoretical aspects of a diagnostic system. Attention to these issues should be useful in assessing current deficiencies of the *DSM-III* system and facilitating substantive advances for future revisions of the manual. A brief history of the developments in psychiatric classification and nosology is provided as a framework for the current discussion.

For many years, the *International Classification of Diseases (ICD)* and its predecessors have provided a statistical classification of mental disorders for the primary purpose of categorizing medical records diagnoses into major groups. Groupings of this type are useful for insurance reimbursement and for international comparisons of treatment rates. However, psychiatric nosologists and clinicians concerned with systematic description and treatment of psychopathology usually have operated on a track relatively independent of the statistical classification specialists. Clinicians, nosologists, and statisticians all recognized the need for greater specification of the statistical classification terms during the *ICD-9* development, which ultimately included the first glossary of terms used in describing symptoms of syndromes. This greater specification did not prevent a wide latitude in criteria for specific disorders within *ICD-9* to accommodate variations in concepts of psychopathology and etiology associated with different countries.

The third edition of the American Psychiatric Association's *Diagnostic and Statistical Manual of Mental Disorders (DSM-III)* represented a further advance in specificity by more explicitly indicating criteria that were necessary for individual diagnoses. Such criteria include the types and numbers of symptoms, the age of onset, duration, and a hierarchy of diagnoses in which a more encompassing or severe diagnosis may exclude another disorder. The combinations of symptoms, duration, exclusion rules, and age of onset have come to be known as operational criteria for making specific diagnoses. As such, these combinations constitute specific hypotheses that the entity so described can have both reliability, in terms of reproducibility of their application, and validity, in terms of the meaningfulness of these categories for predicting clinical course, response to treatment, genetic clustering, and other measures of construct validity covered elsewhere in this volume.

By including such criteria in one volume with an international statistical classification format, an attempt was made to more fully integrate the scientific research fields of psychopathology, nosology, and statistical classification. That such an integration has been controversial is not unexpected. However, it is safe to say that one result has been an entirely new level of appreciation of the importance of specifying diagnostic criteria to increase the clarity of communication in psychiatry's research, clinical, and statistical classification fields.

Nevertheless, some of the criticisms of the *DSM-III* should be addressed in any future revision. In general, the criticisms are aimed not at the concept of explicit criteria themselves but more at the level of evidence required before such criteria are incorporated into a universal classification of mental disorders. For future revisions, it would be particularly helpful if the sources and types of evidence for accepting diagnostic criteria were made more explicit. One common criticism has been that the *DSM-III* criteria are in some cases arbitrary hypotheses based on minimal, if any, research evidence. Although there is nothing wrong with stating a diagnostic hypothesis, the concern is that there should be a clear statement to explain if criteria are theoretical or hypothetical, rather than based on empirical research information.

Hence, in order to enable a more accurate assessment of the diagnostic categories, it would be useful to know the sources of information used in postulating these criteria. For example, do such criteria come from clinical studies of psychopathology, controlled clinical trials of therapeutics, community epidemiologic studies, historic conventions secondary to clinical descriptions, or group-consensus conferences of experts using Delphi techniques to arrive at a best judgment based on accumulated experience?

Another criticism that has arisen from attempts to use the existing *DSM-III* criteria is that sometimes there is the appearance of precision despite the wide latitude that is possible for interpreting these criteria in different ways. Hence, highly structured psychiatric interviews have been shown to interpret the same *DSM-III* criteria in somewhat divergent ways – an inherent critique of their reliability, as well as a recognition of the need for greater specificity of measurement instruments when the specificity of the criteria themselves increases.

Although all of these criticisms cannot be addressed in the three chapters in this Part VII, it is possible to illustrate how a systematic empirical evaluation of the diagnostic hierarchy of *DSM-III* can shed new light on a key component of the *DSM-III* structure. The chapters by Drs. Boyd and Spitzer and their associates specifically address these hierarchical issues and the epidemiologic data base on which this examination depends. As such, they address the larger issue of how the individual diagnostic entities relate to each other as part of an overall diagnostic system. If one were studying only schizophrenia or only anxiety disorders, it would not be immediately apparent that the criteria used for one disorder may have a major impact on another area of psychiatric research. Nosologists are confronted with such issues only when all such disorders are put together in a single diagnostic system and the issues of hierarchies and exclusions become paramount. In this regard, the focus on exclusions demonstrates the continued interest in seeing the *DSM-III* system as a nosologic framework, not simply as a statistical system.

Dr. Barrett provides a somewhat broader framework for examining how statistical, clinical, and research classification systems might coexist. Although *DSM-III* attempts to facilitate attainment of objectives in all three areas, Dr. Barrett focuses more on the statistical classification aspect of its performance. The importance of this aspect must not be underestimated. It was necessary for the *DSM-III* statistical designations to be consistent with the *ICD-9-CM* before the U.S. government would approve *DSM-III* use for Medicare and Medicaid reimbursement purposes. The U.S. government is obliged by virtue of its being a member of the World Health Organization to observe the statistical classification conventions of the ICD. However, it is clear that the entities identified by the same names in the United States and other countries of the world may be substantially different when the latitude for interpretation is significantly diminished by the explicit criteria of *DSM-III*.

In their earliest deliberations, the World Health Organization, ICD, and Division of Mental Health components have recommended the development in the *ICD-10* revision of a tripartite section on mental disorders to address this level-of-evidence concern. At the most basic level would be a statistical classification of disorders that would consist of an agreed listing of mental-disorder names pulled together into groups of disorders with properties in common. At the second level, it is proposed that the current glossary of mental-health terms be expanded to include explicit clinical guidelines or criteria necessary for defining the mental-disorder entity. At a third level, it is proposed that research diagnostic criteria be proposed that may have both a higher degree of specificity and a lower degree of general acceptance in the clinical community because of the current state of research or clinical knowledge supporting such criteria.

In summary, attention to the criticisms of *DSM-III* and basic scientific and nosologic principles should help us address the challenge to improve on its performance in our future efforts at revision. The *DSM-III* evaluation workshop itself continues the scientific approach with an effort to evaluate the performance of *DSM-III* and to refine its properties. An expansion of our empirical data base should make such an exercise less political and more constrained by the empirical realities of the patients our profession seeks to serve.

Darrel A. Regier

25 The exclusion criteria of DSM-III

A study of the co-occurrence of hierarchy-free syndromes

JEFFREY H. BOYD, JACK D. BURKE,
ERNEST GRUENBERG, CHARLES E. HOLZER,
DONALD S. RAE, LINDA K. GEORGE,
MARVIN KARNO, ROGER STOLTZMAN,
LARRY McEVOY, AND GERALD NESTADT

The diagnostic criteria for a disorder in the third edition of the *Diagnostic and Statistical Manual (DSM-III)* often state as a requirement that the disorder is "not due to" another disorder (American Psychiatric Association, 1980). For example, criterion C in the definition of panic disorder states that it is "not due to a physical disorder or another mental disorder, such as Major Depression, Somatization Disorder, or Schizophrenia." Such exclusion criteria are found in 60% of the disorders for which explicit criteria are elaborated in *DSM-III*. Although such exclusion criteria play a prominent role in *DSM-III*, there has been little discussion in the literature of the rationale for them (Treece, 1982; Leckman et al., 1983a,b), and almost no empirical research focused on the

An earlier version of this chapter was published in the *Archives of General Psychiatry* (41:983–989, 1984).

The authors would like to thank Robert L. Spitzer, M.D., Myrna M. Weissman, Ph.D., Gerald L. Klerman, M.D., Lee N. Robins, Ph.D., Marshal F. Folstein, M.D., Larry G. Kessler, Sc.D., Carl Taube, Ph.D., Morton Kramer, Ph.D., and James Barrett, M.D., for their comments on an earlier draft of this chapter.

The authors wish to thank statistical consultants for review of the methods of this article: Ronald Forthover Ph.D., Professor of Biometry, and Eun Sul Lee Ph.D., Associate Professor of Biometry, University of Texas School of Public Health, Houston, Texas.

The Epidemiologic Catchment Area program is a series of five epidemiologic research studies performed by independent research teams in collaboration with staff of the Division of Biometry and Epidemiology (DBE) of the National Institute of Mental Health (NIMH). The NIMH principal collaborators are Darrel A. Regier, Ben Z. Locke, and William W. Eaton; the NIMH Project Officer is Carl A. Taube. The Principal Investigators and Co-Investigators from the five sites are as follows: Yale University, Uo1 MH 34224, Jerome K. Myers, Myrna M. Weissman, and Gary Tischler; Johns Hopkins University, Uo1 MH 33870, Morton Kramer, Ernest Gruenberg, and Sam Shapiro; Washington University, St. Louis, Uo1 MH 33883, Lee N. Robins, John Helzer, and Jack Croughan; Duke University, Uo1 MH 35386, Dan Blazer and Linda George; University of California, Los Angeles, Uo1 MH 35865, Richard Hough, Marvin Karno, Javier Escobar, and Audrey Burnam.

assumptions underlying the use of the *DSM-III* exclusions (Leckman et al., 1983a,b). The purpose of this chapter is to subject the exclusion criteria to empirical examination, using data from the multisite NIMH Epidemiologic Catchment Area (ECA) program (Regier et al., 1982).

The language of *DSM-III* makes a distinction between the "essential features" and "associated features" of a disorder. For example, panic symptoms would be considered an "essential feature" of panic disorder, but an "associated feature" of major depression. This linguistic distinction, however, does not address the question why panic symptoms occurring during an episode of major depression should be considered to be a manifestation of the major depression, not a manifestation of true panic disorder occurring at the same time as major depression (Leckman et al., 1983a).

The use of the phrase "not due to" in *DSM-III* can be confusing, because the phrase is not operationalized in *DSM-III,* nor is it defined in the *DSM-III* glossary. Discussions within the ECA project have attempted to operationalize this phrase as meaning "not always occurring during an episode of." However, some ECA investigators take exception to this operationalization, because they interpret *DSM-III* differently. Some ECA investigators interpret *DSM-III* to mean that a disorder at one period of time might "cause" a disorder at another period of time, even if there is a symptom-free interval of many years in between. These investigators point to the possibility that a disorder such as major depression might recur, and present with panic symptoms when it recurs. In this way, an earlier episode of major depression can "cause" a subsequent episode of panic disorder. Such differences of opinion arise when ambiguous phrases such as "due to" are used in a classification system without providing an operational definition.

FEIGHNER CRITERIA AND RESEARCH DIAGNOSTIC CRITERIA

Exclusion criteria are present in the parent nosologic systems that preceded *DSM-III,* namely, the Feighner criteria (Feighner et al., 1972) and the Research Diagnostic Criteria (RDC) (Spitzer, Endicott, and Robins, 1978). In these diagnostic systems, the exclusions are defined in more operational terms, making it easier to apply them in an unambiguous manner. However, the rationale for the exclusions criteria is explained in the Feighner criteria in a cursory and abbreviated way as follows: "Since similar clinical features and laboratory findings may be seen in patients suffering from different disorders . . . it is necessary to specify exclusion criteria so that patients with other illnesses are not included in the group to be studied" (Feighner et al., 1972). The key to understanding this sentence is in the last phrase, "the group to be studied." The purpose of exclusion criteria here is to ensure that researchers are able to select homogeneous samples of patients.

A classification system must serve the unrelated needs of different masters. Even when classification is for research purposes, different types of research need different levels of exclusivity. For purposes of biological research, exclusion criteria might be desirable as a way to ensure that the patients to be studied are homogeneous with respect to the disorder in question, and therefore most likely to share biologic characteristics. For such research one would prefer to exclude questionable or atypical cases, as well as patients who might have a different disorder. Genetics research asks two different things of a classification system: On the one hand, it is useful to select homogeneous samples of probands from which questionable or borderline cases have been excluded; on the other hand, it is useful to note all disorders found in relatives including the questionable or excluded disorders (Leckman et al., 1983a). For purposes of epidemiologic and nosologic research it is important to assess everyone in a population, and it makes sense to assign multiple diagnoses if these are present. For clinical, as opposed to research, purposes, a classification system is useful if it aids in prognosis and the choice of therapy and serves various accounting purposes. Thus, clinicians will find exclusion rules useful if the rules eliminate from consideration disorders that do not alter the prognosis or treatment of the patient.

DIAGNOSTIC-HIERARCHY RESEARCH IN ENGLAND

There is a European literature that has addressed the question of exclusion criteria or diagnostic hierarchy in other diagnostic systems. The literature from England and Germany provides a rationale for a diagnostic hierarchy, although not necessarily the same hierarchy as is included in *DSM-III*.

Kendell has suggested that the idea of a diagnostic hierarchy arose because in practice clinicians were reluctant to make more than one diagnosis for a given patient (Kendell, 1975; Surtees and Kendell, 1979). A diagnostic hierarchy provides the clinician with decision rules for choosing that one diagnosis. Implicit in the Kraepelinian classification tradition is a hierarchy with the following order: organic mental disorders, nuclear schizophrenia, manic-depressive illness, and neurotic illnesses (Surtees and Kendell, 1979; Roth, 1981). The presence of any disorder from this hierarchy would preclude a diagnosis lower on the hierarchy. This hierarchy is also implicit in the *International Classification of Diseases (ICD)*, and to an extent in diagnostic computer programs such as CATEGO and DIAGNO (Surtees and Kendell, 1979). Such a hierarchy implies that the presence of any disorder can cause manifestations of disorders lower in the hierarchy (Kendell, 1975). Kendell said that "any given diagnosis excludes the presence of symptoms of all higher members of the hierarchy and embraces the symptoms of all lower members." Although such a diagnostic hierarchy is implicit in the work of Kraepelin (Roth, 1981), it was first explicitly articulated by Jaspers (Jaspers, 1962; Kendell, 1975; Surtees and Kendell, 1979). Jaspers assumed that this hierarchy did not necessarily describe a phenomenon of nature, but was a convention adopted to enable psychiatrists to attribute a single diagnosis to each patient (Jaspers, 1962).

Empirical research on diagnostic hierarchies began quite recently with Foulds (Foulds and Bedford, 1975; Foulds, 1976). Foulds's research focused on psychiatric symptoms rather than syndromes. His concept of hierarchy is rather unusual and deviates from the order of the *DSM-III* hierarchy and from the order of the Kraepelinian hierarchy described earlier. Foulds's concept is that delusions of disintegration are at the top of the hierarchy, followed by integrated delusions (delusions of persecution or grandeur, contrition), followed by neurotic symptoms (conversion, dissociative, phobic, compulsive, and ruminative symptoms), followed by "dysthymic states" (anxiety, depression, and elation) (Foulds, 1976).

Foulds created the Delusions–Symptoms–States Inventory (DSSI), which collects symptom-level data relevant to his theory (Foulds and Bedford, 1975; Foulds, 1976). He found that the presence of symptoms from any level of this hierarchy implied the presence of at least two symptoms from lower levels of the hierarchy. For example, someone with delusions of persecution is found to have neurotic symptoms and also anxiety or affective symptoms (Foulds, 1976). The fact that Foulds presented data supporting a hierarchical model that contradicts the hierarchical assumptions of *DSM-III* and also contradicts the hierarchical assumptions of the *ICD* is startling. Foulds's diagnostic hierarchy contradicts *DSM-III* in the sense that *DSM-III* lists affective disorders as higher in the diagnostic hierarchy than disorders such as obsessive–compulsive disorder or phobias, whereas Foulds placed affective symptoms at the bottom of the hierarchy.

Foulds's work was followed by a series of replication studies that confirmed his findings (Bagshaw, 1977; McPherson et al., 1977; Bedford and Presly, 1978; Palmer, Ekisa, and Winbow, 1981), except for manic patients (Bagshaw and McPherson, 1978; Surtees and Kendell, 1979) and some schizophrenics (Surtees and Kendell, 1979). However, Sturt (1981), in reviewing these studies, has argued convincingly that Foulds's particular hierarchical theory is not the only way to interpret these studies. In a convincing analysis of data from the Present State Examination (PSE), Sturt showed that subjects who have rare PSE syndromes, such as delusions, tend to have high total symptom scores. The same is true not only of symptoms but also of syndromes (i.e., CATEGO classes). She showed that Foulds's hierarchy is an example of a more general principle:

Symptoms and syndromes are far from random with respect to each other [but] it does not follow that a particular model with hierarchical classes of symptoms is thereby proven. Any grouping of symptoms and syndromes into classes based roughly on prevalence (i.e. with the higher classes containing the rarer symptoms) would show a certain tendency for subjects displaying symptoms of a high class also to have symptoms of the lower classes, because every symptom shows a highly significant association with total symptom score. (Sturt, 1981)

RESEARCH USING STRUCTURED DIAGNOSTIC INTERVIEWS IN THE UNITED STATES

In the United States, the use of systematic diagnostic interviews has facilitated empirical research on the diagnostic hierarchy of *DSM-III*. Instruments such as the Schedule for Affective Disorders and Schizophrenia (SADS) and the NIMH Diagnostic Interview Schedule (DIS) (Robins et al., 1981a,b) force a comprehensive collection of information, without necessarily following the hierarchical assumptions of a clinician. For example, the SADS was used in a study in New Haven of the familial aggregation of depression (Leckman et al., 1983a,b). In arriving at best-estimate diagnoses in relatives, exclusion criteria were not used. The result was that the exclusion criteria could be subjected to empirical investigation. It was discovered that

relatives of individuals with major depression plus an anxiety disorder are at greater risk for major depression, as well as anxiety disorders, than are the relatives of individuals with major depression without an anxiety disorder. This increased risk appears to be present whether or not the anxiety disorder occurs solely in association with episodes of major depression or is temporally separate. (Leckman et al., 1983a,b)

Studies of the treatment of depression with tricyclics or ECT have similarly found that depression with anxiety is more difficult to treat than depression without anxiety (Roth, 1981). The use of exclusion criteria may obscure the importance of anxiety as defining a possible subtype of major depressive disorders (Leckman et al., 1983a).

PROPOSED TERMINOLOGY

In previous discussion we found semantic confusion arising from use of the words "excluding disorder" and "excluded disorder." For clarity, we use the term "excluded disorder" when a diagnosis such as panic disorder cannot be made because of another disorder. We use the term "dominant disorder" to refer to a diagnosis, such as major depression, that takes precedence over the lesser diagnosis, such as panic disorder.

RATIONALE FOR THE PRESENT STUDY

Although the literature is unclear concerning the rationale for exclusions, a minimal interpretation of the phrase "not due to" in *DSM-III* is that some disorders such as major depression are capable of causing phenomena, or "associated features," that are indistinguishable from the "essential features" of another disorder such as panic disorder. The assumption that one disorder can cause something that looks like the other disorder is amenable to being investigated empirically.

The orientation we use in addressing our data is as follows: If major depression causes phenomena that cannot be distinguished from panic disorder, then people who are in an episode of major depression should have increased odds of having panic disorder, as compared with people who are not in an episode of major depression. The same thing can be stated as a null hypothesis: If the phenomena of panic disorder are not "due to" major depression, then there should be equal odds of having panic disorder among those who are in an episode of major depression and those who are not in an episode of major depression. To state the same null hypothesis in more general terms: If A is the dominant disorder and B is the excluded disorder, then the odds of having disorder B should be no greater among the population who have disorder A than among the population who do not have disorder A.

METHODS

Sampling

Four systematic samples of households were drawn: 4,045 households in New Haven, 3,817 households in Baltimore, 3,778 households in St. Louis, and another 11,276 households in New Haven (Eaton et al., 1982; Regier et al., 1982). One adult over the age of 18 was selected at random from each of the first three household samples and invited to be interviewed. In the Baltimore sample, in addition, every adult age 65 or older was selected. For the first three samples, the response rates were 75.6%, 77.9%, and 79.2%. The larger New Haven sample ($N = 11,276$ households) was screened for subjects age 65 or older, and 2,423 such persons were found, for whom the response rate was 81.4%. The data presented here are based on 11,519 interviews: 3,058 in the first New Haven sample, 1,976 in the second New Haven sample, 3,481 in the Baltimore sample, and 3,004 in the St. Louis sample.

This sample of 11,519 was selected to represent a population of $N = 752,551$ in these communities. Therefore, in order to obtain an estimate of the morbidity among community populations, each person in the sample is weighted to represent between 9 and 650 persons from the community population. Later we discuss the implications of using weighted data.

Diagnostic procedures

Diagnostic information was gathered using the DIS, which is a highly structured interview schedule that is suited for administration by a lay interviewer (Robins et al., 1981a,b). The DIS data were then processed by a diagnostic computer program that was written to simulate *DSM-III* diagnoses. The characteristics of this computer program and the precision or imprecision with which it operationalizes each *DSM-III* diagnosis are reviewed in detail elsewhere (Boyd et al., 1985). A procedural-validity study on the DIS has compared the computer-generated diagnoses from a nonclinician interviewer's administration of the DIS to diagnoses based on the clinical judgment of a psychiatrist who also administered the DIS but was able to ask additional questions to clarify ambiguous points (Robins et al., 1982). That study demonstrated that the specificity of the lay-administered DIS was above 90% for all disorders except simple phobia, for which the specificity was 88%. Schizophreniform disorder was not studied.

An independent study of the DIS compared with the Schedule for Affective Disorders and Schizophrenia (SADS–L) showed very high agreement in another clinical population, of 42 alcoholics, for several disorders, including major depression (Hesselbrock et al., 1982). In addition, a study of the DIS in bilingual populations has demonstrated interrater reliability even across two languages (Burnam et al., 1983). Additional studies comparing the DIS diagnoses in community populations and those generated by several types of clinical interviews have been conducted, and analysis is under way in New Haven, Baltimore, St. Louis, and Puerto Rico. Extensive information will soon be available about the correspondence of DIS diagnoses to those produced by psychiatrists. In the meantime, however, we are calling the diagnoses in this article "DIS/ *DSM-III* disorders" to indicate that the method of examination is the DIS, which is standardized and appears reliable (Robins et al., 1981b; Burnam et al., 1983), but which has not been fully assessed in comparison with a psychiatrist's diagnoses.

For purposes of data analysis in this chapter, disorders were defined without using the exclusion criteria of *DSM-III*. Thus, this chapter is based on hierarchy-free DIS/*DSM-III* syndromes. For example, panic disorder is defined based on *DSM-III* criteria A and B, but without criteria C or D. We consider only disorders that have occurred in the month prior to interview. A one-month time frame has been chosen because sufficient information is available to know that two disorders overlapped temporally.

Statistical methods

The magnitude of the relationship between two DIS/*DSM-III* disorders is quantified by means of an odds ratio. An odds ratio, sometimes referred to as a "cross-product ratio," is calculated as follows: A 2 × 2 table is constructed showing the presence or absence of condition A on the top, and the presence or absence of condition B on the side. The number of persons with each disorder is put in one of the cells of the table. The odds ratio is the product of the number in the upper left cell of the table and the number in the lower right, divided by the product of the other two numbers.

Odds ratios are used because they have become the most widely used measurement of risk in chronic disease epidemiology (Kleinbaum, Kupper, and Morgenstern, 1982). In epidemiologic studies the comparison is typically between a "risk factor" and a presumed later-developing disorder. In this chapter the dominant disorder in *DSM-III* is being tested as the "risk factor" for the excluded disorder.

Because most of the disorders we are studying are rare events in a population survey, the coexistence of two such disorders is an extremely rare event. In order to deal with the problem of rare events, we have pooled data from the three ECA sites in the calculation of odds ratios. The generalizations we arrive at apply to a target population consisting of the combined populations of catchment areas of the New Haven, Baltimore, and St. Louis ECA studies.

If our study were based on a simple random sample, then we could use χ^2 to test whether or not an odds ratio is significantly greater than 1. However, with the complex stratified sampling methods that were used to collect information for the ECA study, an ordinary χ^2 might lead to inaccurate results because it would fail to take into account the effect of the sample design.

As mentioned earlier, our sample of 11,519 is of interest because, as a representative sample, it allows us to estimate the nature of the larger population of 752,551 persons in the three communities. Our sample cannot be treated as if it were a simple random sample of that larger population, because individual subjects had unequal probabilities of being selected. For example, we selected a large oversample of elderly persons in New Haven and Baltimore. In order to estimate the state of affairs in the population, we need to analyze the data with weights that correct for the different sampling probabilities. In this way, the sample can be used as a reflection of the community population from which it was drawn.

To test statistical significance, we used the CPLX program (Fay, 1982), which allows a contingency-table analysis for weighted data and complex sample designs, using a maximum-likelihood approach. For each odds ratio in this chapter, we fit a loglinear model that tests the null hypothesis that the odds ratio is 1. The test statistic is a likelihood-ratio χ^2 based on jackknifed replicate half samples (Fay, 1982).

RESULTS

Disorders subject to exclusion rules

Table 25.1 shows the odds ratios for all those DIS disorders that, according to *DSM-III*, are excluded by a major affective disorder. As seen in the first line of data, the odds ratio relating panic disorder to a major depressive episode is 18.8. This means that someone who is in a major depressive episode is about 19 times more likely to have panic disorder than someone who is not in a major depressive episode. This is statistically significant ($p < .001$). In other words, we must reject the null hypothesis of no relationship between the phenomena of the two disorders.

Similarly, someone in an episode of major depression has 15 times the odds of having agoraphobia as someone not in an episode of major depression ($p < .001$). Table 25.1 shows that major depression also increases the odds of having simple phobia, obssessive–compulsive disorder, schizophrenia, and schizophreniform disorder ($p < .001$).

One question that arises is whether or not one disorder increases the duration of the other disorder. We cannot study the duration of an episode using DIS data, but we can study the number of years from the onset to the end of the disorder. We find that panic disorder does not increase the number of years someone had major depression, nor vice versa. Similarly, none of the disorders in Table 25.1 significantly increases the duration of major depression, or vice versa.

Table 25.2 shows the odds ratios for all DIS disorders that, according to *DSM-III*, are excluded by schizophrenia. The presence of schizophrenia greatly

Table 25.1. *Odds ratios for coexistence of a major affective disorder and a disorder excluded by major affective disorder according to DSM-III (hierarchy-free syndromes occurring in the past month)*

Dominant disorder	Excluded disorder	Odds ratio
Major depressive episode	Panic disorder	18.8***
	Agoraphobia	15.3***
	Simple phobia	9.0***
	Obsessive–compulsive	10.8***
	Schizophrenia	28.5
	Schizophreniform	33.1***
Manic episode	Schizophrenia	89.1***
	Schizophreniform	4.6
	Antisocial personality	6.7*

Note: *p < .05; ***p < .001.

Table 25.2. *Odds ratios for coexistence of schizophrenia and a disorder excluded by schizophrenia according to DSM-III (hierarchy-free syndromes occurring in the past month)*

Dominant disorder	Excluded disorder	Odds ratio
Schizophrenia	Manic episode	89.1***
	Major depressive episode	28.5***
	Obsessive–compulsive	12.3**
	Agoraphobia	20.0***
	Simple phobia	9.1***
	Panic disorder	37.9***
	Antisocial personality	19.3*

Note: *p < .05; **p < .01; ***p < .001.

increases the odds of having major affective disorders, anxiety disorders, or antisocial personality.

Table 25.3 shows the odds ratios for all DIS disorders that, according to *DSM-III*, are excluded by anxiety or somatoform disorders. In each case the excluded disorder has a higher odds of being found in the presence of the dominant disorder than in the absence of the dominant disorder.

The very large odds ratio (96.5) relating somatization disorder and panic is what one would expect. Because of the overlap of the symptoms of panic and somatization disorder (American Psychiatric Association, 1980), it is not surprising to find empirical evidence of a strong relationship between the two disorders.

Table 25.3. *Odds ratios for existence of two anxiety or somatoform disorders related to each other according to the diagnostic hierarchy of DSM-III (hierarchy-free syndromes occurring in the past month)*

Dominant disorder	Excluded disorder	Odds ratio
Agoraphobia	Panic disorder	18.0***
Obsessive–compulsive	Agoraphobia	10.9***
Obsessive–compulsive	Simple phobia	9.7***
Somatization	Panic disorder	96.5**

Note: **$p < .01$; ***$p < .001$.

Disorders not subject to exclusion rules

The question arises whether or not this relationship between dominant and excluded disorders is specific to such disorders. A similar analysis of odds ratios can be performed with DIS disorders that are not mentioned in the *DSM-III* exclusion rules.

Table 25.4 shows the odds ratios for coexistence in the past month of two disorders not related to each other in the *DSM-III* exclusion rules. We find, for example, that the presence of schizophrenia increases the odds of having somatization disorder by 44.4 times ($p < .01$), compared with the odds of having somatization disorder in the absence of schizophrenia. The zeroes in Table 25.4 indicate that we sometimes have empty cells in our tables: No one in the sample had that pair of disorders. The disorders we are discussing are rare events, and the coexistence of two rare events can be an extremely rare event, resulting in empty cells.

The main trend that is evident in Table 25.4 is that the presence of any DIS disorder increases the odds of having almost any other DIS disorder. Schizophreniform disorder and somatization disorder are occasional exceptions to this trend. Schizophreniform disorder is conspicuous on Table 25.4 in that it greatly increases the odds of having obsessive–compulsive disorder, mania, or major depression. However, the procedural-validity study cited earlier (Robins et al., 1982) did not study schizophreniform disorder. The modest agreement found between lay interviewers and psychiatric diagnoses for schizophrenia in a predominantly inpatient population (Robins et al., 1982) may not be generalizable to schizophreniform disorder in a general population sample. The number of cases of schizophreniform disorder is given in Table 25.5.

To facilitate an independent review of these data, a complex set of 2 × 2 tables for this set of pairwise comparisons is presented in Table 25.5. Both weighted and unweighted data are given so that the reader may evaluate our odds ratios.

Table 25.5 consists of a matrix of 2 × 2 tables, each of which is defined by

Table 25.4. Odds ratios for coexistence in the past month of two disorders not related to each other in the DSM-III hierarchy (hierarchy-free syndromes)

	Manic episode	Major depressive episode	Alcohol abuse or dependence	Drug abuse or dependence	Schizophrenia	Schizophreniform	Obsessive–compulsive	Any phobia	Somatization	Panic
Major depressive episode	—									
Alcohol abuse or dependence	14.5***	4.1***								
Drug abuse or dependence	3.4	4.2*	10.7***							
Schizophrenia	—	—	10.1**	7.6*						
Schizophreniform	—	—	0	28.8*	—					
Obsessive–compulsive	17.8***	—	3.4**	4.9***	—	29.8**				
Any phobia	12.7***	—	2.4***	2.5**	—	11.4*	—			
Somatization	11.9*	26.8***	1.6	0	44.4**	0	2.2	38.6***	—	
Panic	24.1***	—	4.3*	4.1	—	0	20.6***	—	—	
Antisocial personality	—	5.1**	15.5***	24.2***	0	0	10.1**	3.0*	0	8.7*

Note: *p < .05; **p < .01; ***p < .001; a dash indicates that the disorders exclude one another in DSM-III.

Table 25.5. Tables for each pair of disorders: sample size (unweighted N) and population estimate (weighted N)

Upper-right triangle of each pairing gives the sample size (unweighted N); lower-left triangle gives the population estimate (weighted N).

		Manic episode		Major depressive episode		Alcohol abuse or dependence		Drug abuse or dependence		Schizophrenia		Schizophreniform	
		+	−	+	−	+	−	+	−	+	−	+	−
Manic episode	+			22	26	10	38	2	46	12	36	1	47
	−			250	11,003	282	10,929	129	11,095	61	11,171	10	11,222
Major depressive episode	+	1,890	15,961			32	238	11	260	23	248	3	268
	−	1,990	722,380			260	10,735	120	10,885	50	10,962	8	11,004
Alcohol abuse or dependence	+	1,141	20,502	1,849	19,793			29	263	13	279	0	292
	−	2,739	714,822	15,962	701,892			102	10,853	59	10,900	11	10,948
Drug abuse or dependence	+	164	9,418	861	8,722	2,182	7,401			5	126	2	129
	−	3,716	727,061	16,892	714,050	19,461	709,351			68	11,063	9	11,122
Schizophrenia	+	1,179	3,593	1,852	2,921	1,071	3,680	417	4,356			0	73
	−	2,700	733,044	15,994	720,068	20,572	713,089	9,165	725,417			11	11,205
Schizophreniform	+	12	492	225	279	0	504	137	367	0	504		
	−	3,868	736,144	17,621	722,708	21,643	716,264	9,445	729,404	4,773	735,746		
Obsessive-compulsive	+	683	8,702	1,834	7,617	852	8,572	593	8,858	623	8,784	139	9,267
	−	3,196	723,889	15,897	711,619	20,791	704,715	9,898	717,642	4,150	722,106	365	725,890

Sample size (unweighted N)

Population estimate (weighted N)

414

Any phobia	+	1,708	42,735	6,430	38,610	2,784	41,713	1,285	43,036	2,020	42,543	213	44,350
	−	2,171	691,327	11,301	682,376	18,859	671,839	8,297	683,631	2,753	689,028	291	691,489
Agoraphobia	+	1,297	19,614	4,701	16,593	1,675	19,257	997	19,952	1,678	19,322	213	20,787
	−	2,583	715,064	13,030	705,009	19,968	694,912	8,586	707,331	3,095	712,865	291	715,667
Simple phobia	+	1,348	36,116	5,293	32,683	2,182	35,318	902	36,357	1,523	35,977	84	37,417
	−	2,531	698,440	12,437	688,797	19,461	678,728	8,681	690,804	3,250	696,088	420	698,916
Somatization	+	52	839	350	541	40	851	0	891	194	698	0	891
	−	3,827	733,423	17,380	720,669	21,603	713,038	9,582	726,147	4,579	731,210	504	735,283
Panic Disorder	+	371	3,204	1,613	3,508	432	3,351	187	3,536	652	3,035	0	3,688
	−	3,509	729,667	17,167	700,594	21,163	709,045	9,338	722,019	4,121	727,367	504	730,982
Antisocial personality	+	132	3,313	437	3,508	1,165	2,781	870	3,075	408	3,538	0	3,945
	−	3,683	713,650	17,167	700,594	18,852	696,777	8,271	708,704	4,247	712,209	504	715,950
Population totals[a] (N = 752,551)		3,880	738,734	17,915	725,509	21,643	718,197	9,582	731,361	4,773	736,250	504	740,518

Note: Plus sign indicates that the disorder was present within the past month; a minus sign indicates that the disorder was absent within the past month.

[a] The numbers do not add up to the totals because of missing diagnoses.

Table 25.5 (*cont.*)

	Obsessive-compulsive +	Obsessive-compulsive −	Any phobia +	Any phobia −	Agoraphobia +	Agoraphobia −	Simple phobia +	Simple phobia −	Somatization +	Somatization −	Panic disorder +	Panic disorder −	Antisocial personality +	Antisocial personality −	Sample totals[a] (unweighted, $N = 11,519$)
Manic episode +	9	39	19	29	17	31	15	33	1	47	5	43	2	44	48
Manic episode −	144	10,965	767	10,359	344	10,794	645	10,488	18	11,118	59	11,056	55	10,802	11,260
Major depressive episode +	27	239	96	170	67	199	78	188	7	259	30	236	5	259	273
Major depressive episode −	127	10,772	698	10,223	300	10,633	588	10,340	12	10,920	37	10,873	52	10,593	11,049
Alcohol abuse or dependence +	17	275	42	250	27	265	33	259	1	291	9	282	21	252	292
Alcohol abuse or dependence −	136	10,708	742	10,103	335	10,522	624	10,228	18	10,838	57	10,778	36	10,572	10,979
Drug abuse or dependence +	10	121	18	113	14	117	13	118	0	131	4	126	11	113	131
Drug abuse or dependence −	144	10,875	767	10,251	350	10,680	644	10,381	19	11,011	62	10,947	46	10,727	11,154
Schizophrenia +	11	62	29	44	25	48	22	51	4	69	10	63	5	66	73
Schizophrenia −	141	10,934	755	10,326	337	10,756	634	10,454	15	11,077	55	11,016	52	10,769	11,216

Table. Comorbidity of psychiatric disorders — Sample size (unweighted N, top) and Population estimate (weighted N, bottom). (N = 752,551)

		Schizophreniform	Obsessive-compulsive	Any phobia	Agoraphobia	Simple phobia	Somatization	Panic disorder	Antisocial personality
Schizophreniform	+	3 / 149	5 / 779	6 / 10,364	5 / 357	6 / 10,798	3 / 653	8 / 10,497	0 / 19
	−	8 / 10,988						0 / 65	0 / 57
Obsessive-compulsive	+	49 / 736	105 / 10,263	33 / 329	121 / 10,682	45 / 613	109 / 10,393	1 / 18	14 / 53
	−		153 / 10,993						
Any phobia	+	3,297 / 6,154	41,220 / 685,707	0 / 367	426 / 10,417	666 / 0	128 / 10,417	12 / 7	28 / 39
	−							782 / 10,406	
Agoraphobia	+	2,128 / 7,323	18,858 / 708,686	21,294 / 23,710	0 / 694,641	251 / 414	116 / 10,436	9 / 10	25 / 42
	−							358 / 10,843	
Simple phobia	+	3,074 / 6,376	34,397 / 693,024	37,977 / 7,063	0 / 694,641	493 / 37,484	657 / 9	10 /	22 / 45
	−						657 / 10,538		
Somatization	+	25 / 9,426	867 / 726,433	635 / 44,405	257 / 693,909	381 / 20,913	510 / 718,051	399 / 701,324	5 / 62
	−							14 / 11,116	
Panic disorder	+	754 / 8,650	3,051 / 722,773	1,418 / 43,338	2,386 / 690,665	1,271 / 19,904	2,533 / 714,717	1,016 / 36,695	2,789 / 697,802
	−	282 / 609	3,522 / 733,643					3 / 54	62 / 10,769
Antisocial personality	+	437 / 8,708	3,509 / 708,550	623 / 42,484	3,322 / 674,724	431 / 9,971	3,515 / 697,853	446 / 35,829	3,499 / 681,873
	−	0 / 891	3,945 / 716,688	162 / 3,494	3,783 / 712,546	57 / 10,856			
Population totals[a] (N = 752,551)		9,450 / 727,527	45,040 / 694,643	21,295 / 719,038	37,977 / 702,200	891 / 739,410	3,805 / 734,729	3,945 / 717,906	

the presence (plus sign) or absence (minus sign) in the past month of one disorder at the top of the table, and the presence or absence of another disorder at the left margin of the table.

There is a diagonal drawn in Table 25.5. Above the diagonal line, the data are unweighted (i.e., we show the actual number of cases in our sample of 11,519). Below the diagonal line, the data are weighted (i.e., we show the estimated number of cases in the community population of 752,551). The odds ratios presented in Tables 25.1–25.4 are based on weighted data (lower half of Table 25.5).

Table 25.5 gives the answer to an otherwise puzzling question: Why are the odds ratios in Tables 25.1–25.4 so high? The answer is that the lower right-hand cell of each 2 × 2 table, which represents the persons with neither disorder, is extremely large. This is because 87% of the people in this community population have no disorder whatsoever. The effect of this large D cell is to inflate the odds ratios, compared with what would be found in a clinical population, in which almost everyone would qualify for at least one diagnosis. In other words, the high values of the odds ratios in Tables 25.1–25.4 result from the fact that we are studying a community population instead of a clinical population.

Figure 25.1 shows graphically the odds ratios in Tables 25.1–25.4. On the left is the distribution of odds ratios for all pairs of disorders that, according to *DSM-III,* are related through the exclusion criteria. On the right is the distribution of the odds ratios for pairs of disorders not mentioned in the *DSM-III* exclusion criteria. There is considerable overlap between the two distributions. When we compare these two distributions using a Wilcoxon rank-sum test (Wilcoxon and Wilcox, 1964) we find that the left-hand distribution is higher ($p <$ .01), which tends to validate the judgment of *DSM-III* concerning which pairs of disorders occur together most often.

Multiple diagnoses

A question arises: If we have shown that one disorder increases the odds of having a second disorder, is there a similar increase in the likelihood of having three or more coexisting disorders? Table 25.6 shows the number of respondents that we observed with multiple disorders. The observed number of subjects is compared with the number we would expect if the same disorders were independently distributed in the population. The expected number is computed by using the prevalence rates for these disorders in the sample and calculating how many people one would expect to have no disorder, one disorder, two disorders, three disorders, and so forth.

We find from Table 25.6 that 87% of the sample had no disorder in the past month. Of the 13% who had at least one disorder, one-fifth had two or more disorders. There are more people with two disorders, and more people with three or more disorders, than one would expect if these disorders were independently distributed (χ^2 = 2208.5, d.f. = 3, $p <$ .0001).

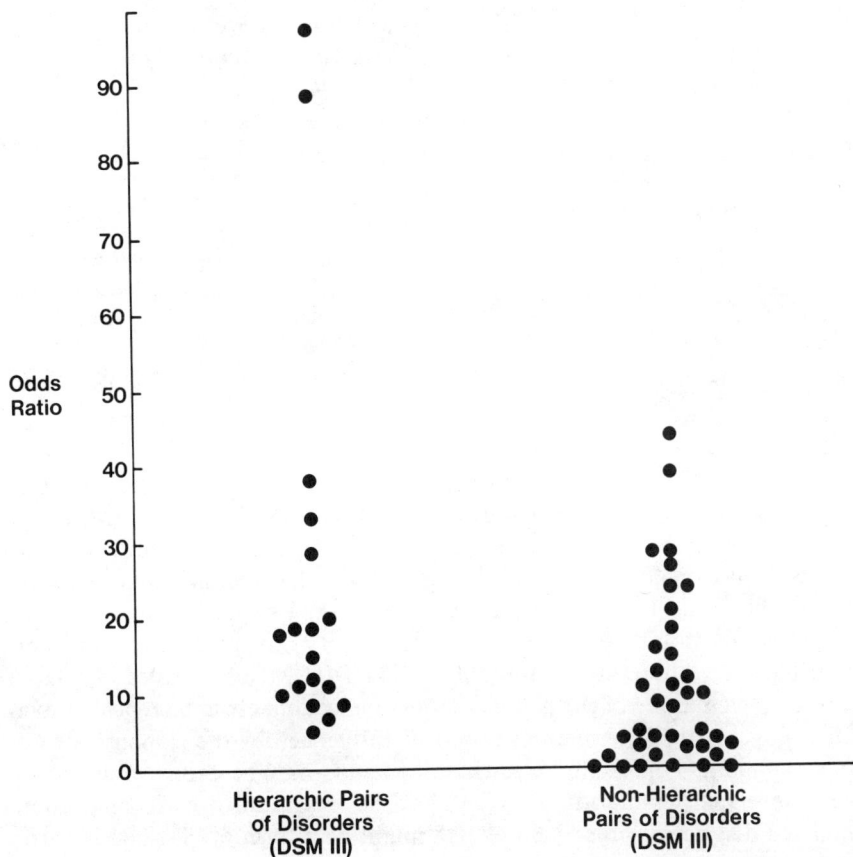

Figure 25.1. Comparison of odds ratios for two groups of paired *DSM-III* disorders.

DISCUSSION

Limitations

The DIS has been found to have specificity of 88% or higher in clinical populations (Robins et al., 1982). However, when any diagnostic instrument is used in the general population, there is a problem caused by the low prevalence of the disorders (Baldessarini, Finklestein, and Arana, 1983). If one shifts from a population in which disorders are common to one in which they are rare, the positive predictive value of a diagnostic instrument drops (Baldessarini et al., 1983). This means that a smaller number of those given the diagnosis actually have the disorder. We do not know if this has happened in the data presented, but it is possible.

Table 25.6. *Observed and expected numbers of persons with multiple psychiatric disorders (ECA data on 11 hierarchy-free syndromes within the past month) (unweighted data)*

Number of coexisting disorders	Number of persons	
	Observed	Expected
0	10,060	9,676.3
1	1,150	1,722.0
2	215	116.5
3 or more	94	4.2
Total	11,519	11,519

Because the DIS is a reliable instrument (Robins et al., 1981b; Burnam et al., 1983), this chapter simply proposes that the ECA data for "DIS/*DSM-III* disorders" show these patterns concerning the co-occurrence of disorders. It may be important to note that it is unlikely that these data can be replicated soon, because the clinical studies in the ECA either used small, less representative sampling designs or used exclusions as interpreted by the psychiatrists in a non-reversible way. Therefore, a study of the *DSM-III* exclusion rules in a large, representative sample of the general population is unlikely to be repeated soon.

It is possible that the findings might be influenced by the response style of the respondent: For example, some respondents may be prone to say yes to many unrelated conditions, and therefore be misclassified as having several unrelated diagnoses. This "halo effect" might be a form of bias that is particularly problematic when using lay interviewers and an instrument such as the DIS that assesses symptoms based on the subject's report rather than a clinician's judgment.

Sturt published a study similar to this one, based on data collected by the PSE, using interviewers with clinical skills, and found the same lack of independence of psychiatric disorders as we found (Sturt, 1981). To quote Sturt's summary: "Neurotic . . . syndromes which are common enough to be found in reasonable numbers in community surveys are not distributed randomly with respect to each other. A subject who exhibits any given . . . syndrome is more likely to show other . . . syndromes as well. This is a very robust finding that one would expect to be replicated." We have replicated this aspect of Sturt's work. If Sturt's findings and our findings are artifactual, then they are robust and reproducible artifacts.

Principal findings

We have found that we must reject the null hypothesis of no relationship between a dominant and an excluded DIS disorder. People with a dominant disorder such as major depression have much higher odds of having the symptoms of an excluded disorder, such as panic disorder, than are people without the dominant disorder. This confirms the clinical impression underlying *DSM-III* that a dominant disorder sometimes presents with symptoms of the excluded disorder. Thus, the beliefs that led to the use of exclusion criteria in *DSM-III* are confirmed by our data.

Surprisingly, we have also found that people with any DIS disorder have significant odds of having almost any other DIS disorder. Our data indicate that there is considerable overlap between the odds ratios of presumably related and presumably unrelated disorders. However, the odds ratios for disorders that *DSM-III* considers to be related are higher ($p < .01$) than the odds ratios for those that *DSM-III* considers to be unrelated. This finding again provides support for the clinical judgments represented in *DSM-III* about which disorders are related to each other.

The ECA data indicate that DIS disorders are not independently distributed in a community population. The lack of independence would be expected for disorders that *DSM-III* defines as related to each other; a similar but attenuated lack of independence is also found for disorders that *DSM-III* defines as unrelated. Furthermore, having one disorder increases the chance of having two, three, or more disorders (Table 25.6).

Similar results have been found in internal medicine. For example, Feinstein discusses the research implications of having patients with two or more unrelated disorders, such as diabetes mellitus and hypertension (Feinstein, 1970).

Exclusion criteria as an empirical question

The data that we have presented in this chapter provide only an initial examination of the assumptions underlying the use of exclusion criteria. They leave fundamental questions unanswered, such as whether or not the exclusion criteria are valid. In order to further investigate the question of validity, different kinds of data would be needed.

Follow-up studies would provide a much more powerful approach to the study of diagnostic hierarchies. If follow-up studies can show that the presence or absence of an excluded disorder occurring with a dominant disorder makes no difference in the outcome for the dominant disorder, then a hierarchical relationship is justified (unless family studies and/or biological studies provide strong evidence to the contrary). This type of reasoning provided much of the justification for the dominance of affective syndromes over schizophrenia, because the appearance of schizophrenialike symptoms in a patient with an affective syndrome appeared to make little difference to the outcome (Pope and Lipinski, 1978). A similar approach ought to be taken with many of the other hierarchical pairs.

In order to demonstrate that disorder *A* can "cause" disorder *B*, there are two central principles that would have to be demonstrated. First, one would need to show that the disorders wax and wane together. This means that for certain patients, disorder *B* occurs only during episodes of disorder *A,* and also that successful treatment of disorder *A* leads to remission of disorder *B.* The second principle is that disorder *B* can be divided into two different disorders. If disorder *B* is divided into two types, the type that occurs during episodes of disorder *A* and the type that is independent of disorder *A,* then the risk factors, genetics, treatment outcomes, and prognoses for the two types would need to indicate that they are different disease entities.

Consider, for example, the evidence that paranoid psychosis can be "due to" amphetamine intoxication. Such psychoses occur during an episode of amphetamine intoxication and remit within a few days (Peterson, 1980). Therefore, the two disorders wax and wane together. Furthermore, paranoid psychosis following amphetamine intoxication is different from other forms of paranoid psychosis in terms of prognosis, family history, premorbid history, and need for long-term antipsychotic medications. Therefore, paranoid psychoses can be divided into different types: those occurring during an episode of amphetamine intoxication, and those unrelated to amphetamines (Peterson, 1980).

CONCLUSIONS

Our study has examined whether or not hierarchy-free DIS/*DSM-III* syndromes occurring in the month prior to interview in a community population are distributed independent of each other. We find three things:

1. Disorders that *DSM-III* says are related to each other in a hierarchical fashion are always strongly associated with each other.
2. Disorders that *DSM-III* says are related to each other are more strongly associated with each other than disorders that *DSM-III* says are unrelated to each other.
3. Nevertheless, there is a general tendency toward co-occurrence of disorders, such that the presence of any DIS disorder increases the odds of having almost any other DIS disorder. This does not mean that most persons in the population have two or more disorders; in fact, 97% of our sample had either no disorder or only one disorder. However, given that only 10% had one disorder, the finding that 3% had more than one disorder is higher than would be expected if the disorders were independent of each other.

When Sturt investigated Foulds's diagnostic hierarchy, she provided an alternative explanation of the data: What appeared at first to be a hierarchy could also be interpreted as a manifestation of a tendency toward co-occurrence of psychiatric disorders (Sturt, 1981).

The present study is not a definitive study of the problem of exclusion criteria. We have, however, identified an operating assumption of *DSM-III* that has not received the kind of empirical research it deserves. Studies have not yet been done to show that certain nonorganic psychiatric disorders can cause other nonorganic disorders. Follow-up studies would be particularly useful in studying diagnostic hierarchies. We have outlined the form that such studies might take. One disorder can be said to be due to another disorder if the two disorders have the same prognosis, if they wax and wane together, and if the excluded disorder has different risk factors and responds to different treatment than it would if it occurred in the absence of the dominant disorder.

REFERENCES

American Psychiatric Association: Diagnostic and Statistical Manual of Mental Disorders, third edition, Washington, D.C., APA, 1980

Bagshaw VE: A replication study of Foulds' and Bedford's hierarchical model of depression. Br J Psychiatry 131:53–55, 1977

Bagshaw VE, McPherson FM: The applicability of the Foulds and Bedford hierarchy model to mania and hypomania. Br J Psychiatry 132:293–295, 1978

Baldessarini RJ, Finklestein S, Arana GW: The predictive value of diagnostic tests and the effect of prevalence of illness. Arch Gen Psychiatry 40:569–573, 1983

Bedford A, Presly AS: Symptom patterns among chronic schizophrenic in-patients. Br J Psychiatry 133:176–178, 1978

Boyd JH, Robins LN, Holzer CE, et al: Making diagnoses from DIS data, in Epidemiologic Field Methods in Psychiatry; The NIMH Epidemiologic Catchment Area Program. Edited by Eaton WW, Kesslor LC. Orlando, Fla, Academic, 1985, pp 209–231

Burnam MA, Karno J, Hoff RH, et al: The Spanish Diagnostic Interview Schedule: reliability and comparison with clinical diagnoses. Arch Gen Psychiatry 40:1189–1196, 1983

Eaton WW, Myers JK, Von Korff M, et al: The design of the ECA surveys: the control and measurement of error. Presented at the annual meeting of the American Public Health Association, Montreal, Quebec, November 17, 1982

Fay III RE: Contingency Table Analysis for Complex Sample Designs (CPLX). Washington, D.C., Bureau of the Census, 1982

Feighner JP, Robins E, Guze SB, et al: Diagnostic criteria for use in psychiatric research. Arch Gen Psychiatry 26:57–63, 1972

Feinstein AR: The pre-therapeutic classification of co-morbidity in chronic disease. J Chronic Dis 23:455–468, 1970

Foulds GA: The Hierarchical Nature of Personal Illness. New York, Academic Press, 1976

Foulds GA, Bedford A: Hierarchy of classes of personal illness. Psychol Med 5:181–192, 1975

Hesselbrock V, Stabenau J, Hesselbrock M, et al: A comparison of two interview schedules: the Schedule for Affective Disorders and Schizophrenia–Lifetime and the National Institute of Mental Health Diagnostic Interview Schedule. Arch Gen Psychiatry 39:674–677, 1982

Jaspers K: General Psychopathology, seventh edition. Translation by Hoenig J, Hamilton MW. Manchester, England: Manchester University Press, 1962, pp 611–612

Kendell RE: The Role of Diagnosis in Psychiatry. London, Blackwell Scientific, 1975, pp 102–103

Kleinbaum DG, Kupper LL, Morgenstern H: Epidemiologic Research, Principles and Quantitative Methods. Belmont, Calif, Lifetime Learning Publications, 1982

Leckman JF, Merikangas KR, Pauls DL, et al: Anxiety disorders associated with episodes of depression: family study data contradict DSM-III convention. Am J Psychiatry 140:880–882, 1983a

Leckman JF, Weissman MM, Merikangas KR, et al: Panic disorder and major depression: increased risk of depression, alcoholism, panic, and phobic disorders in families of depressed probands with panic disorder. Arch Gen Psychiatry 40:1055–1063, 1983b

McPherson FM, Antram MC, Bagshaw VE, et al: A test of the hierarchical model of personal illness. Br J Psychiatry 131:56–58, 1977

Palmer RL, Ekisa EG, Winbow AJ: Patterns of self-reported symptoms in chronic psychiatric patients. Br J Psychiatry 139:209–212, 1981

Peterson GC: Organic mental disorders induced by drugs or poisons, in Comprehensive Textbook of Psychiatry, vol 2, third edition. Edited by Kaplan HI, Freedman AM, Sadock BJ. Baltimore, Williams & Wilkins, 1980, p 1441

Pope HG, Lipinski JF: Diagnosis in schizophrenia and manic-depressive illness: a reassessment of the specificity of 'schizophrenic' symptoms in the light of current research. Arch Gen Psychiatry 35:811–828, 1978

Regier DA, Myers JK, Kramer M, et al: The NIMH Epidemiologic Catchment Area Program: historical context, major objectives, and study population characteristics. Presented at the annual meeting of the American Public Health Association, Montreal, Quebec, November 17, 1982

Robins LN, Helzer JE, Croughan J, et al: NIMH Diagnostic Interview Schedule, Version III. St Louis, Washington University School of Medicine, 1981a

National Institute of Mental Health Diagnostic Interview Schedule, its history, characteristics, and validity. Arch Gen Psychiatry 38:381–389, 1981b

Robins LN, Helzer JE, Ratcliff KS, et al: Validity of the Diagnostic Interview Schedule, Version II: DSM III diagnoses. Psychol Med 12:855–870, 1982

Roth SM: Problems in the classification of affective disorders. Acta Psychiatr Scand [Suppl] 290:42–51, 1981

Spitzer RL, Endicott J, Robins E: Research diagnostic criteria: rationale and reliability. Arch Gen Psychiatry 35:773–783, 1978

Sturt E: Hierarchical patterns in the distribution of psychiatric symptoms. Psychol Med 11:783–794, 1981

Surtees PG, Kendell RE: The hierarchy model of psychiatric symptomatology: an investigation based on Present State Examination ratings. Br J Psychiatry 135:438–443, 1979

Treece C: DSM-III as a research tool. Am J Psychiatry 139:577–583, 1982

Wilcoxon F, Wilcox R: Some Rapid Approximate Statistical Procedures. Pearl River, NY, Lederle Laboratories, 1964, pp 7, 27

26 Revising DSM-III

The process and major issues

ROBERT L. SPITZER AND
JANET B. W. WILLIAMS

The American Psychiatric Association (APA) was wise in recognizing, soon after the publication of *DSM-III* in February 1980, the need for a committee to evaluate it. The fact that the members of this committee themselves were not directly involved in the development of *DSM-III* made good sense, because, inevitably, it is difficult to be objective about the strengths and limitations of one's own offspring. So as to have some direct input from individuals who were involved in the development of *DSM-III*, three consultants (including R.L.S.) who had been members of the Task Force on Nomenclature and Statistics that guided the development of *DSM-III* were appointed to aid the committee in its work.

In March of 1983, the Committee to Evaluate *DSM-III* recommended to the board of trustees of the APA that a new group be created that would work on the "fine tuning" of *DSM-III*. This resulted in the appointment in May 1983 of the Work Group to Revise *DSM-III*, with the understanding that its work would be completed by December 1984. That was intended to allow for publication of *DSM-III-R* (for revision) in mid-1985. Thus, this conference represents the culmination of the work of the Committee to Evaluate *DSM-III* and the early stage of the work of the Work Group to Revise *DSM-III*. This conference is important in the effort to evaluate *DSM-III*, its primary purpose, and it should also provide a firm basis for discussion about possible revisions in *DSM-III*.

This chapter first discusses the formation of the Work Group to Revise *DSM-III*, the early stages of its work, and some likely directions for the next phase of its work. It then discusses an important nosologic issue that bears on the entire *DSM-III* classification: the *DSM-III* diagnostic hierarchies.

THE WORK GROUP TO REVISE *DSM-III*

The initial stages

The members of the Work Group were selected to ensure broad representation of clinical and research perspectives, including psychodynamic, biological, general clinical practice, family systems, epidemiologic, and adminis-

425

trative. In addition, they were chosen to ensure expertise in major content areas of *DSM-III* (child psychiatry, affective disorders, psychotic disorders, anxiety disorders, personality disorders, and multiaxial evaluation). The members of the Work Group are: Robert L. Spitzer, M.D. (chair), Dennis Cantwell, M.D., Allen Frances, M.D., Kenneth Kendler, M.D., Gerald Klerman, M.D., David Kupfer, M.D., Roger Peele, M.D., Judith Rapaport, M.D., Darrel Regier, M.D., Bruce Rounsaville, M.D., George Vaillant, M.D., Lyman Wynne, M.D., Ph.D., Janet B. W. Williams, D.S.W. (consultant), and Steven Sharfstein, M.D. (APA staff liaison).

The Work Group first met briefly during the annual meeting of the APA in May 1983 to review the scope of the revision. Because medical record-keeping systems in this country will continue to utilize *ICD-9-CM,* no changes can be made that would result in incompatibility with that classification (of which *DSM-III,* with a few minor exceptions, is a subset). Therefore, no new categories with official codes that are not now in *ICD-9-CM* can be added. However, it would be possible in the revision to add to *DSM-III* categories that are already in *ICD-9-CM,* such as paraphrenia. New categories that might be added that are not in *ICD-9-CM* would have to share a code number with a category already in *DSM-III.* For example, the inclusion of a category called organic anxiety syndrome would have to be coded as "other organic brain syndrome," and the inclusion of masochistic personality disorder would have to be coded as "other personality disorder."

The Work Group discussed the need, in the revision, for clarifications in the text and diagnostic criteria and inclusion of new data regarding prevalence and sex ratios, as well as the possibility of developing unofficial additional axes that could be included in an appendix (e.g., for dimensions of personality disturbance, social supports, coping mechanisms, and classifying family disorders).

At the next meeting of the Work Group in June, each member reviewed problematic issues and areas of controversy in *DSM-III* within his or her own substantive area. For example, Dr. Klerman noted the broad acceptance of the *DSM-III* distinction between major depression and bipolar disorder, but the concern of many that the definition of a major depressive episode is too broad and that the distinction between a major depressive episode in partial remission and dysthymic disorder is unclear. Dr. Rapaport, discussing the childhood categories, noted the continuing controversy regarding the distinction between the socialized and undersocialized subtypes of conduct disorder and the validity of the new *DSM-III* category of oppositional disorder.

Members of the Work Group had been asked to compile lists of individuals in their fields who might be able to make contributions to the revision. It was decided that at this first step, a broad net would be cast that would include individuals in this country and abroad who had been known to be critical of some aspects of *DSM-III.* By the end of the meeting, a list of approximately 150 individuals had been compiled. Over the next few weeks, additional names were added from a developing bibliography on *DSM-III* (Skodol and Spitzer, in press). In addition, the Work Group identified a number of professional mental health organizations, such as the American Psychological Association and the American Psychoanalytic Association, to whom letters would be sent inviting their input to the revision.

Beginning in early July, a letter was sent to each potential resource person, briefly explaining the scope of the work to be done and including a brief questionnaire asking the respondent to note in what ways (if any) he or she would like to contribute to the revision: reviewing drafts of proposed changes and providing written critiques, suggesting changes (or the need for changes) in specific areas of the text or criteria, and providing data from studies (completed or ongoing) that have implications for the revision.

At the time of this conference, more than 200 letters and questionnaires have been sent out, and the list of potential resource persons is still growing. To date, approximately 160 have responded, and with only a few exceptions, all have indicated interest in reviewing drafts of changes in the text and criteria of *DSM-III*, and in accompanying letters, many have expressed strong approval for the plans to revise *DSM-III* based on experience and data that have accumulated in the several years following its publication. Nearly 40% of the respondents suggested specific changes, or the need for changes, in the text or criteria. Approximately one-third of the respondents indicated that they had done studies with implications for the revision (usually accompanied by descriptions of their studies in the form of articles, preprints, and even some books). Over a quarter of the respondents indicated that they would soon have data that might have implications for the revision. Although some of the suggestions for changes in *DSM-III* that were submitted in response to the questionnaire were clearly beyond the possible scope of this revision (e.g., basic reorganization of the classification), most were appropriate for consideration over the coming months.

The next step

On the basis of initial discussions of the Work Group, the responses to the questionnaires, and the thoughtful critiques of *DSM-III* presented at this conference, the next step will be to gather together ad hoc groups of consultants to work with one or more Work Group members in particular substantive areas of *DSM-III*. The following is a description of the areas that will receive high priority.

Revisions in the diagnostic criteria. Despite extensive field testing of the *DSM-III* criteria prior to their official adoption (Spitzer and Forman, 1979; Spitzer, Forman, and Nee, 1979), experience with them has revealed, as expected, many cases in which the criteria are not entirely satisfactory and need to be revised. First of all, there are ambiguities in the wording. For example, the *DSM-III* criteria for dysthymic disorder state that "during the past two years . . . the individual has been bothered most or all of the time by symptoms characteristic of the depressive syndrome. . . ." The exact meaning of the phrase "most or all of the time" was unclear, because it was not clear whether "most" referred to the proportion of each day or the proportion of days during the two-year period. Clarity and therefore increased reliability probably can be achieved by revising the unclear phrase to "more days than not."

In identifying ambiguities in the diagnostic criteria, the work of investigators involved in translating the *DSM-III* criteria into computer algorithms, such as in the NIMH Epidemiologic Catchment Area program (Regier et al., 1982), and in developing computer diagnostic consultation programs (Erdman et al., 1980) will be extremely useful.

Some diagnostic criteria are clear, but wrong. For example, although the text of *DSM-III* makes it clear that the diagnosis of generalized anxiety disorder is not given if the syndrome is due to a known physical factor (e.g., a drug), this important exclusion is not included in the criteria, but clearly should be. Another example is the *DSM-III* diagnosis of paranoid disorder, which requires persecutory delusions or delusional jealousy. This definition, for no good reason, ignores the historical concept of paranoia that is much broader than that described in *DSM-III*. This limitation of the *DSM-III* criteria for paranoid disorder has been widely criticized both in this country (see Chapter 7) and abroad (Spitzer, Williams, and Skodol, 1983).

The second part of this chapter deals in detail with the issue of the need for revisions in the diagnostic hierarchies of *DSM-III* that are expressed in the criteria in the form of exclusion criteria.

The Work Group recognizes that any changes in the diagnostic criteria must be made only when there are compelling reasons to do so, and that the revised criteria, if at all possible, should be tried out prior to their final inclusion in the revision.

Revisions in the text. The descriptions of the various disorders will need to be revised in accordance with any changes in the diagnostic criteria. In addition, in many cases, factual data regarding prevalence and sex ratio will be available based on studies that have occurred since the publication of *DSM-III*. Clinical experience using *DSM-III* has also indicated the need for amplifications in the discussion of differential diagnosis.

New diagnostic categories. Consideration will be given to addition of several new diagnostic categories. The absence of a specific category for anxiety syndromes due to known organic factors has been noted (Mackenzie and Popkin, 1983) (see Chapter 9). Organic anxiety syndrome could be added to the classification, and, as already mentioned, in order to maintain compatibility, there would have to be instructions to code the category as an "other organic mental syndrome." The exclusion of individuals over the age of 45 with first onset of a psychotic disorder from the category of schizophrenia has been criticized widely (Miller and Cohen, 1982; Spitzer et al., 1983), partly on the grounds that in such cases *DSM-III* forces the diagnosis to the residual category of atypical psychosis, which makes it difficult to separate such cases. A possible solution to this problem would be to add the *ICD-9-CM* category and code number for paraphrenia to the classification. Finally, several psychodynamically oriented clinicians have made a strong case for adding a description of masochistic personality disorder to *DSM-III-R*, and some early work has provided empirical support for a proposed set of diagnostic criteria for the disorder (F. Kass, pers. commun.).

Changes in the multiaxial system. Although the multiaxial system in *DSM-III* is regarded by many as one of its most important features, there have been many criticisms of the structure and content of each of the five axes. Proposals for changes in the five axes that clearly deserve consideration include the following: inclusion of mental retardation on axis II, thus providing construct validity for axis II disorders as being relatively stable and lifelong handicaps (Kendell, 1983); clarifying the criteria for noting an axis III condition or disorder; reconsideration of the axis IV approach to rating the severity of psychosocial stressors; subdividing axis V into separate ratings for social functional and occupational functional, which might allow for incorporation of the level of social support into the social-functioning rating of axis V.

In addition, because of the great interest in developing other axes, which could be included in an appendix to *DSM-R* as optional axes, attempts will be made to develop axes for noting an individual's predominant coping style or use of defense mechanisms (see Chapter 30) and for classifying family psychopathology (see Chapter 31).

Dimensional approach to personality assessment. The limitations of the traditional categorical approach to diagnosis of personality disorders have been noted by several authors (Millon, 1981) (see Chapter 17), with the recommendation that it be replaced with a system that would allow each patient to be evaluated in terms of the severity of disturbance according to a number of personality dimensions. The Work Group will consider adding, in an appendix to *DSM-III-R*, an optional scheme for rating each of the *DSM-III* personality-disorder types as a separate scaled dimension of personality disturbance. Such schemes for rating the *DSM-III* personality disorders dimensionally have been developed by others (Kass et al., 1985; Shea et al., 1987) and seem promising.

Outline for case formulation. A rating of directors of residency training was conducted to assess the impact of *DSM-III* on their training of psychiatric residents (Williams, Spitzer, and Skodol, 1985). Approximately half of the respondents believed that a significant negative effect of *DSM-III* is that it "focuses on signs and symptoms so much that it detracts from a more in-depth understanding of patients' problems." This problem was anticipated during the development of *DSM-III* and was the reason for including a discussion in the introduction to *DSM-III* of the need for other important nondiagnostic information as a basis for treatment planning. Clearly, admonitions alone are not enough.

The Work Group will consider the possibility of developing a comprehensive outline for case formulation that could be included in an appendix. This outline would indicate the areas of information additional to the multiaxial assessment that a clinician should consider in a comprehensive evaluation. Some of these areas would include the new unofficial axes described earlier, such as that for coping styles and family functioning. Input to the development of this case formulation from psychiatric educators will help to maximize the likelihood that such an outline will actually be used by residents in their training. (An ongoing survey of directors of medical-student education in psychiatry conducted by the authors includes a specific question regarding the value of including in *DSM-III-R* such an outline for case formulation. Preliminary results indicate that approximately 50% of the respondents are in favor of such a proposal.)

The process

The ongoing process of the development of *DSM-III-R* will involve, as did the development of *DSM-III,* a large number of individuals and much open discussion of the issues. The scope of the changes must be limited, partly because of limited time and because of the need to maintain compatibility with *ICD-9-CM.* However, many promising ideas that cannot be translated into *DSM-III-R* will certainly be stimuli for development of *DSM-IV.*

DSM-III DIAGNOSTIC HIERARCHIES

In *DSM-III,* the diagnostic classes are hierarchically organized on the assumption that a disorder high in the hierarchy may have symptoms found in disorders lower in the hierarchy, but not the reverse. The hierarchical structure of the classification is operationalized by exclusion criteria, so that a diagnosis (in this case, the "excluded diagnosis") is not given if its inclusion symptoms are considered to be a symptom of a more pervasive disorder (the "dominant disorder").

Data from the NIMH-sponsored Epidemiologic Catchment Area (ECA) program (Regier et al., 1982) have called into question the fundamental assumptions that form the basis of many of the *DSM-III* hierarchies, and particularly those for the anxiety disorders. Boyd and associates (see Chapter 25), using data from this project, found that the presence of a dominant disorder (e.g., major depression) greatly increased the likelihood of the presence of a related excluded syndrome (e.g., panic attacks), as would be predicted by the *DSM-III* hierarchies. However, there was also a tendency for the presence of any *DSM-III* syndrome to increase the likelihood of the presence of almost any other *DSM-III* syndrome. Other research has also challenged the validity of the *DSM-III* hierarchical principle that gives affective disorders precedence over anxiety disorders. Leckman and associates (1983), in a large case–control family study of depression, found that the presence of a history of panic attacks in the probands, whether associated with a major depressive episode or occurring at other times, predicted increased family prevalence of depression, alcoholism, and other anxiety disorders. These data suggest that research, and perhaps clinical practice as well, might be improved by eliminating some of the *DSM-III* diagnostic hierarchies that prevent joint diagnoses of different syndromes when they occur together in one episode of illness.

There are other problems with some of the hierarchical principles embodied in the exclusion criteria for the anxiety disorders. Some exclusion principles are not applied consistently. For example, a psychotic disorder in *DSM-III*, such as schizophrenia, explicitly takes precedence over all of the anxiety disorders except social phobia and posttraumatic stress disorder. In addition, some of the exclusion criteria confuse differential diagnostic issues with hierarchical issues. Thus, the *DSM-III* exclusion criteria for agoraphobia list obsessive–compulsive disorder and paranoid personality disorder. These two diagnoses are noted because it was recognized that individuals with obsessive–compulsive disorder and paranoid personality disorder are sometimes afraid to go out of their houses alone. The need for a differential diagnosis of the symptom of fear of going out of the house should not be confused with a hierarchical principle, because the fear of leaving the house because of fear of sudden incapacitation (the hallmark of agoraphobia) is not a symptom of obsessive–compulsive disorder or paranoid personality disorder.

We have agonized long and hard over the problem of the *DSM-III* hierarchies, attempting to identify general principles for diagnostic hierarchies that will avoid many of the problems previously noted, but will not reduce the classification of mental disorders to a list of symptom complexes or syndromes. We propose (and the Work Group to Revise *DSM-III* will consider) that the following principles for diagnostic hierarchies be consistently applied to all of the *DSM-III* categories:

1. When a syndrome has a known organic cause, the diagnosis of an organic mental disorder takes precedence over the diagnosis of that syndrome outside of the class of organic mental disorders. For example, a manic syndrome that is judged to be due to the use of amphetamines would be diagnosed as an amphetamine-induced organic mental disorder, rather than as an affective disorder; a persecutory delusional syndrome judged to be due to a brain tumor would be diagnosed on axis I as an organic delusional syndrome (with the brain tumor noted on axis III), rather than as a paranoid disorder. This hierarchical principle is fundamental to virtually all classifications of mental disorders.

2. A symptomatically more pervasive disorder preempts the diagnosis of a less pervasive disorder that is based on a symptom that is part of the essential features of the more pervasive disorder. According to this principle, a patient with schizophrenia who has persecutory delusions and hallucinations would not also be diagnosed as having a paranoid disorder. Similarly, a patient with both manic episodes and major depressive episodes would not be given diagnoses of both bipolar disorder and major depression.

3. A diagnosis is not given if its essential features are typically associated features of another disorder whose essential features are also present. According to this principle, chronic dysphoric mood is such a typical associated feature of such chronic disorders as alcohol dependence, agoraphobia, and obsessive–compul-

sive disorder that an additional diagnosis of dysthymic disorder would not be given. Another example would be the presence of generalized anxiety during an acute psychotic episode; generalized anxiety disorder would not be diagnosed in addition to the psychotic disorder. This is the most problematic principle, because it requires knowledge of the relative frequencies of associated features in any given diagnosis.

Table 26.1 shows the *DSM-III* exclusion criteria for anxiety disorders and our proposed revisions based on the foregoing principles. As can be seen, the revised exclusion criteria are unambiguous and, with the exception of the residual category of generalized anxiety disorder, are far simpler than the *DSM-III* criteria. Furthermore, the revised criteria remove the hierarchical principle of a major depressive episode excluding a diagnosis of an anxiety disorder, a principle that the ECA data have called into question. As a consequence, many of the previously excluded diagnoses would, with the revised criteria, be regarded as complications of the dominant diagnosis. Thus, in a case in which recurrent panic attacks followed and were superimposed on a major depressive episode, the panic disorder could be given as an associated diagnosis and conceptualized as a complication of the major depressive episode. Application of these principles would also mean that generalized anxiety disorder could be given as an additional diagnosis to an individual who concurrently has a depressive disorder. This would respond to the criticism of Shader and Greenblatt (1981) that *DSM-III* does not recognize the validity of mixed anxiety/depressive disorders. It is also in accord with the findings of a recent study by Finlay-Jones and Brown (1981) in which it was found that individuals who had experienced both severe loss and severe danger developed mixed depression/anxiety states. Application of the traditional diagnostic hierarchy to these cases would have obscured the mixed nature of the disorder.

What would happen to the combination category of agoraphobia with panic attacks following adoption of the proposed hierarchical principles? We believe that there is sufficient clinical evidence that agoraphobia is usually a complication of recurrent panic attacks to justify the following revision in the *DSM-III* classification of agoraphobia and panic disorder: The category of agoraphobia without panic attacks would be unchanged, but the diagnoses of panic disorder and agoraphobia with panic attacks would be combined into a single category of panic disorder that would have three subtypes:

Panic disorder, uncomplicated
Panic disorder, with limited phobic avoidance
Panic disorder, with agoraphobia (extensive phobic avoidance)

This revision would acknowledge the central role of panic attacks in the typical development of agoraphobia. It would also provide a subtype of panic disorder for cases in which the individual avoids one or more activities because of fear of having panic attacks (e.g., going into restaurants), but in which the phobic avoidance is not as extensive as would be the case with agoraphobia. There is no satisfactory way to diagnose such cases according to *DSM-III*.

Table 26.1. *DSM-III exclusion criteria for anxiety disorders and proposed revisions*

Agoraphobia	
DSM-III:	Not due to a major depressive episode, obsessive–compulsive disorder, paranoid personality disorder, or schizophrenia
Revised:	No exclusions
Social phobia	
DSM-III:	Not due to another mental disorder, such as major depression or avoidant personality disorder
Revised:	Unrelated to fear of having a panic attack or to engaging in a compulsion in a social situation
Simple phobia	
DSM-III:	Not due to another mental disorder, such as schizophrenia or obsessive–compulsive disorder
Revised:	Unrelated to the content of the obsessions of obsessive–compulsive disorder
Panic disorder	
DSM-III:	Not due to a physical disorder or another mental disorder, such as major depression, somatization disorder, or schizophrenia
Revised:	Not due to a specific organic factor (e.g., amphetamine intoxication, hyperthyroidism)
Obsessive–compulsive disorder	
DSM-III:	Not due to another mental disorder, such as Tourette's disorder, schizophrenia, major depression or organic mental disorder
Revised:	No exclusions
Posttraumatic stress disorder	
DSM-III:	No exclusions
Revised:	No exclusions
Generalized anxiety disorder	
DSM-III:	Not due to another mental disorder, such as a depressive disorder or schizophrenia
Revised:	Not due to a specific organic factor (e.g., hyperthyroidism, caffeine intoxication); has not occurred only during the course of an active phase of a psychotic disorder or another anxiety disorder in which generalized anxiety is usually present (i.e., panic disorder, agoraphobia, obsessive–compulsive disorder, or posttraumatic stress disorder)

REFERENCES

Erdman HP, Greist JH, Klein MH, et al: Computer consultation for psychiatric diagnosis, in Proceedings of the Fourth Annual Symposium on Computer Applications in Medical Care, New York, IEEE, 1980

Finlay-Jones R, Brown GW: Types of stressful life events and the onset of anxiety and depressive disorders. Psychol Med 11:803–815, 1981

Kass F, Skodol AE, Charles E, et al: Scaled ratings of *DSM-III* personality disorders. Am J Psychiatry 142:627–630, 1985

Kendell RE: DSM-III: a major advance in psychiatric nosology, in International Perspectives on DSM-III. Edited by Spitzer RL, Williams JBW, Skodol AE. Washington, DC, American Psychiatric Press, 1983

Leckman JF, Merikangas KR, Pauls DL et al: Anxiety disorders and depression: contradictions between family study data and DSM-III conventions. Am J Psychiatry 140:880–882, 1983

Mackenzie TB, Popkin MK: Organic anxiety syndrome. Am J Psychiatry 140:342–344, 1983

Miller NE, Cohen G (eds): Proceedings of a conference on schizophrenia, paranoia, and schizophreniform disorders in later life, June 7–8, 1982, Bethesda, Md, sponsored by the Center for Studies of the Mental Health of the Aging and the Center for Studies of Schizophrenia, NIMH, ADAMHA. New York, Guilford Press (in press)

Millon T: Disorders of Personality. DSM-III: Axis II. New York, Wiley, 1981

Regier DA, Meyers JK, Kramer M, et al: The NIMH Epidemiologic Catchment Area (ECA) program: historical context, major objectives, and study population characteristics. Arch Gen Psychiatry 41:934–941, 1984

Shader RI, Greenblatt DJ: Antidepressants: the second harvest and DSM-III. J Clin Psychopharmacol 1:51–52, 1981

Shea MT, Lass DR, Pilkonis PA, et al. Frequency and implications of personality disorders in a sample of depressed outpatients. J Pers Disorders 1:27–42, 1987 ·

Skodol AE, Spitzer RL: An Annotated Bibiliography of DSM-III. Washington, DC, American Psychiatric Press (in press)

Spitzer RL, Forman JBW: DSM-III field trials, II: initial experience with the multiaxial system. Am J Psychiatry 136:818–820, 1979

Spitzer RL, Forman JBW, Nee J: DSM-III field trials, I: initial interrater diagnostic reliability. Am J Psychiatry 136:815–817, 1979

Spitzer RL, Williams JBW, Skodol AE (eds): International Perspectives on DSM-III. Washington, DC, American Psychiatric Press, 1983

Williams JBW, Spitzer RL, Skodol AE: DSM-III in residency training: results of a national survey. Am J Psychiatry 142:755–758, 1985

27 DSM-III in evolution

JAMES BARRETT

Classification schemes have different purposes. As background for discussion of the excellent presentations in Chapters 25 and 26, I want to describe three purposes, or goals, that provide the basis for grouping particular classification systems. The first group comprises those classifications whose primary use is for research purposes. The principal concern of a *research classification* system is validity for each category. Put another way, the goal of the classification is to come up with categories that will be useful in some way for research purposes, whatever that research may be. Because validation is a primary concern, reliability is essential for the categories. One way to increase reliability is to limit coverage; thus, in a research nosology, one often uses an "other" category as a place to put heterogeneous groups or those groups unrelated to the research involved. Also note that a research classification system need not be accepted by everyone, although it is desirable to have acceptance by the research community working in the same research area.

An example of a classification for research purposes would be Joseph Schildkraut's proposed classification for affective disorders (Schildkraut, 1970). That classification had as an underlying principle the relationships of depression categories to a presumed biochemical abnormality. Other categories, such as drug abuse or schizophrenia, were not covered, because it was a research classification concerned primarily with the affective disorders. Another example, one with somewhat broader coverage, is provided by the Research Diagnostic Criteria developed by Spitzer, Endicott, and Robins (1978). Here the underlying validation principal was clinical course. Based on existing data from clinical and follow-up studies, categories were chosen that were internally consistent, were descriptively clear, and were related to the clinical course. Of necessity in this system there was a large "other psychiatric disorder" category as a repository for individuals who were believed to have something wrong with them but who did not fit the full criteria for any of the defined disorders in the nosology.

A second group of classification schemes is concerned with *statistical classification*. By "statistical classification," I mean that the principal purpose is to classify and count, usually for planning or archival purposes, all disorders present in a given unit, be it mental health center, state, region, or country. The principal concerns of such a system must be that it be comprehensive – all disorders are to be included in it – and that all people involved in treating patients use it. In other words, the principal requirements of a statistical classification are complete coverage and complete acceptance, or compliance. Such a system typically evolves by gathering together individuals with differing points of view, to be sure that all possible categories will be included, and trying to arrive at consensus regarding which categories to include and who should be placed in them. Ideally, such a classification system is also concerned with reliability and with the validity of its categories, but in practice the method of arriving at the categories and at their definitions is through committee work and consensus. Such a system usually is atheoretical, for it must encompass all points of view in the region or country concerned.

The *International Classification of Diseases* and any of the *DSM*s, including *DSM-III*, are statistical classifications. In these remarks, I do not mean to imply that those who drew up those classifications were not concerned with reliability or validity of categories, but I am saying that, in practice, the principal method of developing categories was to obtain consensus among contributors with different points of view. Thus, I am highlighting one immediate difference between a research nosology and a statistical classification. Coverage and reliability tend to be contradictory goals, with the reliability of categories diminishing as coverage increases. The necessity for complete coverage and the requirement that the system be used by everyone (compliance) are the principal features that distinguish a statistical classification from a research nosology.

A third set of classification schemes comprises those that exist primarily for clinical purposes. The principal concern of a *clinical classification* system is clinical utility, or predictive validity. The classification must predict who will respond favorably to what treatment, or, if there are no treatments, it must accurately predict the course of the disorder. Reliability of categories is certainly desirable, and often assumed, but it is not the principal guiding criterion in arriving at the classification categories. And, as with classification systems for research purposes, coverage need not be complete. An "other" category can be used for those conditions for which responses to treatment are uncertain or outcomes are highly variable. What is important is to include, as specific categories, all disorders for which there are known treatments that are efficacious and all disorders whose courses without treatment are relatively invariant. An example of a clinical classification is found in the Feighner criteria, as spelled out in the original article by Feighner and associates (1972) and in the book by Woodruff, Goodwin, and Guze (1974), who state that "Diagnostic categories – diseases, illnesses, syndromes – are included if they have been sufficiently studied to be useful. . . . In choosing the categories, the guiding rule was: diagnosis is prognosis." Repeating, clinical utility is the principal criterion on which the categories of a clinical classification are based.

In presenting these three purposes for classification systems, let me quickly acknowledge that these purposes need not lead to different categories in each system. There can be, and often is, considerable overlap among the three types of systems. In an ideal world, there would be complete overlap. There would be a statistical classification in which each and every category would be clinically precise and reliable and would have meaningful correlates – clinical, biochemical, familial, or any other abstraction believed to be relevant for the category involved. There would be complete coverage; all disorders would have a place, and everyone would agree on the necessity and reasonableness of their inclusion. The categories would have proven usefulness established by carefully designed basic research and clinical research. Such a system would be intrinsically so desirable that everyone would wish to comply with it.

Unfortunately, what I have just described does not accurately characterize the state of the art in psychiatric classification in the 1980s. Hence the need for our 1983 conference, as well as ongoing committees to revise and improve the categories of statistical classification used in *DSM-III*. However, I presented this background overview to highlight the fact that classification schemes do have different purposes and that each should be evaluated or criticized depending on how it meets its own particular purpose. At the present time, research purposes are different in many instances from clinical purposes, and both research and clinical purposes may be at variance with a statistical classification that has to please everyone and be used by everybody, no matter how much its originators may have wished it to be based on reliable scientific categories for which there are good validation data. Many of the *DSM-III* categories do meet such criteria, but others do not, and this fact is my point of departure for discussing the presentations by Dr. Boyd and by Dr. Spitzer. My contention is that their classification schemes are basically aimed at different purposes. The classification principles underlying Dr. Boyd's presentation (Chapter 25) are primarily those of a research classification system. He is concerned with validation of categories and with descriptive consistency (descriptive validity) across national boundaries, goals that are important for epidemiologic and nosologic research. And he is concerned with correlates of different ways of classifying the same individuals, or at least certain individuals, those for whom hierarchical principles have been proposed.

Dr. Spitzer (Chapter 26), on the other hand, at this stage in the development of *DSM-III*, has to be concerned primarily with coverage and with compliance. To be sure, from the outset he and his colleagues were concerned that the categories that evolved by consensus also be clinically useful and suitable for research purposes, probably in that order. Thus, before final acceptance of the present categories in *DSM-III*, he and his collaborators took the unprecedented step of submitting the consensus categories, evolved through the work of his committees, to field trials. Thus, one unique aspect of the development of *DSM-III* categories was the fact that from the outset they were to be modified by feedback from users, users concerned with clinical usefulness and users concerned with research purposes. And here is where these two presentations come together. Dr. Spitzer, having gone through the exercise of obtaining consensus on categories, and having demonstrated reliability for many, and having shown that they will be used, is now seeking feedback, from well-designed clinical studies and basic research studies, on which to base changes in the classification categories, if needed. And it is just such data, using results from the Epidemi-ologic Catchment Area project, a large-scale epidemiologic research project, that Dr. Boyd is trying to provide. The question for us, and indeed for those concerned with revisions in *DSM-III*, is this: What have we learned from Dr. Boyd's results that would suggest, or even require, that we revise *DSM-III*, the statistical classification scheme designed to be used in the United States?

Dr. Boyd's presentation has as a principal finding that if two DIS disorders are related to each other according to *DSM-III* exclusion criteria, then the pres-ence of one, which he and his collaborators call the "dominant" disorder, greatly increases the odds of having the other, the "excluded" disorder. In other words, from their analyses using their diagnostic categories, which they cor-rectly call "DIS disorders" to distinguish them from "*DSM-III* disorders," these DIS disorders were associated; they traveled together, so to speak. Dr. Boyd's interpretation of this finding was to call into question the use in *DSM-III* of diagnostic hierarchies – the *DSM-III* convention whereby when a particular (dominant) diagnosis is present, then other (excluded) diagnoses are not made even though symptoms related to those excluded diagnoses are present.

The hierarchical approach – the decision-making process whereby certain categories are diagnosed first and take precedence over other categories – has a long-standing tradition in both medical and in psychiatric nosology. It was implicit in the clinical descriptions of Kraepelin, in which, for example, in the presence of severe, persistent clouding of consciousness an organic psychiatric syndrome was diagnosed, irrespective of other features such as depressive or paranoid symptoms that might be associated. In Kraepelin's system, schizo-phrenia was given precedence over affective features, and endogenous depres-sive or manic disorder received priority in diagnosis over neurotic syndromes. There is nothing wrong with such hierarchies; they are essential to ordinary clinical practice, but it is worth stating, as does Martin Roth in a recent review, that diagnostic rules are not sacrosanct. The entities have to be treated as hypotheses open to challenge and refutation. He argues, as would many of us, for "a flexible and open hierarchical system" and that "diagnostic entities and the rules that govern their relationship are in the nature of hypotheses derived from clinical observation but open to refutation or modification in the light of fresh findings" (Roth and Barnes, 1981).

It is in this spirit – treating the decision rules, the "exclusionary criteria," of *DSM-III* as hypotheses to be tested – that Dr. Boyd and his associates carried out the analyses related to their presentation in Chapter 25. Returning to these findings, in reviewing their analyses I had a number of concerns. One concern had to do with their method of making their "DIS diagnoses" and whether in some instances that method deviated sufficiently from clinical reality to be sus-pect. A related concern had to do with the interpretation, using that method, that they placed on the coexistence, or comorbidity as they call it, of certain disorders.

Let me illustrate my concern with one aspect of their method by the follow-ing case history. Imagine a man, age 44, who presents with depressive symptoms that have existed for at least six months. They include a persistent depressed mood that is worse in the morning, early morning awakening, loss of appetite, weight loss, loss of interest in usual activities, low energy, feelings of worthlessness, and suicidal ideation. In addition, off and on during the six-month period, he has had somatic delusions, feeling that his insides are rotting and that he has cancer in several of his organs. I selected this case because many clinicians would assign this man a diagnosis of major depressive disorder with melancholia. Somatic delusions are present, but these are consistent with the preceding diagnosis. However, now take away the depressive symptoms. By *DSM-III* decision rules, and I assume also therefore by the DIS diagnostic decision-making program, this patient would now receive a diagnosis of schizophrenic disorder. If one applied the diagnostic program used by Boyd and associates, one that ignores exclusion criteria, this man now would receive two diagnoses, one of major depression, and the other of schizophrenia, and comorbidity of these disorders would be established in this case. However, I doubt very much if such a diagnosis of comorbidity would be made in usual clinical practice. On the basis of outcome studies, somatic delusions that occur in the presence of melancholia have little or no effect on outcome, in that the outcome for such patients is the same as for other melancholics without such delusions. Conversely, in the absence of melancholia, the clinical picture of this man is that of schizophrenia, which would relate to a poor clinical outcome.

The issue here is that the emergence of comorbidity in this case would be an artifact of the scoring program. This particular hierarchy evolved in the first place because the clinical correlates (the course) for somatic delusions plus melancholia were similar to those for melancholia alone and different from those for schizophrenia. The key words are "clinical correlates," and here I am repeating a necessary concept, that of external validating criteria. If there is existing evidence that a hierarchy (exclusionary criteria) will allow the course to be accurately predicted, then that is a strong piece of evidence that the particular hierarchy should be maintained.

An additional concern, also related to the DIS diagnoses, in the material originally presented by Dr. Boyd was that at times there was a confusion, an inappropriate jumping, from the symptom or syndrome level to the level of a specific disorder. In the example given, one of panic anxiety symptoms occurring in major depressive disorder, this appeared to be the case. This point is not very exciting to describe, but let me try to give one example. Boyd and associates (Chapter 25) argued that if major depression causes panic symptoms, then people who are in an episode of major depression should have increased odds of having panic symptoms as compared with people who are not in an episode of major depression. So far, so good. They continue:

The same thing can be stated as a null hypothesis: If the panic *symptoms* are not associated with depression, then there should be equal odds of having panic *symptoms* among those who are in an episode of major depression and those who are not in an episode of major depression. To state the null hypothesis in more general terms: If *A* is the dominant *disorder* and *B* is the excluded *disorder,* then the odds of having disorder *B* should be no greater among the population who have disorder *A* than in the population who do not have disorder *A*. [from Boyd et al.'s original paper, emphasis added; cf. Chapter 25, where this passage has been amended]

Panic symptoms had become equated with panic disorder in this restating of the null hypothesis. Using my earlier clinical example, somatic delusions would become equated with schizophrenia, and this would produce the problem outlined earlier, an artifactual discovery of comorbidity of schizophrenic disorder and major depressive disorder. I rather suspect that this difficulty – confusion of the symptom level of abstraction with the diagnostic-category (disorder) level – may have been operating to produce some of the data in their Table 25.2, such as the coexistence of a manic episode or a major depressive episode with schizophrenia.

In leaving this discussion of Dr. Boyd's presentation, let me put my remarks in perspective. I am not saying that the approach of these authors is critically flawed. I am saying that, in some cases, the comorbidity data shown may be artifactual, related to the scoring algorithms of the DIS ceasing to approximate clinical "truth" for some conditions when the exclusionary criteria were dropped. The importance of Dr. Boyd's presentation is that it quite rightly focuses our attention on how these exclusionary criteria, these diagnostic hierarchies, were arrived at. In the example I gave, accept, for the sake of argument, that they were arrived at by solid, carefully done follow-up studies. However, I suspect that some, if not many, of the exclusionary criteria in *DSM-III* are not based on such solid evidence, but rather reflect the consensus view of the particular committee that arrived at that criterion. Dr. Boyd's presentation highlights the point that in revising *DSM-III,* for each disorder with exclusion criteria it is important to examine the clinical evidence on which the exclusionary criteria are based. Separate those disorders whose exclusionary criteria are based on solid clinical research from those that are not. Subject the latter to the same field-trial method used in the evolution of *DSM-III* categories to test the reliability of the consensus categories. We should not do away with hierarchies, or exclusion criteria, but treat them in the same fashion as any other of the operational defining criteria. See if they make a difference in terms of outcome in clinical field trials. I emphasize that this approach is not the same as manipulation or rescoring of DIS symptom data. That approach can result in artifacts produced by the scoring system, as I believe to be the case for some of the comorbidity data in Dr. Boyd's presentation. What we need are some external validating criteria against which various combinations of symptoms and syndromes, in association with specific disorders, can be assessed.

Dr. Spitzer's presentation (Chapter 26) covered two separate major topics. One was the process of revision planned for *DSM-III*. He described forming a Work Group "to ensure broad representation." Areas to be represented that he specifically mentioned were: "psychodynamic, biological, general clinical practice, family systems, epidemiologic, and administrative." This Work Group, among other tasks, has been asked to compile lists of others who might contribute to revisions – the phrase used was that "a broad net would be cast." This description of the revision process emphasizes the point made earlier that a primary focus of *DSM-III* is as a statistical classification – coverage must be broad, and consensus is a principal method of arriving at categories. Concerning that process of consensus, I want to repeat that one unique aspect in the development of *DSM-III* was the inclusion of field trials. The developers of the categories were not permitted simply to say, "That's it; we agree; well done, lads," with the system then cast in cement for the next 10 years, but those consensus categories were to be tested for reliability and usability before they actually became part of the official nosology. I would like to urge that the same method be continued and strengthened during this revisionary process. Targeting smaller-scale clinical studies at nosologic issues related to particular disorders, rather than large, all-inclusive trials, would be one such strengthening. Testing the exclusionary criteria for particular disorders, as was suggested in the discusion of Dr. Boyd's presentation, in outcome studies targeted at those disorders would be one such example.

In this process, however, there is one problem that has no easy solution: Some categories are of greater scientific interest than others. The "consensus" categories for the affective disorders or for schizophrenia will receive careful attention and validation work, with regular interplay between those using them for research and those using them for clinical purposes. Some other categories, I suspect, will not receive the same attention. They are there because someone argued eloquently for them, and thus, under the coverage rule, they are included. Many psychiatrists do not care that much one way or the other about them, and thus the stimulation to do the evaluation (validation) work may be minimal or absent. I rather suspect that "tobacco dependence disorder" or "egodystonic homosexuality" will be such categories, diagnoses for which no one really wants to bother with the careful validation work that would be required.

A second major topic in Dr. Spitzer's presentation concerns specific areas in which revisions are already known to be needed. In addition to particular areas of the text where there are known inconsistencies, he suggests changes in the multiaxial system, such as adding a sixth axis. In this process, I would like to see included an open discussion of the principles underlying each axis. The inclusion of an axial system was another unique aspect of *DSM-III*. Although this concept had been suggested in the past, by Essen Möller, Wing, Rutter, and Strauss, to name a few, an axial system had never before become part of an official statistical classification system. The axial system of *DSM-III*, in contrast to *DSM-I* or *DSM-II*, which tended to force patients into various mutually exclusive categories, permits a given individual to be characterized on separate conceptual dimensions believed to have prognostic or theoretical implications.

With respect to axis II, although in his presentation Dr. Spitzer states that axis II disorders are to reflect "relatively stable and lifelong handicaps," comments and discussion at this conference have reflected ambiguity and disagreement about the conceptual underpinning of this axis, and it would be helpful to review it. Even if there is not agreement about what that conceptual basis should be, having in the open what it is, what was agreed on, at least will permit changes to be understandable and to be debated on some common basis. For example, is the presence of a "disorder" its primary concept, or should axis II be used as a descriptor for a character style (a dimension) that is on a continuum from normal to pathological? Axis II is an important axis; in relation to the defining criteria for its categories, it needs as much attention as axis I, but it has not received it to date.

In conclusion, I would like to emphasize again that statistical classification systems are different from research classification systems, which in turn are different from clinical classification systems. In the ideal world they would be one and the same. The development and evolution of *DSM-III*, a statistical classification system, have been guided from the outset by attempts to make it a true clinical classification system, one that will be widely used and will reflect, based on evidence, true prognostic implications. Its very success, however, carries with it some dangers. I think it has been seized uncritically by some, with each of the categories reified to a degree never intended by Dr. Spitzer and by the original committee members. At a recent APA annual meeting, in the course of a debate about *DSM-III*, it was referred to as a "textbook of psychiatry." It is not, nor was it ever intended to be. Using state-of-the-art methods from the late 1970s, it is a carefully arrived at statistical classification system that its authors believed would also be useful, or at least many of its categories would be, for clinical and research purposes. To quote Roth and Barnes again: "The dangers of a prestigious and in many ways valuable work such as the DSM-III is that it will be invested with a spurious final authority and create a closed system where the need in many places is for specific investigations." *DSM-III*, as Dr. Spitzer has continually reinforced in his writing, was never intended to be a "final authority" or a "closed" system. The developers of *DSM-III* have made a promising beginning, but further work remains to be done.

REFERENCES

Feighner JP, Robins E, Guze SB, et al: Diagnostic criteria for use in psychiatric research. Arch Gen Psychiatry 26:57–63, 1972

Roth M, Barnes TRE: The classification of affective disorders: a synthesis of old and new concepts. Compr Psychiatry 22:54–77, 1981

Schildkraut JJ: Neuropsychopharmacology and the Affective Disorders. Boston, Little Brown, 1970

Spitzer RL, Endicott J, Robins E: Research diagnostic criteria: rationale and reliability. Arch Gen Psychiatry 35:773–782, 1978

Woodruff RA, Goodwin DW, Guze SB: Psychiatric Diagnosis. Oxford University Press, 1974

DARREL A. REGIER

The provocative presentation by Boyd and associates (Chapter 25) was recognized as having major implications for the future revision of *DSM-III*. One participant characterized the elaborate structure of *DSM-III* as being like a house of cards in which one of the principal cards of diagnostic hierarchies has suddenly been removed. This somewhat facetious remark illustrated the importance of empirical data for an evaluation of *DSM-III* hypotheses, an importance that, in fact, had already resulted in Dr. Spitzer's suggested reformulation of exclusion-criteria principles, as reflected in Chapter 26.

As one would suspect, given the importance of such empirical data, there were considerable questions about the applicability of community epidemiological data and the instrumentation used in obtaining these data. An empirical question was raised about the possibility of particularly puzzling cases in community samples yielding false-positive answers on multiple diagnostic areas in the questionnaire. If this occurred, the correlation of these errors would produce a pattern of high levels of association between multiple disorders. In reply to this question, it was noted that the DIS showed a high level of specificity for disorders when compared with a clinician reappraisal and that there was no empirical evidence for a yea-saying bias.

The high odds ratios reported by Boyd were also the subject of some discussion. The hypothesis was advanced that they might partially be explained by inclusion of the large number of subjects with no disorders in the community. An analysis of only those subjects who have at least one disorder to see if there is more specific clustering of related disorders might provide a somewhat different picture. The observation was made that the data may not be that different from data that would be obtained from a study of other chronic diseases. In response to both issues, Boyd referred to a preliminary analysis of the Health and Nutrition Examination Survey data performed by the National Center for Health Statistics showing similar odds ratios between all physical disorders, with the ratios being on the order of 2:1 to 3:1, as opposed to the mental-disorder ratios of 20:1 to 30:1.

Dr. Robins presented a somewhat different perspective that started with the *DSM-III* structure itself. Dr. Robins noted that because *DSM-III* does not put in exclusions for all disorders known to be highly related (e.g., alcohol and drug abuse), it should not be surprising to find a high degree of correlation between many disorders. In preliminary analyses of her own ECA data, she found that some disorders that are not highly correlated on a clinical basis, such as mania and major depression, had lower odds ratios than other related disorders. Because these correlations were found across multiple sites, she dismissed the possibility that the finding was due to random error.

Finally, it was pointed out that there are limitations to a cross-sectional study of correlations between multiple disorders. A much more powerful demonstration of the probability of association between multiple disorders would be to see if they wax and wane together over a longitudinal time frame. The etiologic significance of this association also is not clear, because one disorder could be caused by the other, multiple disorders could be precipitated by a common etiologic agent, or multiple disorders could occur in the presence of a preexisting generalized vulnerability.

As mentioned previously, Dr. Spitzer's presentation had already been influenced by the findings of Boyd and associates, and much of the discussion focused on his plans for a revision of the hierarchy principle incorporated in *DSM-III*. He acknowledged that the hierarchy rules for individual diagnoses and for the entire system could well stand more systematic scrutiny than they received in the *DSM-III*. Several of the comments have already been incorporated into the published version of his chapter, and the initial recommendation of using a different term than "dominant disorder" has been taken to reflect the recommendation that the concept of "more symptomatically encompassing disorder" would provide greater clarity.

The reasons for hierarchies in the past that included the Jaspers and Kraepelin goals of explaining as many patient symptoms as possible under one parsimonious diagnosis were reviewed. It was noted, however, that previous discussions in the workshop had held that it was important not to lose data on some features of disorders that could meaningfully subdivide disorders along a variety of other possible criteria – including longitudinal course and treatment response. In addition, the sequence in which symptoms occur can cause some difficulty with a hierarchy. For example, although dysthymia may be a common component of alcohol dependence/abuse, it should not be incorporated under alcoholism if the dysthymia preceded any abuse of alcohol. The point was also made that we are in more danger of losing important clinical information by imposing hierarchies than we are of having some excessive redundancy that hierarchies are designed to eliminate.

Presenting a different viewpoint, the premise was advanced that one value of hierarchies is to preclude inappropriate labeling of patients with certain stigmatizing disorders. For example, where severe organic disorder exists, it is important to note that, so as not to give conduct disorder or antisocial personality diagnoses to children when such behavior can be explained by organic causes.

In addition to the study of hierarchies, there was extensive discussion of the process of revising *DSM-III* and of the reasons for such revisions. A theme that was raised concerned changing the diagnostic criteria at a time when many research investigators are using such criteria. The resultant discontinuity between their results and those from studies using the new criteria would be likely to cause confusion in the field. The comment was made that there must be good scientific reasons, not simply economic reasons, for any such revision.

At the other end of the spectrum concern was expressed that failure to change the criteria over the next seven or more years before *ICD-10* and *DSM-IV* come out could result in a disservice to the research and clinical community in cases in which clear deficiencies in the existing diagnostic criteria have already been identified. An alternative viewpoint was that scientists would continue to develop their own research diagnostic criteria that in many cases would go beyond anything that *DSM-III* could possibly do. This reflected an earlier comment concerning ongoing investigations attempting to validate *DSM-III* categories that require investigators to collect more data than are called for in *DSM-III*. It was suggested that revisions should be recommended only in areas in which a really convincing case can be made that the nosology is getting in the way of clinical practice.

Another clinical concern raised was that the current *DSM-III* often is not comprehensive enough in its coverage to classify all patients and that future revisions should address this issue. Finally, it was pointed out that many schools of medicine are using *DSM-III* as a textbook, and it is seen not simply as a statistical classification but as a repository of the current best knowledge on psychopathology. As a result, revisions will be important for a wide range of professions, even though it will be necessary to keep these revisions within certain fine-tuning boundaries permitted by the *International Classification of Diseases* statistical conventions.

In addition to the informal discussions summarized earlier, Dr. Barrett (Chapter 27) provided a formal critique of Chapters 25 and 26 that stimulated many of the comments made by participants. Although some of his comments have subsequently been addressed by revisions in those chapters, the text of his comments is included in its entirety.

PART VIII

The multiaxial approach

The introduction of a multiaxial system of classification in *DSM-III* represented a major innovation. Multiaxial evaluation provides a vehicle for describing different aspects of a patient's condition in order to improve our understanding of the condition and thereby to improve its treatment. *DSM-III* contains five axes. Personality and specific developmental disorders are listed on axis II, whereas axis I includes the remaining clinical syndromes as well as conditions not attributable to a mental disorder that are the focus of attention or treatment. The third axis is for physical disorders or other conditions potentially relevant to the understanding or management of the patient. The first three axes are grouped together to provide the official *DSM-III* diagnosis. Two additional axes are included to provide supplemental information that might help treatment planning and outcome prediction. On axis IV, the severity of psychosocial stressors associated with the patient's condition is recorded, and axis V records the patient's highest level of adaptive functioning during the past year. These latter two axes are for use only in special clinical and research settings, a limitation founded on concern about confidentiality.

This Part VIII contains an appraisal of the value, usefulness, and acceptance of multiaxial evaluation, with the purpose of suggesting ways to strengthen it, if, indeed, there is a need to do so. Juan Mezzich and his associates provide a review of the current literature, ongoing research, and current thinking about multiaxial evaluation as a facilitator of clinical decision making and discuss the development of innovative multiaxial systems with promising clinical utility. An examination of recent literature and ongoing research relevant to the development of and need for a psychodynamic axis as an integral component of a multiaxial approach to diagnosis is the focus of the presentation by George Vaillant. Lyman Wynne addresses the importance of strengthening the multiaxial approach through focusing greater attention on social context and relational systems, with special emphasis on the health dysfunction of the family.

Richard Finn

29 *On the clinical utility of multiaxial diagnosis*

Experience and perspectives

JUAN E. MEZZICH, HORACIO FABREGA,
AND ADA C. MEZZICH

This chapter addresses the clinical value of the *DSM-III* multiaxial system, first by reviewing patterns underlying the development of multiaxial schemata, then by discussing recent research findings of both survey and clinical-appraisal types, and finally by formulating some proposals for improving multiaxial diagnosis in general and the *DSM-III* system in particular.

A REVIEW OF CONCEPTS AND PATTERNS

An examination of the roots of the word "diagnosis" reveals two meanings that have striking relevance for major themes in current diagnostic work. The first, "to distinguish," pertains to the process of thoughtfully sorting out categories in order to accurately identify the patient's disorder, and it is reflected in the current endeavor to develop more explicit and specific criteria for assignment of diagnostic labels. The second meaning, "to know thoroughly," applies to the concern for understanding the patient's condition as comprehensively and effectively as possible, and it is reflected most clearly in the multiaxial model. This model attempts to tease out the key elements of the patient's condition and evaluate them in isolation from one another.

Multiaxial thinking can be traced back to the Hippocratic concern for remaining close to the patient, which is therefore clinical, par excellence, in contraposition to a Platonic abstraction of the definition of disease. At the turn of the century, this controversy was enlivened by Hoche's (1912) argument for separating syndrome and cause versus Kraepelin's (1902) all-encompassing disease-entity model. In 1947, Essen-Möller and Wohlfahrt proposed the first formal multiaxial system, which involved separation between the type of mental reaction and etiology, as a suggested amendment to the Swedish classification of mental disorders.

Elaborating, in various ways, on Essen-Möller's dichotomy, a number of multiaxial systems have been developed in different regions of the world. A recent review of the literature revealed 15 published multiaxial systems, originating from Brazil (Leme Lopes, 1954; Rocha, 1977), France (Sadoun, Casadebaig, and Hatton, 1976), East Germany (Kreyssig, 1978), West Germany (Helmchen, 1975; von Cranach, 1977), Japan (Kato, 1977), Norway (Retterstøl and Dahl,

1983), Poland (Bilikiewicz, 1970), Sweden (Essen-Möller, 1961, 1971, 1973, 1982; Ottosson and Perris, 1973), the United Kingdom (Wing, 1970; Rutter, Shaffer, and Sturge, 1975b), and the United States (Strauss, 1975, American Psychiatric Association, 1980). These systems are outlined in Table 29.1.

Further documenting the international anchorage of the multiaxial model, 16 unpublished multiaxial systems, originating from Australia, Austria, Brazil, the People's Republic of China, Cuba, Denmark, Egypt, Nigeria, Pakistan, Peru, Poland, Spain, Taiwan, and Turkey, have been called to our attention.

The types of axes included in proposed multiaxial systems may provide an indication of the aspects of the patient's condition that are considered to be of high clinical value internationally. An examination of these patterns, based on the published (more formalized) multiaxial systems listed in Table 29.1, elucidates two broad and pervasive themes, namely, phenomenology and etiological or associated factors. However, there is considerable variance regarding specific axes. Psychiatric syndromes or symptoms have the highest frequency of inclusion (14 of the 15 systems). Other axes and their frequencies are as follows: cause specified by clinician (9 systems), personality disorders (7), physical disorders (6), intelligence level (5), duration and course of illness (4 each), psychosocial stressors (4), psychopathological severity/psychoticism (presence and degree of psychotic symptoms) (4), adaptive functioning (2), and speed of illness onset (2).

The kinds of axes listed speak of the diversity of the patient's condition. Such richness has to be balanced with the limited number of axes that can be included in a system that is to be manageable in regular clinical work. The number of axes most frequently composing the multiaxial systems presented in Table 29.1 was five (included in six systems), followed by four and three (in four systems each).

AN INTERNATIONAL CONSULTATION ON MULTIAXIAL DIAGNOSIS

In an attempt to explore the international experience with traditional and multiaxial systems and the views of a panel of expert diagnosticians on the most appropriate number and types of diagnostic axes, an international consultation on multiaxial diagnosis (ICMD) was conducted by mail during the first half of 1983 under the sponsorship of the World Psychiatric Association (Mezzich, Fabrega, and Mezzich, 1985). By July 1983, 164 experts, representing 50 countries and spanning the six World Health Organization (WHO) regions, had completed the study. These diagnosticians were distributed around the world as follows: 38 from the Americas, 55 from Europe, 14 from Africa, 12 from the eastern Mediterranean, 34 from Southeast Asia, and 11 from the western Pacific. Their mean theoretical orientation profile was 39% biological, 22% psychodynamic, 21% social/community, 11% behavioristic, and 8% "other." Their mean profile of professional activities included 44% clinical practice, 22% research, 21% teaching, and 12% administration. The average age distribution

Table 29.1. *A comparative synopsis of published multiaxial diagnostic systems*

System	Phenomenology	Etiological or associated factors	Time frame	Adaptive functioning	Other
Essen-Möller and Wohlfahrt (1947), Essen-Möller (1961, 1971)	I. Syndrome A. Specific syndrome B. Gross syndrome (psychosis; neurosis; transient mental decompensation; habitual abnormality, including personality disorder & mental retardation; unspecified mental disorder)	II. Etiology			
Leme Lopes (1954)	I. Syndrome	III. Etiological constellation			
Bilikiewicz (1970)	II. Pre-morbid personality III. Functional syndrome	I. Psychoorganic illness, process, or deficit			
Wing (1970)	II. Pre-morbid personality III. Psychiatric condition III. Mental subnormality (I.Q. also coded)	I. Cause (organic or psychological) IV. Additional physical illness or handicap			
Ottosson and Perris (1973), von Knorring et al. (1978)	I. Symptomatology	IV. Etiopathogenesis Somatogenic Histogenic Chemogenic Hereditary Psychogenic Sociogenic Characterological Multifactorial Cryptogenic	III. Course Episodic Periodic, same disorder Periodic, diff. disorder Chronic stable Chronic progressive		II. Severity Healthy Nonpsychotic Psychotic Occasionally psychotic

Table 29.1 (*cont.*)

System	Phenomenology	Etiological or associated factors	Time frame	Adaptive functioning	Other
Helmchen (1975)	I. Symptomatology	II. Etiology A. Disposition B. Precipitation C. Fixation	III. Time A. Onset age B. Onset speed C. Duration D. Course		IV. Intensity (of axes I and II) V. Certainty (of axes I, II, and III)
Rutter et al. (1975)	I. Psychiatric syndrome II. Specific delays in development III. Intellectual level	IV. Medical conditions V. Abnormal psychosocial situations			
Strauss (1975)	I. Symptoms	III. Associated factors A. Environmental stresses B. Physical illness C. Drug/alcohol abuse	II. Duration and course of symptoms A. Duration Long term Moderate duration Recent onset B. Course Remittent Fluctuating Continuous	IV. Personal relations (5-point scale) V. Work functioning (5-point scale)	
Sadoun et al. (1976)	I. Basic diagnostic reference; syndromes II. Intelligence level III. Associated disturbances	IV. Etiological factors			
Rocha (1977)	I. Symptoms II. Pathogenic levels	IV. Etiology			

von Cranach (1977)
- I. Symptomatology
- II. Acuity of episodes
- III. Personality (personality proper, intellectual level, age)
- IV. Etiology
  - A. Biological
  - B. Psychosocial
- V. Personality disorder

Kato (1977)
- I. Illness (medically evaluated)
- II. Caseness (culturally evaluated)
- III. Course of illness
  - Episodic
  - Intermittent
  - First episode
  - Chronic

Kreyssig (1978)
- I. Nosologic
- II. Syndromatological
- III. Somatic
- IV. Sociodynamic
- V. Psychodynamic

DSM-III, APA (1980)
- I. Clinical psychiatric syndrome (some categories subclassified according to duration, course, and severity)
- II. Personality disorder (adults) or specific developmental disorder (children)
- III. Physical disorder
- IV. Psychosocial stressors severity (7-point scale)
- V. Highest level of adaptive functioning in past year (7-point scale)

Retterstol & Dahl (1983)
- I. Clinical diagnosis
- II. Predisposing personality
- III. Current life stress/situation

Source: adapted from Mezzich (1984).

of their patients was 8% children, 17% adolescents, 62% adults, and 12% geriatrics.

The findings most relevant to the subject of this chapter are summarized next. Regarding the use of standard diagnostic systems, only a slightly smaller number of the participants used *DSM-III* (71%) than used *ICD-9* (77%). Thirty-four percent of the users rated *DSM-III* highly in terms of clinical usefulness, whereas only 23% rated *ICD-9* that way.

The most frequent recommendations for improvement of diagnostic systems offered by 121 of the participants included use and refinement of multiaxial diagnosis (30%), advances in the diagnostic evaluation process (26%), development of internationally useful diagnostic systems (22%), better descriptions of diagnostic categories (18%), and empirical evaluation of diagnostic systems (12%).

The use of some form of multiaxial diagnosis appeared to be widespread, as this was reported by 83% of all participants and ranged from 77% in Africa to 100% in the western Pacific. By far, the most frequently used specific multiaxial systems were *DSM-III* and close derivatives (58%), followed by the pentaxial system developed by Rutter and associates (1975b) for child psychiatry (10%).

The multiaxial approach was considered to be very useful by 68% of the respondents, somewhat useful by 30%, and not useful by 2%. The principal ways in which multiaxial systems were found useful were by providing a comprehensive evaluative formulation (37%), by facilitating treatment planning and management (28%), by allowing greater comparability of diagnoses (15%), by teasing out key diagnostic elements (12%), and by enhancing the usefulness of diagnosis for different purposes (12%).

The main difficulties reported in the use of multiaxial systems were unclear or problematic definitions (32%), cumbersome or time-consuming usage (28%), and clinician resistance (11%).

The number of axes most frequently considered to be feasible or manageable for use in regular clinical work was five (31%). Only 21% of the respondents considered it feasible to use six or more axes.

A list of 21 potential axes was presented to the participants for judging their value for four diagnostic purposes: (1) describing the clinical condition, (2) making treatment decisions, (3) predicting illness outcome, and (4) advancing theory development. Table 29.2 lists the axes rated as best, along with the percentages of respondents who rated them as somewhat important or very important, first across diagnostic purposes, and specifically (and particularly pertinent to this chapter) for making treatment decisions. There was, with few exceptions, considerable concordance in the rankings of the axes according to various diagnostic purposes.

In addition to noting the highest-rated axes, it is of interest to review the ratings obtained for alternative forms of axes IV and V of *DSM-III*. First, Table 29.3 shows the frequencies with which two aspects of psychosocial stress were rated as important by the ICMD participants. "Specific psychosocial stressors" was rated higher for each of the diagnostic purposes, obtaining an overall

Table 29.2. *Axes most frequently rated as important for various diagnostic purposes by ICMD participants*

Potential axes	Overall purposes (%)	For treatment decisions (%)
Psychiatric syndromes	95	98
Physical disorders	91	96
Course of illness	89	96
Personality disorders	87	89
Specific psychosocial stressors	85	87
Duration of illness	83	92
Speed of illness onset	78	79
Current adaptive functioning	77	86
Psychoticism	77	86
IQ/mental retardation	77	85
Specific development delays	77	80

Table 29.3. *Frequencies with which "specific psychosocial stressors" and "overall stressor severity" were rated as important by ICMD participants*

Axes	Diagnostic purposes (%)				Overall frequency (%)
	Clinical description	Treatment decision	Prediction of outcome	Theory development	
Specific psychosocial stressors	79	87	88	85	85
Overall stressor severity	67	78	83	70	75

importance frequency of 85%, as opposed to 75% for "overall stressor severity" (*DSM-III* axis IV). Table 29.4 shows the frequencies with which two facets of adaptive functioning were rated as important. "Current adaptive functioning" was rated higher regarding clinical description and treatment decisions, reflecting immediate utility, whereas "highest level of adaptive functioning in the past year" (*DMS-III* axis V) was rated higher regarding prediction of outcome and theory development, with the overall rating slightly favoring "current functioning." These findings are all the more remarkable because they indicate that the alternatives tended to be preferred to the official forms of these two *DSM-III* axes by diagnosticians who, on the whole, were quite impressed with *DSM-III*.

Some additional axes or combinations of axes were suggested by some of the panelists after they rated the standard list of 21 axes. The most frequent pro-

Table 29.4. *Frequencies with which "highest functioning in past year" and "current functioning" were reported as important by ICMD participants*

Axes	Diagnostic purposes (%)				Overall frequency (%)
	Clinical description	Treatment decision	Prediction of outcome	Theory development	
Highest functioning in past year	69	82	90	57	75
Current functioning	84	86	85	51	77

posals included (1) an additional axis on family structure and functioning, suggested by 13 participants, (2) the combination of course, duration, speed of onset, and age at onset of the illness, suggested by 11 participants, and (3) the combination of personality, specific developmental disorders, and IQ, suggested by 9 participants. Less frequent suggestions involved an additional axis on biological markers or vulnerability (7 proponents), the combination of type and overall severity of psychosocial stressors (7), and the combination of highest level of functioning in the past year and current functioning (5).

EMPIRICAL ASSESSMENTS OF THE MULTIAXIAL APPROACH

First, we present an overview of the literature on evaluation, with clinical cases, of the reliability and perceived usefulness of certain multiaxial systems, followed by a report concerning the ongoing experience at the University of Pittsburgh.

Studies by Rutter, Shaffer, and Shepherd (1975a), Mattison and associates (1979), Spitzer, Forman, and Nee (1979), and Mezzich and Mezzich (1979) on the comparative interrater reliabilities of multiaxial systems, conducted around the times of their introductions, have yielded similar results for their entire syndromic axes, as opposed to whole traditional uniaxial systems. However, multiaxial systems have tended to have greater comparative reliabilities when the evaluation has focused on specific syndromes or on particularly complex cases. In comparison with other axes, facets of adaptive functioning have tended to show high reliability, whereas those involving psychosocial stressors have been found to be low. It is likely that with additional diagnostic training and experience and with the use of structured or semistructured evaluation procedures, the interrater agreement among clinicians using systems such as *DSM-III* will increase.

Regarding perceived usefulness, a number of studies (Rutter et al., 1975a;

DIAGNOSTIC SUMMARY

I. Clinical psychiatric syndromes *(Instructions and codes on back of pages 6 and 7)*

Main Formulation:	Codes	Alternatives to be ruled out	Codes
1.			
2.			
3.			
4.			

II Personality and specific developmental disorders *(Instructions and codes on back of pages 6 and 7)*

Main Formulation:	Codes	Alternatives to be ruled out:	Codes
1.			
2.			

III. Physical Disorders *(Instructions on back of page 7)*

Main Formulation:	Codes	Alternatives to be ruled out:	Codes
1.			
2.			
3.			
4.			

IV. Psychosocial stressors *(Instructions on back of this page)*   Codes

A. Ranked list: 1.
                         2.
                         3.
                         4.

B. Overall stressor severity:	1 None	2 Minimal	3 Mild	4 Moderate	5 Severe	6 Extreme	7 Catastrophic	0 Unspecified

V. Highest level of adaptive functioning during the past year *(Instructions on back of this page)*

	1 Superior	2 Very Good	3 Good	4 Fair	5 Poor	6 Very Poor	7 Grossly Impaired	0 Unspecified

VI. Current functioning: *(Instructions on back of this page)*

		Superior	Adequate	Slightly Impaired	Moderately Impaired	Markedly Impaired	Unspecified
	A. Occupational	1	2	3	4	5	0
	B. With family	1	2	3	4	5	0
	C. With other indiv. & groups	1	2	3	4	5	0

Figure 29.1. IEF diagnostic summary.

Cantwell et al., 1979; Spitzer and Forman, 1979; Mezzich, 1980) have found that multiaxial systems have generated better impressions than traditional systems among clinicians appraising clinical cases.

Since 1980, *DSM-III* has been systematically used at the Western Psychiatric Institute and Clinic (WPIC) of the University of Pittsburgh School of Medicine. WPIC is a large, comprehensive institution that serves as both a community mental health center and a regional referral facility. It handles approximately 1,900 inpatient admissions and 100,000 outpatient visits per year, providing specialized child, adolescent, adult, and geriatric programs for a psychiatric population presenting a wide variety of forms and levels of psychopathology.

Experience with *DSM-III* at WPIC has involved the use of a special format for multiaxial formulation (Mezzich, Coffman, and Goodpastor, 1982) (Figure 29.1) that is part of the Initial Evaluation Form (IEF) (Mezzich et al., 1981, 1983), a semistructured psychiatric evaluation procedure used with all patients seen at the WPIC.

For each of the three typological axes of *DSM-III*, the format provides specific spaces for a main formulation of diagnostic terms and codes, as well as for alternatives to be ruled out. Several slots are provided in each axis for listing disorders in order of priority for evaluation and care. The coding of each standard diagnostic category includes fields for a five-digit code plus an optional

Table 29.5. *Frequencies with which mental-retardation patients (N = 190) had concomitant diagnoses on axes I and II*

	N	%
Axis I concomitant diagnoses	138	73
Axis II positive diagnoses	15	8

field and code that were developed to identify the category as a "principal" and/or a "provisional" diagnosis.

For axis IV, slots are provided first for specifying and ranking up to four psychosocial stressors in decreasing order of importance. These are then coded using a set of categories of stress extended from those mentioned in *DSM-III*, on the basis of two years of experience with the IEF. Identification of specific stressors is a prerequisite to using the scale of matching stressors for rating overall stressor severity. To facilitate the recording (circling) and visual inspection of this rating, the terms and codes for all levels of the scale are arranged on one line in the format.

Similarly, for axis V, all levels of functioning are specified and arranged on one line to facilitate their circling.

Current functioning, a sixth axis used with the IEF, is separately rated for occupational functioning, functioning with family, and functioning with other individuals and groups.

The manual for the IEF and the back of the IEF's diagnostic page contain detailed instructions for rating axes IV, V, and VI, which are in line with, but more specific than, those included in *DSM-III*.

A large data base is being developed to include all new patients seen at WPIC and evaluated with the aforementioned format and procedure. Two examples of the use of this data base, pertinent to the appraisal and revision of *DSM-III*, are presented next.

Of the 5,573 new patients presenting for care at WPIC from August 1, 1980, through November 30, 1982, 190 received a diagnosis of mental retardation, which is an axis I diagnosis in *DSM-III*. As Table 29.5 shows, 73% of these mentally retarded patients received one or more concomitant diagnoses on axis I, whereas only 8% of them had a positive diagnosis in axis II. Aside from conceptual considerations, these differential overlap findings suggest that mental retardation may more appropriately be housed on axis II.

An empirical study (Mezzich et al., 1984), directly relevant to assessment of clinical utility, was used to assess the comparative values of the five axes of *DSM-III* and a sixth axis on current adaptive functioning to predict admission decisions. This study was based on all 745 patients who presented during a six-month period at the Diagnostic and Evaluation Center, a 24-hour walk-in

Table 29.6. *Significant correlations between diagnostic categories and axes and inpatient disposition*

Axis	Diagnostic variables	r
I	Clinical psychiatric syndromes	
	Organic mental disorders	0.14
	Psychotic disorders not elsewhere classified	0.15
	Anxiety disorders	−0.12
	Adjustment disorders	−0.20
	Non-mental-disorder conditions	−0.13
	All psychotic disorders	0.18
II	Personality disorders present	−0.13
III	Physical disorders present	0.06
IV	Overall psychosocial stressor severity	0.12
V	Highest level of adaptive functioning in past year	0.27
VI	Current adaptive functioning	0.45

clinic, and the main entry point for inpatient and outpatient care at WPIC. As shown in Table 29.6, a diagnosis of psychotic disorder was found to be significantly associated with hospitalization, whereas anxiety disorders, adjustment disorders, personality disorders, and non-mental-disorder conditions were associated with outpatient referral. However, the strongest correlations with hospitalization were observed for current adaptive functioning (axis VI) and, to a lesser extent, for highest level of adaptive functioning in the past year (axis V).

Other clinical-utility studies being planned with the WPIC patient data bases will assess the relationships among diagnostic axes, on one hand, and the length of hospitalization and treatment-modality choice, on the other.

A PROPOSAL FOR IMPROVING THE USEFULNESS OF A MULTIAXIAL FORMULATION

On the basis of the comparative and evaluative analyses presented in preceding sections of this chapter, it appears that the following prospective axes have high standing among experts, as well as promise of usefulness:

1. Psychiatric syndromes
2. Personality disorders
3. Physical disorders
4. Course of illness (episodicity, duration, etc.)
5. Specific psychosocial stressors
6. Current adaptive functioning
7. Psychopathological severity/psychoticism
8. Specific developmental disorders

9.   IQ/mental retardation
10.   Etiology specified by clinician

Views and findings outlined earlier in this chapter suggest that the number of axes feasible for regular clinical work may be around five. This would require either very seriously considered selection decisions or innovative arrangements for development of improved multiaxial systems. As one option, a small group of axes could be selected to serve as a core or standard diagnostic system, and remaining axes could be considered as special, for use with particular populations or situations.

Alternatively, integrative and economizing arrangements could be considered. For example, personality disorders, specific developmental disorders, and mental retardation (numbers 2, 8, and 9, respectively, in the preceding list) could be housed in one axis involving long-standing or stable behavioral conditions.

An even more innovative and potentially powerful arrangement would make use of extended codes to add axes such as course of illness, psychopathological severity, and etiological formulation (numbers 4, 7, and 10, respectively) to the characterization of another axis such as psychiatric syndromes (number 1). The latter arrangement, in addition to its economizing intention, would also respond to the observation that some axes, such as course of illness and etiology, appear to have clear-cut meaning when referring to a specific syndrome (say a depressive condition). This would seem to be especially true if the patient presents more than one syndrome (which is the case for at least 25% of the patients presenting for care at WPIC).

Making use of these integrative arrangements, a new multiaxial system is proposed and delineated in Table 29.7, side by side with the current axes of *DSM-III*, in order to show some lines for possible revision. The suggested revisions for axes II, IV, and V may be easier to implement than those for axis I.

In addition to the core or standard set of axes, additional axes may be considered for special populations or for complex situations (e.g., depression, chronic pain, or violent delinquent adolescents, all of which have been subjects of recent multiaxial proposals). The option of additional axes could also be the way to accommodate certain clinical aspects of far-reaching importance, such as family concerns and psychodynamic factors. Alternatively, the possibility could be explored of integrating these aspects into more established axes. For example, psychodynamic defenses could be included in a fuller characterization of personality patterns, and special family situations could be housed in a revised axis IV.

In an attempt to further appraise the implications and potential value of the proposed revisions, one may consider some of the administrative challenges facing psychiatry today. For example, the American Psychiatric Association and some insurance organizations have proposed a coding system for claims reporting that would contain six categories that are largely characterized by levels of psychopathological disturbance and social dysfunction. The use of such a cod-

Table 29.7. *On revising the DSM-III multiaxial system*

Axis	Current *DSM-III*	Proposed revision
I	Psychiatric syndromes	Psychiatric syndromes, qualified by severity/psychoticism, course, and etiology (expanded code)
II	Personality & specific developmental disorders	Stable behavioral handicaps (personality, specific developmental disorders, mental retardation)
III	Physical disorders	Physical disorders (better instructions)
IV	Overall severity of psychosocial stressors	Specific psychosocial stressors/ situations (including lack of supports)
V	Highest level of adaptive functioning in past year	Current adaptive functioning

ing system could be greatly facilitated by a revised axis I, which would consider psychopathological severity, and, especially, by a revised axis V, which would assess *current* impairment in adaptive functioning.

Another illustrative challenge, exemplified by the development of the so-called diagnostic-related groups, is the concern for predicting the length and cost of hospitalization. Although specific psychiatric syndromes seem to be poor predictors in this regard, more promising variables may include the degree of impairment in adaptive functioning (a revised axis V) and lack of support systems (which could be housed as an abnormal psychosocial situation within a revised axis IV).

ADDITIONAL PERSPECTIVES

Complementing the development of innovative multiaxial systems with promising clinical utility, definitive efforts are needed to evaluate in a rigorous way the reliability and various aspects of the validity of such proposals. The latter should include assessment of the perceived suitability and usefulness of the proposed axes among experienced clinicians and their impact on treatment decisions such as inpatient versus outpatient disposition, formulation of problem lists, and use of specific treatments. Critical evaluations should also address the ability of axes, individually and in combination, to predict illness course and outcome.

Another important perspective for future work on multiaxial systems involves international considerations. This is important because of the insights that are likely to continue to be derived from an acquaintance with and a study of proposals generated in various parts of the world, and also because of the desirability of greater compatibility between future national systems, such as *DSM-IV,* and the next revision of the *International Classification of Diseases.*

REFERENCES

American Psychiatric Association: Diagnostic and Statistical Manual of Mental Disorders, third edition. Washington, DC, APA, 1980

Bilikiewicz T: Die Atioepigenese in der psychiatrischen Forschung. Nova Acta Leopoldina, Neue Folge, vol 35, no 193, 1970

Cantwell DP, Mattison R, Russell AT, et al: A comparison of DSM-II and DSM-III in the diagnosis of childhood psychiatric disorders, IV: difficulties in use, global comparison and conclusions. Arch Gen Psychiatry 36:1227–1228, 1979

Essen-Möller E: On classification of mental disorders. Acta Psychiatr Scand 37:119–126, 1961

Suggestions for further improvement of the international classification of mental disorders. Psychol Med 1:308–311, 1971

Standard lists for three-fold classification of mental disorders. ACTA Psychiatr Scand 49:198–212, 1973

Gutenberg and the ICD-9 of mental disorders. Br J Psychiatry 140:529–531, 1982

Essen-Möller E, Wohlfahrt S: Suggestions for the amendment of the official Swedish classification of mental disorders. Acta Psychiatr Scand [Suppl] 47:551–555, 1947

Helmchen H: Schizophrenia: diagnostic concepts in the ICD-8, in Studies in Schizophrenia. Edited by Lader MH. Br J Psychiatry Special Publication No 10, 1975, pp 10–18

Hoche A: Die Bedeutung der Symptomenkomplexe in der Psychiatrie. Z Gesamte Neurol Psychiatrie 12:540–551, 1912

Kato M: Multiaxial diagnosis in adult psychiatry. Paper presented at the Symposium on Multiaxial Diagnosis, VI World Congress of Psychiatry, Honolulu, Hawaii, 1977

Kraepelin E: Clinical Psychiatry. New York, Macmillan, 1902

Kreyssig M: Soziodynamische Aspekte im Rahmen der mehrdimensionalen Diagnostik psychischer Erkrankungen. Psychiatr Neurol Med Psychol (Leipz) 30:577–585, 1978

Leme Lopes J: As dimensões do diagnóstico psiquiátrico. Rio de Janeiro, Agir, 1954

Mattison R, Cantwell DP, Russell AT, et al: A comparison of DSM-II and DSM-III in the diagnosis of childhood psychiatric disorders, II: interrater agreement. Arch Gen Psychiatry 36:1217–1222, 1979

Mezzich AC, Mezzich JE: Perceived suitability and usefulness of DSM-III vs DSM-II in child psychopathology. J Am Acad Child Psychiatry 24:281–285, 1985

Mezzich AC, Mezzich JE, Coffman GA: Reliability of DSM-III vs DSM-II in child psychopathology. J Am Acad Child Psychiatry 24:273–280, 1985

Mezzich JE: Multiaxial diagnostic systems in psychiatry, in Comprehensive Textbook of Psychiatry, fourth edition. Edited by Kaplan HI, Sadock BJ. Baltimore, Williams & Wilkins, 1984

Mezzich JE, Coffman GA, Goodpastor SM: A format for DSM-III diagnostic formulation: experience with 1,111 consecutive patients. Am J Psychiatry 139:591–596, 1982

Mezzich JE, Dow JT, Rich CL, et al: Developing an efficient clinical information system for a comprehensive psychiatric institute, II: initial evaluation form. Behav Res Methods Inst 13:464–478, 1981

Mezzich JE, Evanczuk KJ, Mathias RJ, et al: Admission decisions and multiaxial diagnosis. Arch Gen Psychiatry 41:1001–1004, 1984

Mezzich JE, Fabrega H, Mezzich AC: An international consultation on multiaxial diagnosis, in Psychiatry – The State of the Art. Edited by Pichot P, Berner P, Wolfe R, et al. New York, Plenum, 1985

Mezzich JE, Slayton RI, Dow JT, et al: A semi-structured psychiatric evaluation procedure. Paper presented at the Symposium on New Developments in Systematic Clinical Evaluation, 136th annual meeting of the American Psychiatric Association, New York, May 1–6, 1983

Ottosson JO, Perris C: Multidimensional classification of mental disorders. Psychol Med 3:238–243, 1973

Retterstøl N, Dahl AA: Scandinavian perspectives on DSM-III, in International Perspectives on DSM-III. Edited by Skodol A, Spitzer RL. Washington, DC, American Psychiatric Press, 1983

Rocha Z: Disturbios do comportamento na clinica diaria (abordagem diagnostica pluridimensional). Neurobiologia (Recife, Brazil) 40:269–296, 1977

Rutter M, Shaffer D, Shepherd M: A Multiaxial Classification of Child Psychiatric Disorders. Geneva, World Health Organization, 1975a

Rutter M, Shaffer D, Sturge C: A Guide to a Multiaxial Classification Scheme for Psychiatric Disorders in Childhood and Adolescence. London, Institute of Psychiatry, 1975b

Sadoun R, Casadebaig F, Hatton F: Studies of the infant population placed in charge of the A. Binet Mental Health Center in 1970 and 1971. Social Psychiatry (Berlin) 11:179–205, 1976

Spitzer RL, Forman JBW, Nee J: DSM-III field trials, I: initial interrater diagnostic reliability. Am J Psychiatry 136:815–817, 1979

Spitzer RL, Forman JBW: DSM-III field trials, II: initial experience with the multiaxial system. Am J Psychiatry 136:818–820, 1979

Strauss JS: A comprehensive approach to psychiatric diagnosis. Am J Psychiatry 132:1193–1197, 1975

von Cranach M: Categorical vs multiaxial classification. Paper presented at the VI Symposium on Multiaxial Diagnosis, VI World Congress of Psychiatry, Honolulu, Hawaii, 1977

von Knorring L, Perris C, Jacobsson L: Multiaspects classification of mental disorders: experiences with clinical routine work and preliminary studies of inter-rater reliability. Acta Psychiatr Scand 58:401–412, 1978

Wing L: Observations on the psychiatric section of the International Classification of Diseases and the British Glossary of Mental Disorders. Psychol Med 1:79–85, 1970

30 An empirically derived hierarchy of adaptive mechanisms and its usefulness as a potential diagnostic axis

GEORGE E. VAILLANT

In no area of psychiatry is the need for a synthesis of frames of reference greater than in the field of personality disorders. In this field there are two views especially that need integration so that a given individual can be viewed along different axes. First, there is the descriptive and objective classification system of axis II of *DSM-III*. Second, there is the dynamic, intrapsychic, and far more subjective classification system of psychoanalysis, with its commitment to ego mechanisms of defense. Should defense mechanisms be part of the *DSM-III?* I think that the answer is yes.

We know all too little about how, within their own minds, individuals mold and rearrange external reality that they cannot bear. The closest that we have come to understanding this process is by studying those intrapsychic processes encompassed by the psychoanalytic metaphor – ego mechanisms of defense (Freud, 1937; Meissner, 1980). Others have called the process repression (Freud, 1906), denial (Hackett, Cassem, and Wishmie, 1968) or (unconscious) coping mechanisms (Haan, 1963). Such innate adaptive processes refer to largely unconscious regulatory mechanisms that allow individuals to reduce cognitive dissonance and to minimize sudden changes in internal and external environments by altering how these events are perceived.

There is accumulating evidence that individual differences in defense or coping styles make a major contribution to individual differences in responses to stressful environmental stimuli (Hackett, Cassem, and Wishmie, 1968; Cochlo, Hamburg, and Adams, 1974; Kobasa, 1979; Vaillant, 1979). However, as is the case with both immune mechanisms and homeostasis, deployment of ego mechanisms of defense is based largely on processes outside of voluntary control. Defense mechanisms are as distinct from the *conscious* coping strategies outlined by Lazarus (1966) or from the voluntary use of social supports advocated by Caplan and Killela (1976) as the release of antibodies is distinct from the taking of antibiotics (i.e., a coping strategy) or as the clotting of blood is distinct from seeking a paramedic with a tourniquet (i.e., a social support).

An earlier form of this chapter appeared in ACTA Psychiatrica Scandinavica (Supp. 319) 71:171–180, 1985. Copyright 1985 Munksgaard International Publishers Ltd., Copenhagen, Denmark.

Ego mechanisms of defense imply integrated and synthetic psychological processes. Their use usually alters the individual's perception of both internal and external reality. Such an alteration often compromises other facets of cognition. Awareness of instinctual "wishes" is usually diminished, and alternative – sometimes antithetical – wishes may be passionately adhered to.

Some inferred purposes of ego mechanisms of defense are as follows:

1. to keep affects within bearable limits during sudden alterations in one's emotional life,
2. to restore psychological homeostasis by postponing or deflecting sudden increases in biological drives,
3. to attain a time out to master sudden changes in self-image that cannot be immediately integrated,
4. to manage conflicts with important people, living or dead, from whom one cannot bear to take leave,
5. to resolve cognitive dissonance,
6. to adapt to sudden, unanticipated changes in external reality.

If defenses are to be included in a revised version of *DSM-III*, several steps are necessary. First, a consensually valid, mutually exclusive set of definitions must be provided. In the past, there have been many different names for defense mechanisms, but little effort to provide consistent definitions. This was one reason that defense mechanisms were excluded from *DSM-III*. However, parallel with publication of *DSM-III*, a hierarchy of defenses and definitions have been accepted by leading textbooks of psychiatry (Kolb, 1977; Kaplan and Sadock, 1981). Second, it must be demonstrated that defenses can be identified reliably and that such identification provides prospective validity. Only in the last 20 years have investigators, on the basis of empirical, usually longitudinal, research (Weinstock, 1967; Semrad, Grinspoon, and Feinberg, 1973; Haan, 1977; Vaillant, 1976), overcome problems of rater reliability and arranged defense mechanisms along an axis of theoretical psychopathology.

This chapter has two purposes. First, I wish to underscore the existing empirical data that support the validity and reliability of defense mechanisms in diagnosis. Second, I wish to review our published work in detail in the hope that further empirical studies can build on its strengths and rectify its limitations.

Table 30.1 shows the validation for Meissner's (1980) hierarchy of defense mechanisms in previous studies and summarizes the data to be presented later. Each study employed quite different global mental health measures. Initially, Haan's work (1963, 1969) provided empirical support for her hierarchy by showing that for members of the Berkeley Growth Studies, "coping" mechanisms (those in parentheses in Table 30.1 under "mature defenses") were significantly correlated with upward social mobility, with adult increases in IQ, and with three other measures of positive midlife outcomes. In her work, "defense" mechanisms (those listed in parentheses under the "neurotic" and "immature" headings) were negatively correlated with adaptive outcomes.

To quantify adaptive outcomes in a sample of 95 college men selected for

Table 30.1. *Correlations of adaptive styles with global measures of mental health in prior studies*

Term from *Comprehensive Textbook of Psychiatry*[a]	Haan (1963)[a]	Adult Adjustment Scale (Vaillant, 1976)[a]	Global Assessment Scale (Battista, 1981)	HSRS (present study)
I. Mature defenses				
Anticipation (objectivity)[b]	Coping	.34	.50	.40
Suppression (suppression, concentration)	Coping	.57	.25	.55
Altruism	Coping	.10	.19	.46
Sublimation (substitution, sublimation)	Coping	.04	.26	.45
Humor (playfulness)	Coping	–	–	.33
Asceticism	–	–	–	–
II. Neurotic (intermediate) defenses				
Intellectualization (isolation)	Defending	−.14	.29	.06
Repression (repression)	Defending	.04	.04	.04
Reaction formation (reaction formation)	Defending	−.13	–	.00
Displacement (displacement)	Defending	−.16	−.16	.12
Externalization, inhibition, sexualization, somatization, controlling, rationalization	–	–	–	–
III. Immature defenses				
Passive-aggression or masochism (repression)	Defending	−.19	.07	−.47
Hypochondriasis	–	−.23	−.04	−.52
Acting out	–	−.37	−.22	−.27
Dissociation (denial)	Defending	−.24	−.40	−.39
Projection (projection)	Defending	−.41	−.22	−.46
Schizoid fantasy	–	−.28	−.60	−.55
Blocking, introjection, regression	–	–	–	–

Note: A dash indicates that a specific term was not rated.
[a]Psychotic or "narcissistic" defense (i.e., mechanisms associated with frank psychosis) have been excluded [e.g., denial of external reality, delusional thinking, distortion (hallucinations)].
[b]Terms in parentheses are Haan's terms for equivalent mental processes.

mental health, Vaillant (1976) used a 32-item scale reflecting objective success in working and loving. In their work, both Haan and Vaillant capitalized on the fact that outcome and defensive style can be relatively reliably determined by comparison of behavioral outcomes in longitudinally studied samples.

Battista (1982) used the Global Assessment Scale (GAS) (Endicott et al., 1976) as an outcome measure and a cross-sectional design in assessing 78 psychiatric inpatients. He estimated defense style by means of an ego-function inventory that rated each of 30 defenses on a 5-point Likert-type scale.

In another study not summarized in Table 30.1, Bond and associates (1983) correlated a self-administered questionnaire on self-perception of defensive style to 209 patients and nonpatients. Factor analysis revealed four clusters of defenses that Bond correlated with an independent questionnaire measure of ego adaptation and with Loevinger's (1976) sentence-completion test of ego maturity. Projection, passive aggression, dissociation, and acting out all loaded highly together in the cluster that correlated most negatively with their estimates of ego strength and ego maturity (schizoid fantasy and hypochondriasis were not sought). Humor, suppression, and sublimation all loaded highly together in the cluster that correlated most positively with estimates of ego strength and ego maturity (altruism and anticipation were not sought).

PRESENT STUDY

My own most recent strategy was to take a sample of relatively unselected junior-high-school boys (Glueck and Glueck, 1950) and follow them for 35 years, and in that way behaviorally identify from a community sample a subsample who appeared to suffer personality disorders. Then the entire sample of men were assessed by *independent* sets of raters along three contrasting diagnostic axes. The first axis was each man's global psychiatric impairment as measured by the Health-Sickness Rating Scale (HSRS) of Luborsky (1962). The second axis was whichever *DSM-III* axis II diagnosis, if any, the man met. The third axis was the maturity and nature of each man's predominant defense mechanism, as first described by Freud (1937) and redefined and ordered by Vaillant (1971) and Meissner (1980).

The sample consisted of 392 inner-city boys chosen by the Gluecks as control subjects in their prospective study of juvenile delinquents. Both method and sample have been extensively described elsewhere (Vaillant and Milofsky, 1980; Vaillant and Vaillant, 1981). Between 1940 and 1945, these men were selected in junior high school as nondelinquent. They were matched with severely delinquent boys in terms of residence in high-crime neighborhoods, ethnicity, and intelligence. At that time, these boys and their families were studied intensively.

The men in the sample were reinterviewed at ages 25 (circa 1955), 32 (circa 1962), and 47 (circa 1977). Because the men were studied first as controls for a study of delinquency (Glueck and Glueck, 1968) and then for a study of alcoholism (Vaillant, 1983), data relevant to personality disorder were systematically gathered.

Early-life ratings

Judgments regarding childhood were based on interviews with the boy, his parents, and his teacher and on a search of social service records. Judges were blind to all postadolescence information. Among hundreds of variables examined, the following scales seemed most relevant:

1. *Multiproblem family membership.* This judgment required the presence of 10 or more items on a 25-concrete-item scale of childhood weaknesses (Vaillant and Milofsky, 1980) that encompassed the Gluecks' more subjectively defined delinquency-prediction scale (Glueck and Glueck, 1950). Sample items were "contact with nine or more social agencies" and "raised for more than six months apart from *both* parents."
2. *Childhood emotional problems.* This judgment meant that the boy was very shy or dissocial or that he manifested tics, phobias, bed wetting beyond age 8, severe feeding problems, or other noted problems.
3. *Emotional maturity.* Psychiatrist's subjective impression in 1940–5 (Vaillant, Bond, and Vaillant, 1986).
4. *Restlessness.* Teachers' and parents' subjective impressions in 1940–5 (Vaillant et al., 1986).
5. *Social class of parents.* Based on the Hollingshead and Redlich 5-point scale (1959).
6. *IQ.* On entrance to the study, each core-city child was given the Wechsler–Bellevue Intelligence Test.

Adulthood ratings

Judges were kept blind to all information collected before subjects reached age 30 and rated the men primarily on the basis of the recent semi-structured two-hour interview. Judgments regarding HSRS, axis II diagnosis, and defensive maturity were each made by one or two independent raters who did not access the other two variables.

1. *Maturity of defenses.* This nine-point scale was based on the hierarchy outlined by Vaillant (1971) and by Meissner (1980). The assessment was based on a two-hour interview at age 47. To quantify clinical impressions, the following procedure was observed: 1–5 points were assigned for the relative tendency to employ mature defenses (sublimation, suppression, anticipation, altruism, and humor), 1–5 points for the relative tendency to deploy neurotic (intermediate) defenses (displacement, repression, isolation, and reaction formation), and 1–5 points for the relative tendency to deploy immature defenses (projection, schizoid fantasy, masochism, acting out, hypochondriasis, and neurotic denial/dissociation). It was required, however, that the three ratings always sum to 8. This meant that a nine-point range with normal distribution was obtained by subtracting the 1–5 rating for immature defenses from the 1–5 rating for mature defenses (e.g., the score for men who used mostly mature defenses was 4, and that for mostly immature defenses was −4). Interrater reliability for this scale was $r = .84$. Ratings for individual defenses were less satisfactory, but agree-

Table 30.2. *Association of maturity of defenses with psychosocial outcome (percentage)*

Outcome variable	Maturity of defenses		
	Immature (N = 73)	Neurotic (intermediate) (N = 164)	Mature (N = 70)
HSRS (85–100) (i.e., healthy)	1	14	71
Generative (Erikson stage VII)	4	24	70
Income $20,000+	7	24	43
Good object relationships	5	21	38
HSRS (0–65) (i.e., impaired)	54	9	0
Sociopath	21	2	3
4+ years unemployed	44	10	4
Social class V	21	4	1
Never married	22	7	0

ment as to whether a given defense was present or absent was 75% or higher. In this chapter, a defense is considered to have been present only if one rater called it major and the other rater called it definitely present or major.

2. DSM-III *axis II diagnosis. DSM-III* criteria were observed. Each subject could receive 0, 1, or 2 diagnoses. Rater reliability is discussed elsewhere (Drake and Vaillant, 1985).

3. *HSRS.* This scale is described in detail elsewhere (Luborsky, 1962). The raters used 34 case illustrations as guides to place each subject on a 100-point continuum that ranged from total institutional dependence (rating of 0–25) to no psychological dysfunctions and multiple manifestations of positive mental health (rating of 90–100). Interrater reliability for this scale was r = .89.

The rater who judged HSRS also rated the men on Robin's (1966) 19-item scale of sociopathy and on the five-point scale of Hollingshead and Redlich (1959) for social class.

Results

Among the 456 boys selected by the Gluecks 35 years previously, we were able to obtain separately rated measures of maturity of defenses and *DSM-III* axis II personality diagnoses and measures of global mental health for 307 individuals. Major sources of attrition were death, incomplete interviews, and breach of blindness for one clinical judge. No subject was completely lost, and only four men were unlocated within the last five years.

Table 30.2 documents that the 70 men employing the theoretically most mature defenses were also those who were psychosocially the healthiest. In contrast, 39 of the men with severe psychological impairment – those men whose

Table 30.3. *Childhood predictors of defensive maturity (percentage)*

Childhood variable	Maturity of defenses		
	Immature (N = 73)	Neurotic (intermediate) (N = 164)	Mature (N = 70)
Social class V	26	24	32
Multiproblem family membership	14	10	12
Emotional problems	36	29	26
<10 grades of school	42	26	30
Emotional maturity	20	31	43
Very restless	38	27	25
IQ > 100	22	36	39

HSRS global mental-health scores were under 66 – had defenses that fell in the bottom quartile for maturity. Most of their identified defenses were drawn from the immature category, and few, if any, from the neurotic and mature end of the theoretical hierarchy outlined in Table 30.1.

Virtually none of the men with immature defenses and 70% of the men with mature defenses had achieved Erikson's adult life tasks of intimacy and generativity (Vaillant and Milofsky, 1980). Men with mature defenses were 6 times more likely to be making above-average incomes and were 7 times more likely than men who used immature defenses to have warm relationships with a wide variety of people. Men with immature defenses were 11 times more likely to have been unemployed for four or more years, and they accounted for 75% of the men who could be classed as sociopaths.

It is tempting to view mature defenses as a by-product of middle-class socialization or, at the very least, of loving parents. However, Table 30.3 suggests that there was not a strong association between the maturity of defenses and the quality of the men's childhoods. Because all of the men had been raised in inner-city neighborhoods and because *parental* social class did not affect defensive style, the association of low *adult* social class with immature defense deployment seemed a result, not a cause, of immaturity of defensive style.

There was no difference in terms of maturity of defenses between men who came from multiproblem families and those who did not. Low IQ, a history of emotional problems in childhood, and limited education were only weakly correlated with immaturity of defenses.

As Table 30.4 suggests, projection, fantasy, and hypochondriasis were particularly common in the most psychologically impaired; passive-aggression and dissociation or neurotic denial were seen in those men who were severely impaired and in those who were somewhat less impaired. Conversely, the mature defenses of altruism and suppression were rarely seen in men with psychosocial impairment from emotional reasons.

Table 30.4. *Association of individual defenses with global mental health, HSRS*
(percentage)

	Impaired		Healthy	
Major defense	0–65 (N = 55)	66–70 (N = 35)	71–84 (N = 143)	85–99 (N = 74)
Projection	30	17	7	0
Fantasy	19	11	1	0
Hypochondriasis	21	11	1	0
Passive-aggression	32	36	15	1
Dissociation	55	36	15	1
Altruism	0	3	6	35
Suppression	2	14	27	59

Table 30.5. *Association of individual defenses with axis II personality disorders*
(percentage)

N	Disorder	Pro-jection	Fan-tasy	Passive-aggress.	Acting out	Dissoc.	Hypo-chondr.	Predom. Immature defenses
233	None	7	2	12	12	7	2	10
74	Personality disorder	27	15	34	27	32	17	66
12	Avoidant	17	8	25	17	25	17	58
18	Schizoid	17	33	11	6	17	17	39
23	Dependent	26	17	30	30	56	26	78
18	Narcissistic	39	17	33	61	83	11	78
8	Antisocial	38	0	25	75	63	0	75
6	Paranoid	100	17	33	75	33	33	100
14	Passive-aggressive	14	7	64	21	43	0	71

What about adaptive style and axis II personality disorders? As Table 30.5
indicates, of the 307 individuals with complete data sets, 232 received no axis
II diagnosis. The 10% of men without an axis II diagnosis but with immature
defenses were virtually all men manifesting severe axis I disorders. An individual was considered to use a given defense if one blind rater scored it "major"
and the other blind rater called it "present" or "major." Immature defenses
were seen three to eight times as frequently among those 74 men with axis II
disorders as among those without. The 12 avoidant personalities, while using

generally immature defenses, did not appear to "specialize" in any defense. As might be expected, the 18 schizoid subjects were more likely to use fantasy, the 14 passive-aggressive personalities turned anger against themselves, and the 6 paranoid personalities used projection. The men described as dependent tended to use dissociation or neurotic denial. It is interesting that in terms of defense style, narcissistic personalities could not be distinguished from antisocial characters. Both the narcissistic and antisocial characters seemed to use projection, acting out, and dissociation. However, narcissistic personalities did receive far lower scores on the Robins scale of deviant behaviors than did those who met axis II criteria for antisocial personalities.

Success at human relationships, social class, percentage of life spent employed, and meeting the criteria for *DSM-III* axis II personality disorders represent external behaviors. In contrast, defense mechanisms reflect intrapsychic ways of processing conflicts and sudden changes in reality. As such, then, axis II and the dimension of defensive maturity are quite separate, if highly correlated, axes. However, much further work is needed to remove assessment of ego defenses from the "halo effects" produced by external behavior. It remains to be shown that maturity of defenses predicts, rather than is merely associated with, psychological health.

Various techniques have been used to validate the concept of defenses. The relatively successful techniques (e.g., Haan, 1963; Vaillant, 1971) have employed taking the long view and strategies for qualitative research (Runyan, 1982) as opposed to quantitative research. In such studies, defenses can be rated on the basis of redundancy and by "triangulation" rather than by self-assessment or projective techniques. By "triangulation," I mean combining subjective report (e.g., autobiography), overt behavior (e.g., biography), and creative product (e.g., symptom) to identify distortions of inner and outer reality by ego mechanisms. In assessing defenses, projective techniques have not lived up to their promise. However, I have administered Bond and associates' (1983) self-assessment questionnaire of defensive styles to my subjects and thereby replicated the assessment of defensive style based on the clinical interview (Vaillant et al., 1986).

A second difficulty in assessing defenses is that they are metaphors. Ego defenses are a shorthand way of describing cognitive styles. Like creativity and facial recognition, defense mechanisms reflect concepts that do not easily yield to being broken into component parts, but are nevertheless valid aspects of personality that can be appreciated better from a distance rather than by too close inspection. Like facial recognition, defenses have not yielded to rating scales, to close experimental analysis, or to precise description. Like assessment of beauty or creativity, what description of defensive style loses in reliability, it gains in validity.

SUMMARY

Assessment of predominant ego defenses – an essentially psychoanalytic view of intrapsychic processes – corresponded well with independent assessment of *DSM-III* axis II personality disorders based on a descriptive view and an assessment of external behaviors. I believe that such concordance means that psychiatrists should learn to value defensive style in clinical assessment more than they do and that assessment of defensive style should be added as axis VI to *DSM-IV*.

One reason why the concept of unconscious adaptive styles is such an important one – in spite of the difficulty that we may have in studying them objectively – is that such mechanisms help to explain the phenomena of recovery from mental illness and of the so-called invulnerable child. Like the immune system, the human ego continues to provide human beings with better therapy than the best trained physician or the most up-to-date pharmacy.

A second important reason for including defensive style in diagnosis is to make therapeutic management more rational. A major difficulty in the treatment of psychiatric patients is that their behavior appears irrational. Systematic identification of a patient's defensive style provides professionals a logical means of understanding and of circumventing what seems most unreasonable about their patients. In this regard, a diagnostic axis that would include defenses very likely would be even more useful than axis II.

APPENDIX

The following examples illustrate both the inferred intrapsychic mechanisms and the objective criteria excerpted from the interview protocols by the blind raters to illustrate classification of a defense as "major." Clearly, the ratings did not depend heavily on assessment of social class, education, or intelligence. These two defenses, *schizoid fantasy* and *suppression*, were chosen because they were among the most important defenses for maturity ratings and also among the most ambiguous. The material presented reflects those portions of the interview transcript selected by the rater to justify identifying a defense as "major."

Essential to schizoid fantasy is to create one's gratifying interpersonal relationships inside one's head. Essential to suppression is stoicism, minimizing distress, and postponing gratification without repressing awareness of the impulse.

Schizoid fantasy: case A. This is a man with 11 grades of school, a good childhood environment, and parents in social class V. He works in a library. He "enjoys a vicarious sense of prestigiousness from the slight association that he has with professors and doctors." "I just like the academic atmosphere," he says, "I just sort of feel a part of it." When asked about his future, "I will still be at the library, maybe something on the academic level. I'm still interested in photography ... I've had so many cameras." He talked with a "tinge of grandiosity as he began to talk about certain cousins in the 'old country' who were all '8 feet tall.'" Age 47 and unmarried, he blamed religious prejudice. He said he had had little to do with non-Jewish girls. When asked about girls, he recalled a girl at school 35 years ago, in 1942, on whom he had had a crush and of whom he had thoughts of marrying. He thought that she had married someone else. There had been no one since. He does not drive, does not have a driver's license, although he says he might be interested in getting a license in the future. He said he knew "intuitively" how to drive a car and did not require driving lessons. He does not entertain much, but relaxes in his spare time, listens to the radio or to records by himself.

Schizoid fantasy: case B. This is a man with 9 grades of school, a so-so childhood environment, and parents in social class IV. He works as a security night guard. He entered into the job for "no special reason" but because he was "fascinated by it." When asked of any difficulty in his job, he remarked that alertness is the top priority. He said he gets along with people and illustrated this by a story of striking up a conversation with people on a park bench during a vacation in California. Mostly he works alone. If living his life over, he had thought of being a physical therapist or a lawyer wanting to help people. He was interested in journalism and he occasionally thought of writing a book. He took an electronics course, but nothing came of it. He said his family is very close. (In fact, his parents were divorced 25 years ago and had just remarried each other in New Mexico; he lives in Rhode Island.) He said he was not particularly close to any one relative: "They are all the same – cousins, aunts, and everybody." He has had no children. Then he said if he had had children, he might have had a son killed in Vietnam or a "daughter to worry me sick." Instead, he and his wife have a dog and a cat. He says of his dog, "You could swear he was human." He said of his cat, "He has a mind of his own." He and his wife get along although they should not, he says, because "I am a Scorpio and she is a Leo." When troubled, or angry, he runs up to the attic to listen to his CB radio, on which he has a police scanner. After 5 to 10 minutes, his anger passes. He never did have a special friend. He says he is not a loner, but that he just does not happen to see anyone. There is no one outside his family to whom he would go for help because he "never needs people." He and his wife mostly "keep to ourselves" and "don't need anyone." His hobbies include CB radio, photography, shooting targets (not animals), and fishing. He also likes war movies, and he jogs around the house.

Suppression: case C. This is a man with 11 grades of school, a so-so childhood environment, and parents in social class IV. His main job is "keeping the peace between customers and the boss." In his role as diplomat, he finds that he often has to "bite his tongue." He has been married for 26 years and says "nothing really bothers him" about his wife. "She's my whole life, I get to love her more every day.... The family just doesn't disagree about much ... nothing major." He and his wife both agree that they have worked hard on their marriage but "after 26 years it's beautiful." He and his wife remember that they had thoughts of separating in the first year of their marriage. When he feels bad, he tries to "think positive," and then he tries to "take care of whatever the problem is." For instance, when he is overwhelmed with bills, he just starts to pay them one at a time. Believing that he was losing control of his alcohol use, he stopped drinking 19 years ago. He says he has not been sick a day in his life. Hearing this, his wife groaned and said "He would go into work even if he was bleeding." When he gets a cold, he does not believe in staying home; as he always says, "I have to work."

Suppression: case D. This is a man with 9 grades of schools, a so-so childhood environment, and parents in social class V. This man was not able to report having had any serious problems with other men in his shop. When he gets troubled, he tries not to show it and "to take things in stride." In this way, he maintains an even temperament "at least on the outside." At work, he is known as the man with "no emotions" because he never looks rattled. "I want to make sure I know what I am hollering about before I start hollering." "I guess I just don't want to make a fool of myself – if you get mad first and then find out you are wrong, well, then it's too late." He did speculate first that his style might have been the reason for his ulcer problem. When he is especially troubled, he talks things over with his wife, and they try to settle it together. When he gets very angry, he becomes quiet. He never raises his voice, and tries to avoid blowing his top. Sometimes he will sit and play music on his record player until he cools off. He generally tries to avoid fights. On the other hand, he says that he has never backed down from a fight if it got to a point where it could not be avoided without losing face.

REFERENCES

Battista JR: Empirical test of Vaillant's hierarchy of ego functions. Am J Psychiatry 139:356–357, 1982

Bond M, Gardner ST, Christian J, et al: Empirical study of self-rated defense style. Arch Gen Psychiatry 40:333–338, 1983

Caplan G, Killela M: Support Systems and Mutual Help. New York, Grune & Stratton, 1976

Coehlo G, Hamburg D, Adams J (eds): Coping and Adaptation. New York, Basic Books, 1974

Drake RE, Vaillant GE: A validity study of axis II of the DSM-III. Am J Psychiatry 142:553–558, 1985

Endicott J, Spitzer RL, Fleiss JL, et al: The Global Assessment Scale: a procedure for measuring overall severity of psychiatric disturbance. Arch Gen Psychiatry 33:766–770, 1976

Freud A: Ego and the Mechanisms of Defense. London, Hogarth Press, 1937

Freud S: My views on the part played by sexuality in the aetiology of the neuroses, in The Complete Psychological Works, vol 7. Translated by Strachey J. London, Hogarth Press, (1906) 1953

Glueck S, Glueck E: Unraveling Juvenile Delinquency. New York, The Commonwealth Fund, 1950

Delinquents and Nondelinquents in Perspective. New York, The Commonwealth Fund, 1968

Haan NA: Proposed model of ego functioning: coping and defense mechanisms in relationship to IQ change. Psychol Monogr 77:1–23, 1963

Tripartite model of ego functioning values and clinical research applications. J Nerv Ment Dis 148:14–30, 1969

Coping and Defending. San Francisco, Jossey-Bass, 1977

Hackett TP, Cassem NH, Wishmie HA: The coronary care unit – an appraisal of its psychologic hazards. N Engl J Med 279:1365–1370, 1968

Hollingshead AB, Redlich FC: Social Class and Mental Illness. New York, Wiley, 1958

Kaplan HI, Sadock BJ: Modern Synopsis of Comprehensive Textbook of Psychiatry, III. Baltimore: Williams & Wilkins, 1981

Kobasa SC: Stressful life events, personality and health: an inquiry into hardiness. J Pers Soc Psychol 37:1–11, 1979

Kolb LC: Modern Clinical Psychiatry. Philadelphia, WB Saunders, 1977

Lazarus RS: Psychological Stress and the Coping Process. New York, McGraw-Hill, 1966

Loevinger J: Ego Development. San Francisco, Jossey-Bass, 1976

Luborsky L: Clinicians' judgments of mental health. Arch Gen Psychiatry 7:407–417, 1962

Meissner W: Theories of personality and psychopathology: classical psychoanalysis, in Comprehensive Textbook of Psychiatry, III. Edited by Kaplan HI, Freedman AM, Sadock BJ. Baltimore, Williams & Wilkins, 1980

Robins LN: Deviant Children Grown Up: A Sociological and Psychiatric Study of Sociopathic Personality. Baltimore, Williams & Wilkins, 1966

Runyan WM: Life Histories and Psychobiography: Explorations in Theory and Method. Oxford University Press, 1982

Semrad EV, Grinspoon L, Feinberg SE: Development of an ego profile scale. Arch Gen Psychiatry 28:70–77, 1973

Vaillant GE: Theoretical hierarchy of adaptive ego mechanisms. Arch Gen Psychiatry 24:107–118, 1971

Natural history of male psychological health, V: the relation of choice of ego mechanisms of defense to adult adjustment. Arch Gen Psychiatry 33:535–545, 1976

Health consequences of adaptation to life. Am J Med 67:732–734, 1979

Natural History of Alcoholism: Causes, Patterns, and Paths to Recovery. Cambridge, Mass, Harvard University Press, 1983

Childhood environment and maturity of defense mechanisms, in Human Development: An Interactional Perspective. Edited by Magnusson D, Allen V. New York, Academic Press, 1984

Vaillant GE, Bond M, Vaillant CO: An empirically validated hierarchy of defense mechanisms. Arch Gen Psychiatry 43:786–794, 1986

Vaillant GE, Milofsky ES: Natural history of male psychological health, IX: empirical evidence for Erikson's model of the life cycle. Am J Psychiatry 137:1348–1359, 1980

Vaillant GE, Vaillant CO: Natural history of male psychological health, X: work as a predictor of positive mental health. Am J Psychiatry 138:1433–1440, 1981

Weinstock A: Longitudinal study of social class and defense. J Consult Psychol 31:539–541, 1967

31 *A preliminary proposal for strengthening the multiaxial approach of DSM-III*

Possible family-oriented revisions

LYMAN C. WYNNE

Stephen Fleck (1983) has recently commented: "The major advance represented by DSM-III is the multiaxial approach, which recognizes that no matter what *sine qua non* cause or mechanism we may discover, the treatment of the patient will require multifaceted understanding and measures. Familial disturbance is among those factors that need to be assessed and addressed therapeutically if indicated." On the other hand, family therapists universally agree that the *form* of the multiaxial approach in *DSM-III* is far too poorly worked out to be of practical diagnostic and therapeutic use.

This conclusion is supported by the results from a survey recently conducted among senior psychiatrists and other mental health professionals who are members of the American Family Therapy Association (AFTA). *DSM-III* was widely regarded by these family therapists as useful for diagnosis of *individual* disorders, but as woefully incomplete for assessing and planning effective and comprehensive treatment that would include a family orientation. *DSM-III* was viewed as overfocusing or even misdirecting attention almost exclusively on the individual-system level, all too often promoting neglect of observations relevant to diagnosis and to efficacious and efficient interventions. Despite the broadened potential scope of the multiaxial approach, *DSM-III* inadequately addresses the issue of assessment of the *relational context* of individual disorders and persons.

DSM-III AND SYSTEMS THEORY

In theory, the multiaxial approach of *DSM-III* has the potential to provide a framework for comprehensive, integrated assessment and treatment across different conceptual levels. Multiaxial evaluation in *DSM-III* builds on a central principle of general systems theory: Nature can be viewed as a hierarchy of levels of organization, with more complex, larger units superordinate to less complex and smaller units. This formulation has been in use in biology for a long time, going back to the work of the biologists Paul Weiss (1925) and Ludwig von Bertalanffy (1952, 1968) (Figure 31.1).

Many psychiatrists with an interest in the family context, such as Fleck (1976, 1983) and Wynne (1968; Wynne, Jones, and Al-Khayyal, 1982), have noted the

Biosphere
↕
Society–nation
↕
Culture–subculture
↕
Community
↕
Family
↕
Two-person
↕

┌─────────────────────────────┐
│   │
│   Person   │
│   │
│   (experience and behavior) │
│   │
└─────────────────────────────┘

↕
Nervous system
↕
Organs/organ system
↕
Tissues
↕
Cells
↕
Organelles
↕
Molecules
↕
Atoms
↕
Subatomic particles

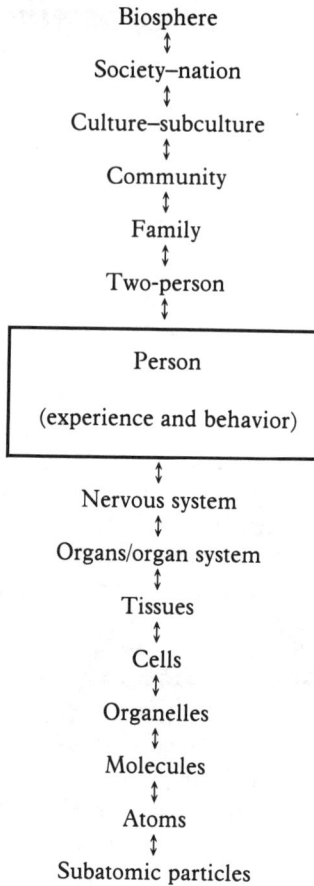

Figure 31.1. Systems hierarchy (levels of organization). *Source:* Engel (1980). *Am J Psychiatry* 137:535–544, 1980. Copyright 1980, the American Psychiatric Association. Reprinted by permission.

advantages, on both theoretical and therapeutic grounds, of integrated assessments on the biologic, personal, and interpersonal levels. It should be clear that recognition of family and other interpersonal contexts in no way negates or minimizes the importance of biologic links to personal disorder and health. Engel (1977, 1980) has eloquently argued that a biopsychosocial model, based on the concept of a systems hierarchy, is crucial for a scientifically sound and therapeutically effective medical model.

What is distinctive about the general systems view is that each level in the hierarchy is regarded as an organized whole, with distinctive proper ties and characteristics that are not reducible to other levels. Nevertheless, all system levels have semipermeable boundaries across which they are linked to one another. Thus, the cell, the organ, the person, the family, and the community all constitute levels in this hierarchy of organization, and each has distinctive and unique qualities. The methods and rules of study of the person as person are not reducible to study of the cell as cell, or organ as organ, and the family as family cannot be reduced to the study of person as person. The concept of influence from one system level to another in the hierarchy of open linked systems means, clinically, that the presenting problems of an individual identified patient may be the starting point for treatment of family dysfunction and, conversely, that intervention at the family level may ameliorate individual disorders.

Marriage and the family constitute the smallest, relatively enduring social units in these concentric contexts of general systems theory. Beyond the nuclear family, larger systemic organizations can be identified: networks of extended families, social and occupational networks, and organizations and networks linked to diverse religious, ethnic, and other value systems (Parsons, 1965; Speck and Rueveni, 1969; Spiegel, 1971; Beels, 1978; McGoldrick, Pearce, and Giordano, 1982; Landau, Griffiths, and Mason, 1982; Bloch, 1983). Within the nuclear family, individual persons constitute subsystems that in turn have functional subsystems: biochemical, neurophysiologic, behavioral, psychodynamic, and so forth. In short, the "family *is* context and *has* context" (Bloch, 1980).

FAMILY ASSESSMENT AND AXES I, II, AND III

In a preliminary way, let us consider how the five axes of *DSM-III* presently deal with the family and the relational context. *DSM-III* currently makes assessments explicitly at two major system levels, biologic and personal, but not at dyadic or family levels. On axis III, the level of "physical disorders or conditions" in physiologic systems is well established. More complexly, axes I, II, and V all deal with the person, or personality, as a system level. These three axes each focus on different components of the person level of functioning. "In DSM-III each of the mental disorders is conceptualized as a clinically significant behavioral or psychological syndrome or pattern that occurs *in an individual*. . . . A common misconception is that a classification of mental disorders classifies individuals, when actually what are being classified are disorders that individuals have" (American Psychiatric Association, 1980, p. 6; italics added). This formulation is most accurately applicable to axis I, whereas axis II emphasizes more enduring behavioral patterns that characterize the person as a whole.

To be sure, indications can be found in *DSM-III* that the psychosocial context, particularly the family, needs to be assessed in order to make most diagnoses, even on axis I. For example, an essential diagnostic criterion for schizophrenia is "deterioration from a previous level of functioning in such areas as work, social relations, and self-care" (American Psychiatric Association, 1980, p. 189). Major prodromal residual symptoms in schizophrenia include "social isolation or withdrawal" and "marked impairment in role functioning" (American Psychiatric Association, 1980, p. 189).

Whereas biologic systems are assessed distinctively on axis III, relational systems, including family systems, are assessed in a highly inadequate and fragmentary manner. Using axes I and II, only a disjointed aggregation of inferences derived from individual diagnoses can be made. For example, marital conflict often is a presenting problem and can be taken to be the focus for treatment planning even when the husband may also have a diagnosable problem of alcohol abuse, the wife may have diagnosable depression, and one or more children may have a conduct disorder or other problems. Diagnosing and treating any one of these family members in isolation will constitute a highly piecemeal approach to difficulties in contextual, relational systems. The most noisy or visible disorder is apt to be given exclusive or predominant attention, and undiagnosed relational problems that have evoked or at least have helped to perpetuate the individual difficulties are likely to be neglected.

A central point is that the quality and severity of the family-system problem cannot be deduced from individual *DSM-III* diagnoses on axes I, II, and III. Even when individual family members have clear-cut *DSM-III* diagnoses, they often function within the family-system setting in ways that are unexpected in light of their individual diagnostic labels. The level of family dysfunction regularly will be either overestimated or underestimated from a knowledge of individual diagnoses. In a current study of 145 families (each of which had a parent hospitalized for psychiatric illness) that were followed for 10 years in the Rochester Risk Research program, we have been repeatedly surprised at the many instances of relatively healthy family relationships despite a well-documented history of parental illness. Even psychotic individual illness, especially if this has been episodic and not affectively constricted, does not necessarily produce serious family-level dysfunction. If an ill parent and a "corrective" spouse have been able to work out an effective marital coalition, the offspring are by and large free of disturbances or may even have superior competence when assessed independently in the school or by clinicians or psychological testers (Wynne et al., 1982; Wynne and Cole, 1983).

In contrast, many couples and families now seek help for relational difficulties without specifying any single family member as the identified patient, and without individual symptoms as the focal presenting complaint. Later, individual diagnoses may be found to be applicable for one or more family members, but not at the point of entry into the assessment process. However, the individually based medical and psychiatric tradition has skewed the public to believe that in order to receive help they must report individual symptoms. The result too often is neglect of the relational difficulties that constitute the presenting problem as perceived by the family members. One example of the difference that the expectations of mental health staff make on what problems are diagnosed and treated was reported by McPartland and Richart (1966), who showed that psychiatrists tend to inquire about and to treat certain symptoms and disorders and to ignore and leave untreated the problems for which the patient and/or family sought help. In their study, the broader problem, often a relational one, was instead reported independently to social workers in the same setting. At follow-up, the individual symptoms often were found to have been relieved, but the presenting problem for which they had sought help was unchanged.

At present, family dysfunction, even when it is the most pressing reason for seeking help from a mental health professional, cannot be reported usefully within the *DSM-III* format of axes I–III. In most instances in which family or marital therapy is undertaken, an individual family member can legitimately be given a reimbursable *DSM-III* diagnosis, but to do so clearly misrepresents the actual clinical problem. As a result, family and marital therapists are placed in a bind that is unsatisfactory ethically, scientifically, and fiscally. There are now 11,000 members of the American Association for Marriage and Family Therapy, with their primary clinical activities in this field, plus unnumbered thousands of psychiatrists, psychologists, and other mental health professionals who see couples and families more selectively. At present, there is no way of knowing how frequently interventions by mental health professionals take place at the level of family or other relational systems. Neither primary nor secondary attention to the family level is presently reported even when it can be carefully assessed.

THE V CODES

In those exceptional situations in which no individual family member meets the criteria for an axis I or II diagnosis, but in which there may be a disruptive life-cycle developmental crisis or other family dysfunction, *DSM-III* provides an unsatisfactory reporting device: the V codes. These codes, for "conditions not attributable to a mental disorder that are a focus of attention or treatment," include the labels "marital problem" (V61.10), "parent-child problem" (V61.20), and "other specified family circumstances" (V61.80). Although the V codes are global, they could serve the purpose of preliminary screening if they were used uniformly whenever family dysfunction is "a focus of attention or treatment." However, the text of *DSM-III* specifies that the V codes are a last resort, to be "noted because, after a thorough evaluation, no mental disorder is found. In other instances the scope of the diagnostic evaluation has not been adequate to determine the presence or absence of a mental disorder." To be sure, a third circumstance is mentioned: "Finally, an individual may have a mental disorder, but the focus of attention or treatment is on a condition that is not due to the mental disorder. For example, an individual with Bipolar Disorder may have marital problems that are not directly related to manifestations of the Affective Disorder but are the principal focus of treatment" (American Psychiatric Association, 1980, p. 331).

These strictures, plus the pragmatic fact that treatment for V codes is not reimbursable, discourage their use and invite record-keeping based only on individual diagnosis, even when this is not the treatment focus. Clearly, the diagnostician is powerfully penalized by nonreimbursement when concluding that only a V code is applicable. Even in research and in special settings in which reimbursement may not be a decisive issue, the V codes have at best been viewed as having a residual, nonsystematic conceptual relationship to the rest of *DSM-III*. For purposes of family diagnosis, they are stepchildren deeply hidden in the shadows. Especially troubling is the fact that developmental crises in the family life cycle and other family-level dysfunctions may be seriously disturbing to all or nearly all of the family members and yet not be diagnosable initially on axis I or II. Later on, one or more family members may be predictably likely to develop progressive psychiatric symptoms. At least some of these potentially disturbed outcomes could well be attenuated, if not prevented, by earlier attention to the family-level dysfunction (Goldstein, 1983).

THE CATEGORY OF ADJUSTMENT DISORDER

Terkelsen (pers. commun.) has proposed that some of the need for family assessment could be met by adding a subcategory under the heading of adjustment disorder, namely, "adjustment disorder with disturbance of family (or other primary interpersonal) relationships." This would be parallel to category 309.23, adjustment disorder with work (or academic) inhibition. Terkelsen believes that the addition of this subcategory might "facilitate the authenticity of clinical assessment and intervention at the level of discourse without relegating it to a V Code, which is of no use in the interface with third-party payers" (K. Terkelsen, pers. commun.). It is possible that the *ICD-9* code number "309.29, Adjustment Reaction, Other," might be used to redefine a category with a label of this kind.

This proposal is interesting and deserves consideration as having merit for certain cases. However, such a diagnostic category would involve several difficulties, especially if it were the main locus for assessing family dysfunction in *DSM-III*. First, it would constitute another global reference to families without providing details. This could be justified if it were accompanied by a definite expectation that relational disturbances would be assessed separately in their own right. Second, it can be argued that interpersonal disturbances always will be associated with one of the individual symptomatic disturbances of "emotions and conduct" specified in the existing subcategories of adjustment disorder. This makes "disturbance of family relationships" redundant, but "work inhibition" may occur as an isolated symptom.

Third, a more serious problem is that the overall category of adjustment disorder is defined in *DSM-III* on terms that are too narrow for use with a full range of disturbances of family and other interpersonal relationships. Adjustment disorder is defined as "a maladaptive reaction to an identifiable psychosocial stressor, that occurs within three months of the onset of the stressor," and "the disturbance will eventually remit after the stressor ceases or, if the stressor persists, when a new level of adaptation is achieved" (American Psychiatric Association, 1980, pp. 300–1). These time stipulations are not applicable to most family circumstances, in which stressful conditions usually accumulate insidiously over time, and their onset usually cannot be readily identified in the way that physical trauma can. Even for specific events such as divorce, the disturbance in marital and family relationships typically long antedates this legal landmark. Furthermore, the concept of a stressor ceasing within three months, as specified in *DSM-III*, is not meaningful in family interactional terms. Once again, a divorce may technically end one type of stressor, but other stressors, such as disputes over custody of children and visitation rights, may continue unabated. From the standpoint of family assessment, it is just as important diagnostically and therapeutically to describe the family setting qualitatively as it is to describe the symptomatic manifestations of the individual family members. Family problems may be associated with a variety of diagnosable individual disorders, often of a more severe and enduring nature than is applicable to adjustment disorders. Hence, diagnostic reliance on a category of adjustment disorder with disturbance in family relationships would underestimate the extent to which other individual problems are linked to family dysfunction.

Finally, the *DSM-III* concept of adjustment disorder as a reaction to a stressor emphasizes the unidirectional impact of external psychosocial stressors on individual functioning. Family-systems formulations, on the contrary, all recognize that there may be multidirectional and circular chains of effects, so that the individual has an impact on the family, as well as vice versa. However, adjustment disorder could be provided with a conceptually more sophisticated definition if a subcategory were to be formulated as a link between diagnosis at the personal and family levels of functioning applicable at least to certain mild cases.

AXIS V

In one respect, axis V is parallel to axis I and axis II. All three axes make assessments at the personal level of organization. However, in rating "highest level of adaptive functioning in the past year," axis V is a positive complement to the diagnosis of disorder in axes I and II. Axis V provides a partial corrective to the imbalance of earlier diagnostic systems that failed to evaluate *assets* of the individual. These assets are crucial components in a comprehensive diagnosis that is prognostically relevant to treatment, rehabilitation, and prevention of relapses. Unfortunately, axis V at present provides only a crude quantitative rating of "highest level of adaptive functioning in the past year." This does not deal with the qualitative aspects of adaptation nor with the individual's *current* level of adaptation. (See the proposal by Mezzich for rating current functioning, Chapter 29.)

The present instructions for axis V recommend that adaptive functioning be assessed in three contexts: social relations ("with particular emphasis on family and friends"), occupational functioning, and use of leisure time. Although these instructions provide an entry point for assessing the social context, no format for recording qualitative data and only very general criteria for evaluating these three areas are currently given in *DSM-III*. Conceptually, the focus remains on the functioning of the individual and does not shift to the family as a distinctive system level.

AXIS IV

The axis of *DSM-III* that gives attention most explicitly to social context is axis IV, Severity of Psychosocial Stressors. In describing this axis, the text usefully states: "Although a stressor frequently plays a precipitating role in a disorder, it may also be a consequence of the individual's psychopathology – e.g., Alcohol Dependence may lead to marital problems and divorce, which can then become stressors contributing to the development of a Major Depression" (American Psychiatric Association, 1980, pp. 26–7). Nevertheless, the concept of stressors is poorly elaborated in the actual ratings. The family and other relational contexts of the individual are not conceptualized in their systemic qualities. Therefore, only a haphazard and unreliable beginning for family assessment is produced.

As in axis V, the ratings of axis IV are only in terms of a global seven-point scale of severity. This means that a host of qualitatively different stressful conditions are lumped together without providing any cues as to treatment implications. *DSM-III* mentions in the text: "In addition to the severity rating, in certain settings it may be useful to note specific psychosocial stressors" (p. 27). It seems unlikely that this axis will prove useful unless a better conceptual framework is provided. Also lacking is any schema or format for classifying and recording stressors. (Mezzich has suggested a useful format in Chapter 29.) It is noteworthy, but not surprising, that none of the respondents in the AFTA survey found either axis IV or axis V, in their current state, to be of any practical value.

One conceptual shortcoming of axis IV is that only stressors, not psychosocial supports, are presently assessed. Yet these supports, or their lack, may be prognostically and therapeutically crucial. Both stressors and supports optimally should be assessed in each major relational system, usually starting with the family and the workplace. Additionally, other, less established social groups may be more relevant in some instances, for example, in the relational systems of an unemployed patient without a family and living in a halfway house. How to do justice to the complexity of the social context and not create a descriptive format that is unwieldy is a real dilemma, but clearly this problem deserves further exploration and field trial.

One approach would be to broaden the present emphasis of axis IV on "severity of psychosocial stressors" and identify axis IV as a "family axis," or more accurately as an axis for assessing *relational systems*. At a higher conceptual level, this then would parallel axes I, II, and III. Such an evaluation would need to be a compromise between having enough detail to be enlightening and sufficient brevity to be of practical utility for clinicians. In order to facilitate use by the general clinician of today, it may be necessary to devise a format for assessing the relational context that is essentially at the level of screening, with many more details specified in supplementary "axes" to be used when family therapy and other psychosocial interventions are undertaken.

FORMS OF RELATIONAL ASSESSMENTS

At least four approaches to more detailed assessment of family and other relational systems can be considered: (1) narrative case formulation, (2) global rating of family health or dysfunction, (3) family typology, either of families as systems or of problems as seen at the family level, and (4) dimensionalized family assessment.

Case formulations

These would include attention to social context and could be quite immediately usable on a general basis. Spitzer has suggested that an explicit format for making a case formulation in *DSM-III-R* would serve some of the needs for a broader-based evaluation than is possible with the present labels of axes I–III. Unless axes IV and V were made substantially more detailed, supplementation of these coded ratings would still be necessary. A format for case formulation could readily include a description of the stressors and supports in the social context that appear to be most relevant to the predisposing, precipitating, and perpetuating factors in the illness. Also, the transactional qualities, in which "causal" effects operate in reciprocal and spiral fashion over time, could be briefly identified. Such systemic factors clearly are relevant to the ease or difficulty with which interventions can be effective.

Although qualitative case formulations have many advantages for clinical use, they are difficult to implement in a consistent or standardized manner. They would not well facilitate comparative study and research on different conditions and treatments.

Global ratings of interpersonal and occupational functioning

These could be introduced quite easily as a revision of axis IV. Probably social and occupational functioning, minimally, need to be rated separately. Examples of global family ratings that have been used successfully are found in the Beavers–Timberlawn Family Evaluation Scale (Lewis et al., 1976) and in the General Functioning Scale of the McMaster Family Assessment Device (Epstein, Baldwin, and Bishop, 1983).

Typological and dimensionalized family assessment

In the family-research literature, there have been many alternative proposals for classification of families. For examples of clinically relevant family typologies and dimensional classifications, see Ackerman (1958), Beavers and Voeller (1983), Epstein and associates (1983), Ford and Herrick (1976), Gehrke and Kirschenbaum (1967), Lewis and associates (1976), Minuchin (1974),

Olson, Russell, and Sprenkle (1983), Ravich and Wyden (1974), Reiss (1981), Richter (1974), Sager (1977), Stierlin (1972), and Voiland (1962).

Fisher (1977) reviewed a number of these family schemes. His review suggests that the family typologies are nearly all quite ad hoc. Such a classification could begin with such major problems as "abusing families," "emotionally over-involved (enmeshed) families," and so on. At present, there seems to be little readiness in the family field to agree that one family typology of this sort is superior to another. Therefore, it would be useful for a group of family clinicians and researchers to try out more systematically the use of selected, readily agreed on family categories. The possibility that such an effort could be relevant to a revision of *DSM-III* would constitute a timely stimulus to undertake effective collaboration.

Alternatively, or additionally, along with selected ad hoc categories, agreement on a conceptually comprehensive *dimensional* framework that could meet with widespread acceptance would be useful in family assessment. Three proposals that are currently undergoing trials have been published and discussed by Beavers and Voeller (1983), Epstein and associates (1983), and Olson and associates (1983). A review and critique of these schemes is beyond the scope of this chapter.

Another kind of framework worthy of consideration uses the concept of the family developmental life cycle. In this formulation, marriages and families pass through a definable series of stages, with the transition points being likely times of crises and dysfunction. The simplest version of the family life cycle involves five main stages: the newly married couple, the family with young children, the family with adolescents, launching children out of the family, and the family in later life. For alternative variations for assessing the family life cycle, see Carter and McGoldrick (1980), Duvall (1967), Fleck (1983), Haley (1973), Hill and Rodgers (1964), and Grunebaum and Bryant (1966). Family researchers and therapists have regularly found that both individual and family dysfunctions predictably occur at points of crisis in the family life cycle. Specification of a workable life-cycle schema for general use could be the shared task of interested consultants concerned with *DSM-III-R* and *DSM-IV*.

SUMMARY

I strongly recommend that the multiaxial approach of *DSM-III* be strengthened through greater attention to relational systems and the social context, with special emphasis on the health and dysfunction of the family. Axes I, II, and III appear inappropriate for this aspect of mental health assessment. Restructuring of axis IV should be considered. Current social functioning, especially familial and occupational functioning, could be globally rated in a two-track revision of axis IV that would attend to social supports as well as psychosocial stressors. In addition, explicit provision for narrative comments about the social context could be included in a narrative case formulation that might be a routine part of future assessments. Finally, more detailed evaluation of relational systems will still be needed by family and marital therapists. One or more task forces of family therapists and researchers should review and develop assessment alternatives, explore their feasibility in field trials, and make recommendations for possible use in *DSM-III-R* and/or *DSM-IV*.

REFERENCES

Ackerman NW: The Psychodynamics of Family Life. New York, Basic Books, 1958

American Psychiatric Association: Diagnostic and Statistical Manual of Mental Disorders, third edition. Washington, DC, APA, 1980

Beavers RW, Voeller MN: Family models: comparing and contrasting the Olson circumplex model with the Beavers systems model. Fam Proc 22:85–98, 1983

Beels C: Social networks, the family, and the schizophrenic patient. Schizophr Bull 4:512–521, 1978

Bloch DA: The future of family therapy, in Dimensions of Family Therapy. Edited by Andolfi M, Zwerling I. New York, Guilford Press, 1980, pp 273–280

Family systems perspectives on the management of the individual patient, in Psychiatry Update: The American Psychiatric Association Annual Review, vol II. Edited by Grinspoon LG. Washington, DC, APA, 1983, pp 203–215

Carter EA, McGoldrick M (eds): The Family Life Cycle: A Framework for Family Therapy. New York, Gardner Press, 1980

Duvall ER: Family Development. Philadelphia, Lippincott, 1967

Engel GL: The need for a new medical model: a challenge for biomedicine. Science 196:129–136, 1977

The clinical application of the biopsychosocial model. Am J Psychiatry 137:535–544, 1980

Epstein N, Baldwin LM, Bishop DS: The McMaster Family Assessment Device. J Marr Fam Ther 9:171–180, 1983

Fisher L: On the classification of families: a progress report. Arch Gen Psychiatry 34:424–433, 1977

Fleck S: A general systems approach to severe family pathology. Am J Psychiatry 133:669–673, 1976

A holistic approach to family typology and the axes of DSM-III. Arch Gen Psychiatry 40:901–906, 1983

Ford FR, Herrick J: Family rules: family life styles. Am J Psychiatry 44:61–69, 1976

Gehrke S, Kirschenbaum M: Survival patterns in family conjoint therapy. Fam Proc 6:67–80, 1967

Goldstein MJ: Family interaction: patterns predictive of the onset and course of schizophrenia, in Psychosocial Intervention in Schizophrenia. Edited by Stierlin H, Wynne LC, Wirsching M. Berlin, Springer-Verlag, 1983, pp 5–19

Grunebaum HV, Bryant CM: The theory and practice of the family diagnostic: theoretical aspects and resident education. Psychiatr Res Rep 20:150–162, 1966

Haley J: Uncommon Therapy. New York, Ballantine Books, 1973

Hill R, Rodgers RH: The developmental approach, in Handbook of Marriage and the Family. Edited by Christensen HT. Chicago, Rand McNally, 1964, pp 171–211

Landau J, Griffiths J, Mason J: The extended family in transition: clinical implications, in The International Book of Family Therapy. Edited by Kaslow F. New York, Brunner/Mazel, 1982, pp 360–369

Lewis J, Beavers WR, Gossett JT, et al: No Single Thread: Psychological Health in Family Systems. New York, Brunner/Mazel, 1976

McGoldrick M, Pearce JK, Giordano J: Ethnicity and Family Therapy. New York, Guilford Press, 1982

McPartland TS, Richart RH: Social and clinical outcomes of psychiatric treatment. Arch Gen Psychiatry 14:179–184, 1966

Minuchin S: Families and Family Therapy. Cambridge, Mass, Harvard University Press, 1974

Olson DH, Russell CS, Sprenkle DH: Circumplex model of marital and family systems, VI: theoretical update. Fam Proc 22:69–83, 1983

Parsons T: Social Structure and Personality. London, Free Press, 1965

Ravich RA, Wyden B: Predictable Pairing. New York, Wyden, 1974

Reiss D: The Family's Construction of Reality. Cambridge, Mass, Harvard University Press, 1981

Richter HE: The Family as Patient. New York, Farrar Straus & Giroux, 1974

Sager CJ: A typology of intimate relationships. J Sex Mar Therapy 3:83–112, 1977

Speck RV, Rueveni U: Network therapy, a developing concept. Fam Proc 8:182–190, 1969

Spiegel JP: Transactions. New York, Science House, 1971

Stierlin H: Separating Parents and Adolescents. New York, Times Book Corp, 1972

Voiland AL: Family Casework Diagnosis. New York, Columbia University Press, 1962

von Bertalanffy L: Problems of Life. New York, Wiley, 1952

General Systems Theory. New York, Braziller, 1968

Weiss P: Tierisches Verhalten als "Systemsreaktion": Die Orientiering der Ruhestellungen von Schmetterdingen (Vanessa) gegen Licht und Schwertkraft. Biol Gen 14:168–248, 1925

Wynne LC: Methodologic and conceptual issues in the study of schizophrenics and their families. J Psychiatr Res 6:185–199, 1968

Wynne LC, Cole RE: Rochester Risk Research program: A new look at parental diagnoses and family relationships, in Psychosocial Intervention in Schizophrenia: An International View. Edited by Stierlin H, Wynne LC, Wirsching M. Berlin, Springer-Verlag, 1983, pp 25–48

Wynne LC, Jones JE, Al-Khayyal M: Healthy family communication patterns: observations in families "at risk" for psychopathology, in Normal Family Processes. Edited by Walsh F. New York: Guilford Press, 1982, pp 142–164

32 *Overview*

RICHARD FINN

Mezzich's proposed axes modifications and the many options and alternatives he offers could greatly help those who will work on revisions and new editions of the diagnostic manual. If, as he suggests, five axes are the practical limit, inclusion of the many meritorious suggestions for new and revised axes will require a creative and innovative effort. The potential magnitude of such a task was highlighted by the myriad suggestions for modifications that emerged during the course of the discussion of the chapters included in this part.

Citing a report by an ad hoc committee of the American Psychoanalytic Association, the notion was put forth that the current structure of axis I and axis II introduces an artificial separation between common psychopathological entities that are manifested by different behaviors. If one accepts that premise, the possibility exists of combining the two into a single axis that captures all psychiatric disorders. A new axis II could then be used to describe defensive styles or note the level of personality function. The recommendation could be considered along with a suggestion by Karasu and Skodol (1980), who have called on researchers to construct a standardized psychodynamic evaluation for use in such a new axis. Also discussed were the advantages and disadvantages of axes describing specific and general cognitive impairments, rating the degree of substance use or misuse, and incorporating the psychiatric coding system for insurance-claims reporting published by the American Psychiatric Association and the Health Insurance Association of America. The latter is a method of reporting the medical necessity for treatment without revealing diagnoses or other information found in the current classification system and is discussed in greater detail in Chapter 35 by Sharfstein. Other recommendations that were discussed included that of Alarcon (1983) for inclusion of transcultural factors and that of Schover and associates (1982) for specific descriptions of sexual problems and dissatisfactions. It was also suggested that a series of research axes would provide a useful adjunct to a multiaxial system. Such axes would be used for concepts that have yet to achieve professional consensus, but in which systematic collection of data could lead to further advances in knowledge. The range of suggestions indicates a lack of consensus within the field about what, for classification purposes, represents "clinically useful information."

UTILIZATION STUDIES OF MULTIAXIAL EVALUATION

Expert opinions on the need for new axes and for alterations in the current axes, sound as they may be, must be balanced by study of the actual use of multiaxial evaluation. The Multiaxial Evaluation Committee of the *DSM-III* Task Force has only the field-trial data to balance its opinions. After nearly four years of *DSM-III* use, a wealth of data is not available. There have been only six small studies on this point. Their sample sizes were small, but the results invite larger, more representative studies that can be used for statistical analysis.

In the first, Williams, Spitzer, and Skodol studied axis use in residency training through a survey of directors of psychiatric residency training in the United States. Ninety percent of the 190 directors responded. Fifty percent of the respondents reported that their residents used only axes I, II, and III; 25% reported that their residents used all five axes; the remaining 25% reported that their residents used the axes in varying patterns. From this it can be said that in 75% of the programs, the residents get a consistent experience with using axes I, II, and III, but in only 25% do they get a consistent experience with axes IV and V. If this training pattern continues, we can expect a growing number of recently trained psychiatrists without experience or professional investment in axes IV and V.

The second study was a survey at St. Elizabeth's Hospital in Washington, D.C. Dr. Roger Peele, chairman of psychiatry at the federal mental hospital, asked staff psychiatrists there what they wanted to see happen to axes IV and V in future. Forty-nine percent of the respondents wanted both axes retained, and 41% wanted both removed.

In the third study, 37% of Brooklyn Psychiatric Society members responded to a survey about the usefulness of multiaxial evaluation. Fourteen percent of the respondents said that it was highly useful, 46% thought it was moderately useful, 35% thought it was not useful, and 5% had no opinion.

Regarding a survey of mental health staff members in student health services, Robert L. Arnstein reported to the American College Health Association that only 38% of the respondents used *DSM-III,* 32% used another system, and 30% used no system regularly. Among *DSM-III* users, all used axis I, "most" axis II, "some" axis III, but "few" axes IV and V.

The last two studies were surveys of the members of the Assembly of District Branches of the American Psychiatric Association and of participants at an annual scientific meeting of the Iowa Psychiatric Society. The same questionnaire was used in the two surveys, which were conducted in the fall of 1983. The Assembly sample numbered 132, the Iowa sample 79.

The survey instrument (Table 32.1) asked four questions. The first asked the respondents how they used each of the *DSM-III* axes in their inpatient and outpatient practices; the choices given were "always," "sometimes," or "never." Table 32.2 compares the responses of the Assembly members and the Iowa participants.

Table 32.2 shows the overwhelming acceptance and use of axes I and II in

Table 32.1. *Survey instrument*

Name _____ City _____ State _____

1. I use this axis in my practice:

   a. *Inpatient*   *Always*   *Sometimes*   *Never*
      Axis I   _____   _____   _____
      Axis II   _____   _____   _____
      Axis III   _____   _____   _____
      Axis IV   _____   _____   _____
      Axis V   _____   _____   _____

   b. *Outpatient*
      Axis I   _____   _____   _____
      Axis II   _____   _____   _____
      Axis III   _____   _____   _____
      Axis IV   _____   _____   _____
      Axis V   _____   _____   _____

2. In a future DSM-IV, I want:

	Continued	*Altered*	*Removed*	*Don't care*	*Other* (please specify)
Axis I	____	____	____	____	_____
Axis II	____	____	____	____	_____
Axis III	____	____	____	____	_____
Axis IV	____	____	____	____	_____
Axis V	____	____	____	____	_____

3. If you want new axes, please describe them.

4. Do any third-party payers, peer review or audit agencies, etc., *require* multiaxial diagnoses?

   _____ yes _____ no. If so, please name them.

Please leave this at the front of the auditorium. Thanks.

---

both inpatient and outpatient practices of the Assembly and the Iowa respondents. Axis III lagged only a little behind. This is not only a demonstration of the usefulness of the first three axes but also a demonstration of the success of multiaxial evaluation as an operational procedure in the diagnostic process. Whatever the reason for these successes, it did not carry over to the use of axes IV and V. Table 32.2 shows a considerable drop in their use, most notably by the Iowans. Still, use in the 56%–60% range for the Assembly and in the 30%–37% range for the Iowans is remarkable given the *DSM-III*'s stated limitations on axes IV and V uses in "special settings" only. Certainly, in Iowa, there were few, if any, respondents who practiced in such "special settings."

A breakdown was done for the Iowa respondents into four groups: private practice, government-supported hospital practice, outpatient clinic practice,

Table 32.2. *Comparison of axis use by members of the APA Assembly and of the Iowa Psychiatric Society*

	Always or sometimes (%)		Never (%)		No response (%)	
	APA	IPS	APA	IPS	APA	IPS
Inpatient						
Axis I	94	99	3	1	3	0
Axis II	92	96	5	4	3	0
Axis III	84	86	11	14	5	0
Axis IV	60	37	30	51	10	12
Axis V	56	36	33	53	11	11
Outpatient						
Axis I	97	99	2	1	1	0
Axis II	93	97	5	3	2	0
Axis III	84	80	9	17	7	3
Axis IV	59	35	29	51	12	13
Axis V	58	30	30	57	12	13

and other or unspecified. (A similar breakdown for Assembly respondents could not be done.) Table 32.3 examines axis use by the two largest Iowa groups, private and government-hospital practitioners. Table 32.3 shows the major reason for the high rate of nonuse of axes IV and V by the Iowa respondents: the high rate of nonuse in private practice. At the same time, the rate of nonuse of axes IV and V by Iowa hospital respondents was slightly higher than the nonuse rate for all Assembly respondents, as shown in Table 32.2. Unexplained is the high rate of nonresponse by Iowa hospital psychiatrists.

The second survey question asked respondents what they wanted to see happen in future diagnostic manuals to the axes as they are in *DSM-III*. They were asked if they wanted each axis continued as is, altered in some way, or removed for some reason, or perhaps they had another opinion or "don't care." Table 32.4 compares the responses of the Assembly and Iowa groups. The two groups were of one mind about the future of axes I, II, and III; their responses were quite similar. But in regard to axes IV and V, the two groups diverged. There was strong support from both Assembly and Iowa groups for continuing axes I, II, and III as they are in *DSM-III*. Assembly support for continuing axes IV and V, however, dropped almost by half, and Iowa support was less than half of that. In the Assembly, there was an even split between those who supported continuing axes IV and V as is and those who did not. The Iowa outcome was not equivocal, with three-quarters of the respondents not supporting the continuation of axes IV and V as they are now.

A breakdown of the Iowans (Table 32.5) shows strong support in private and

Table 32.3. *Comparison of axis use by Iowa Psychiatric Society members in private or government-hospital practice*

	Always or sometimes (%)		Never (%)		No response (%)	
	Priv.	Hosp.	Priv.	Hosp.	Priv.	Hosp.
Inpatient						
Axis I	97	100	3	0	0	0
Axis II	94	100	6	0	0	0
Axis III	75	100	25	0	0	0
Axis IV	28	49	66	34	6	17
Axis V	25	49	69	34	6	17
Outpatient						
Axis I	97	100	3	0	0	0
Axis II	97	100	3	0	0	0
Axis III	72	96	28	0	0	4
Axis IV	22	47	72	31	6	23
Axis V	22	47	72	31	6	23

Note: Private practice, $N = 32$; hospital practice, $N = 29$.

Table 32.4. *Comparison of Assembly and Iowa respondents' opinions about the axes in future diagnostic manuals*

Axis	Continue (%)		Alter (%)		Remove (%)		Don't care (%)		No response (%)	
	APA	IPS	APA	IPS	APA	IPS	APA	IPS	APA	IPS
I	86	90	6	4	1	0	2	2	5	4
II	79	80	8	8	2	1	5	8	5	4
III	77	77	3	4	4	2	8	11	7	5
IV[a]	44	18	7	10	12	23	26	44	10	5
V[a]	43	21	7	6	11	24	27	44	11	5

[a]Two Assembly responses to a fifth alternative, "other," are not included.

hospital practice for continuing axes I and II, with only a slight drop in private-practice support for axis III. Table 32.5 shows that support for axes IV and V dropped markedly in both groups, with only 13% of private practitioners wanting them continued. One-quarter of both groups wanted these two axes removed, and half the private-practice respondents and nearly 40% of the hos-

Table 32.5. *Comparison of Iowa private and hospital practitioners' opinions about the axes in future manuals*

Axis	Continue (%) Priv.	Hosp.	Alter (%) Priv.	Hosp.	Remove (%) Priv.	Hosp.	Don't care (%) Priv.	Hosp.	No response (%) Priv.	Hosp.
I	88	86	3	7	0	0	6	0	3	7
II	78	83	6	3	0	3	13	3	3	7
III	69	93	3	0	3	0	19	0	6	7
IV[a]	13	28	3	7	25	24	50	38	9	3
V[a]	13	31	3	3	25	24	50	38	9	3

[a]A fifth alternative, "other (specify)," drew no response.

pital respondents did not care what would happen to these axes. The Iowa private-practice group made the least use of axes IV and V and gave the least support for their continuation. This could very well have come about from the use limitations on axes IV and V stated in *DSM-III*. By obeying the instructions, these private practitioners may have found that they could get along without the two optional axes, and this could explain why they wanted to keep it that way.

A breakdown of Assembly respondents by type of practice was not possible, but other figures can be considered. The Assembly Task Force on Private Practice defined private practice in its 1981 report. Using that definition, the percentages of private practitioners in various groups were as follows: APA members, 1981, 50%; APA Assembly, 1979, 46%; Iowa Psychiatric Society, 1983, 42%; Iowa survey responders, 40%. Assuming the 1979 percentage holds for the 1983 Assembly, the use of and opinions about the future of axes IV and V by Assembly private practitioners must be much different from those for the Iowa private practitioners, if Iowa hospital practitioners and hospital practitioners nationwide behave similarly. What cannot be determined is whether or not either private-practice group is representative of APA members in private practice.

The third survey question asked respondents if they wanted any new axes. Many took this opportunity to discuss alterations in existing axes as well. In Iowa, 9% volunteered not wanting any new axes. In the Assembly group, there were 36 suggestions, 17 for new axes and 19 for alterations. In the Iowa group there were 11 suggestions, 2 for new axes and 9 for alterations. In the Assembly group, 16 of the 19 suggestions for alterations, and in Iowa 7 of the 9 suggestions for alterations, focused on axes IV and V. Seven of the 47 suggestions were directed at somehow adding severity of illness or level of impairment to multiaxial evaluation. Descriptions of defense mechanisms or defensive styles and of family or support-system factors were also mentioned by a similar number of respondents.

The last survey question asked respondents to name any requirements for the use of multiaxial evaluation per se. Only 6% of each survey group knew of any such requirements. When this is considered in conjunction with the reports of axis use in Table 32.2, it seems undeniable that the high rate of use of multiaxial evaluation by the respondents was not caused by outside coercion, but rather came from individual decisions about the utility of the method. This underscores the importance of periodic appraisal of the current status of multiaxial evaluation, including not only expert opinion about improvements that could be made but also studies of the actual use of the method in clinical practice, teaching, and research.

The findings of the six surveys can be summarized as follows:

1. There is broad acceptance and voluntary use of multiaxial evaluation.
2. There is widespread support for continuing multiaxial evaluation in future diagnostic manuals.
3. There is a very high percentage use of axes I and II, and almost as much of axis III, but considerably less use of axes IV and V, although at a rate much greater than expected considering the stated limitations on their use.
4. Very strong support exists for continuing axes I, II, and III in future manuals as they are in *DSM-III*. There is much less support for continuation of axes IV and V, with a strong suggestion that the decisions of private practitioners and psychiatric educators need further study.

CONCLUSION

I would like to close with a brief discussion of what may become the most pressing problem for those who will revise multiaxial evaluation: its relationship to developing prospective-payment systems and to older reimbursement systems becoming more concerned with their financial integrity than they are with covering the costs of medical care for those who hold contracts with them. During the discussion, Mezzich, in response to a question from Mel Sabshin, said that he believes multiaxial evaluation as it is in *DSM-III* is not suitable for prospective-payment systems, because it emphasizes clinical syndromes that are not as predictive of length of stay as are the severity of illness, the impairment in adaptive functioning, and the quality and quantity of support systems.

If this means that is it possible that our patients will be denied the treatment they need or the reimbursement they cannot pay out of their pockets or from their savings because we did not take the steps we could have taken in revising multiaxial evaluation, then we have little choice. Those of us who want a new axis VI or a modified axis IV, or whatever, may have to sacrifice what we want.

Modifying multiaxial evaluation for *DSM-III*, revised, or *DSM-IV* will be much more difficult than creating it for *DSM-III*. Many of the decisions made by the *DSM-III* Task Force about multiaxial evaluations were arbitrary – there was no other way – but now, with more data about its utility, with more experience with it in practice, and with increasingly rigorous external demands, we must remember what Simons told the conference about modifying multiaxial evaluation: "We are all concerned that these changes will be thought through carefully."

REFERENCES

Alarcon RD: A Latin American perspective on DSM-III. Am J Psychiatry 140:102–105, 1983

Fleck S: A holistic approach to family typology and the axes of DSM-III. Arch Gen Psychiatry 40:901–906, 1983

Karasu TB, Skodol AE: VIth axis for DSM-III: psychodynamic evaluation. Am J Psychiatry 137:607–610, 1980

Schover LR, Friedman JM, Weiler SJ, et al: Multiaxial problem-oriented systems for sexual dysfunctions, an alternative to DSM-III. Arch Gen Psychiatry 39:614–619, 1982

PART IX

Clinical, educational, and administrative applications of DSM-III

The introduction to *DSM-III* states that it "had to be, first of all, clinically useful, while also providing a basis for research and administrative use." Many would add that it should be valuable for educational purposes as well. Most of this volume has been devoted to the value of *DSM-III* as a tool in conducting research and the value of research in the continuing development and refinement of *DSM-III* and its successors. This final Part IX focuses on other applications of *DSM-III*. Paul Chodoff discusses the use of *DSM-III* in the clinical practice of psychiatry in a private-practice outpatient setting, the setting in which most American psychiatrists spend most of their time. Richard Simons reviews *DSM-III* and the teaching of psychiatry to residents and medical students. Finally, Steve Sharfstein analyzes the relationship between psychiatric diagnoses and strategies of third-party payment and reimbursement for psychiatric services, an area of great interest in contemporary psychiatric administration.

One theme emerges repeatedly in each of these chapters and in the discussions that followed their presentation: There is much that is important about psychiatric patients that is not included in their *DSM-III* diagnoses. Dr. Chodoff tells us what is important to the practitioner; from Dr. Simons we hear what is important to the teacher and the student; and Dr. Sharfstein tells us what is important to the third-party payer and the psychiatric administrator. They each want to expand *DSM-III* so that it will be more valuable in treating patients, teaching students, and administering psychiatric service systems. In the discussion, there was consideration of the appropriate limits of diagnosis, of what kinds of data are best included within the diagnosis and what are best left out and incorporated in an extradiagnostic formulation. Which of these suggestions promise improvement and which threaten other features of the nomenclature is a major theme of the discussion.

Robert Michels

33 *DSM-III and the psychiatric practitioner*

PAUL CHODOFF

In this chapter I undertake a critical discussion of the applicability and usefulness of *DSM-III* to primarily office-oriented psychiatric practices in which, although drugs are prescribed as indicated, psychotherapy is the principal treatment modality employed. The psychotherapy dispensed in such practices ranges from supportive to the more intense and insight-oriented variety including psychoanalysis. This kind of practice is engaged in by a large number of American psychiatrists who earn their livings through fees for their services, abetted by third-party reimbursement, rather than from institutional or academic salaries. Although my own practice differs in some respects from those of others in this group, I have no reason to believe that these differences are crucial. I consider that my experience with *DSM-III* is reasonably representative.

My presentation is based on my practice experience generally, and specifically on a review of the *DSM-III* diagnoses of all patients seen during the months of April, May, and June 1983. Patients diagnosed included those with whom I had an ongoing therapeutic relationship as well as those seen for consultation with a view to recommending appropriate treatment regimes either with myself or other psychiatrists. My practice load during that period included 34 separate individuals. Of these, 28 were in treatment; the other 6 were for consultations and were seen only once or twice. I was able to make *DSM-III* diagnoses in five of these consultations; I did not understand one well enough to make a diagnosis. I made all appropriate axis I and axis II diagnoses in each instance. In only one case was there a relevant axis III entry. I also undertook to grade the conditions that I was seeing on a scale of 1 for mild, 2 for moderate, and 3 for severe (grade 4 would require hospitalization).

Table 33.1 groups the 34 patients by number with all relevant diagnoses. Of the 33 cases in which diagnoses were made, 26 were diagnosed on axis I and 26 on axis II. In 19 instances, a majority, there were diagnoses on both axes. I believe that the frequency of axis II diagnoses is a characteristic feature of the kind of practice I am describing. It differentiates such patients from those seen in inpatient (and possibly clinic) settings. In seven cases, axis II diagnoses stood alone. In three of the consultations, axis II diagnoses might have been added to those in axis I if I had known the patients better. Two patients with anxiety

499

Table 33.1. *All diagnoses (by patient)*

Case[a]	Axis 1	Axis 2	Severity
1	300.40	301.89	3
2	V62.81		1
3		301.89	2
4	300.30	301.40-301.22	3
5	309.00	301.89	2
6	305.2-302.83	301.89	2
7	309.00-V62.20	301.89	1
8	300.40	301.89	2
9		301.89	3
10	302.00	301.50	2
11	309.28	301.40	2
12	309.00-V62.20		1
13		301.89	2
14	302.71	301.89	2
15		301.81	3
16	302.83	301.89	3
17	309.28-V61.10	301.89	2
18	302.00-309.00		1
19	309.00	301.89	2
20	292.84	301.20	2
21 (C)		301.40	2
22	305.6	301.81	2
23		301.89	2
24 (C)		301.83	3
25	300.02		2
26	309.00	301.82	2
27	302.74-302.75	301.89	2
28 (C)	302.00-302.74		2
29 (C)	300.40	301.89	3
30	309.00	301.89	2
31 (C)	300.60		2
32	V62.81	301.89	1
33	300.01		2
34 (C)	799.90	799.90	

[a](C), consultation.

disorders (one with panic disorder and one with generalized anxiety disorder), seen at relatively infrequent intervals and treated primarily with medication, also were not diagnosed on axis II. This illustrates the significant point, to which I shall return later, that when the principal mode of treatment is exploratory psychotherapy, personality factors assume major importance. This is, of course, also true for those axis I disorders treated primarily with psychotherapy, in which case the therapist quickly becomes concerned with the personality attributes of the patient and thus is likely to add an axis II diagnosis.

Table 33.1 shows my estimation of the severities of the conditions I was treating (5 at grade 1, 21 at grade 2, and 7 at grade 3). I believe this has some usefulness for diagnostic purposes. The one patient for whom there was a significant axis III item suffered from a carcinoma that affected her psychological functioning. I made no effort to undertake axis IV or V ratings. I question the reliability of the criteria used for these axes. Also, the process of assessing the strengths and weaknesses of patients and the environmental forces impinging on them is so intrinsic to evaluation and treatment as to render artificial its separation out in formal diagnostic terms.

Table 33.2 is a tabulation of all axis I diagnoses (including 799.90 for the patient I was unable to diagnose). Although I treat patients with primary affective and schizophrenic disorders, none were under my care during the three months included in the survey. The diagnoses include a fair sprinkling of other conditions, with a predominance of adjustment and psychosexual disorders (9 each). It will be noted that I have included five V-code diagnoses. In one case this was the only diagnosis made. In the others, although I may not have been strictly following the rules (the presence of a mental disorder presumably would rule out a V-code diagnosis), I believed that these designations had some usefulness in indicating the reasons for which the patients had consulted me and the changes they hoped for as a result of treatment.

Although making these axis I diagnoses sometimes created uncertainty in my mind, on the whole I found the criteria for them reasonably satisfactory and applicable. They seem to answer satisfactorily the stated purpose of *DSM-III*, to diagnose the conditions from which individuals suffer, rather than the individuals themselves. In addition to their role in pointing to treatment decisions, at times the power of these diagnoses to organize a symptom picture was helpful. Thus, a young woman described certain distressing complaints that at first sounded depressive or possibly delusional. On listening further, it became apparent that these were depersonalization symptoms and that she suffered from the rather rare depersonalization disorder. This realization was reassuring and enabled me to make a satisfactory disposition of her case. However, when significant personality factors intrude on the relatively firm ground of axis I diagnosis, the judgment becomes less clear. Thus, one patient flattered my diagnostic acumen by offering the probability that he was suffering from a major affective disorder as a complication of antihypertensive medication. He responded to tricyclic medication and reassurance, but then, as his depressive symptoms were succeeded by demoralization, isolation, and a fear of returning to work, he revealed himself as a superficially affable schizoid personality, and I became somewhat less confident about my original diagnosis.

In view of the close relationship between medical diagnosis and treatment planning, we may ask how useful these axis I diagnoses were for this purpose. The well-trained psychiatric practitioner today has a number of options and is not restricted either to automatic prescription of insight-oriented psychother-

Table 33.2. *Axis I diagnoses (including V codes)*

Diagnosis	Code	No.
Substance-induced disorders	292.84	1
Substance-use disorders	305.6	1
	305.2	1
Affective disorders	300.40	3
Anxiety disorders	300.01	1
	300.02	1
	300.30	1
Dissociative disorders	300.60	1
Psychosexual disorders		
Psychosexual dysfunctions	302.74	2
	302.75	1
	302.71	1
Paraphilias	302.83	2
Other psychosexual disorders	302.00	3
Adjustment disorder	309.00	7
	309.28	2
V codes	V61.10	1
	V62.20	2
	V62.81	2
Additional codes	799.90	1

apy, as was true of a previous generation, or, one may hope, to automatic drug prescription. I have found that selection among these options is facilitated by reference to axis I criteria and the experience that has been garnered from their application. Thus, I referred one case to a sex therapist for consideration of his inhibited orgasm and recently (not during the three-month period being audited) have also referred two patients with fairly specific phobic disorders for behavioral therapy.

I have found some weaknesses in axis I. I am not comfortable with the controversial dysthymic disorder (in fairness, I was also often dissatisfied with the *DSM-II* depressive neurosis). The criteria for this condition are difficult to

Table 33.3. *Axis II diagnoses*

Diagnosis	Code	No.
Schizoid	301.20	1
Schizotypal	301.22	1
Histrionic	301.50	1
Narcissistic	301.81	2
Borderline	301.83	1
Compulsive	301.40	3
Avoidant	301.82	1
Atypical, mixed, or other personality disorder	301.89	17

apply. They often merge into those not uncommon characterological depressions that need to be distinguished from any variety of primary affective disorders.

I also have some doubts about the criteria for the famous 302.00 diagnosis: ego-dystonic homosexuality. In my fairly considerable experience with male homosexual patients, acceptance and rejection of their sexual orientation usually are far too complexly intertwined to allow for any easy distinction between syntonic and dystonic attitudes.

Table 33.3 lists the 27 axis II diagnoses made for the 34 patients seen during the index period. I have already indicated that greater knowledge of some of the patients seen in consultation might have increased this number. It also might have been increased, as is discussed later, if a different decision had been made with regard to the level at which personality difficulties that are the focus of treatment become a personality disorder. Patients with personality difficulties and with formal personality disorders compose the bulk of my psychotherapeutic practice (Chodoff, 1982), and I believe this to be true also of my colleagues with similar practices (Gedo, 1979). It is in connection with making axis II diagnoses that adequately label these patients and differentiate them from each other that *DSM-III* faces a considerable challenge, and it is to the problems posed by personality diagnosis that I devote the remainder of my discussion.

A glance at Table 33.3 demonstrates immediately that although I could make a variety of specific personality disorder diagnoses by employing axis II criteria, in the majority of these patients (17 as opposed to 10) I had to affix the label 301.89: atypical, mixed, or other personality disorder.

Why was I driven to this somewhat unsatisfactory expedient, and why did I find axis II diagnoses substantially harder to establish than axis I diagnoses? Psychiatric diagnosis in general faces difficulties not present with the diagnosis of medical and surgical conditions, which often can be made on the basis of more objective criteria than those available for psychiatric disorders. These depend largely on different varieties of observable behavior. Axis II diagnosis adds additional uncertainties and ambiguities. These problems are of two kinds.

First, at what level does a personality distortion, one, say, responsible for a persistent conflict with authority figures, become severe enough to receive a 301 designation? We are told that a personality disorder should be diagnosed only when personality traits are "inflexible and maladaptive and cause either significant impairment in social or occupational functioning or subjective stress." A determination of this kind is clearly a judgment call on the part of the diagnosing psychiatrist. One must find one's way within a large gray area with difficult distinctions between "normalcy" and significant personality distortion, and between the latter and personality disorder. Let me cite some illustrative cases. A young man found himself unable to make a decision whether or not to commit himself to the young woman with whom he was living. He was seriously concerned about this dilemma. It loomed large in his current life and had serious implications for his future. There was no question that his indecisiveness was related to prior determining influences stemming from his developmental history, and thus it was not totally rational, but had a psychopathological component. On the other hand, he was not significantly anxious or depressed; he functioned quite adequately and was a well-put-together individual. Did the presence of a rather consistent psychopathological pattern warrant a 301.89 diagnosis? I decided not, and left him entirely with a V-code diagnosis.

In two other instances, also with V-code entries into treatment, the situation was similar. In both, there was a somewhat greater degree of subjective distress and the responsible psychopathological patterns were more entrenched and of greater scope. With these patients I used the 301.89 designation, but as can be seen, the degree of confidence with which I made these diagnostic judgments was not of a high order.

The reality here, of course, is that nobody is perfect. H. S. Sullivan said that we are all more simply human than otherwise. To be human is to be imperfect. None of us functions in a conflict-free realm, a state not only impossible of achievement but also impossible of consensual definition. If present, such a state would be inhuman. I want to say emphatically that this does not mean that the patients I am describing were not in need of psychotherapeutic attention. They were, and they could benefit from it. The patient I described earlier to whom I gave only a V-code designation got substantial help for a significant problem.

Although the patients I have described constitute a troubling conceptual problem for psychiatric nosology, I do not want to exaggerate their frequency. The defects of most of those who come to my office because of personality malfunctioning are severe enough to satisfy comfortably the overall criteria for inclusion in *DSM-III* personality disorders. Here, however, we are faced with the second area of difficulty in utilizing axis II. As can be seen by the preponderance of 301.89 diagnoses, it is no easy matter to place people suffering from significant personality distortions within the other 11 listed 301 designations. I personally believe that some of these diagnoses are more satisfactory than others. Particularly the avoidant and passive-aggressive disorders seem to constitute rather meager descriptions of one particular trait in an individual's makeup. As such, they are not as comprehensive and satisfactory as the more rounded and inclusive aggregate of characteristics that define, say, the compulsive, the histrionic, and the narcissistic disorders. But the relative strengths and weaknesses of these disorders is only part, and the less serious part, of the problem. For human nature is quantitative, not qualitative, as far as personality attributes are concerned. The ingredients going into the personality soup are generally the same, although, there are marked differences in the proportions in which these ingredients are distributed. The spectrum of psychopathology has an analogy in the visible spectrum of light. That we designate particular colors at particular wavelengths does not at all mean that there are not other colors with or without specific names at other points in the wavelength continuum. In a similar manner, certain patients will demonstrate a cluster of qualities that enables us, with a reasonable degree of confidence, to designate them as, say, schizoid or paranoid. Unfortunately, and more frequently, the qualities defining an individual's psychopathological state will overlap with and merge with the qualities descriptive of another personality disorder, or will not in fact fit any of them. Occasionally this difficulty can be surmounted by making more than one personality disorder diagnosis. This was done in case 4, a patient who suffered from both compulsive and schizotypal personality disorders. Often, however, this is not possible, and the attempt to do so is a futile denial of the impossibility of extracting some kind of order from what may be a personality chaos. As an example, I understand that at St. Elizabeth's Hospital, John Hinckley has been given four different personality diagnoses.

I have indicated that, in my practice, axis I diagnoses satisfied reasonably well the *DSM* purpose of designating the condition rather than the person. That this cannot be done nearly so readily for axis II adds another complexity to the problem of personality diagnosis. In cases that fall within this purview, we often find ourselves trying to describe the person rather than the condition. This process confronts us with the puzzling and humbling need to acknowledge that sometimes the more one knows about a person, the harder it is to diagnose the person. A principal reason that psychotherapeutic practitioners may find it difficult to adhere to the *DSM-III* intent in this regard is the connection to which I have already alluded between personality disorders and psychotherapy.

Certain therapeutic implications flow from an axis I diagnosis as we choose among psychotherapy, drugs, ECT, and behavioral or sex therapy. However, when a label of personality disorder is applied to a patient in my practice, the prescription is usually for psychotherapy, sometimes supportive in nature, but often insight-oriented. There are, of course, exceptions: I use psychotropic drugs in a supplementary fashion when necessary in a minority of these cases, and in the course of treating one borderline-personality patient it was necessary to hospitalize her nine times in two years. And there are those who would accord drugs a more primary role in some 301 disorders. Thus, MAOIs have been advocated for the avoidant personality disorder (Klein et al., 1980). But for the large majority of 301 cases seen in practices like mine, the equation between personality disorder and psychotherapy is relevant. With many of the axis I diagnoses, psychotherapy is also indicated, but in these instances the personality aspects of the individual responsible for the particular symptomatic state come to the fore, and, as I have suggested, they may then receive an additional axis II diagnosis. Thus, whenever psychotherapy is the indicated modality, interest focuses on the individual psychodynamics and the personality makeup of the patient. Such an interest is, in a sense, diametrically opposed to the usual diagnostic concern to make class distinctions by finding the commonalities in certain states. To apply psychotherapy satisfactorily, we want to know not so much what makes people alike, but rather what makes them different, what makes them individuals. This endeavor requires not so much a medical diagnosis, but rather a formulation, a psychodynamic and psychogenetic understanding of what makes that particular patient tick. When we look at patients in this way, with so detailed a scrutiny, the details we unearth make it difficult to assume the somewhat more distant posture that facilitates the forest-over-trees judgment enabling a particular personality disorder diagnosis.

Personality diagnosis in "medical" terms thus is of limited usefulness for psychotherapeutic prescription. This limitation and the failure to distinguish between medical diagnosis and psychodynamic formulation have led to some of the dissatisfaction of psychoanalysts with *DSM-III*. An appreciation of the diagnosis–formulation distinction would be helpful in resolving some of these objections, but certain troubling, probably structural, incompatibilities about the application of essentially medical criteria to personality diagnosis will remain.

Granting these intrinsic difficulties in personality diagnoses for *DSM-III* purposes, I believe that measures can be taken to improve their reliability and usefulness. One corrective step would be to acknowledge that, for whatever reason, we have been perhaps too global in our ambitions to find a medical diagnosis for every applicant for our services, particularly when those services are psychotherapeutic. I would like here to quote from an article by an English observer of *DSM-III:*

It might have been wiser to admit that DSM-III, like most other psychiatric classifications, is not really a classification of mental disorders at all. It is a classification of the problems psychiatrists are consulted about; and if in practice shy adolescents and surly teenagers come, or are brought, to see psychiatrists, then an appropriate pigeonhole must be found for them. But it should not be assumed that just because a consultation has taken place, a mental disorder is necessarily present. [Kendell, 1980]

Psychiatry is not the only branch of medicine to have this problem. There is reason to believe that a substantial number of patients of internists and family practitioners present themselves for purposes other than treatment of medical illnesses. That psychiatrists have difficulty in accepting that this is true also for a minority of psychiatric patients may be evidence of a certain defensiveness about the extent to which psychiatric patients conform to the medical model. Most of them do, but some do not, and we should acknowledge this. One consequence of such acknowledgment would be to free the framers of *DSM-III* or of a future *DSM-IV* from the necessity of finding a name for the problems of everyone who consults a psychiatrist. It would also confer legitimacy on people who come to us for what can be called problems in living. Here, like the young man described in my previous vignette, I designate individuals whose psycho-pathological patterns, exerting adverse effects on their comfort and relation-ships and requiring skilled psychotherapeutic attention, do not constitute a per-sonality aberration so severe as to be considered a disorder. An unapologetic resort to V-code labels for such cases might clear the air.

Another way in which personality diagnosis may be improved is by introduc-ing a measure of severity, as in the Table 33.1 ranking of patients on a severity scale. To return to the analogy between the spectrum of psychopathology and the spectrum of visible light, colors differ not only in wavelength but also in intensity. Although we do not have a measure so specific as the square of the amplitude of the wavelength to determine intensity in psychopathology, the judgment of the therapist about the severity of the condition being treated should be reasonably reliable. It should introduce a useful element into person-ality diagnosis, possibly also in some axis I instances. If it were judged that good reasons exist to adhere as closely as possible to medical-model considerations, I could envisage 301.89 diagnoses at the lowest level of severity to be another way of including the problems-in-living category that I have described. Inci-dentally, it seems to me that Otto Kernberg's work (1967) in equating the bor-derline personality disorders with levels of organization rather than with partic-ular clusters of symptoms is a step in this direction.

The use of personality-trait designations rather than disorder designations is another possibility already present in *DSM-III* to increase diagnostic flexibility with regard to the less severe personality aberrations. This device might have value in making more complete certain axis I diagnoses. However, choosing among traits would run into the same difficulties as choosing among disorders. Furthermore, for patients presenting because of personality problems, an exclu-sive trait designation would not constitute a diagnosis.

Another ambitious approach to improving the specificity of axis II diagnoses (as well as of *DSM-III* diagnosis generally) is being undertaken by some psy-choanalysts who are, for various reasons, dissatisfied with the diagnostic scheme. By penetrating below the level of observable behavior, as with the use of patho-logical findings in medical and surgical diagnosis, they suggest basing class dis-tinctions among psychiatric disorders on psychopathological rather than behav-ioral commonalities. The establishment of patterns and hierarchies of ego defenses, as suggested by Vaillant and Drake (1985), and certain characteristic pathological psychodynamic patterns could replace the more observable but overlapping behavior phenotypes for purposes of classification. This effort can be seen as a more sophisticated reworking of the early Freud–Abraham classi-fication of mental illness in terms of stages of psychosexual development. These psychoanalytic attempts are interesting and certainly to be encouraged. Person-ally, I believe that they will run into difficulties, for two reasons. First, I suspect that psychopathological patterns and defense structure will prove to be even more overlapping and nonspecific than observable behavior. Second, I suspect that making diagnoses on the basis of such criteria will be beyond the capacity of some psychiatrists and will require, at best, rather prolonged evaluation.

On the more immediately practical level, I believe that personality diagnosis can be improved by eliminating or consolidating some of the present designations and also by introducing others. I have already indicated my dissatisfaction with passive-aggressive and avoidant personality patterns as being each too thin to bear the weight of specific diagnoses. I would retain the other 301 entities now in use, but I believe additional ones could be introduced with profit. For instance, it would be helpful to have criteria, under the name of the masochistic personality disorder, for those individuals who persistently find ways to spoil and take no satisfaction in anything good that happens to them, for whom behavior akin to the negative therapeutic reaction is characteristic, and who seem perversely to glory in their misery. There are also people (including, as I have suggested, some with the diagnosis of dysthymic disorder) who could usefully bear the designation of depressive personality. Otto Kernberg (1981) has also suggested criteria for a putative masochistic-depressive rubric. Another possibility is immature or infantile personality, which incidentally might include some of those patients now diagnosed as having passive-aggressive personality disorders. This designation, additionally, might sharpen the criteria for histrionic personality disorder and eliminate some of the confusion between "oral" hysterics and borderlines. I am aware that there may be practical difficulties in introducing new personality disorders because of the need to remain cognate with *ICD-9*, but if these difficulties can be surmounted, I believe that practical and helpful improvements can be made in axis II.

I close with a few remarks about the general utility of *DSM-III* for a practitioner like myself. I have already discussed the applicability of the manual to treatment prescription and its limitation with regard to patients for whom psychotherapy is the main treatment modality. However, this limitation certainly is not absolute. The harvest of articles on psychotherapeutic treatment of the compulsive, histrionic, borderline, and narcissistic personality disorders indicates that there is some prescriptive purpose in establishing criteria for these conditions and thus providing a focus for the gathering of data on treatment methods.

But diagnosis has other purposes than therapeutic prescription. It provides a shorthand for discussion with our colleagues, labels for hospital and third-person records, and data for research on the causes, incidences, and prognoses for the conditions we treat. If we have aspirations to scientific as well as professional status, we need ways of ordering the data that come into our ken, and although it has weaknesses and can be improved, *DSM-III* represents the current state of the art as far as psychiatric diagnosis is concerned.

Finally, a nonspecific advantage of the promulgation of *DSM-III* is the way in which it has introduced a veritable firestorm of discussion and controversy into the field. It has opened up a cleansing debate about many areas within the psychiatric universe that previously had been passed over with silence or rationalizations.

REFERENCES

Chodoff P: Assessment of psychotherapy. Arch Gen Psychiatry 39:1097–1103, 1982

Gedo J: A psychoanalyst reports at mid-career. Am J Psychiatry 136:646–649, 1979

Kendell RE: DSM-III: a British perspective. Am J Psychiatry 137:1630–1631, 1980

Kernberg O: Borderline personality organization. J Am Psychoanal Assoc 15:641–685, 1967

    Problems in the classification of personality disorders. Presented at Clinical Grand Rounds, New York Hospital, Cornell Medical Center, Westchester Division, September 11, 1981

Klein DF, Gittelman R, Quitkin F, et al: Diagnosis and Drug Treatment of Psychiatric Disorders: Adults and Children, second edition. Baltimore, Williams & Wilkins, 1980

Vaillant GE, Drake RE: Maturity of ego defenses in relation to DSM-III axis II personality disorders. Arch Gen Psychiatry 42:597–601, 1985

34 *Applicability of DSM-III to psychiatric education*

RICHARD C. SIMONS

The topic that I discuss involves the applicability of *DSM-III* (American Psychiatric Association, 1980) to psychiatric education. Although psychiatric education is a broad field, from undergraduate courses on college campuses to postgraduate courses for practicing physicians and mental-health professionals, I limit my remarks to the two groups of students with whom I have had the most contact: medical students and psychiatric residents. Because systematic evaluations of the use of *DSM-III* in psychiatric education are still in their beginning stages (Webb et al., 1981; Williams, Spitzer, and Skodol, 1985), and because ultimate assessment of the meanings of those data will no doubt be quite difficult and complex, I present here only my own personal impressions and observations – with all limitations of such an approach. I do not attempt to discuss all of the various advantages and disadvantages of *DSM-III*. These have been eloquently addressed by others, most notably by Klerman and Spitzer on one side and by Vaillant and Michels on the other side at the May 1982 annual meeting of the American Psychiatric Association in Toronto (Klerman et al., 1984). I restrict myself only to the positive and negative effects of *DSM-III* that I have seen thus far in the education of medical students and psychiatric residents.

POSITIVE EFFECTS OF *DSM-III* ON PSYCHIATRIC EDUCATION

To my mind, the single most important contribution of *DSM-III* to psychiatric education is the multiaxial classification (Frances and Cooper, 1981), which explicitly asks the medical student and the psychiatric resident to

The initial version of this chapter was presented at the conference on "*DSM-III:* An Interim Appraisal," sponsored by the Committee to Evaluate *DSM-III*, held at Washington, D.C., October 13–15, 1983. A revised version was presented at the panel on "Psychoanalytic Contributions to Psychiatric Nosology" held at the spring meeting of the American Psychoanalytic Association, Denver, Colorado, May 16–19, 1985 and published in the *Journal of the American Psychoanalytic Association,* Volume 35, 1987.

evaluate the multiple factors that need to be taken into consideration in the diagnostic assessment of every psychiatric patient:

1. the clinical syndrome that may be present (axis I),
2. the personality disorder or specific developmental disorder that may also be present (axis II),
3. the physical disorders and conditions that may be present (axis III),
4. the presence and severity of any psychosocial stressors (axis IV),
5. the highest level of adaptive functioning during the past year (axis V).

All of us – but I think especially the beginning medical student and the beginning psychiatric resident – are sometimes overly eager to find the single all-encompassing diagnosis that will sum up and explain the bewildering interaction of psychopathology and strength in any given patient. That is one reason, in my opinion, for the almost epidemic popularity of the diagnosis of borderline personality disorder in recent years (see Chapter 17). It seems to cover so much, and yet on closer examination that diagnosis may not accurately identify the clinical syndrome that may be present (e.g., an affective disorder), or the mixture of personality traits or even personality disorders that may be present, or the creative and adaptive assets that may also exist in certain areas of functioning. With its multiaxial classification, *DSM-III* asks the student to move away from the easy but ultimately dehumanizing catchall of single and simplistic diagnostic labels and to consider instead the much more complex but also much more uniquely human assessment of multiple levels of psychopathology, personality structure, physical condition, environmental stress, and adaptive functioning.

A survey of 214 directors of residency training in this country conducted by Williams and associates (1985) on the impact of *DSM-III* on residency training suggests that in this relatively short period of time we may already be seeing a more comprehensive approach to patient evaluation through the use of the multiaxial system. Whatever ambiguities may exist within and between the various axes, I believe that our task as educators should be to support and strengthen the multiaxial system, and valuable recommendations (see Chapters 26 and 29) have already been made in this regard as part of the process of evaluating and revising *DSM-III*.

The other invaluable contribution of *DSM-III* to psychiatric education is the one that has already been widely recognized and discussed (Kendell, 1980; Spitzer, Williams, and Skodol, 1980), namely, the attempt to place psychiatric diagnosis on a sound descriptive basis, hopefully with increasing precision and specificity and reliability of the operational criteria for each mental disorder. The survey by Williams and associates (1985) previously cited suggests a number of highly positive effects on residency training from this emphasis on operational criteria. Of the 97% responding to the questionnaire, over 80% reported that *DSM-III* "facilitates learning basic elements of psychopathology," "encourages residents to pay attention to specific patient behaviors," "offers a common language for diagnostic discussions," and "helps in formulating differential diagnoses."

However, this second contribution of *DSM-III* to psychiatric education may paradoxically be working against the first contribution of the multiaxial system. At least that has been my experience and the experience of a number of my colleagues. It is now not uncommon for some medical students and psychiatric residents to become so preoccupied with the lists of diagnostic criteria in *DSM-III* that the latter becomes quite literally their textbook of psychiatry, despite Spitzer's warning that " . . . DSM-III is not a textbook, since it does not include information about theories of etiology, management and treatment. It should also be noted that the DSM-III classification of mental disorders does not attempt to classify disturbed dyadic, family, or other interpersonal relationships" (American Psychiatric Association, 1980, p. 9).

NEGATIVE EFFECTS OF *DSM-III* ON PSYCHIATRIC EDUCATION

There is also evidence for this negative educational effect of *DSM-III* in the survey by Williams and associates (1985). Over 50% of the respondents to the questionnaire reported that *DSM-III* "focuses on signs and symptoms so much that it detracts from a more in-depth understanding of patients' problems," "gives the false impression that our understanding of mental disorders is more complete than it actually is," and "promotes a mechanistic cookbook approach to assessing patients." I do not believe that the authors of *DSM-III* intended for this to happen. In fact, in the Introduction to *DSM-III*, Spitzer made the following statement:

A common misconception is that a classification of mental disorders classifies individuals, when actually what are being classified are disorders that individuals have. . . . Another misconception is that all individuals described as having the same mental disorder are alike in all important ways. Although all the individuals described as having the same mental disorder show at least the defining features of the disorder, they may well differ in other important ways that may affect clinical management and outcome. [American Psychiatric Association, 1980, p. 6]

Nevertheless, an appreciation of the uniqueness of the individual patient and the various ways in which that patient attempts to integrate complex levels of adaptive and maladaptive functioning (an appreciation that should come about through consistent use of the multiaxial system) is not always gained. And what happens instead in case write-ups and in clinical presentations by the beginning student may be a chillingly fragmented and impersonal listing of diagnostic details in a patient who is not only nameless but also faceless and personless. It is as though Spitzer's admonition is ignored, and instead Schopenhauer's warning is reenacted: "When the counting begins, the understanding stops." In their review of *DSM-III*, Cooper and Michels (1981, p. 128) predicted

... that *DSM-III* will be difficult to teach, particularly to students who have had little clinical experience or personal familiarity with psychiatric patients.... Although the individual categories in *DSM-III* may be descriptively valuable, the beginning student may find that he or she is trying to remember details and lists without simple rules of organization.

In part, their prediction may already be coming true for an entire generation of students. But I also believe that *DSM-III* holds out the promise of truly advancing and stimulating psychiatric education for medical students and psychiatric residents by asking them to first observe *what* the various struggles are that seem to be occurring in the lives of their patients, as reflected in specific symptoms and behaviors (the descriptive model), before prematurely leaping to various theories that attempt to explain *how* those symptoms occur (the dynamic model) or *why* they came to be (the developmental-genetic model) (Table 34.1).

THE DATA OF UNCONSCIOUS MENTAL FUNCTIONING

When I try to make a case come alive for a student using the *DSM-III* criteria, I find myself confronted with what I believe to be the single most fundamental failing of *DSM-III*: the failure to consistently view the data of unconscious mental functioning as descriptive data without which it is impossible to make a complete diagnostic assessment of any patient, rather than as data that are synonymous with certain psychodynamic and psychoanalytic theories regarding the etiology of various clinical syndromes and personality disorders. I would once again agree with Cooper and Michels: " ... the concept of unconscious conflict is not merely the province of a special theoretical view. Furthermore, the ubiquity of unconscious conflict makes clear that it should be considered descriptive rather than etiologic" (1981, p. 129). Dreams provide an example par excellence of ubiquitous, universal unconscious mental functioning. But that does not mean that the dream state can be causally explained solely on the basis of unconscious conflict or regression to the primary process. Neurophysiological mechanisms and neurochemical transactions must also be taken into consideration. Multiple personalities, fugue and amnesic states, hypnotic phenomena, slips of the tongue, and other parapraxes are further dramatic examples of unconscious mental functioning. But, once again, one would have to look beyond unconscious psychodynamic factors to causally explain any of these various behaviors. To return again to the multiaxial classification, how can recent adaptive functioning be assessed or even described without taking into consideration unconscious personality traits, unconscious mechanisms of defense and coping style, and unconscious patterns of perception, cognition,

Table 34.1. *Evaluation of the psychiatric patient*

Models	Descriptive	Dynamic	Developmental-genetic
Biological	*Physical exam* Current physical strengths Current physical disorders or conditions (*DSM-III* axis III)	Biological factors in mental illness	History of genetic and other constitutional factors History of physical illness, injuries, operations, medications
Psychological	*Mental-status exam* Current psychological strengths and adaptive functioning (*DSM-III* axis V) Presence of one or more mental disorders (*DSM-III* axis I and axis II)	Psychodynamic factors in mental illness Learning factors in mental illness	Developmental factors and experiences in infancy, childhood, adolescence, and adulthood
Sociocultural	*Life setting* Current psychosocial supports (*DSM-III* axis V) Current psychosocial stressors (*DSM-III* axis IV)	Sociocultural factors in mental illness	Family history Racial, religious, cultural, and socioeconomic background

Source: Simons (1985, p. 539), by permission of Williams & Wilkins.

and learning? I would submit that all of these data belong to what Waelder (1962) has called the primary level of clinical observation, not to the other levels of inference that are more removed from the observational data (i.e., the levels of clinical interpretation, clinical generalization, clinical theory, and metapsychology).

I recognize that there will be many who will disagree with this position and claim that the assumption of unconscious mental functioning represents a level of inference beyond the observational data, indeed, one that has not yet achieved consistent interrater reliability. The incorporation of an outline for case formulation as an appendix in *DSM-III*, as recommended by Spitzer and Williams (see Chapter 26), might help to begin to move us toward such reliability in the assessment of unconscious data. So also might Vaillant's proposal (see Chapter 30) for an additional axis in *DSM-III* or a glossary of defense mechanisms that would attempt to assess an individual's predominant coping styles and psychological response patterns.

It is not that *DSM-III* has failed totally to view the data of unconscious mental functioning as descriptive data that exist at the level of clinical observation. But the acceptance by *DSM-III* of such data as part of its diagnostic criteria is so clearly begrudging, as in the case of conversion disorder, and so obviously neglected with many other disorders, that the overall result is quite puzzling. As W. C. Fields said in describing a certain city that shall remain unidentified: "It's not too hot. It's not too cold. It's too medium." I would hope that eventually unconscious mental functioning can be accepted in our psychiatric nosology without the implication of adherence to any of Freud's psychoanalytic theories, just as the acceptance of reinforcement and avoidance-reaction patterns should be possible without the implication of adherence to any of Skinner's behavioral theories. Or, to take another example of a process that is present both in normal development (self–object differentiation) and in certain pathological conditions (borderline personality disorder), surely the mechanism of projective identification can be described without the implication of adherence to any of the theories of Melanie Klein, Kernberg, or Kohut. In general, I am in agreement with the efforts of the authors of *DSM-III* to be atheoretical in regard to etiology. But being appropriately humble about our lack of certainty in regard to the multiple causes of many, if not all, of the mental disorders does not require taking a narrow and restricted view of the observational data that will be necessary to advance our knowledge. Nor does it require sacrificing clinical validity and clinical relevance on the altar of interrater reliability.

I now attempt to support this basic criticism of *DSM-III* by presenting a concept (i.e., masochism) that has been discussed at all of the levels of inference that Waelder has delineated: the levels of clinical observation, clinical interpretation, clinical generalization, clinical theory, and metapsychology. I hope to demonstrate that the concept of masochism has diagnostic and clinical relevance at the level of clinical observation, entirely apart from its meaning and importance at any of the other levels of inference. I then try to demonstrate the extension of that diagnostic and clinical relevance in two conditions of great interest to medical students and psychiatric residents, namely, anorexia nervosa and the somatoform disorders.

FORMS OF MASOCHISTIC BEHAVIOR

To begin my discussion of the various forms of masochistic behavior, I first turn to Freud's seminal paper, "The Economic Problem of Masochism" (Freud, 1924). In that paper, Freud described three forms of masochism: erotogenic masochism, feminine masochism, and moral masochism. To read that paper is both illuminating and disturbing – illuminating because of Freud's rich clinical observations of various masochistic phenomena, disturbing because of Freud's repetitive weaving back and forth between all of the levels of inference described by Waelder without his making clear distinctions at any given point

Forms of Masochistic Behavior

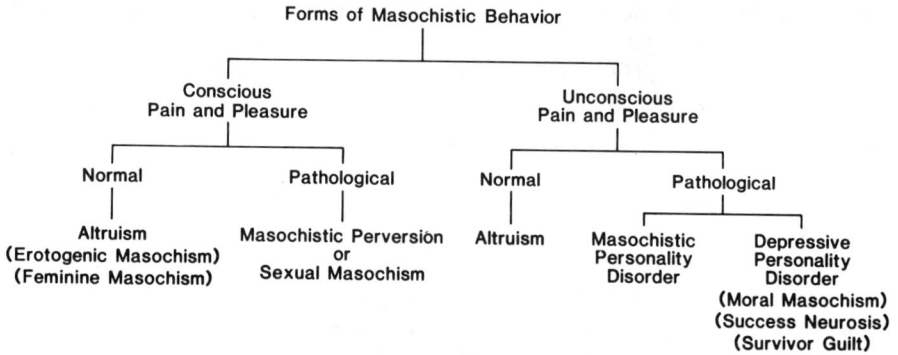

Figure 34.1. Forms of masochistic behavior. Copyright 1983 by Richard C. Simons.

between one level and the other. At the level of metapsychology, Freud attributes the origins of masochism to his metapsychological concepts of the death instinct, the repetition compulsion, the constancy principle, and the Nirvana principle. At the level of clinical theory, he explains certain forms of masochism as regressions away from the oedipal conflict and toward earlier anal-sadistic fixations. At the level of clinical generalization, he implies that masochistic phenomena have a higher incidence among women than among men. And at the level of clinical interpretation, he attributes other forms of masochism as being due to a libidinization of suffering and a reinstinctualization of aggression in the relationship between the ego and superego. No wonder that there is so little mention of masochism anywhere throughout *DSM-III!*

However, if one accepts a distinction between conscious mental functioning and unconscious mental functioning at the level of clinical observation, then masochism, in my opinion, should occupy a much more significant place in *DSM-III,* because I am convinced that masochistic phenomena are among the most common that we encounter in our psychiatric practices – and are among the most commonly overlooked and misdiagnosed. And I believe that this can be done without necessarily adhering to any of Freud's interpretations, generalizations, theories, or metapsychological speculations about masochism. Recognizing at the onset that there is a good deal of overlap with mixed clinical pictures among the various forms of masochistic behavior that I am about to describe, and recognizing also that the terms "normal" and "pathological" represent relative concepts that always exist on a continuum, nevertheless I believe that masochistic behavior can be usefully separated into behavior in which there is a predominantly conscious link between pleasure and pain, and behavior in which that link is predominantly unconscious. Furthermore, I believe that both forms of masochistic behavior exist in a normal form and a pathological form (Figure 34.1).

We see normal masochistic behavior that is conscious at every stage of development, where the conscious pleasure of advancement and individuation is accompanied by the conscious pain of loss and separation, and where the pleasures of certain impulses and wishes have to be painfully disavowed in order for other pleasures and gratifications to be achieved. This might be one somewhat broader way of viewing Freud's category of erotogenic masochism, which Loewenstein (1957, p. 226) also described rather broadly as a "fundamental property of the human mind, of experiencing as pleasurable some painful processes." Loewenstein also offered a more drive-oriented definition of erotogenic masochism:

In its individual development the aggressive drive is very closely bound up with the libidinal development. During this development, both active and passive forms of these fused drives manifest themselves. Thus the passive forms, i.e., the erotogenic masochism, according to the stage of libidinal development, take on the shape of the wish (or fear): to be devoured, to be beaten, to be castrated. [Loewenstein, 1957, p. 226]

I would add, in the case of the little girl, to be genitally penetrated and mutilated rather than castrated.

Freud's category of feminine masochism could be subsumed here as well, provided that by that confusing and often misleading term one referred only to those *normal* psychosexual experiences in the life of a woman in which consciously experienced pleasure is linked with consciously experienced pain or discomfort (i.e., menarche and possibly some subsequent menses, first intercourse if the hymen is still intact, and childbirth). There are no such unique and ubiquitous psychosexual experiences in the life of a man in which consciously experienced pleasure and gratification are so predictably and causally linked with consciously experienced pain or discomfort. However, if by the term "feminine masochism" one implies that the character structure of women is inherently masochistic in a pathological sense, then I would strongly disagree. Blum (1976), Bernstein (1983), and others have already written about this issue from the perspective of psychoanalytic theory, as has Caplan (1985) from a feminist perspective. In my own clinical experience, I find masochistic behavior and masochistic personality traits to be just as common among men as among women, despite the fact that such behavior and traits are unfortunately diagnosed far more frequently in women than in men. The same is true in my clinical experience for histrionic behavior and histrionic personality traits.

Finally, I believe that altruism that is consciously directed could be considered as still another form of normal masochistic behavior in which pain and sacrifice and possibly even death are consciously accepted in return for the gratification of living (and possibly dying) for something or someone beyond oneself. Clearly, all of the foregoing assumes that we have accepted the phenomenon of masochism (the coexistence of pain and pleasure) as normal and universal and have moved away from the pejorative but common assumption that masochism is inevitably pathological. We need to remind ourselves that precisely the same holds true for the phenomenon of narcissism – that it exists in both conscious and unconscious forms, as well as in both normal and pathological forms. Hillel captured more succinctly than anyone the essence of both healthy narcissism and healthy masochism in the form of altruism: "If I am not for myself, who will be? But if I am for myself alone, what am I? And if not now, when?"

There is, of course, a pathological form of masochistic behavior in which there is a conscious link between explicitly *sexual* pleasure on the one hand and pain and suffering on the other, and *DSM-III* indeed does justice to this disorder (Figure 34.1). Prior to *DSM-III*, it was known as masochistic perversion. With *DSM-III*, it is listed among the paraphilias as sexual masochism. Much could be said about this disorder, in which conscious pain and suffering are necessary conditions for the individual to be able to achieve conscious sexual arousal and orgasm. It is a disorder that probably is more common than we realize, but that discussion would take us too far afield.

What is not too far afield is the one sentence that *DSM-III* devotes to unconscious masochistic behavior. On page 274, under the discussion of sexual masochism, the following sentence appears: "Masochistic personality traits, such as the need to be disappointed or humiliated, are distinguished from Sexual Masochism by the fact that they are not associated with sexual excitement." The statement is true as far as it goes, but that is my whole point: It does not go far enough, and in failing to do so, it leaves behind an entire population of patients who occupy our medical clinics, our hospital wards, our psychiatric outpatient offices, and, yes, even our analytic couches. It is not just that masochistic personality traits are "not associated with" sexual excitement. The more central distinction is that the link between pleasure and pain has become unconscious and no longer explicitly sexual, and this is a much more active and specific and pathological process than is indicated by the words "not associated with."

What are the consequences for *DSM-III* of the failure to make this crucial distinction? It is possible that in some forms of altruism the link between pleasure and pain is predominantly unconscious (Figure 34.1). Although this may have significance for a broad theoretical understanding of masochism, what is more relevant for our discussion here is the existence of a pathological masochism in which the link between pain and pleasure has become unconscious rather than conscious (Figure 34.1). I believe that there are at least two diagnostic categories that can be clinically distinguished from each other, and I believe these distinctions have important therapeutic and prognostic implications. In the masochistic personality disorder – in my opinion a very common condition in either pure form or mixed with other personality disturbances – the inner struggle is externalized and then acted out with the external world. This is the individual whose provocative behavior tortures and blackmails others and eventually leads to retaliation in one form or another. These are the chronic and perpetual "victims" who are not aware of their repetitive activities in maintaining a victimized role. I emphasize "repetitive" to distinguish these individuals from the tragically large number of people in our society (most of them children and women) who are truly trapped in a victimized role from which they are unable to extricate themselves because of social, economic, religious, or psychological reasons. Not infrequently, these victims of spouse abuse or child abuse are realistically afraid of even greater violence or physical harm if they try to seek help or leave their victimized situations. To mindlessly call such individuals "masochistic" simply adds insult to injury.

In sharp contrast, persons suffering from a masochistic personality disorder repeatedly (but nevertheless unconsciously) seek out their tormentors, or else place themselves in situations of suffering and humiliation from which they would be able to extricate themselves if they chose to do so. This is Terry Dunn from Judith Rossner's *Looking for Mr. Goodbar*, Geoffrey Firmin from Malcolm Lowry's *Under the Volcano,* and Edith Wharton's *Ethan Frome.* These are the patients whose provocatively self-defeating and self-destructive behavior has been vividly described in the psychoanalytic literature by Reich (1933), Reik (1941), Fenichel (1945), Berliner (1947), Bergler (1949), Brenman (1952), Eidelberg (1954, 1959), Brenner (1959), Cooper (1978), Katz (1978), Glenn (1984), and Maleson (1984), among many others. They are the patients who unconsciously provoke their therapists to give up on them or to sadistically abuse them with premature and unempathic interpretations or to pejoratively dismiss them with the misdiagnosis of borderline personality disorder or passive-aggressive personality disorder. The underlying dynamics may be quite different from one patient to another. In one case, guilt may be predominant. In another case, fears of separation may be the crucial dynamic issue. In still another case, identification with an abusing or abused parent may be the central unconscious factor at work. But whatever the unconscious motives may be in each individual case, the final behavioral outcome is achievement of what Theodor Reik (1941) called "victory through defeat," and often the defeat is a failed psychiatric treatment. Whereas if the therapist could accurately diagnose the unconscious masochistic behavior that the patient is externalizing and reenacting in the treatment situation, followed by recognition of the therapist's own unconscious counterreaction to that unconscious masochistic provocation, the treatment might well be saved. In many stalemated treatments about which I have been asked to consult, just such an interaction was at work, but went unrecognized and undiagnosed.

By not listing masochistic personality disorder as a disorder in its own right in the category of the personality disorders, by not listing it in its index of diagnostic terms, and by giving it only the most cursory recognition in one word under "other personality disorder" (*DSM-III,* p. 330: "*Other Personality Disorder* should be used when the clinician judges that a specific Personality Disorder not included in this classification is appropriate, such as Masochistic, Impulsive, or Immature Personality Disorder"), I believe that *DSM-III* has perpetuated our professional denial of this serious, sometimes life-threatening, disorder.

In his presentation on the applicability of *DSM-III* to clinical practice (see Chapter 33), Chodoff made a similar plea for a separate listing of masochistic personality disorder:

For instance, it would be helpful to have criteria, under the name of the masochistic personality disorder, for those individuals who persistently find ways to spoil and take no

Table 34.2. *Traits of the depressive personality (according to Schneider and Akiskal)*

1. Quiet, passive, and nonassertive
2. Gloomy, pessimistic, and incapable of fun
3. Self-critical, self-reproaching, and self-derogatory
4. Skeptical, hypercritical, and complaining
5. Conscientious and self-disciplining
6. Brooding and given to worry
7. Preoccupied with inadequacy, failure, and negative events to the point of a morbid enjoyment of one's failures

Source: after Schneider (1958, 1959).

satisfaction in anything good that happens to them, for whom behavior akin to the negative therapeutic reaction is characteristic, and who seem perversely to glory in their misery.

The other form of pathological unconscious masochism that requires our attention is that of Freud's category of moral masochism, which he first described in those patients who appear to be "wrecked by success" (Freud, 1916), and which he eventually came to understand more completely through his conceptualization and recognition of an unconscious sense of guilt and an unconscious need for punishment. In moral masochism, the conflict is internalized, rather than externalized as with the masochistic personality disorder. One clinical manifestation of this moral masochism may be the "success neurosis" so widespread in our culture, in which the unconscious meanings of success bring anxiety and guilt instead of pleasure and happiness. Recently, Schafer (1984) has offered a number of clinical examples of such patients who spend their lives in the pursuit of failure, the avoidance of success, and the idealization of unhappiness.

Another clinical manifestation may be the intense and prolonged "survival guilt" that is in part responsible for the impaired self-esteem, the depressive mood, and the suicidal behavior of many bereaved patients who remain in a state of pathological mourning, but whose condition unfortunately often remains undiagnosed as such. Granted, these patients do not provoke aggression from the outside in the same self-destructive way that the patient suffering from a masochistic personality disorder does. But their suffering is no less severe simply because they are their own punishers and tormenters. And their guilt may frequently end in the extreme self-punishment of suicide.

Perhaps the most common clinical manifestation of moral masochism is the depressive personality disorder described by Schneider (1958, 1959). The traits of the depressive personality according to Schneider's typology, as modified by Akiskal (1983), are listed in Table 34.2.

In my opinion, self-torturing that leads to self-defeat is the hallmark of the depressive personality disorder, in contrast to the self-defeating retaliation provoked from others that is so characteristic of the masochistic personality disorder. As I have already stated, I believe there are important clinical distinctions (with important therapeutic implications) between the masochistic personality disorder and the depressive personality disorder, even though one may often see mixed pictures of the two disorders in actual clinical practice. In fact, Kernberg (1970) has referred to a "depressive/masochistic character type," and Gunderson (1983, p. 31) agrees with Kernberg " ... that DSM-III omits a clinically valuable depressive/masochistic character type for which neither the avoidant nor the dependent categories can be expected to compensate." It may well be that the term "self-defeating personality disorder" could provide a broad descriptive category within which the specific subtypes of masochistic personality disorder and depressive personality disorder might be delineated and subsumed.

Regarding the frequency of mixed conditions in clinical practice, it is of interest that in an article on the teaching and learning of *DSM-III* by Skodol, Spitzer, and Williams (1981), the one case vignette that the authors chose to present as an example from the *DSM-III Case Book* (Spitzer et al., 1981) was that of a 28-year-old chronically depressed woman with seriously impaired self-esteem and persistent dissatisfaction in her marriage, her job, and her social relationships, despite two extensive periods of psychotherapy. The authors diagnosed the patient as suffering from a dysthymic disorder and then made what to my mind is a helpful closing comment: "We would not quarrel with a clinician who wished to note, in addition, on Axis II, Atypical or Other (Masochistic) Personality Disorder, in order to emphasize the presence of many self-defeating personality features, such as the patient's lack of assertiveness and her tendency to be excessively critical of herself and others" (Spitzer et al., 1981, p. 1585). On the basis of the clinical material presented, I would suggest that this patient was indeed suffering from a chronic depression as well as a self-defeating personality disorder with both masochistic and depressive features. I would also suggest that there is diagnostic and therapeutic value in distinguishing between the patient's depressive personality traits (i.e., her excessive criticism of herself) and the patient's masochistic personality traits (i.e., the externalization of that self-criticism onto relationships with others, leading to provocation of anger and criticism toward the patient by her husband, her supervisors at work, and at least some of her social acquaintances).

THE DIAGNOSTIC CATEGORY OF DYSTHYMIC DISORDER

At the present time, *DSM-III* has abandoned the diagnosis of depressive personality disorder in favor of the new diagnosis of dysthymic disorder within the affective disorders. Figure 34.2 presents a current classification of the affective disorders into primary and secondary affective disorders, and Figure 34.3 presents the *DSM-III* classification of the primary affective disorders.

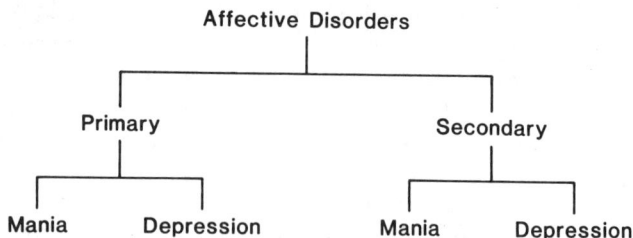

Figure 34.2. Classification of the affective disorders, following Robins and Guze (1972), Klerman and Barrett (1973), and Krauthammer and Klerman (1978). *Source:* Simons (1985, p. 701), with permission of Williams & Wilkins.

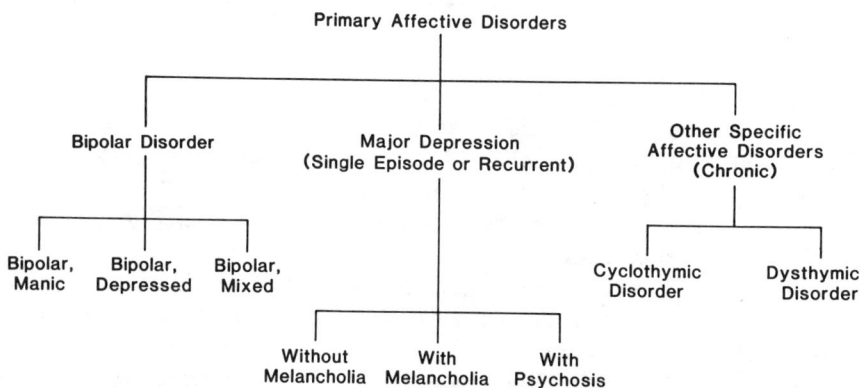

Figure 34.3. Classification of the primary affective disorders according to *DSM-III*, modified from Andreasen (1983) and Klerman (1983). *Source:* Simons (1985, p. 702), with permission of Williams & Wilkins.

A number of authors have been critical of the overinclusiveness of the DSM-III category of dysthymic disorder. In an extensive review of his own work and that of others, Akiskal (1983, p. 19) concluded that "although the concept of dysthymia as introduced in DSM-III is less nebulous than that of neurotic depression, the findings . . . suggest that chronic depressions are 'the final clinical pathway' of many conditions, including primary affective, neurotic, and characterological disorders." Frances has made the same point:

Dysthymic disorder probably includes an extremely heterogeneous group of patients. They may have vegetative symptoms indicative of an affective disorder; psychological conflicts that make them pessimistic, self-defeating, and unhappy; a chronically difficult life situation; or various mixtures of the above. DSM-III would have been more consistent had it selected one way to handle both the schizophrenic and the affective spectrum disorders. If dysthymic disorder must be included in the affective section, it should have required as an essential criterion the presence of vegetative symptoms; this is not the case now. Nonvegetative chronic depression should have appeared separately under one or another title (I would have preferred depressive or masochistic personality) in the personality disorders section. [Frances, 1980, p. 1052]

And Chodoff (see Chapter 33) has made essentially the same observation: "The criteria for this condition [dysthymic disorder] are difficult to apply and often merge into those not uncommon characterological depressions that need to be distinguished from any variety of primary affective disorders."

If current field trials should be successful in establishing operational criteria for self-defeating personality disorder, hopefully with both masochistic and depressive subgroups, then we would be in a better position to substantiate the criticisms of Akiskal, Frances, Chodoff, and others that dysthymic disorder is a heterogeneous, overinclusive category that is not clinically useful. I agree with their criticisms. It is my belief that there are at least four clinically distinct subgroups within dysthymic disorder that need to be distinguished from each other, because the therapeutic approaches to them may be (and usually are) quite different. Only the first of these subgroups actually belongs in the category of dysthymic disorder:

1.   patients with a *true affective disorder* in a mild or attenuated form that is less severe than a major depression,
2.   patients with a *somatoform disorder* (such as hypochondriasis) that is a depressive equivalent presenting with somatic symptoms rather than a mood disturbance,
3.   patients with a *self-defeating personality disorder* (with either masochistic or depressive features or both) presenting with an impaired sense of self-esteem and various maladaptive personality traits rather than a mood disturbance,
4.   patients with an *adjustment disorder with depressed mood,* in which the psychosocial stressor may not be clearly identifiable or may not have been accurately diagnosed.

Examples of type 4 might include states of pathological mourning following a loss (where survivor guilt and anniversary reactions are prominent), as well as the paradoxical depressions following a success seen in the "success neurosis" and "those wrecked by success."

I have tried to indicate why I believe that recognition of unconscious masochistic behavior is important for the general practice of psychiatry and for effective psychiatric treatment of many patients. Our psychiatric residents need to be able to diagnose masochistic personality disorder, depressive personality disorder, and the other clinical subgroups within dysthymic disorder so that they can then effectively treat these common, serious, sometimes life-threatening conditions. Let me now give two further clinical examples that demonstrate the importance of these same concepts in the education of our medical students. The two conditions that I use as examples are anorexia nervosa and the somatoform disorders.

ANOREXIA NERVOSA

The incidence of anorexia nervosa (and the related eating disorder of bulimia) has risen dramatically in recent years, for reasons that are far from clear, at least to me. And for reasons that are equally unclear, this disorder that was so rare when I was in medical school and psychiatric residency that I never saw a single case seems to be a topic of endless fascination to today's medical student. In the human-behavior course that I coordinate for second-year medical students, I can expect at least two or three honors papers being written every year on this disorder. I cannot say the same about any other topic in the course. On several occasions, students writing the papers have revealed to me that they themselves have had this illness, or have had a friend or sibling or lover who has suffered from it. This is not the place to discuss in any detail the fascinating features of this life-threatening illness, except to say that it is an illness that defies easy diagnostic categorization. It combines the delusional body image of some schizophrenic patients, the ruminations (about food) and the ritualistic doing (gorging) and undoing (purging) of some obsessive–compulsive patients, the repudiation of femininity of some transsexual patients, the pathological mourning for the childhood or adolescence that is being lost of some bereaved patients, the frantic effort to freeze time and place and person of some organic patients, the extraordinary efforts to control the environment of some histrionic and passive-aggressive and dependent personalities, the hyperactivity and euphoric denial of some manic patients, and the suicidal drive of some depressive patients. *DSM-III* either explicitly describes or at least implicitly hints at all of the foregoing. But there is no mention of the profound unconscious masochistic behavior that should be considered in the diagnostic description of this disorder and that surely is an important factor to be considered in the always difficult and all too often unsuccessful treatment of these self-destructive patients.

I would again say that adding this unconscious dimension to the descriptive criteria for this illness in no way implies any theoretical commitment in regard to the etiology of the condition. Hilde Bruch (1978) has argued eloquently for various intrapsychic conflicts and family conflicts as causative of the illness, and she has also speculated that social and cultural factors (i.e., the current emphasis on thinness as beautiful, and the expanded sexual and career choices brought about by the women's liberation movement that may overwhelm many girls and women who have not been prepared for such choices) may explain the marked increase in the incidence of the illness in recent years. Intriguing reports are appearing in the literature suggesting disturbances in the hypothalamic–pituitary–adrenal axis and in certain neurotransmitter levels as possible primary dysfunctions in the illness (Gerner and Gwirtsman, 1981; Gold et al., 1983; Gwirtsman et al., 1983) rather than as simply secondary to the physiological effects of starvation and weight loss. Winokur, March, and Mendels (1980) have postulated that there may be a subgroup of patients with anorexia nervosa whose relatives have an increased incidence of primary affective disorder and who may therefore have a genetic loading for affective disorder that is manifested through the anorexia nervosa. The final answer is far from complete in regard to the complex multifactorial etiology of anorexia nervosa. But the descriptive presence of unconscious masochistic behavior in this condition is surely unarguable.

SOMATOFORM DISORDERS

The somatoform disorders are another group of disorders of great interest to medical students, and rightly so, in view of the prevalence of these conditions in any general medical practice. I personally am not persuaded that *DSM-III* has established clear and clinically valid diagnostic criteria among the various somatoform disorders. To imply that somatization disorder or Briquet's syndrome is common, and that conversion disorder is relatively uncommon, seems to me to be quite arbitrary and unsupported, but obviously this is related to the equally arbitrary decision that conversion disorder is not to be diagnosed when conversion symptoms are limited to pain. Psychogenic pain disorder is no doubt deserving of a separate diagnostic category, but why is there no acknowledgment of the fact that acute psychogenic pain may sometimes be the final outcome of a conversion disorder, and that chronic psychogenic pain may sometimes be the final outcome of hypochondriasis? Furthermore, there is only the briefest discussion of psychogenic pain disorder and hypochondriasis under the differential diagnosis of conversion disorder. Yet these are three conditions of enormous importance to the general medical and surgical practitioner in which differential diagnosis and the presence of mixed clinical pictures may have extremely important therapeutic and prognostic implications (Barsky and Klerman, 1983; Hackett, 1983; Lazare, 1983).

In the Introduction to *DSM-III*, Spitzer stated: "In DSM-III there is no assumption that each mental disorder is a discrete entity with sharp boundaries (discontinuity) between it and other mental disorders. . . ." (American Psychiatric Association, 1980, p. 6). I do not believe that statement of principle has been fully realized with regard to the somatoform disorders. I would agree with the observation of McKegney (1982, p. 282) that "the separation of Psychogenic Pain Disorder and Conversion Disorder is confusing, both clinically and theoretically." I would also agree with the conclusion of Leigh and his colleagues that because all pain has a psychogenic component, regardless of the extent of the organic disorder, "no purpose is served by the diagnosis of Psychogenic Pain other than to attach stigma to the patient. A more appropriate diagnosis would be Chronic Pain Syndrome in Axis III, with Psychological Factors Affecting Physical Condition or, in cases where definite psychopathogenesis can be demonstrated, Conversion Disorder–Pain, in Axis I" (Leigh et al., 1982, pp. 285–6). The proposal of Williams and Spitzer (1982) that the *DSM-III* category of psychogenic pain disorder be changed to "idiopathic pain disorder" may be a helpful step in the direction proposed by Leigh.

In his Founders Award Lecture, "Systems Thinking in Psychiatry: Some

Theoretical and Clinical Implications," Marmor (1983, p. 834) made the following point:

> Another implication of systems thinking is that the growing tendency to think in terms of distinct and sharply demarcated phenomenological entities, as exemplified in DSM-III, deserves some skeptical evaluation despite its usefulness pragmatically.... I am not implying that there are no qualitative differences between various psychopathological states but only that there are no rigid lines of demarcation between them.

Although Marmor's observation is relevant for all psychopathological syndromes, it seems to me to be particularly apt in regard to the somatoform disorders. By placing the various somatoform disorders in apparently distinct and separate diagnostic categories, without really addressing the significant overlap that often occurs clinically among all of these conditions, I believe that *DSM-III* has made matters more difficult and confusing for our medical students and our fellow physicians, with very little gain. But I believe that *DSM-III* could have helped our medical students and our medical and surgical colleagues considerably by emphasizing the unconscious masochistic behavior that, for me, forms such an essential feature of the descriptive criteria not only for many of the somatoform disorders but also for many of the factitious disorders. These are all disorders which often lead to noncompliance with medical advice (Mackenzie, Popkin, and Callies, 1983), provocation of the physician into unnecessary medical and polysurgical interventions (Menninger, 1934; Engel, 1959), and even outright rejection of the patient and refusal by the physician to provide any further treatment (Spiro, 1968).

CONCLUSION

In response to an editorial by Wortis, Michels (1983, p. 518) wrote the following:

> On to a DSM-IV that serves the entire spectrum of American psychiatry – neuroses as well as psychoses, character types as well as organic syndromes, the findings of Freud as well as those of Kraepelin, and the study of the mind as well as that of the brain. There are indeed many areas which novelists, or for that matter neurochemists, understand better than psychiatrists do; let us construct a nomenclature that will allow all of them to speak to each other.

Marmor made the same point when he warned against the fallacies of biological, psychological, and sociological reductionism (i.e., a tendency to think of causation in linear, unifactorial terms) and urged instead "an awareness of the pluralistic, multifactorial origins of psychopathology" that "broadens our understanding and increases our therapeutic potential" (Marmor, 1983, p. 837).

I believe that our best hope for achieving what Michels and Marmor have urged is for us to make every effort to broaden the base of observational data that enter into our operational diagnostic criteria, without making reductionistic, unifactorial assumptions from those data that lead to premature closure in regard to etiology. In some respects, *DSM-III* has moved us away from that important goal, as I have tried to indicate in this chapter. Yet despite its failings, *DSM-III* nevertheless does hold out the promise of placing psychiatric diagnosis on a stronger clinical basis through its multiaxial classification and on a stronger scientific basis through its more precise and verifiable diagnostic criteria. I would only hope that *DSM-IV* pays as much descriptive attention to the softer and darker undertones of the human condition as it does to the brighter and more readily registered surface notes, so that "music heard so deeply that it is not heard at all" may once again become part of our diagnostic nomenclature.

REFERENCES

Akiskal HS: Dysthymic disorder: psychopathology of proposed chronic depressive subtypes. Am J Psychiatry 140:11–20, 1983

American Psychiatric Association: Diagnostic and Statistical Manual of Mental Disorders, third edition. Washington, DC, APA, 1980

Andreasen NC.: The diagnosis and classification of affective disorders, in The Affective Disorders. Edited by Davis JM, Maas JW. Washington, DC, American Psychiatric Press, 1983, pp 135–149

Barsky AJ, Klerman GL: Overview: hypochondriasis, bodily complaints, and somatic styles. Am J Psychiatry 140:273–283, 1983

Bergler E: The Basic Neurosis: Oral Regression and Psychic Masochism. New York, Grune & Stratton, 1949

Berliner B: On some psychodynamics of masochism. Psychoanal Q 16:459–471, 1947

Bernstein I: Masochistic pathology and feminine development. J Am Psychoanal Assoc 31:467–486, 1983

Blum HP: Masochism, the ego ideal, and the psychology of women. J Am Psychoanal Assoc [Suppl] 24:157–191, 1976

Brenman M: On teasing and being teased. Psychoanal Study Child 7:264–285, 1952

Brenner C: The masochistic character: genesis and treatment. J Am Psychoanal Assoc 7:197–226, 1959

Bruch H: The Golden Cage: The Enigma of Anorexia Nervosa. Cambridge, Mass, Harvard University Press, 1978

Caplan PJ: The Myth of Women's Masochism. New York, Dutton, 1985

Cooper AM: The masochistic-narcissistic character. Bull Assoc Psychoanal Med 17:13–17, 1978

Cooper AM, Michels R: DSM-III: an American view. Am J Psychiatry 138:128–129, 1981

Eidelberg L: The masochistic character, in A Comparative Pathology of the Neuroses. New York, International Universities Press, 1954, pp 174–180

Humiliation in masochism. J Am Psychoanal Assoc 7:274–283, 1959

Engel GL: "Psychogenic" pain and the pain-prone patient. Am J Med 26:899–918, 1959

Fenichel O: The Psychoanalytic Theory of Neurosis. New York, WW Norton, 1945, pp 363, 499

Frances A: The DSM-III personality disorders section: a commentary. Am J Psychiatry 137:1050–1054, 1980

Frances A, Cooper AM: Descriptive and dynamic psychiatry: a perspective on DSM-III. Am J Psychiatry 138:1198–1202, 1981

Freud S: Some character types met with in psycho-analytic work: those wrecked by success, in The Standard Edition of the Complete Psychological Works of Sigmund Freud, vol 14. London, Hogarth Press, (1916) 1957, pp 316–331

The economic problem of masochism, in The Standard Edition of the Complete Psychological Works of Sigmund Freud, vol 19. London, Hogarth Press, (1924) 1961, pp 159–170

Gerner RH, Gwirtsman HE: Abnormalities of dexamethasone suppression test and urinary MHPG in anorexia nervosa. Am J Psychiatry 138:650–653, 1981

Glenn J: Psychic trauma and masochism. J Am Psychoanal Assoc 32:357-386, 1984

Gold PW, Kaye W, Robertson GL, et al: Abnormalities in plasma and cerebrospinal-fluid arginine vasopressin in patients with anorexia nervosa. N Engl J Med 308:1117–1123, 1983

Gunderson JG: DSM-III diagnoses of personality disorders, in Current Perspectives on Personality Disorders. Edited by Frosch JP. Washington, DC, American Psychiatric Press, 1983, pp 20–39

Gwirtsman HE, Roy-Byrne P, Yager J, et al: Neuroendocrine abnormalities in bulimia. Am J Psychiatry 140:559–563, 1983

Hackett TP: Chronic pain, in Inpatient Psychiatry: Diagnosis and Treatment. Edited by Sederer LI. Baltimore, Williams & Wilkins, 1983, pp 168–181

Katz JB: Masochism as resistance and defense, in The Human Mind Revisited. Edited by Smith S. New York, International Universities Press, 1978, pp 217–244

Kendell RE: DSM-III: a British perspective. Am J Psychiatry 137:1630–1631, 1980

Kernberg OF: A psychoanalytic classification of character pathology. J Am Psychoanal Assoc 18:800–822, 1970

Klerman GL: The nosology and diagnosis of depressive disorders, in Psychiatry Update, vol 2. Edited by Grinspoon L. Washington, DC, American Psychiatric Press, 1983, pp 356–382

Klerman GL, Barrett JE: The affective disorders: clinical and epidemiologic aspects, in Lithium: Its Role in Psychiatric Research and Treatment. Edited by Gershon ES, Shopsin B. New York, Plenum Press, 1973, pp 201–236

Klerman GL, Vaillant GE, Spitzer RL, et al: A debate on DSM-III. Am J Psychiatry 141:539–553, 1984

Krauthammer C, Klerman GL: Secondary mania. Arch Gen Psychiatry 35:1333–1339, 1978

Lazare A: Conversion symptoms, in Inpatient Psychiatry: Diagnosis and Treatment. Edited by Sederer LI. Baltimore, Williams & Wilkins, 1983, 157–167

Leigh H, Price L, Ciarcia J, et al: DSM-III and consultation-liaison psychiatry: toward a comprehensive model of the patient. Gen Hosp Psychiatry 4:283–289, 1982

Loewenstein RM: A contribution to the psychoanalytic theory of masochism. J Am Psychoanal Assoc 5:197–234, 1957

McKegney FP: DSM-III: a definite advance, but the struggle continues. Gen Hosp Psychiatry 4:281–282, 1982

Mackenzie TB, Popkin MK, Callies AL: Clinical applications of DSM-III in consultation-liaison psychiatry. Hosp Community Psychiatry 34:628–631, 1983

Maleson FG: The multiple meanings of masochism in psychoanalytic discourse. J Am Psychoanal Assoc 32:325–356, 1984

Marmor J: Systems thinking in psychiatry: some theoretical and clinical implications. Am J Psychiatry 140:833–838, 1983

Menninger KA: Polysurgery and polysurgical addiction. Psychoanal Q 3:173–199, 1934

Michels R: Letter to the editor. Biol Psychiatry 18: 517–518, 1983

Millon T: Disorders of Personality. DSM-III: Axis II. New York, Wiley, 1981

Reich W: The masochistic character, in Character Analysis, third edition. Translated by Wolfe TP. New York, Simon & Schuster, (1933) 1949, pp 208–247

Reik T: Masochism in Modern Man. New York, Farrar & Rinehart, 1941

Robins E, Guze SB: Classification of affective disorders, in Recent Advances in the Psychobiology of the Depressive Illnesses. Edited by Williams TA, Katz MM, Shield JA. Washington, DC, U.S. Government Printing Office, 1972, pp 283–293

Schafer R: The pursuit of failure and the idealization of unhappiness. Am Psychologist 39:398–405, 1984

Schneider K: Psychopathic Personalities. Translated by Hamilton MW. Springfield, Ill, Charles C Thomas, 1958

Clinical Psychopathology. Translated by Hamilton MW. New York, Grune & Stratton, 1959

Simons RC (ed): Understanding Human Behavior in Health and Illness, third edition. Baltimore, Williams & Wilkins, 1985

Skodol AE, Spitzer RL, Williams JBW: Teaching and learning DSM-III. Am J Psychiatry 138:1581–1586, 1981

Spiro HR: Chronic factitious illness: Munchausen's syndrome. Arch Gen Psychiatry 18:569–579, 1968

Spitzer RL, Skodol AE, Gibbon M, et al: DSM-III Case Book. Washington, DC, American Psychiatric Association, 1981

Spitzer RL, Williams JBW, Skodol AE: DSM-III: the major achievements and an overview. Am J Psychiatry 137:151–164, 1980

Waelder R: Psychoanalysis, scientific method, and philosophy. J Am Psychoanal Assoc 10:617–637, 1962

Webb LJ, Gold RS, Johnstone EE, et al: Accuracy of DSM-III diagnosis following a training program. Am J Psychiatry 138:376–378, 1981

Williams JBW, Spitzer RL: Idiopathic pain disorder: a critique of pain-prone disorder and a proposal for a revision of the DSM-III category psychogenic pain disorder. J Nerv Ment Dis 170:415–419, 1982

Williams JBW, Spitzer RL, Skodol AE: DSM-III in residency training: results of a national survey. Am J Psychiatry 142:755–758, 1985

Winokur A, March V, Mendels J: Primary affective disorder in relatives of patients with anorexia nervosa. Am J Psychiatry 137:695–698, 1980

35   Third-party payments, cost containment, and DSM-III

STEVEN S. SHARFSTEIN

Mental disorders are not reimbursed by third-party payers in the same degree or manner as general medical disorders. A recent 300-plan survey of insurance programs conducted by the American Psychiatric Association (APA) demonstrated that only 6% of these plans provide the same inpatient and outpatient coverage for mental disorders as for other conditions. Fifty-nine percent provide equivalent inpatient benefits, but reduced outpatient mental health benefits. Three percent provide equivalent outpatient benefits, but reduced inpatient benefits. Thirty percent provide reduced inpatient and outpatient coverages. The reduced coverages include a variety of mechanisms ranging from total exclusion of benefits to greater limits on dollars expended, increased deductibles, greater copayments, and additional day or visit limits (Muszynski, Brady, and Sharfstein, 1983). As a result, private third-party insurance is twice as readily available for general medical care (26%) as for psychiatric care (13%) (Sharfstein, 1978).

Furthermore, Medicare, the U.S. national health program for the elderly and disabled, restricts outpatient coverage to 50% of physician charges or $250 in a calendar year, whichever is less, and inpatient coverage to 190 days lifetime in a psychiatric hospital. As a result, only 2% of Medicare expenditures are psychiatric (U.S. Department of Health and Human Services, 1980). Because Medicare is the U.S. flagship on entitlement for and accessibility to medical care, these mental health care limitations are significant national policy statements. Further, current efforts to contain Medicare costs through prospective payments for diagnosis-related groupings (DRGs) create a new role for diagnosis in Medicare and psychiatry.

The purpose of this chapter is to examine whether or not and how *DSM-III* has made or could make a difference in third-party coverages. Issues of equity and parity are at stake (Goldman, Sharfstein, and Frank, 1983), but in this era of cost containment, issues of accountability and confidentiality must be addressed as well. Risking the reader's disinclination to read further, I answer the key question at the outset: *DSM-III* has made very little difference in extending or expanding third-party coverage and will continue to have a small role in whatever changes occur in third-party opportunities throughout the 1980s. On the other hand, DRGs and cost-containment strategies will compel

530

a reevaluation of *DSM-III* and its role in psychiatry. Why I feel this way is the subject of this chapter.

The first section reviews the overt, traditional, often-stated problems of the third-party carriers regarding reimbursement for mental disorders and describes how *DSM-III* could have a role in creating a more favorable reimbursement climate. The second section considers the need for an acknowledged (i.e., consensually validated) system of reliable and valid diagnoses and an ability to estimate the numbers of individuals at risk for mental disorders and treatment, areas in which *DSM-III* provides clear advantages for reimbursement purposes. Further issues of confidentiality and accountability and the possible interaction of *DSM-III* with the APA coding system for mental disorders are discussed in the third section. The fourth section provides a review of DRGs under Medicare and the impact of this system on individuals with mental disorders, a challenging and potentially interesting application for *DSM-III*. The fifth section examines the basic political, sociological, and cultural issues involved in the choices for improving third-party coverages for mental disorders and suggests that economic pressures create a climate for diagnostic change and improvement.

TRADITIONAL DILEMMAS OF COVERING PSYCHIATRIC DIAGNOSES IN THIRD-PARTY PROGRAMS

Greater limitations on coverage for mental disorders, in comparison with general medical disorders, are the rule, not the exception. These limitations have been in place since the invention of third-party insurance in the 1930s. There is evidence that the limits are increasing today, even to the extent of not covering short-term treatment, and thereby creating an economic barrier to early access. For example, in 1981 and 1982 the Federal Employees Program (FEP) Blue Cross/Blue Shield cut its psychiatric-care benefits by increasing copayments for mental disorders and by adding limits to outpatient visits and inpatient days (Sharfstein and Taube, 1982).

Third-party insurance coverage for illness ("health insurance" is a misnomer) is an effort on the part of the community to pool the resources of individuals to provide timely access for the individual when medical care is needed. It is also an effort on the part of providers to create a predictable source of financial support and avoid being put in the ethical and economic dilemma of denying access to needed care because of an individual's inability to pay the bill. It is an effort on the part of the group to spread the financial risk for individuals so that the impact of cost of care is not felt at the receipt of such care by the sick person, and to create no disincentive on the part of the provider to deliver needed care.

One can see from the foregoing economic and ethical perspective that in order for insurance to be acceptable and effective, certain medical and economic objectives and assumptions must be approximated. At the core of an insurance system and its feasibility as a means of payment for medical and mental disorders is the capacity of physicians and psychiatrists to represent their treatments as medically necessary and appropriate. Although this is possible to a considerable extent, the medical model for mental illness breaks down at significant points. Continuing questions from the third-party carriers about the illnesses we treat, the treatments we use, and the length and scope of our services have led to our current inequality of coverage and our inability to capture a fair share of the insurance market.

Insurance carriers and third-party policymakers are part of the society in which we live. Mental illness and substance abuse in our culture are not seen or understood in the same way as physical disorders. Mentally ill individuals often are viewed as being responsible for bringing on their anxiety states, depressions, or alcohol problems. It is an inaccurate cultural stereotype, often portrayed in the entertainment media, that relatively healthy people seek mental health care for self-actualization or self-fulfillment purposes rather than because they have developed an incapacitating serious illness with suffering that requires care and treatment.

Furthermore, psychiatric services contrast with general medical services in that a higher proportion of the overall cost is paid by the public sector, chiefly state and local governments. Almost two-thirds of all mental-care costs are paid by this sector, compared with less than one-third for all other health care (Sharfstein, 1982b). The public institution and the traditional custodial care provided there raise a fixed and ugly image in the public eye. Despite recent improvements in care and evidence of the improved effectiveness of psychiatric treatments, many people believe that serious mental illness is incurable and is a drain on society's public and private resources. An additional issue for support for mental treatment relates to the fact that much mental illness (especially the most severe disorders) involves primarily the lower social classes in our society.

Thus, at one extreme, private insurance companies are wary of mental coverage because of the "moral hazard" of people bringing a mental illness on themselves or seeking self-actualization or self-fulfillment in mental treatment. At the other extreme, they are wary of thousands of "incurables" who languish in custodial care. The insurers believe that either extreme threatens to bring financial ruin to a third-party carrier (Sharfstein, 1978). Furthermore, the health-insurance industry is competitive, and consumer-demand issues are critical. Perhaps the best way to underscore this point is to quote from the senior director of program development for Blue Cross/Blue Shield in Chicago (Sharfstein, 1982a):

Some mental health benefit programs have been reduced by accounts either as one way to reduce overall costs or to find monies for new coverages of greater preference. Benefits for outpatient psychotherapy appear particularly vulnerable. We sense that some accounts believe that much of the utilization is for non essential, high cost services, i.e., not for treatment of illness per se but rather for self-fulfillment and self-actualization. These benefits are also viewed as disproportionately expensive given the size of the utilizing population compared to the size of populations using benefits for, as example, dental or vision care. . . . The decision [to cut back benefits] is determined by observations of preferences of federal employees expressed by enrollment trends under competing options with varied features and some market research.

The medical director of the Aetna insurance company underscored the heart of the dilemma of the third-party carrier relating to the diagnostic issue (Guillette, 1979):

Good criteria must be developed to assist the carrier in evaluating diagnoses and treatment. At the present time, the criteria for diagnosis, treatment, and determination of recovery vary widely so that effective peer review is almost impossible.

The psychiatric profession is repeatedly criticized for imprecise diagnoses. When such diagnoses are to protect a patient – a benign diagnosis or a more serious one – I can appreciate your problem. We, however, have to base our review of the case on the diagnosis given to us. We don't expect to see a situational adjustment reaction treated the same as schizophrenia.

A bigger problem is the willingness of some psychiatrists to put an insurance-acceptable diagnosis on a condition that is not considered a covered diagnosis. Examples of this category include the problems of living: floundering marriages, trouble raising children, and the difficulties in finding meaning in life. We can understand why a person would go to an analyst to get rid of such unpleasant or unwanted human behavior or to find themselves, but insurance was never intended to cover this type of "nonpsychiatric problem."

Medical insurance should only be asked to cover medical mental disorders. Insurance is meant to pay for the sick, not the discontented who are seeking an improved lifestyle. We need your help in differentiating between those who have mental disorders and those who simply have problems.

Let us take a closer look at the diagnostic dilemma.

DIAGNOSTIC RELIABILITY AND VALIDITY AND THE CAPACITY TO DEFINE AN EPIDEMIOLOGY HELPFUL TO THE INSURANCE ACTUARY

Insurance rules for coverage of mental care include the capacity to define with some precision the illness and type of treatment, including the frequency of use, duration of care, and cost per unit, to allow some degree of expectation and expertise in predicting episode costs and calculating premium rates. Other insurance rules expect that the losses will be infrequent, beyond the control of the insured and definitive in scope (Follmann, 1970).

Therefore, at the core of the insurance system is the need for definitions of risk and illness. Estimations of benefit expenditures (and premium rates) require that the covered conditions be definable with some precision both in the individual and in relation to an expected incidence in the community. The capacity for an epidemiology, therefore, is an important, if not essential, component of the ability of the insurance industry to cover mental conditions. A definable onset and end of illness (the average episode) need to be specified to some degree. Indeed, by providing an arbitrary limit on visits and days, an insurance company is trying to define its expected losses related to treatment for mental disorders.

It is clear that predictable incidences for an understood course of illness, treated and untreated, are key elements in the ultimate definition of financial risk for the third-party insurance carrier. These are also basics for the medical model and for insurance expectations, which derive from the medical model and its assumptions. Adequate consensus on diagnoses among psychiatrists is critical. This consensus must be adequately communicated to third-party administrators as well.

An additional issue is documentation of the "medical necessity" for the available treatments for specific disorders. Can we define with any specificity the nature and onset of mental conditions and predict with certainty the results for these conditions, with or without treatment? As we know, many mental disorders are not acute illnesses. Perhaps they are more analogous to chronic medical illnesses and disabilities, such as diabetes, rheumatoid arthritis, and hypertension, which often have an insidious onset and a long-term, even lifelong, course. However, these chronic medical conditions are more clearly defined, in terms of both etiopathogenesis and epidemiology.

If *DSM-III* is sufficiently precise to lead to much greater reliability and validity of psychiatric diagnoses, more precise descriptions of clinical courses, with and without treatment, and a more clearly defined epidemiology, then substantial gains will accrue in regard to better insurance coverage for mental disorders.

CONFIDENTIALITY AND ACCOUNTABILITY

To what extent does communication of clinical information from the psychiatrist to the third-party carrier compromise the privacy of the physician-patient relationship? Most mental health professionals insist on a need for strict confidentiality in order for psychotherapy to proceed. If there are many questions concerning the medical necessity for treatment, its length and intensity, and the qualifications of the provider, to what extent and how often must this information be provided to an insurance company or third-party carrier? When does providing this information interfere with the treatment itself? These are issues of intense debate in psychiatry and medicine.

One initiative of the APA and the insurance industry is a coding system for insurance-claims reporting (APA, 1982). This code was developed prior to the publication of *DSM-III*. A task force consisting of APA members and insurance-agency representatives, including the medical directors of several large insurance companies, designed a system using a specific code aimed at fulfilling the insurance agencies' needs for some information, while not revealing specific diagnoses or underlying information that could be misused or otherwise be damaging. The diagnostic system is formulated to divide reportable conditions into six general categories. The categories are an attempt at synthesis of diagnosis with varying degrees of impaired function. This gives the insurance carrier a general notion of the medical necessity for treatments being provided, and if there are questions on the specific treatments or specific diagnoses, these can be referred for peer review.

It has been proposed that in any revision of *DSM-III,* an APA code system be adopted as a separate axis utilizing this specific code system. It would provide an option for reporting psychiatric insurance claims and be part of the overall diagnostic process. Incorporation of the code system into *DSM-III* would make it clear that this code system is not a substitute for diagnosis or other material in case of peer review (Johnson, 1983). Concerns about the use of diagnostic information provided to the insurance company have led providers to report inaccurate diagnoses. Findings from two studies on the utilization of mental benefits in the Blue Cross/Blue Shield FEP in 1977 suggested that diagnostic information submitted to the carrier on claim forms was inaccurate and was of little use for claims or peer review. Submission of inaccurate information compromises the credibility of psychiatry in the eyes of the third-party carrier (Sharfstein, Towery, and Milowe, 1980).

DIAGNOSIS-RELATED GROUPINGS UNDER MEDICARE

Because of rising medical costs, the federal government enacted, with extraordinary speed, legislation amending Medicare that reversed key economic incentives that had driven the behavior of hospitals for the past three decades. The government will replace a cost-reimbursement system with a prospective-payment method based on DRGs. The DRG system, it is hoped, will compel physicians and hospital administrators to work together to more closely moderate expenditures, because hospitals – not the government nor the patient – will be at risk for costs above Medicare's prospective per-case rate based on DRGs.

DRG is a classification scheme invented and tested at Yale University that features 467 diagnostic groupings that include all general hospital inpatients in one of a number of "dynamic, comparable, mutually exclusive, statistically stable, clinically coherent, commonly reproducible and anatomically organized partitions" (Connecticut Hospital Association, 1983). The system is being implemented and was proposed by the administration on the notion, according to one commentator, that "health care is more nearly an economic product than a social good" (Iglehart, 1983).

Between 5% and 6% of the total DRG-related Medicare expenditures must be used to make supplemental payments for typical or "outlier" cases. The principal problem with the nine psychiatric diagnostic categories in the DRG system is that the variabilities in costs and lengths of stay are so great that there will be many outlier cases. As a result, psychiatric hospitals and separate inpatient psychiatric units in general hospitals are initially exempt from this system. However, the law provided that a study be submitted by the Department of Health and Human Services no later than October 1985 on whether or not and how these exempt diagnoses should be included. As of this writing, the Health Care Finance Administration and the National Institute of Mental Health are collaborating on a research proposal that will test different methods for developing a prospective-payment system based on a revised set of DRGs. This study, commissioned by the Office of Technology Assessment and its new advisory body constituted by the legislation, will help determine the shape of psychiatric diagnoses under a prospective-payment scheme.

One key issue is whether *DSM-III* helps or hurts. It probably does not help very much, because diagnosis, no matter how valid or reliable, will never be the key variable in determining length of stay or overall costs.

Many of the problems with the DRG approach with general medical diagnoses apply to psychiatric care. The principal problem is that charges per discharge diagnosis vary considerably across hospital settings and geographic regions. This is so most likely because diagnosis is not a good predictor of utilization and cost. The issue of severity of illness is more important as a predictor (Horn, 1983). One of the dangers of the DRG system has been termed "DRG creaming," with hospitals picking only those patients that are more manageable and can be treated preferentially within the cost parameters. In psychiatry, socially obnoxious patients and poor, depressed, or schizophrenic patients clearly would not be desirable types of patients to admit to a hospital in the system. It has been public policy to move chronically ill individuals to short-term general hospital units rather than state mental hospitals for their acute psychotic episodes. A DRG approach could reverse those incentives.

A related issue is called "DRG creep," or the manipulation or misuse of the DRGs in order to sustain reimbursement. An example would be that "chest pain of unknown cause" might be "upgraded" to "rule out myocardial infarction," because that discharge diagnosis is reimbursed at a more preferential rate. A further issue is cost shifting from the Medicare patients to nongovernment payers and the overall creation of a two-class system of care, with inhibition of the use and introduction of new technology to hospitals because of high costs.

Although the 467 diagnostic groupings were created in order to simplify a system of prospective payment, the system is indeed very complicated and will generate much paper, software packages, and controversy.

For psychiatric patients, possibly key predictors of the cost of hospitalization are the nature and extent of the support system available to that person outside the hospital. How does one build the notion of community support into a DRG and *DSM-III?*

A final thought on DRGs: There have been numerous studies demonstrating that patients with mental disorders are high users of medical care. In a classic study, "High-Cost Users of Medical Care" in the *New England Journal of Medicine* in May 1980, Zook and Moore (surgeons) studied 42,800 discharges in six contrasting hospital populations in 1976. They demonstrated that the high-cost group (13% of patients) consumed as many resources as did the low-cost 87%. Repeated hospitalizations for the same diseases were more characteristic of these very expensive patients than were single-cost intensive stays, intensive care, or prolonged single hospitalizations – the key elements of cost containment in DRGs. The most powerful predictor of these high-cost patients were "harmful personal habits," including consumption of alcohol, use of drugs, obesity, persistent refusal to follow physician advice regarding illness, and heavy smoking. These behavioral indices correlate closely with a secondary diagnosis of mental disorder (Zook and Moore, 1980).

The DRG system, however, will provoke a spate of studies of varying conceptual orientations on the problem of the accuracy, reliability, and validity of diagnostic "groupings." This could have a payoff through refinement of psychiatric nosology. A diagnostic system with the power to predict length of stay in hospitals surely will be an improvement and a welcome addition to current diagnostic concepts. The economics of medical care will push the diagnostic issue to the front burner for the entire profession and for psychiatric patients.

In summary, then, the DRG approach is a special challenge to psychiatric care. Special attention needs to be directed to the severity of illness and the nature of the support systems that will be necessary if the DRG approach is to be developed in an equitable manner for psychiatric patients.

POLITICAL ISSUES: EVEN WITH THE BEST DIAGNOSTIC SYSTEM, CHOICES REMAIN TO BE MADE

DSM-III represents a substantial improvement in the confidence of the psychiatric community in the reliability and validity of psychiatric diagnoses. As such, it extends belief in the legitimacy of psychiatric practice to the community as a whole. At present, this has not extended to the public policymakers. As evidence accumulates on more precise diagnostic systems with replicability, an epidemiology will emerge that will help with prediction of risk and cost for the third-party carrier. Special opportunities accrue with prospective-payment systems based on DRGs for psychiatric care as these will inevitably develop in the next couple of years.

Although the diagnostic issue is one that is often cited by the third-party carrier as a prime reason for discriminating mental disorders, even in Voltaire's "best of all possible worlds," that is, the best diagnostic system with "perfect" reliability and validity, this alone will not turn around the prospects for third-party payments. The high costs of treatment for mental disorders, the low level of overt consumer demand, and the ongoing stigma related to mental illness lead to a low value in our society in the care and treatment of the mentally ill (Foley and Sharfstein, 1983).

Choices will be made in the process of development of public policy incorporating human and economic values, and even personal perspectives. For example, mental illness in the family of a president could provide much stronger impetus for establishing a better cultural climate for reimbursement. The choices remain complex and compounded by human emotion.

REFERENCES

APA: Psychiatric Coding System for Insurance Claims Reporting. Washington, DC, American Psychiatric Association and Health Insurance Association of America, 1982; prepared by the Task Force for the National Field Trial of the Insurance Code Project (American Psychiatric Association) and the Medical Relations Committee of Consumer and Professional Relations (Health Insurance Association of America).

Connecticut Hospital Association: A DRG Primer. Hartford, CHA, 1983

Foley HA, Sharfstein SS: Madness and Government: Who Cares for the Mentally Ill? Washington, DC, American Psychiatric Press, 1983

Follmann JF Jr: Insurance Coverage for Mental Illness. New York, American Management Association, 1970

Goldman HH, Sharfstein SS, Frank RG: Equity and parity in psychiatric care. Psychiatr Ann 13:488–491, 1983

Guillette W: Is psychotherapy incurable? National Association of Private Psychiatric Hospitals Journal 9:30–32, 1979

Horn SD: Measuring severity of illness: comparisons across institutions. Am J Public Health 73:25–31, 1983

Iglehart JK: Medicare begins prospective payment of hospitals. N Engl J Med 308:1428–1432, 1983

Johnson RG: unpublished letter, written while chairperson, Subcommittee for Insurance Code System, to Gary L. Tischler, chairperson, Committee to Evaluate DSM-III, June 30, 1983

Muszynski S, Brady J, Sharfstein SS: Coverage for Mental and Nervous Disorders: Summaries of Private Sector Health Insurance Plans. Washington, DC, American Psychiatric Association, 1983

Sharfstein SS: Third-party payers: to pay or not to pay. Am J Psychiatry 135:1185–1188, 1978

    Competition for catastrophe: insurance for psychiatric care. Compr Psychiatry 23:430–435, 1982a

    Medicaid cutbacks and block grants: crisis or opportunity for community mental health? Am J Psychiatry 139:466–470, 1982b

Sharfstein SS, Taube CA: Reductions in insurance for mental disorders: adverse selection, moral hazard, and consumer demand. Am J Psychiatry 139:1425-1430, 1982

Sharfstein SS, Towery OB, Milowe ID: Accuracy of diagnostic information submitted to an insurance company. Am J Psychiatry 137:70–73, 1980

US Department of Health and Human Services: Toward a National Plan for the Chronically Mentally Ill. Washington, DC, DHHS, 1980

Zook CJ, Moore FD: High-cost users of medical care. N Engl J Med 302:996–1002, 1980

ROBERT MICHELS

The discussion of Dr. Chodoff's chapter underlined several of his major points. He had found in his office practice that axis I diagnoses were relatively easy to make and that they were clinically helpful in that they called attention to important treatment and management issues. However, he also had found that for most of the patients in his practice, the most important clinical problems and the most important themes of treatment related either to axis II conditions or to V-code situations, rather than to their axis I mental disorders. Furthermore, when he attempted to make axis II diagnoses, well over half of his patients had mixed rather than specific disorders. There was discussion of the criteria for specific personality disorders and the need to enrich them, and also of the value of additional specific axis II disorders, particularly the masochistic personality. The possibility of including features relevant to psychotherapy, those considered more "internal" or "psychodynamic" in the definition of personality disorders, was raised, as was the possibility of including some severity criteria that would aid in differentiating severe disorder from mild disorder and both from qualitative variations of normal. Case formulations were discussed, along with the appropriate limits of the concept of diagnosis – which data about the patient are best included within the diagnosis and which are best left to an extradiagnostic formulation. Dr. Chodoff responded to a question by reporting that he had stopped using *DSM-III* diagnoses for his patients when he completed his study; he had not found the process of sufficient clinical value.

Dr. Simons emphasized the value of broadening the data base for diagnoses so that more information of value to physicians and students could be encompassed. He particularly emphasized the need for adding a category of masochistic personality. There was considerable discussion of the impact of *DSM-III* on medical-student teaching. The consensus was that it enriched the students' awareness of phenomenology and increased their precision and sophistication as clinical observers. It was also clear that most students liked it. Some believed that there were problems of balance created by having so effective a text in one area of psychiatry, phenomenology and diagnosis, with students paying less attention to other aspects of their patients and of psychiatry. This was seen as a side effect of success, not reflecting the intention of *DSM-III*'s architects. One suggestion was that any introductory advice or instructions

539

to medical students be included in the popular mini-D, as well as in the longer version, with the hope that more students might then be exposed to it.

Dr. Sharfstein's contribution initiated the most heated and controversial discussion of the day. He emphasized that whatever the preference of the profession or the caveats that accompany its publications, the outside world is interested in psychiatric diagnoses for more than scientific or clinical reasons. Private insurers, government agencies, and others concerned about the cost of health care have placed major hopes for cost control on a prospective-reimbursement system that is based on diagnoses. The nationwide plan to implement this system, although largely excluding psychiatry, had gone into effect only a few days before the conference. Those who were most closely associated with the development of *DSM-III* emphasized that administrative and fiscal considerations had never entered their thinking and that the integrity of the nomenclature might be endangered if it were to be constructed with thoughts of reimbursement policy. Dr. Sharfstein emphasized that our diagnoses would be used in social and fiscal decisions, and the only question was whether we considered this fact in constructing them or ignored it and left it in the hands of others. One discussant suggested that severity factors might be particularly important in predicting costs of psychiatric treatment.

The discussion emphasized that psychiatric diagnoses can be of interest to a great many people and can be used for a great many purposes. Although it seems clear that diagnoses must be based on the traditional kind of criteria and that their ultimate validity and credibility are dependent on their scientific foundation, it is also apparent that other social factors and other applications might be considered in the construction of a diagnostic system. Clinical usefulness, educational value, and even administrative implications are relevant factors in designing a nosology.

Index

The term "external validity" indicates sections, passages, and paragraphs addressed to distinguishing the disorder from other disorders. "Internal validity" indicates sections, passages, and paragraphs addressed to defining, describing, and clarifying the disorder.